The Making of DSM-III®

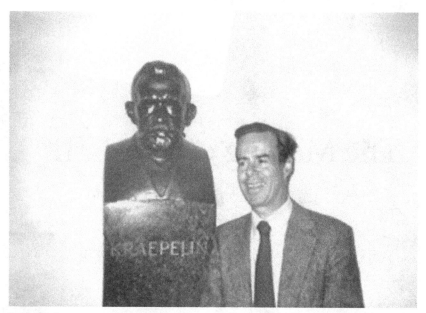

Robert Spitzer next to a bust of Emil Kraepelin in the Max-Planck-Institute for Psychiatry in Munich. Courtesy Dr. Janet B. W. Williams

The Making of DSM-III®

A Diagnostic Manual's Conquest of American Psychiatry

Hannah S. Decker, PhD

Professor of History
University of Houston
Houston, TX

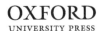

OXFORD
UNIVERSITY PRESS

OXFORD
UNIVERSITY PRESS

Oxford University Press is a department of the University of Oxford.
It furthers the University's objective of excellence in research, scholarship,
and education by publishing worldwide.

Oxford   New York

Auckland   Cape Town   Dar es Salaam   Hong Kong   Karachi
Kuala Lumpur   Madrid   Melbourne   Mexico City   Nairobi
New Delhi   Shanghai   Taipei   Toronto

With offices in

Argentina   Austria   Brazil   Chile   Czech Republic   France   Greece
Guatemala   Hungary   Italy   Japan   Poland   Portugal   Singapore
South Korea   Switzerland   Thailand   Turkey   Ukraine   Vietnam

Oxford is a registered trademark of Oxford University Press in the UK and certain other
countries.

Published in the United States of America by
Oxford University Press
198 Madison Avenue, New York, NY 10016

Library of Congress Cataloging-in-Publication Data
Decker, Hannah S.
The making of DSM-III : a diagnostic manual's conquest of
American psychiatry / Hannah S. Decker.
p. ; cm.
Includes bibliographical references and index.
ISBN 978–0–19–538223–5 (alk. paper)
I. Title.
[DNLM: 1. Diagnostic and statistical manual of mental disorders.
2. Psychiatry—history—United States.   3. History, 20th Century—United States.
4. Mental Disorders—classification—United States.   WM 11 AA1]
616.89—dc23
2012039676

To Norman, who has been my loving and steadfast companion in everything

Winokur, Robins and I suddenly realized we were now in a position to try to shape the department in the direction we thought it should go. We didn't want a psychoanalytic department, we wanted a broad research effort, and we wanted to put tremendous emphasis on improving the diagnostic system in psychiatry....It was a very exciting and heady time. We thought, and it wasn't totally exaggerated, that maybe if we were lucky and lived long enough, we could really make a dent in American psychiatry.

—Samuel B. Guze
Department of Psychiatry, Washington University
c. 1959

Unfortunately for us all, DSM-III in its present version would seem to have all the earmarks for causing an upheaval in American psychiatry which will not soon be put down.

—Boyd L. Burris, President
Baltimore-DC Psychoanalytic Society
1979

CONTENTS

ILLUSTRATIONS

ACKNOWLEDGMENTS

The research for this book, the largest project of my scholarly career, has taken place over the span of several years, and in that time I have had the help of numerous individuals to whom I owe a large debt of gratitude. As I pondered how best to publicly celebrate these persons and express my thanks, I realized that I had received several forms of assistance. Many people had graciously agreed to be interviewed, some at length, and were receptive to continued contact via e-mail or the phone. I was fortunate to have dealt with individuals who repeatedly gave me the benefit of their professional skills, without which any research is doomed. Persons in several fields read my work and offered their suggestions for improvement. Confronted at times with thorny issues relating to the furtherance of my work, I turned to colleagues who were generous with both their concern and advice. Finally, administrators at the University of Houston supported my project and provided me with both research leaves and grants.

I have listed the many people I have interviewed after the endnotes, and I would like to take this opportunity to thank every one of them again for speaking to me, some several times. I would also like to add a few remarks. This book could not have been written without the cooperation of Robert Spitzer and his wife, Janet Williams. Dr. Spitzer also provided me with much material relating to DSM-III that I could not have otherwise gotten. One of his most generous acts was to inform me that I could find very personal information about him from his school records and a revealing interview of him when he was fifteen, in a book by the famous sociologist, David Riesman, *Faces in the Crowd*, where Dr. Spitzer is disguised as "Henry Friend." Moreover, I would like to thank Roger Peele, who has had a distinguished career in psychiatric administration and played an important role in trying to broker a satisfactory solution to the issue of what place "neurosis" would have in the final version of DSM-III. In addition to sharing his thoughts in an interview and in e-mails, Dr. Peele magnanimously supplied indispensable information about the APA Assembly meeting where the crucial vote on the acceptance or rejection of DSM-III took place.

During the many days I spent at the Melvin Sabshin Library and Archives of the American Psychiatric Association in Arlington, VA, the Archivist and Librarian, Gary McMillan, generously took time from his busy duties to aid me in making the most efficient use of my time. He was a gracious and knowledgeable host and continued to help me on occasion over the next two years, especially when it came time to apply for and receive permission from the APA to publish my findings and to use copyrighted material. I also want to thank other archivists, librarians, and editors who assisted me in obtaining the photographs used in this book: Philip Skroska, Archivist, Visual and Graphic Archives, Becker Medical Library, Washington University, St. Louis; Sonya

Rooney, University Archivist, Washington University Libraries; Eve Vagg, Director of the Photography and Illustration Department at the New York State Psychiatric Institute; Ronald H. Sims, Special Collections Librarian, Galter Health Sciences Library, Feinberg School of Medicine, Northwestern University; and Lizabeth Fleenor, Director of Communications and Managing Editor, *Missouri Medicine*.

At the University of Houston, the librarians in the Inter-Library Loan Department were indispensable to my conducting my research over the years; I cannot say enough laudatory things about them. Also, Jennifer Lazarro, former Instructional Designer in the College of Liberal Arts and Social Sciences, provided expert and always cheerful technical assistance.

Allen Frances, Gerald N. Grob, and Bennett Simon read all or parts of my manuscript, and I benefitted no end from their erudition. I want to thank them again for their fruitful observations and opinions, but I alone am responsible for all interpretations and whatever errors I may have made. For stylistic advice I want to thank Carol Herrnstadt Shulman, Will Decker, Russell Harper, and Ruth Decker Harper.

There have been a few times in the long course of my research and writing when I was at a critical crossroad. I was fortunate at these moments to have the opinions and guidance of Susan Kellogg, a good friend and colleague at the University of Houston; Joyce Seltzer, Senior Executive Editor at the Harvard University Press; and Bennett Simon, clinician and historian of psychiatry and psychoanalysis at Harvard, whom I have already thanked for his reading of sections of my manuscript. I remain the thankful recipient of their time and counsel.

I want also to express my appreciation to Stuart Yudofsky, Chair of the Menninger Department of Psychiatry at the Baylor College of Medicine in Houston, for his willingness to promote my work.

For the material furtherance of my project, I would like to thank first of all John Antel, Provost at the University of Houston, who while he was Dean of my college generously took the time to learn about my undertaking and supported me with grants and leaves at a time when I was in the early and middle stages of research and writing. Then I have to thank the present Dean of my college, John Roberts, and former Associate Dean, Kathleen Brosnan, for their support, also with a grant and a leave, at the end stage of my work.

Special thanks go to Caroline Nilsen, a graduate student in history at the University of Houston who was an outstanding research assistant during the final stages of my work. Caroline was both creative and clever in achieving our goals and brought to her duties intelligence and diligence. Some day she will be a great researcher for her own work.

Finally, I have been the beneficial recipient of excellent editorial direction at Oxford Univeristy Press from both David D'Addona and Craig Panner. Both guided me, and David worked closely and efficiently with me in the final months of converting a manuscript into a book. I also want to express my appreciation to Emily Perry, Production Editor, and Jerri Hurlbutt, Copy Editor.

Yet, there is still more to say. There is one person who has been intimately involved with my work in all of the categories of assistance I described in the beginning. That is my husband of many years, Norman Decker, and I cannot thank him enough. He has read everything I have written and offered cogent advice on substance and style. He has given astute advice on organizational matters. At times of crisis he has been unfailingly supportive. He has even rendered crucial technical assistance when my computer smarts failed. For many years we have closely shared with each other our passions and knowledge in history, social issues, and politics, as well as in psychoanalytic and psychiatric history and in psychiatric diagnosis and treatment. We have had a fruitful and enjoyable partnership in all our endeavors over the years, and I dedicate this book to him with great fullness of heart.

Grateful acknowledgement is made to the following for permission to reprint previously published material:

Permission from Transaction Publishing Company to reprint material from *Asylums: Essays on the Social Situation of Mental Patients and Other Inmates* by Ervin Goffman. Chicago: Aldine Publishing, Copyright © 1961.

Permission granted by Hodder Education to print previously published material from *The Psychopharmacologists III: Interviews* by David Healy. London: Arnold and New York: Oxford University Press, Copyright © 2000 Arnold.

Oxford University Press on behalf of the Maryland Psychiatric Research Center and the Schizophrenia International Research Society for permission to reprint copyrighted material from "Feighner et al., Invisible Colleges, and the Matthew Effect," *Schizophrenia Bulletin*, Vol. 8. No. 1, pp. 1–6 by Roger K. Blashfield and Comments on the article by John S. Strauss, pp. 8–9 and R.E. Kendell, pp. 11–12.

Also to Roger K. Blashfield, John S. Strauss, and Ann Kendell for permission to publish the material in the above-named *Schizophrenia Bulletin*.

Material from *Faces in the Crowd: Individual Studies in Character and Politics* (Abridged Edition) by David Riesman in collaboration with Nathan Glazer. New Haven and London: Yale University Press, Copyright ©1965.

Material from the *American Journal of Psychiatry*, Copyright © 1976 by the American Psychiatric Association.

Material from the *Diagnostic and Statistical Manual of Mental Disorders, Third Edition* (DSM-III), Copyright © 1980 by the American Psychiatric Association.

"The Psychiatric Works of Emil Kraepelin: A Many-Faceted Story of Modern Medicine," by Hannah S. Decker, *Journal of the History of the Neurosciences*, September 2004, reprinted by permission of the publisher, Taylor & Frances (Taylor & Frances Ltd, http://www.tandf.co.uk/journals).

"How Kraepelinian was Kraepelin? How Kraepelinians are the neo-Kraepelinians?—from Emil Kraepelin to DSM-III," (SAGE Journals Online http://online.sagepub.com), by Hannah S. Decker. The final, definitive version of this paper has been published in *History of Psychiatry,* Vol. 18, No. 3, 2007 by SAGE Publications Ltd./SAGE Publications, Inc., All rights reserved. © 2007.

INTRODUCTION

This work has had a long and circuitous gestation. It began with a study of Emil Kraepelin, the great German psychiatric classifier, and then crossed the ocean as an investigation of his heirs, the American neo-Kraepelinians. It culminated in this book, on the third edition of the American Psychiatric Association's (APA) *Diagnostic and Statistical Manual of Mental Disorders*—DSM-III.

DSM-III was a sweepingly revisionist work and ultimately created a revolution within psychiatry. Temporally, the saga in this book proceeds from one revolution in psychiatric classification to another and from Emil Kraepelin to Robert Spitzer, the leader of the task force that produced DSM-III. Together these two men are the commanding bookends of twentieth-century descriptive psychiatry.

DSM-III also affected many areas of everyday medical, psychological, legal, and economic life in ways that previous diagnostic manuals had not. Consider, for an instant, the enormous ramifications of the placement of Post-Traumatic Stress Disorder (PTSD) in DSM-III. In one overarching diagnosis it gave legitimacy to the fact that victims of rape, assault, military combat, airplane crashes, fires, floods, bombing, and torture can suffer psychological trauma with symptoms that are debilitating and life changing and that should not be denied.

The epigraph of the book bespeaks one of the historic clashes that unfolds in these pages, a battle between the phenomenologists, descriptive psychiatrists, on the one hand and the psychoanalysts and psychodynamically oriented psychiatrists on the other. The two groups in opposition to each other were the descendants of the two giants of psychopathological thought of the early twentieth century, Kraepelin and Sigmund Freud, both born in 1856. At the beginning of the making of DSM-III in 1974, the adherents of Freud dominated American psychiatry. Yet little-known researchers at Washington University in St. Louis, the neo-Kraepelinians, fervently hoped for a psychiatry in which only empirical studies and exact description of signs and symptoms would reign. In the late 1950s they thought they might be "lucky" to make "a dent" in the psychoanalytically ruled field. Yet just twenty years later the president of the Baltimore-DC Psychoanalytic Society expressed profound fears that the researchers would indeed prevail, bringing with them "an upheaval in American psychiatry" that would spell the end of the analysts' dominion. At the start of our story, neither group could have predicted the swift movement of events that brought about revolutionary change. It is precisely these events that this book chronicles.

FROM A DENT TO AN UPHEAVAL

This book is the story of the writing of a classification, DSM-III, and the leadership of one psychiatrist, Robert Spitzer, as he took on himself the radical revision of an existing nosology. But since nothing suddenly appears completely formulated, we can only understand the composition of the classification within the context of the psychiatry that preceded it. This means examining American psychiatry since the end of World War II in 1945. After the war there was a period of psychoanalytic dominance, but in the 1960s and 1970s psychiatry was broadly maligned. Thus one of the reasons the APA wanted to produce a revised manual was to counteract this antipsychiatry movement and show that psychiatry was a truly scientific discipline worthy of wide respect.

The section on historical background also includes an assessment of the contributions of Kraepelin, the great classificatory separator of the psychoses and master of description. Another part of the background is a discussion of Spitzer's neo-Kraepelinian forebears, the iconoclastic research psychiatrists at Washington University in St. Louis in the 1950s and 1960s.

To understand Spitzer's leadership, we will first study Spitzer the man, as he developed from childhood and adolescence into adulthood and established himself professionally. We will then scrutinize the small group of men and women he selected to work on the new manual, the "Task Force." At times this group assumed a surprisingly powerful independent role. The largest part of the book will be spent observing Spitzer, the Task Force, and the special Advisory Committees as they debated and developed the many dozens of diagnoses that found a home in DSM-III.

Two chapters of this last section are devoted to the tension-filled clash between the dominant analysts, whose rule was ebbing, and the ascending descriptive psychiatrists, represented by Spitzer and the Task Force. There are ironic aspects to this battle. There is no doubt that Spitzer was committed to an empirically based manual. He wanted to get rid of the diagnosis Neurosis found in DSM-II since it implied psychoanalytic etiology. He felt there was no place for etiology unless it was clearly demonstrable, as with organic brain disorders. He also did not want to include in the manual the role of unconscious conflict in the production of psychopathology, arguing there was no observable evidence to support this concept. Moreover, if everyone suffered from intrapsychic conflict, as the analysts asserted, that phenomenon, Spitzer maintained, could not be the basis for diagnosing psychopathology in patients. Ironically, while Spitzer was a graduate analyst, he dismissed analytic concepts. However, he was not totally opposed to accommodating the psychoanalysts to a degree, as long as the essential empirical quality and orientation of DSM-III were not compromised.

There were two occasions when it appeared to Spitzer that it might be possible to recognize some psychodynamic thinking. Perhaps there could be a separate axis in the new five-part multivariable (multiaxial) diagnostic system where the clinician could cite the coping mechanisms of a given patient on one of the axes. Or there could be a sixth axis dedicated to concepts of psychoanalytic ideas regarding etiology. If the Archives tell the whole story, such solutions to the ongoing clashes with the analysts were acceptable to Spitzer but not, as it turned out, to the Task Force. Spitzer had chosen these men and women precisely for their commitment to empiricism and now, in another ironic twist, their devotion to hard facts and measurable data outdid his. Thus, the rejection of psychoanalysis in DSM-III turned out to be complete. But the upheaval of psychoanalysis, while inevitable, did not have to occur as swiftly as it did. Fate can have a caustic edge.

DSM-III became what it was not only because of Spitzer's forceful leadership, as remarkable as it was. Spitzer had a troika of influential support. First, he had behind him the backing of many individuals on the APA Board of Trustees. Even before Spitzer's appointment, the Trustees met in a specially called session in 1973 to discuss what could be done to counter the poor public image of psychiatry among the American public. In the previous decade a strong antipsychiatry movement had arisen. By 1973, judges were overruling expert testimony of psychiatrists in courts who recommended commitment for individuals with severe mental disorders. The judges decided in favor of lawyers' arguments for the patient's "constitutional right to treatment," arguably unavailable in large state hospitals. Although a new DSM had appeared only five years earlier, some among the Trustees thought that perhaps a newly written manual stressing the medical aspect of psychiatry might bolster the professional image of their field.

Moreover, in 1974 the Board appointed a new medical director, Melvin Sabshin (1925–2011). Sabshin said forthrightly that he wanted to return psychiatry to its medical roots. He wished to do away with both the influence of psychoanalysis and the activism of those psychiatrists who put curing social ills before their strictly medical roles. Sabshin was also a man who was adept at quietly influencing events. Finally, given a free hand to choose the committee members of the DSM-III Task Force, Spitzer appointed a group with strong empirical interests who decisively backed him up. This cohort of Trustees, Sabshin, and the Task Force supported Spitzer in his quest to advance empiricism in American psychiatry.

THE DSM

The APA has published the DSM since 1952. DSM-I and DSM-II (1968) were small, spiral-bound books, each a little over 130 pages. DSM-III (1980), the DSM of this book, was a large, heavy, bound volume of almost 500 pages with 265 diagnoses. Little attention was paid to the first two DSMs, which were published mainly for psychiatrists in state mental hospitals who were interested in compiling a variety of statistical information on their patients' lives and deaths. At their height, the state hospitals had a population of over half a million. It was estimated that by 1960, one out of every three hundred individuals in the United States had spent some time in a mental institution. But because of a policy of "deinstitutionalization," those days were ending by the time Spitzer and his task force held their first meeting in 1974.

No longer intended primarily for use in state hospitals, DSM-III was meant instead for psychiatrists in private practice, mainly seeing patients one on one, and for research psychiatrists in academic institutions, carrying out a host of studies on many patients at a time. Beyond this new usage, the revised manual had a fresh format centered on diagnosing patients via a system of specific "diagnostic criteria" covering the signs and symptoms of particular mental disorders. It was a descriptive manual with no reference to etiology except for the organic brain disorders. Psychoanalytically based etiologies, or indeed any psychodynamic thought regarding unconscious phenomena, which had found some place in DSM-II, were omitted. There were other new features as well, such as lengthy discussions of most disorders and a five-category multiaxial diagnostic system. However, it was only with much effort and emotional commitment, drawing on remarkable reserves of energy and leadership, that Spitzer was able to get his vision of a psychiatry that relied on empirical findings translated, however imperfectly, into DSM-III and approved by the APA hierarchy. Fortunately, papers regarding the development of DSM-III are in the Archives of the APA's Melvin Sabshin Library so it is possible to reconstruct much of the making of the new manual.

Since 1980, the uses of the DSMs have multiplied. Consider the following sampling: It is used by all workers in the mental health field—psychiatrists, psychologists, social workers, counselors of every stripe—to diagnose mental disorders. To get reimbursed from health insurance companies, DSM diagnoses and codes must be submitted. Medical students, psychiatry residents, and psychology interns learn diagnostic psychiatry from the manual. Applications for research grants risk losing their funding if they do not use the manual's diagnoses and language. Lawyers, judges, and prison officials use the manual throughout the judicial system. Parents can get free special services for their children in public schools if their child's diagnosis is in the DSM. As an example of how deeply the DSM penetrates into everyday life, regard, for a moment, labor and employment law. The DSM affects what accommodations need to be made by employers for mentally disabled workers, under the Americans with Disabilities Act. Claims citing mental disorders under the Family Medical Leave Act and workers' compensation laws are adjudicated using the current DSM. The Cato Institute (a libertarian think tank) recently called attention to these legal and business implications of the DSM. As can be seen, the DSM has an impact on almost every aspect of society here and abroad—the DSM has been translated into many languages. Thus, the way in which any DSM is constructed, beginning with the third edition, is a vital matter, as borne out in the extensive and sometimes passionate controversies that have swirled around the making of DSM-5, due out in 2013.

PSYCHIATRY

Before leaving this overview of major themes in the book, a few observations about psychiatry as a scientific field are in order. Psychiatry faces great challenges in diagnosing and understanding mental pathology. To begin with, an infinite number of variables go into the making and continued existence of the human brain and personality. The factors affecting any human being are an interactive, ever-evolving mixture of genes, biological processes, experiences, surrounding environments, and thoughts, feelings, and passions, some being below the level of awareness. It is possible that no two consecutive moments of life are identical. The isolation and treatment of psychopathology under these circumstances is a daunting task. Moreover, deciding what is "normal" and what is "pathological" is at times difficult because so much of mental disorder and normal variation exists on a wide spectrum. Finally, psychiatrists and psychologists, though advancing on many fronts, do not yet know the etiologies of many of the mental conditions they are called on to treat. Given these circumstances, imagine the challenges of devising a new classification, a *nosology*, of mental disorders, which in essence is the formulation of many diagnoses and their placement in relation to one another.

Another professional challenge is that for the past 200 years, since the birth of modern psychiatry, the leaders in the field have alternated their basic approach. Psychiatry has swung between emphasizing material (somatic) paths and non-material (psychological/experiential) avenues to knowledge. Psychiatry began as a medical specialty as it ousted religious beliefs in sin as the origin of mental pathology. In its early years, the new field placed stress on "moral" treatment, basically a psychological approach that viewed the environment and the emotions as crucial to the formation of psychopathology. After a few decades, c. 1840–1850, a rebellion against this approach occurred, on the grounds that little useful knowledge had been accumulated while employing non-material investigations and beliefs. Thus, the newcomers to psychiatry denounced the principles of their forebears and swung sharply to a hard-line material approach that emphasized data collection and accepted only empirically derived knowledge. Whatever had been learned in the previous generation was generally ignored or even condemned. But then the empiricists ran into dead ends in their research and treatments, and another swing occurred at the end of the nineteenth century. Freudian psychology, a non-material view of the origins of psychopathology, moved front and center.

Swings such as these have continued to our day, retarding (although not totally halting) progress in psychiatry. Only a philosophy that welcomes both material and non-material positions will hasten progress in diagnosing and treating human beings. The cyclical nature of psychiatric progress is an important focus of this book, since the development of DSM-III strongly affected the cycle with its material approach to understanding human psychopathology.

DETAILED MAP OF THE BOOK

This work is divided into three overarching sections. Section I, "The History," deals with the historical prelude. Section II, "The People," is devoted to learning about the lead players, Spitzer and the eight original members of the Task Force. Section III, "The Making," the longest section, encompasses the construction of the manual.

In Section I, Chapter 1 presents a history of American psychiatry from 1945 to the beginning of the Task Force's work on DSM-III. The coverage of this first chapter forms a triptych: the first part is on the dominance of psychoanalysis, the second part describes the antipsychiatry movement, and the third part covers two climactic events of 1973. Chapter 2 is a crucial look backward to the descriptive psychiatry of Emil Kraepelin that presaged that of psychiatrists who followed him in this country. Chapter 3 includes a discussion of the philosophy and contributions of these men— the neo-Kraepelinians—who sparked the revolution of DSM-III.

In Section II, Chapter 4 introduces us to Spitzer, who ignited the revolution first conceptualized by the neo-Kraepelinians. Bearing in mind Spitzer's pivotal role in the history of psychiatry, we follow him from childhood on. Chapter 5 offers a scrutiny of the professional lives of Spitzer's hand-picked task force.

Chapter 6, which begins Section III, contains necessary introductions to two vital topics: the history of classification in psychiatry in the nineteenth and twentieth centuries, and the problem of constructing a new classification that would improve the abysmal reliability of many psychiatric diagnoses. (Two or three psychiatrists interviewing the same patient often could not agree on the same diagnosis.) In Chapter 7 we plunge into the making of DSM-III during the first year and a half. This is a time when the Task Force and Advisory Committees worked with relatively little outside interference, although Spitzer quite faithfully publicized their work from the start. During this early stage of the development of DSM-III, he made presentations at the annual spring meetings of the APA in May 1975 and May 1976. He also published periodic news articles on DSM-III in *Psychiatric News*, the APA's biweekly newspaper, openly inviting comments. To this publicity he added articles published in psychiatric journals as well as book chapters on his activities. Chapter 8 presents a pivotal event, a conference in 1976 on "DSM-III in Midstream." Here a preliminary draft of DSM-III was presented for discussion and debate by a gathering of almost one hundred psychiatrists, psychoanalysts, and psychologists. It is worth observing that, on the whole, Spitzer was committed to transparency. At all times he mounted attempts to inform and educate American psychiatrists on what he was about. He never shied away from the discussions and challenges that such information might bring. (This way of interaction with the profession led him to criticize strongly in 2007 the manner in which the makers of DSM-5 approached their task, which he regarded as secretive.)

After the Midstream Conference, the whole dynamic of making the DSM-III changed. Now the criticism, which had been moderate up to that time, rose to a new pitch. The pace of events quickened, and the concerns of the many players heightened. From the standpoint of this book's structure, there were times when Spitzer was juggling many issues at a time, thus a chapter may encompass several small subjects, or a given topic may extend over more than one chapter.

Following the Midstream meeting, Chapters 9 through 12 unveil the specific diagnostic, theoretical, technical, political, philosophical, and even economic concerns and battles that occupied Spitzer and the Task Force over the next three years, from the summer of 1976 to the spring of 1979. These four chapters are drawn to a close with the climactic Chapter 13, on the last few weeks before DSM-III was up for approval in May 1979. The decisive vote, which Spitzer was not sure he would win, came at the end of a tense and dramatic session of the APA's Assembly of Delegates.

The reader should note that several chapters contain Pictorial Essays that present many of the lead players of the book in historical synopses. These Essays can be located at the pages specified in the list of Illustrations following the Table of Contents.

AUTHOR'S COMMENTS

Knowing full well that it may be impossible to fully please more than one audience, I have nevertheless written this book for three constituencies: (1) historians of psychiatry, medicine, society, and ideas; (2) clinicians and researchers in psychiatry who take an interest in the history of their disciplines and the contributions of their colleagues; and (3) lay readers who, for whatever reason, are intrigued by the ongoing critiques and defenses of modern psychiatry and who want to know the bases of those views. Of course, in a number of cases, these audiences overlap.

I have striven for both breadth and depth, but where there was a clash or a choice between them, I have opted for depth. Thus, there are aspects of the development of DSM-III that this book does not cover. The chapters that follow deal only with adult psychiatry, not child or adolescent psychiatry. With one exception, none of the organic brain disorders are dealt with since many of their etiologies are known and thus do not pose the same challenges as do the other mental disorders. The lone exception to this is Tobacco Dependence, a pioneering diagnosis in DSM-III and one specifically targeted by the tobacco companies for elimination or alteration while it was being formulated. Further, since there are 265 diagnoses in DSM-III, I have not attempted to write about the judgments that went into the conceptualization and development of diagnostic criteria for all of them. I have concentrated on certain situations that were controversial, on diagnoses that were contentious, and on areas that seemed to pique special interest. There are also some additional brief subjects.

For those interested in specific diagnoses not covered here, there are papers on a variety of diagnoses in the APA Archives in Arlington, VA, in the DSM Collection that invite future research. Whole books on the diagnoses Social Anxiety Disorder and Depressive Disorders have already appeared, and a volume on Autism is planned. A useful supplement to this book, for questions regarding specific facts about DSM-III, is a fourteen-page, 1980 article timed to coincide with the publication of the new manual, by Robert L. Spitzer, Janet B. W. Williams, and Andrew E. Skodol, "DSM-III: The Major Achievements and an Overview," in the *American Journal of Psychiatry*.

This book relies on over one thousand documents from the APA DSM-III Archives, many person-to-person interviews, telephone interviews, e-mails, and numerous secondary sources. Yet I look upon my book as having laid a trail that others can also traverse. It is my hope that this book will spur additional scholars to investigate the making of DSM-III, a path-breaking and revolutionary work—for good or ill—or explore Spitzer's 1987 revision, DSM-III-R, which is not covered here. There are also gaps to be filled in beyond the papers in the APA Archives; while the documents are copious, they do not exhaust the possibilities of other information. The varied reaction to DSM-III, once it appeared, is a subject waiting to be fully researched. I foresee the possibilities of comparative work on DSM-III, III-R, IV (1994), IV-T-R (2000) (IV-T-R is almost double the size of III), and 5.

I welcome all corrections that might further illuminate the subjects I cover here. There have been times when I wondered whether this book should be regarded like a giant Wikipedia article, open to additions and alterations, although I would hope only by legitimate parties. This book went to press five months before the published edition of DSM-5 was due to appear, so it is possible that some references to DSM-5 may be dated.

I regard my book as an introduction to a crucial time in the history of American psychiatry, when so much was up in the air and unsettled. True, there were a number of large trends that were hurtling forward, but the direction in which events would travel was not preordained. In this regard, we will see that much was shaped by the particular personalities of the individuals who played major roles in our story. The configuration of any revolution throughout history is always formed at the point where pre-revolutionary circumstances and the path of the chief actor collide.

SECTION I
The History

1

A PIVOTAL THREE DECADES:
AMERICAN PSYCHIATRY
AFTER WORLD WAR II

Chronicle I: "Weller than Well"

Before World War II (1939–1945), American psychiatry was dominated by asylum psychiatrists who found it useful to employ the ideas of Emil Kraepelin (1856–1926), a famous German psychiatrist widely known for his emphasis on categorization, description, and diagnosis.[1] This thinking was preferred because little was known about the causes of severe mental illness, and there was very limited treatment. After the war, while most European psychiatrists continued to follow Kraepelin, U.S. psychiatrists mainly turned away from his approach, accepting psychological causes of mental illness and advocating psychotherapeutic treatment. One of the main reasons for this decisive departure from Kraepelinian psychiatry was the experience of U.S. psychiatrists during the war. They had seen with awe that psychiatrists who were also psychoanalysts often successfully treated soldiers sent back from the front line with acute cases of "combat neurosis," the shell shock of World War I and the post-traumatic stress disorder (PTSD) of Vietnam. The soldiers were able to emerge from their debilitating shock and return to the front.[2] This was a therapeutic intervention that was largely unknown during the First World War. A theory emerged from the observation that soldiers treated promptly near the front had higher rates of recovery than those of soldiers treated in the rear. Mentally ill civilians, it was hypothesized, would probably do better if treated quickly in the community rather than being sent to remote hospitals, where they were likely to languish.

The war also lessened the belief in Kraepelinian doctrine, founded on the traditional medical model of disease, which postulated that there was a sharp line between the mentally ill and the mentally well. Based on the soldiers' exposure to combat, the conclusion was drawn that anyone with severe enough trauma could become mentally ill, and thus there was a fluid boundary between mental health and mental illness. Moreover, Sigmund Freud (1856–1939) had theorized that the mental life of all people ranged along a continuum, with health at one end and illness at the other. The views of Adolf Meyer (1866–1950), the Swiss-born leader of American psychiatry, were sympathetic to this outlook. Meyer also believed that social issues had to be addressed to understand and help the mentally ill,[3] "[h]ence early treatment in [the] community...might prevent the onset of severe mental diseases that required institutionalization."[4]

When the army's psychiatrists returned home after World War II, many were determined to become psychoanalysts. Psychoanalytic institutes were thus oversupplied with candidates who, when they graduated, generally went into private practice and into academia, often holding voluntary appointments in the psychiatry departments of medical schools, where they taught impressionable residents. Psychoanalysis in the United States was also strengthened by the many European analysts who had fled the Nazi terror and filled posts in local departments of psychiatry. Most department chairs of psychiatry in the 1960s were held by psychoanalysts. The belief was strong that analysis could alleviate most mental illnesses, even though Freud had declared that the psychoses are not amenable to psychoanalytic treatment.[5]

OPTIMISM VIA PSYCHOANALYSIS AND ENVIRONMENTAL CHANGE

Indicative of the strength and influence of roseate psychoanalytic thinking at its apex was the widely read book, *The Vital Balance*, published in 1963 and soon going into a second printing. Written by the well-known psychoanalyst, Karl Menninger, it proposed to "expand and document" the takeover of a "static and...hopeless" psychiatry by psychoanalysis.[6] It preached against the overreliance on classification and diagnosis and declared "there is only one class of mental illness—namely mental illness" (p. 9). Menninger advanced the analytic viewpoint that giving a specific diagnosis to a mentally ill person was not necessary because some form of mental illness was present in human beings most of the time. He and other analysts could point to Freud's *The Psychopathology of Everyday Life* to support this idea.[7] Therefore, he concluded, "current nosologies and diagnostic nomenclature are not only useless but restrictive and obstructive" (p. 33).[8] Yet in matters of development of personality, Menninger was sophisticated, advocating a "psycho-socio-physio-chemical concept" (p. 49).

The book gave detailed advice to readers on how to cope with the stresses of "everyday human life" and mental "dysorganization" (a term Menninger meant to cover all traditional mental disorders) in order "to maintain the vital balance" (p. 125). Included was a forty-three page idealistic chapter on psychoanalytic treatment which talked of a "patient-doctor relation [as] affected by...'intangibles' of love, faith, and hope" (p. 357). Moreover, psychoanalysis envisioned not only "cure" but also prevention of mental illness. It was even possible to transcend the vital balance to achieve "a state of being 'weller than well'" (p. 401). (The psychoanalysts may have been in a dominant position, but they were making promises they could never possibly fulfill.)

With this broad belief in the possibility of cure as well as prevention, many psychiatrists began to see their role as solving the social problems that made for unhealthy and even impoverished environments for so much of society. A new definition of mental illness encouraged psychiatric dealing with unemployment, poverty, racism, and slums.[9] Psychiatrists even pressured their professional organizations to take stands against U.S. involvement in Vietnam and on issues like school segregation; they "marched with Martin Luther King on psychiatric grounds."[10]

It was argued optimistically that early intervention in the community or with psychotherapy in a private-practice setting might prevent acute mental illness from moving on to an incurable psychotic state. There thus appeared new roles for psychiatrists. Robert H. Felix (1904–1990), the persuasive first director of the National Institute of Mental Health (NIMH) from the end of World War II until 1964, urged psychiatrists to "go out and find the people who need help and—that means, in their local communities."[11] (Whatever Felix envisioned for the role of the NIMH, it has been tremendously successful, perhaps even beyond his wildest dreams. The NIMH, under important leadership and through support of diverse theoretical initiatives, has become the U.S. government's investment in the mental health of its citizens.)

In the early 1970s, the Tremont Crisis Center in the South Bronx was an example of a center bringing psychiatric help to the community. It was a storefront clinic where psychiatric residents, nurses, and social workers formed a "team," a concept then beginning to gain popularity. The psychiatrist in charge, Ed Hornick, cut a colorful figure with an earring and a cloak, challenging conventional notions of professional dress. First-year residents were immediately introduced to the history of their field. For example, they read some of Freud's famous early cases because the psychiatrists running the introductory course went of their way not to teach beginning residents with a "textbook-here-is-the-truth" approach. Everything was fluid; there was no last word. The residents would learn by discussing primary sources.[12]

But before community mental health centers were established, organized psychiatry had undergone a transition. The American Psychiatric Association (APA) had long been dominated by psychiatrists who worked in institutional settings. In 1940, on the eve of U.S. involvement in World War II, two-thirds of its members were asylum psychiatrists.[13] After the war a group of psychoanalytically disposed psychiatrists were determined to change the APA, which to them seemed to be stodgy and apathetic. Calling themselves the Group for the Advancement of Psychiatry (GAP), they were able to influence the APA to shift its focus toward the resolution of significant social problems. In 1950, GAP issued a report entitled *The Social Responsibility of Psychiatry: A Statement of Orientation*,[14] One could argue that this marked the beginning of the "social psychiatry" of the 1960s and 1970s. The federal government had also become interested in social issues. In 1949 the NIMH was created with an initial goal to support research in the social bases of mental disorders; biological research took a back seat.[15] Felix, as director of the NIMH and knowledgeable about organizational politics, was very active in attempts to convince Congress and philanthropic agencies that mental illness could be prevented if only the environment were sufficiently altered.

GAP and the NIMH were thus committed to resolving problematic environmental factors. This position was greatly at variance with the stance that had influenced American psychiatry in the earliest days of its founding in the first quarter of the nineteenth century.

At that time, alienists (as psychiatrists were originally called) believed that mentally ill people would get better if they were taken out of vexatious living conditions—the earlier the better for a good result. The alienists practiced "moral treatment," often taking patients into their own homes, which is how mental asylums frequently began. After the Civil War, a second phase began when moral treatment shifted to custodial care, under the influence of a belief in the heredity of mental illness, diminished hopes for effective treatment, and severe overcrowding in state institutions.

President Harry S. Truman (in office from 1945 to 1953) supported the creation of the NIMH. Moreover, in May 1948, just before the annual meetings of the APA and the American Psychoanalytic Association (APsaA), William Menninger, Karl's brother and president of the APsaA, was able to secure a personal meeting with the president. Menninger asked Truman to send "a message of greeting" to the upcoming meetings of the two organizations. The message Truman sent was indicative of the respect that many lay people had for psychiatry and psychoanalysis after the war: "Never have we had a more pressing need for experts in human engineering. The greatest prerequisites for peace...must be sanity...which permits clear thinking on the part of all citizens. We must continue to look to experts in the field of psychiatry and other mental sciences for guidance."[16] When Menninger gave his presidential address before the APsaA, he demonstrated his support of Truman's expectations of psychiatry and psychoanalysis:

> In an unhappy and unsettled world-wide situation, in the face of the need of psychiatric services and the training demands, can any member possibly justify in any conceivable way, the devotion of his entre ability to the treatment of eight or ten patients a year? Insofar as members of this association permit themselves such a misuse of their talents or the commercialization of their science, they threaten all psychoanalysis.[17]

Menninger had referred to "training demands," and GAP turned its attention to medical education immediately. First there was a push to increase the time devoted to psychiatric learning in medical schools, which grew fourfold between 1940 and 1966.[18] Then, for medical students, it was important that they be taught the principles of "psychodynamic psychiatry" (as psychoanalytically-oriented psychiatry is called); for psychiatry residents the emphasis needed to be on "individual therapy [and] the underlying unconscious significance of mental illness." After giving further thought to the teaching of residents, GAP decided that their education should be more comprehensive so that they would have "a broad perspective of Man in transaction with his universe"[19] Aside from a small group of biological psychiatrists, Kraepelin was ignored, and the medical model appeared moribund.

MENTAL INSTITUTIONS IN AMERICAN LIFE

At the same time that American psychoanalysts were trying to ensure that the next generation of psychiatrists would be psychoanalytically oriented and were turning their attention to social problems, change was overtaking state-hospital psychiatry. By 1960, 1 out of every 300 Americans had been involuntarily confined to a public institution at any given time.[20] State asylums, with their large chronic population, had an atmosphere that ranged from discouraging to depressing to horrific. Being the single most expensive item in state budgets, legislatures typically underfunded them; thus the hospitals did not attract professional and auxiliary staffs who were motivated to provide a therapeutic environment.[21] Most American physicians tended to look down on the psychiatrists who worked in state hospitals, condemning them for the backward and unscientific medicine they practiced. Moreover, spurred by the civil rights movement, activists sought to move hospitalized mental patients into local communities to treat them there. The 1962 novel, *One Flew Over the Cuckoo's Nest*, by Ken Kesey, only compounded the inhumane image of mental hospitals. However, the activists overlooked the important fact that chronic patients often remained hospitalized because they had become elderly and sick and had nowhere else to go.[22]

Still, criticism of the state hospitals—and by connection, state policies—was frequent. On the heels of war victory in 1945 came a spate of exposés of conditions in state hospitals. Titles such as *The Shame of the States, Snake Pit,* and *Bedlam 1946* attracted a wide readership and spawned cries for reform.[23] Where the states had failed, it was thought, the federal government could succeed. There were some preparatory experiences: the New Deal under Franklin D. Roosevelt had enlarged the role and services of the federal government, and World War II had bred "total war," in which the national government had mobilized the war front and the home front, increasing federal powers and dictates.

Now, after the war, people highly placed—the Secretary of Education and Welfare, Abraham A. Ribicoff (1910–1998); Felix of the NIMH; and his deputy director, Stanley Yolles (1919–2001)—worked toward developing community mental health centers funded by the federal government, anticipating the demise of the state hospital system within a generation. They were helped both by the spirit of the New Frontier of John F. Kennedy (in office from 1960 to 1963) and the American public's growing comfort with the legitimacy of psychotherapy in everyday life.[24] President Kennedy, in his address to Congress in 1963, proposed a radically optimistic federal health program: "The new knowledge and the new drugs acquired and developed in recent years…make it possible for most of the mentally ill to be successfully and quickly treated in their own communities and returned to a useful place in society." Such "breakthroughs," he added, "have rendered obsolete…a prolonged or permanent confinement in huge, unhappy mental hospitals."[25]

An important theoretical shift had occurred. During the first half of the nineteenth century, psychiatrists thought that mentally ill people could be cured if they were removed from their noxious environments. Then psychiatrists became pessimistic about this approach and lost their belief in the possibility of a cure. They came to espouse a belief in the inheritance of mental illness, for which they saw only custodial care, which in most cases became increasingly bleak. Now, in the 1950s and 1960s and even later, optimism returned, with the goal of reforming the noxious environment in order to prevent mental illness. It is impossible to overstate the belief among so many psychiatrists of that era that the prevention of serious mental disease was achievable.

With psychiatrists riding the crest of a long wave, the possibility of a crash seemed remote. They were busily and, for the most part, happily analyzing their patients, seemingly oblivious to the fact that they were not—even later in community mental health centers—treating the sickest patients. Based on their neurotic patient population, their theoretical position was that demarcating the well from the sick, and hence constructing diagnoses that would clearly distinguish between the two groups, was secondary to discovering the psychological meaning of various symptoms. Moreover, the principles of psychodynamic psychiatry were gaining increasing acceptance in American culture. An example of this is the special issue of the widely read *Atlantic Monthly*, which called itself a "Magazine of Literature, Science, Art, and Politics." The thick special supplement, appearing two years before Menninger's popular book, was entitled "Psychiatry in American Life," and by psychiatry the editor meant "the Freudian Revolution."[26]

DARKENING HORIZONS

At the height of this psychiatric optimism and psychodynamic thinking came a warning from within the psychoanalytic fold. Roy R. Grinker, Sr. (1900–1993), a prestigious voice, had founded the Department of Psychiatry at the University of Chicago and was the founding editor of the American Medical Association's *Archives of General Psychiatry*. He was also a prolific author. In 1965, Grinker spoke before the APA, chiding his colleagues on a number of fronts. He pointed out that the

> brave outpost [of the early psychoanalysts had] become a crumbling stockade of proprietary dogmatism [which] maintain[ed] itself aloof from the progress of behavioral science and look[ed] askance at conceptions of rigor. [More precisely,] studies of the various treatments for mentally ill patients require the establishing of diagnostic categories, defining the methods applicable to each and developing criteria for results [because] with rare exceptions, psychoanalytic reporting confuses cause, content, meaning and results. [He lectured that] rather than being humble about their therapeutic results and more concerned with investigating, psychiatrists ha[d] attempted to extend their influence to many levels of larger and larger group behaviors. [Finally,] public expectations [of a cure for mental illness] ha[d] been reinforced by extravagant promises by psychiatrists themselves in their search for support.[27]

But in 1965, Grinker stood almost alone among the self-assured psychoanalysts, who ignored his jeremiad.

Yet challenging voices could be heard. American psychiatry and psychodynamic thought and treatment were beginning to be called into question and even openly attacked in a variety of ways. In one area, biological psychiatrists chafed under the Freudian approach, which did not encourage empirical research and found the use of the medical model not necessary. Since 1946 the Society for Biological Psychiatry had wanted to link "psychological concepts [to] the anatomical structures that made these concepts possible." Although not in the mainstream of American psychiatry, they began to publicize themselves in the 1950s through professional talks and in articles in the *American Journal of Psychiatry*. To them the brain was the organ of the mind, thus they favored somatic therapies. They attacked psychodynamic thinking and, in a lecture at the APA, derided psychoanalysis as a religion instead of being a science.[28]

A contemporaneous medical trend favored these empiricists. After World War II, controlled clinical trials became the gold standard for evaluating therapies, existing ones, or new ones. Groupings of individuals sharing the same diagnosis were randomly assigned to a treatment group or to a control group. The treatment group received the therapy being tested in the trial, and the controls got another kind of treatment or nothing at all. (If it was a drug trial, the control group received placebos.) Clearly, it was very difficult for psychodynamic psychiatrists to put their therapy to such a test, as they treated patients one on one and did not have the efficacy of their treatment evaluated through these procedures. Moreover, as we have seen, the psychoanalysts in particular eschewed diagnosis; clinical trials, by contrast, relied on a diagnostic classification.[29] For many years, analysts ignored this medical approach as unnecessary to their enterprise, but their procedures could not remain aloof from such a strong challenge forever. An intimation of this future came in a study published in 1967 by Benjamin Pasamanick and colleagues, on the feasibility of treating individuals with schizophrenia who lived in their own homes and received drug therapy. Pasamanick, a career researcher, tested via controlled clinical trials whether severely mentally ill patients could remain in the community without the need for hospitalization. He obtained excellent results and used the opportunity to argue that the education of psychiatric residents was largely obsolete because they were not being properly trained to deal with the kinds of circumstances his study had shown were possible.[30]

From another perspective, a few psychiatrists, soon to be loudly heard, attacked the idea that mental illness was real. Moreover, social critics and academics were starting to claim that psychiatric problems were not medical but social, political, and legal. They argued that "since no pathophysiologic basis can be found to explain mental illnesses, these disturbances cannot be called diseases in the conventional medical sense." Psychiatry began to lose sole jurisdiction over psychotherapy as clinical psychologists became increasingly successful in their struggle to get licensing laws for themselves, thus strengthening their legitimacy.[31] In addition, social psychiatry's focus on "the role of family life, poverty, and racial discrimination" in the origins of mental illness and the stress on community-based treatment for psychiatric disorders had opened the door to criticism by an "antipsychiatry" movement.[32] The critics asked, if psychopathology is caused by harmful environmental conditions, then how can psychiatry claim to be a part of medicine?

Chronicle II: "Psychiatry Kills"

When the APA met in Miami for its 1969 annual meeting, the delegates needed only to look up to see a small plane going back and forth pulling a banner that read "Psychiatry Kills."[33] What lay behind these words?

The antipsychiatry movement was not a simple affair. It had two branches, each of which can be viewed separately but which also interacted with each other.[34] To begin with, the antipsychiatrists challenged the very distinction between mental illness and sanity, accusing psychiatrists of playing a social role to control people who were merely "different," not necessarily mad at all. The antipsychiatrists wanted to abandon the whole process of psychiatric diagnosis, treatment, and prognosis, thereby rejecting the traditional medical model. They also attacked the conventional goals of curing sick people by placing them in hospitals in order to treat them. Confusingly, some of the goals of antipsychiatry were shared by psychiatrists who still regarded themselves very much a part of their profession. Some psychiatrists had moved away from the medical model. Antipsychiatrists also advocated what came to be called "deinstitutionalization," an awkward word that meant getting patients out of state hospitals and into care in the community; ideally, this meant the very emptying of state asylums. (We shall return to this very important subject.)

Eschewing traditional diagnosis and treatment, the antipsychiatrists evolved new and different ways of dealing with what the psychiatrists regarded as illness. As one sociologist has written, "at one stage in the development of anti-psychiatry, for example, 'schizophrenia' was conceived as a voyage into 'inner space' and its 'treatment' [in an alternative] therapeutic community consisted in supporting the voyager through their [sic] voyage rather than attempting to 'cure' them of it."[35] From the vantage point of antipsychiatrists, physicians who helped patients adjust to noxious societal norms were actually harming their patients' very being.

The antipsychiatry movement was also part of a broader rebellion against contemporary Western society, which was seen as oppressive in a number of ways. Antipsychiatrists attended meetings side by side with radicals who fought against a variety of social ills. One such meeting on the "Dialectics of Liberation" included Herbert Marcuse, the Marxist social critic; Stokely Carmichael of the Black Panther Party; Paul Goodman, the author of *Growing up Absurd*, and a peace activist; and Paul Sweezy, the Marxist economist.[36] Antipsychiatry should thus also be seen as part of the counterculture of the 1960s and early 1970s, whose members inveighed against established authority, protested the war in Vietnam, and rose up on college campuses.

Finally, the public image of psychiatry in the 1960s and 1970s was gravely affected by the writings of a few prominent individuals. Here it is important to explore the ideas of the antipsychiatry movement fully in order to gain a sense of the extent to which psychiatry was thrown on the defensive by tightly constructed arguments and at times overwhelmed. We should note also the extent to which the antipsychiatrists referred to each other's work; they did not operate in isolation. We will begin with the ideas of Erving Goffman (1922–1983), a Canadian-born, American sociologist whose assault on state hospitals helped stir up strong feelings over the treatment of patients in large public mental hospitals.

PROMINENT ANTIPSYCHIATRSTS: ERVIN GOFFMAN

In 1954, the year after receiving his Ph.D. degree, Goffman went to Washington to do research at the NIMH in "socio-environmental studies," just what Robert Felix had in mind. Goffman observed the wards at the NIMH Clinical Center and spent a year at St. Elizabeth's Hospital, a public mental institution, which had a large census of over 7,000 patients. He wrote that his goal was "to learn about the social world of the hospital Inmate" and that he had tried to avoid social contact with the staff.[37] Goffman admitted that he came to St. Elizabeth's "with no great respect for the discipline of psychiatry," although he did record that the hospital and NIMH administrations had been very open and helpful. Nevertheless, he did not have the goal of giving a balanced account of psychological medicine. He wrote that "to describe the patient's situation faithfully is necessarily to present a partisan view." He excused this admitted bias, claiming that "the imbalance is at least on the right side of the scale, since almost all professional literature on mental patients is written from the point of view of the psychiatrists, and he [Goffman], socially speaking, is on the other side."[38]

The book he wrote about his observations, *Asylums* (1961), attracted much attention. It coalesced with larger beliefs held by mental health experts, patient advocacy groups, and federal politicians that community mental health centers could better deliver psychiatric care. The book also offered a justification to state legislators who were only too happy to close down costly state psychiatric hospitals, although the book was not their primary spur.[39]

Goffman's gifted prose style made him a compelling, even captivating, writer. This had the effect of making him appear as a quite reasonable and common-sensical social critic. Many reviewers remarked on his distinctive writing style, as well as his effective use of sarcasm and satire.[40] This, of course, increased the success of his arguments. In the discussion that follows here, all observations, opinions, and contentions are Goffman's own, unless otherwise indicated.

Goffman began his book with the view that the "craziness" attributed to a mental patient was due more to the diagnostician's "social distance from the situation that the patient is in" rather than to mental illness. Furthermore, a person's perception of losing his or her mind was based on having cultural and social stereotypes about so-called symptoms, which might simply be "a temporary emotional upset in a stressful situation."[41] How these upsetting situations were dealt with depended on what Goffman called "career contingencies," such factors as socioeconomic class, visibility of the "offense," and nearness to a mental institution. "Mental patients…suffer not from mental illness, but from contingencies"[42] In other words, according to Goffman, a psychiatric diagnosis did not arise from disorders within a person but was determined by circumstances outside of that individual.

Goffman took the position that often a "prepatient" was railroaded into the hospital by someone the person trusted, who then teamed up with the mental health

professional against him or her. Moreover, "the prepatient starts out with at least a portion of the rights, liberties, and satisfactions of the civilian and ends up on a psychiatric
ward stripped of almost everything."[43] In order to come up with a justification for the
hardships about to be inflicted on the prepatient, the medical staff would devise a case
history demonstrating "that all along [the prepatient] had been becoming sick...and
that if he had not been hospitalized much worse things would have happened."[44]

Once the prepatient became an inpatient, Goffman went on, what that person now
had to endure was what befell all those in "segregated establishments," such as prisons
and concentration camps: "mortifying experiences."[45] The patient's movement was
impeded, his or her individuality was crushed, and the person was subjected to the
arbitrary authority of all who worked there. These conditions were indicative of being
in a "total institution."[46] Once in the asylum, the patient, or "inmate," the term preferred by Goffman, had to learn the "ward system," a scheme by which the patient was
either rewarded or punished according to his or her behavior. While these controls and
privations might often be due to a variety of nonmedical circumstances, the patient
was told they were a consequence of his or her actions, which had the effect of chipping
away at self-regard. Ostensible individual or group psychotherapy, Goffman believed,
then became "arranged confessional periods." Furthermore, when patients described
themselves or their situation, the staff would discredit these statements in order to
make patients easier to manage and the patients "insightfully" adopted the hospital's
view of them.[47]

The case record, Goffman declared, showed only the patient's upsets and failures
and never described the times when he or she managed well. The hospital charts also
belittled patients via snide remarks made by the staff about their appearance and
manner. If one looked at almost anyone's life, Goffman charged, one could find sufficient grounds for commitment.

A "moral loosening" occurred in the presence of long-term commitment, Goffman
argued. So, for example, there was a "marriage moratorium." Patients who were already
married and received visits from spouses had extramarital hospital romances that
drew little negative attention or few sanctions. Goffman's conclusion was that mental
institutions encouraged amoral behavior. Patients learned to manipulate the system
and drop the old moral self they had before their hospital stay. They acted in ways that
society might find shameful but that in an institution were accepted; this was another
aspect of the "total institution."

Goffman pursued his indictment further via a sociological study of the relationships between the professional provider and the client in Western society. He sought
to establish that the specially skilled and moral provider acts in the best interest of the
client and that there is mutual respect between the client and provider. It is telling to
note that Goffman supported his contentions regarding the doctor–patient relationship by referring to articles by the antipsychiatrist Thomas Szasz, who had already
published widely before writing his famous book, *The Myth of Mental Illness* (see
below).[48] Goffman also attacked hospitals for operating for reasons other than healing:
Hospitals could have profit motives; they had training programs that affected patient
treatment adversely; they conducted research with agendas and designs that came

before patient care; and they constructed rules for patient management that served the interests of the staff.

Goffman then arrived at his main theme: testing the model of the skilled provider against the reality of the institutional psychiatrist. Here it is of interest how the antipsychiatry critics' assertions often overlapped. Even before publication of the French philosopher and historian Michel Foucault's (1926–1984) critique of the medicalization of insanity, *Madness and Civilization* (1964), Goffman wrote that in the Western history of persons who acted unconventionally, the eighteenth century saw the introduction of "the medical mandate over these offenders....Inmates were called patients, nurses were trained, and medically styled case records were kept."[49] Like the sociologist Thomas Scheff (see below), Goffman challenged the psychiatric position that patients with "functional psychoses"—this term was used to describe serious mental illnesses of unknown etiology, mainly schizophrenia or bipolar disorder—were being handled according to the medical model. Goffman argued that protecting the community from danger and nuisance was an important task of the public mental hospital but was not necessarily a medical service to the patient.

Another problem in comparing the model of skilled provision of expertise with that of the asylum had to do with the nature of involuntary commitment. Once in the hospital, patients found themselves, in almost every element of daily life, under the rule of the psychiatrist, whose "role is unique among [professional] servers, no other being accorded such power." Goffman especially pointed to conditions on the back wards, where "diagnosis...may be medical, while treatment is not."[50] Under the "ward-system," if patients were quiet they received privileges, if they were noisy they were punished. Since this system actually had little medical success, it could not justify institutional psychiatry.[51] And when patients were discharged, they found themselves back in the bizarre world to which their psychotic "symptoms" had been a response.[52] Goffman concluded that the medical model was not applicable to the mental hospital.

Not only did mental patients not receive medical treatment, but psychiatrists could only keep their self-respect through various career stratagems: They could leave the hospital for private practice, abandon the wards for administration, experiment with "new...unproved" family psychotherapy or therapy with the staff, or turn to research. However, if a psychiatrist decided to remain a ward doctor, he or she could only convince him- or herself of the legitimacy of this occupation by constructing for the patient a case record that showed how all of the patient's past had been pathological and then slapping a hazy and debatable diagnostic label on the patient to further corroborate that the patient was ill. So, if negative interpersonal events took place on the ward, Goffman maintained, they were translated in such a way that they became a function of the patient's basic character—for example, an altercation between a staff member and the patient became the latter's "aggressivity." Again, Goffman relied on Szasz, who had pointed out that this process "has similarities to the earlier view that the mental patient has a devil or evil spirit within him that must be and need only be exorcised."[53] The process turned a social problem into a personal psychological problem. Goffman related that he saw a black patient complain to a therapist about racial issues at St. Elizabeth's, which was partly segregated. The therapist told the man that he should ask himself instead why he alone—among all the black patients—was complaining, and what this told him about his personality.

Goffman declared that while prescribing medicine might be a legitimate function of the psychiatrist, doing psychotherapy might not be, because the social perspective had been omitted. The psychiatrist could call sudden changes for the worse "relapses or regressions" and sudden changes for the better "spontaneous remissions," when the reality was that the psychiatrist might not know what caused the changes.[54]

Finally, in order to establish that the hospital actually helped patients, the staff had to conjure up a specious medical construction, Goffman argued. The "ward system," which Goffman felt he had exposed for what it really was, had been transformed, he asserted, into a psychiatric medical service, since the institution had to justify its existence. "Regimentation" was redefined as a framework that allayed the patient's insecurity. "Sleeping dormitories" were called "wards" simply because they had hospital beds. Time spent in "isolation or the hole" was redescribed as a period when the patient could safely deal with acting-out impulses. "Admission wards" were called "acute services," while "back wards" were called "chronic services." Patients ready to leave were placed in the convalescent ward and then released "discharged as cured" or "discharged as improved," to maintain that "the hospital [had] had a hand in the curing or improving."[55] These medicalization efforts had the effect of saying that a medical service had been provided when, in truth, that was not the case, Goffman concluded.

Since American psychiatry in the 1950s and 1960s had little effective way of dealing with the functional psychoses, except with limited medication, this limitation opened the door to attacks on the very existence of the field, based on the contention that its actual practice did not fit the medical model.[56] And, as we shall see in Chapter 2, biologically oriented research psychiatrists attacked the dominant psychosocial/dynamic psychiatry for the same reason. It did not fit the medical model.

Goffman's sharply worded book gave an emotional cast to simultaneous federal policy-makers' views that preferred local community mental health care over that of large state institutions. The book and its title, *Asylums*, conjuring up past, unenlightened times, also met the desires of patient advocacy groups for reform. Moreover, the prospect of large monetary savings dangling before their eyes, state legislators only too happily reduced the census of mental patients or closed hospitals entirely.

THOMAS SZASZ

The same year that Goffman published *Asylums*, Thomas S. Szasz (1920–2012), an American psychiatrist and psychoanalyst born in Hungary, published a book with the startling title, *The Myth of Mental Illness*.[57] Szasz prefaced his book by pointing out that mental illness was said to be the nation's leading health problem; there were over half a million people in psychiatric hospitals. At the same time, psychotherapy was increasing rapidly, although it was "impossible" to know what psychotherapy really was because the term encompassed almost all human interactions. Furthermore, Szasz posed the question, what is it exactly that psychiatrists do? He announced that one goal of his book was to destroy the concept of mental illness and show psychiatry to be a "pseudomedical enterprise."

Szasz's book won him renown—if not notoriety—and soon residents flocked to Syracuse, where he was on the psychiatry faculty at the State University of New York (SUNY) Upstate Medical Center, to study with him. He was known to be an exciting teacher and taught advanced courses about psychoanalytic theory and contemporary psychiatric thinkers.[58] At the same the time he was publishing prolifically, starting in the late 1950s with articles in first-rate journals and then books at good presses.

Szasz equated psychiatry with alchemy and astrology, all "pseudo sciences," and practitioners of psychiatry with alchemists and astrologers, because neither group ever fully disclosed what they did. Psychiatrists might declare that they dealt with mental illness and mental health, but suppose there were no such things, Szasz provocatively pondered. Psychotherapists and psychoanalysts—again, all psychiatrists—who declared themselves to be scientists, actually did no scientific work. They acted as if they were physicians or biologists when, in reality, contended Szasz, the work of analysts and psychotherapists had more in common with that of logicians, those who studied signs (semioticians), and sociologists. Yet psychiatrists claimed they were working with the medical model. But the job of medicine was to study and alter "the physiochemical structure and function of the human body."[59] Psychiatrists, claimed Szasz, were "shackled" to an obsolete conceptual framework. Hence, psychotherapy "should be systemized as a theory of human relationships, involving special social arrangements and fostering certain values and types of learning."[60] Szasz was arguing that one did not have to be a physician to do psychotherapy.

Moreover, Szasz maintained that psychiatrists were using an outmoded concept: Freud's theory that "a single type of antecedent cause [unconscious forces] is sufficient explanation of virtually all subsequent human events." Marxism, he claimed, operated under the same fallacy, except that the single cause was economic conditions. Although Szasz was trained as a psychoanalyst, he asserted that Freud's claim was "an unsupported and…false theory of personal conduct."[61] Unfortunately, most American culture and science erroneously and unsophisticatedly accepted this, at a great cost, because "dynamic psychiatry [was a] means for obscuring and disguising moral and political conflicts as mere personal problems."[62] Actually, Szasz declared, people and society change, so human nature, regardless of what Freud and Marx said, changes too. Therefore, the laws of psychology needed to be formulated together with the laws of sociology.

According to Szasz, what psychiatry really did was to clarify and explain the kind of games people play with each other: "The analyst seeks to unravel the game of life that the patient plays."[63] Therefore, there needed to be a "long overdue *rapprochement* between psychiatry…and philosophy and ethics." As well as games, psychiatrists dealt with such questions as "How does man live?" and "How ought man to live?," which are philosophical and ethical. Therefore, their methods and theories were not the same as those of the natural sciences, Szasz declared. Psychiatrists could not solve moral problems by using medical methods. So-called psychopathology was more akin to a language than to an illness, so psychiatrists could not talk in terms of "treatment" and "cure."

Psychoanalysis had become so involved with intrapersonal problems, maintained Szasz, that it had fallen to other groups to deal with what he called "sociohistorical" issues. One group was the dissident schools of psychoanalysis (in 1961 Szasz had to mean those who were not members of the American Psychoanalytic Association) and another was the social psychiatrists. Szasz challenged the notion that psychoanalysis should be involved with the intrapersonal realm. From the earliest days of psychoanalysis, he argued, it was "concerned with man's relationship to his fellow man, and to the group in which he lives."[64] Making psychoanalysis medical obscured these concerns.

Another leitmotiv running through Szasz's book was announced in the book's subtitle: *Foundations for a Theory of Personal Conduct*. Szasz had a libertarian stance that stressed the freedom of the individual; people should take responsibility for their own lives, and society should respect their autonomy. Psychiatrists, therefore, should not assume that there is something "wrong" with odd behavior, and individuals should not be subject to involuntary hospitalization. One of Szasz's indictments of mental hospitals gained renown: "Involuntary mental hospitalization is like slavery. Refining the standards for commitment is like prettifying the slave plantations. The problem is not how to improve commitment, but how to abolish it."[65] Thus, if a person commits a criminal act and is found guilty, he or she should be punished without resort to an insanity defense. If a person is unhappy, it is up to that person to try to know more about him- or herself, about relations with others, and about possible goals in life. Szasz was once asked, "What if a person has no resources to pay for psychotherapy?" He replied, "He should get a job."[66]

Szasz and Goffman saw eye to eye on many reasons for a person ending up in a mental hospital. Like Goffman, Szasz contended that it was important to know "the sociology of the judge"—the judge being anyone who had the power to decide if someone was admitted to a public institution. Szasz asked, "What sorts of persons have the social power to make their judgments heard and to implement them? How do social class standing and the political makeup of society affect the roles of the judge and the potentially sick person?"[67] Szasz found validation for his views in national politics. He pointed out that before the Civil War there was the medical diagnosis of "drapetomania," the tendency of slaves to run away, and that in the former U.S.S.R. the desire to emigrate was officially designated "schizophrenia."[68]

Although there were certain biological fixed behaviors, Szasz admitted, a person's psychology was determined by his or her social environment. "Accordingly," Szasz claimed, "anthropology, ethics, and sociology are the basic sciences of human action since they are concerned with the values, goals, and rules of human behavior."[69] Arguing like Thomas Scheff (see below) about the process of labeling, Szasz declared that the type of behavior earlier called "witchcraft" was the same as what was now called "mental illness." He contended that psychiatrists were "morally judgmental and socially manipulative" in order to hold power over non-psychiatrists and patients.[70]

Through the experiences of childhood and religious teachings, human beings were commanded "to behave childishly, stupidly, and irresponsibly," what Szasz called an "exhortation to helplessness." Further, the Church and medicine taught that the "disabled...the sinful, the weak, and the sick...should be helped." At this juncture, Szasz's libertarian leanings came into play. He pointed out that those who manage well and are self-reliant do not need to be helped. Yet, "they may even be taxed, burdened, or coerced in various ways. The *rewarding of disability* (italics in the original)—although necessary in certain instances—is a potentially dangerous social practice."[71]

In summing up his arguments, Szasz stated emphatically that problems in living were not the same as diseases of the body. This was of great importance because proclaiming problems in living to be mental illness had political consequences. A citizen "undermine[d] the principle of personal responsibility upon which a democratic political system is necessarily based, by assigning to an external source (i.e., the 'illness') the blame for antisocial behavior."[72] Additionally, to hold an "illness" at fault for one's problems "preclude[d] an inquiring, psychoanalytic approach" to these problems. The challenge to science, Szasz concluded, was to rethink the entire issue of mental illness so that it could be placed under a new category, "the science of man." We might note that the phrase had a convincing ring, yet since Szasz said that psychiatry and psychoanalysis were not supposed to be sciences, what did he mean?

This might be a good place to interpolate that Szasz's assertions were sweet words for the health insurance companies, who argued that since "problems in living" were not mental illness, their treatment should not be reimbursed. And Szasz kept these arguments front and center—and therefore applicable—as he continued to write steadily over the years. Moreover, Szasz's beliefs that one did not have to be a physician to do psychotherapy accorded with the opinions of clinical psychologists and social workers, groups that were growing in number. Over the years, psychotherapy as a treatment had become more accepted by many individuals, so psychiatrists' practices were quite full, and the psychotherapeutic services of psychologists and social workers were increasingly sought. A turf war developed between psychiatrists, wary of the encroachments on their practices by these nonmedical groups, and the psychologists and social workers, who contended that mental disorders were not medical.[73] This was to become a central issue for the American Psychological Association during the making of DSM-III.

A decade after Szasz published *The Myth of Mental Illness*, he joined forces with L. Ron Hubbard (1911–1986), the leader of the Church of Scientology, a group with an extreme antipsychiatry bias, to form the Citizens Commission on Human Rights (CCHR). The CCHR holds that so-called mental illness is not a medical disease, that psychiatric medication is fraudulent and dangerous, and that the psychiatric profession should be condemned.

THOMAS J. SCHEFF

Another powerful voice of the antipsychiatry movement was an American sociologist, Thomas J. Scheff (b. 1929), who argued against the validity of the medical model on the grounds that there was "no rigorous knowledge of the cause, cure, or even symptoms of functional mental disorders. Such knowledge as there is, is clinical and intuitive, and thus not subject to verification by scientific methods."[74] Scheff then quoted psychiatric authorities to buttress his argument.[75] It is important to note the frequency with which the charge was made that psychiatry had no right to claim it was operating within the medical model. In 1973, when the American Psychiatric Association decided to revise its current diagnostic manual, one of the mandates it gave the DSM-III Task Force was to establish American psychiatry firmly within medicine.

In keeping with his assertion that psychiatry was ignorant of the etiology and treatment of many mental disorders, Scheff criticized psychiatric theory (by which he meant psychoanalytic thought) for not incorporating social factors into the understanding of mental disorder. The medical model focused "attention on individual differences rather than on the social system in which the individual is involved."[76] Scheff lauded the work of the sociologists Edwin M. Lemert (1912–1996), Kai T. Erikson (b. 1931), and Erving Goffman and of the psychiatrists Szasz, R.D. Laing (1927–1989), and Aaron Esterson (1923–1999) for trying to bring social processes into their theories without neglecting individual aspects. Regardless of Scheff's seemingly balanced statement, we shall see that, with the exception of Erikson, these men were solidly part of the antipsychiatry camp, although some resisted the label.

Scheff proposed a "social system" model of mental illness, saying it had dual advantages: It would be a framework for empirical research and would be "free of the questionable assumptions of inherent pathology in psychiatric symptoms."[77] He then created a new vocabulary that renamed "mental illness," the "mentally-ill" person, and "symptoms." *Mental illness* became "residual deviance," the *mentally ill person* was a "residual rule-breaker," and *symptoms* were "rule-breaking." The new terms, he argued, would eschew any presumption of illness. Therefore, symptomatic behavior was merely violating agreed-upon rules of the group.

Scheff offered a sociological theory of mental illness which postulated "that most chronic mental illness is at least in part a social role, and that the societal reaction is usually the most important determinant of entry into that role."[78] He used a concept of "deviance" that relied on the prior work of the sociologist Howard Becker (b. 1928). Deviance was the quality of people's reaction to an act, rather than "a characteristic of the act itself."[79] Like Szasz, Scheff stated that mental illness was no different from what other societies have called witchcraft or spirit possession, each a form of rule-breaking for which society originally had no name.

Arriving at the crux of his position, Scheff argued that the population at large had stereotyped views of mental disorder that they had learned in childhood and that were reinforced by the mass media. People then "exaggerated" and even distorted the extent of the violation of societal norms. This pattern of exaggeration Scheff designated "labeling."[80] The term became widely known. To underscore his approach, Scheff quoted what Goffman had written about hospital charts, that the case file of a person in an asylum only recorded instances of the person's "symptoms" and never the "occasions when the patient showed capacity to cope honorably and effectively with difficult life situations."[81] Scheff declared that the "societal reaction of [sic] rule-breaking is to seek signs of abnormality in the deviant's history to show that he was always essentially a deviant."[82] When a person's deviance becomes a public issue, society and that person react according to the traditional stereotypes of insanity. The deviant's rule-breaking adjusts and hardens to fit everyone's expectations, and the person is labeled mentally ill. "*Among residual rule-breakers, labeling is the single most important cause of careers of residual deviance*" (Scheff's own italics.) In subsequent editions of *Being Mentally Ill*, Scheff ameliorated his critique, having been confronted with the increasing prominence of biological psychiatry and psychopharmacology, which brought psychiatry more in line with the medical model. He also recognized that mental illness ("deviance") had to be looked at from more than one vantage point.[83]

Scheff's work had a great impact, providing, as it did, a theoretical substructure for antipsychiatry with his labeling theory. He also gave an academic imprimatur to civil libertarians' crusades to prevent a "deviant's" commitment to an asylum. Moreover, Scheff's pronouncements added to the momentum of discharging mental patients from state hospitals and bringing them into the community, a cause, as we have seen, promoted by many psychiatrists themselves. Seven years after Scheff first promulgated his labeling theory on the grounds that physicians know very little about supposed mental illness, a Stanford psychologist and lawyer, David Rosenhan (1929–2012) (see below), startled America by attempting to show—with an ingenious experiment—that psychiatrists could not tell the difference between the sane and the insane.

R. D. LAING

Scheff, Goffman, and Szasz were joined by R. D. Laing (1927–1989), a Scottish psychiatrist and psychoanalyst whose name came to be conspicuously associated with the antipsychiatry movement, although he did not start out as an antipsychiatrist. His initial psychiatric interest was in schizophrenia, and he brought to the study and comprehension of this condition his existential philosophy.[84] He envisioned his first book, *The Divided Self: A Study of Sanity and Madness*, as the initial publication in a series entitled "Studies in Existential Analysis and Phenomenology." It was the "task of existential phenomenology," he argued, "to articulate what the Other's 'world' is and his way of being in it."[85]

In keeping with his existential orientation, Laing insisted that a troubled human being be seen as a "person" who has "desires, fears, hopes or despair" rather than an "organism" who has psychopathology, for example, "depersonalization." An existentialist formulation of depersonalization would be that sufferers are in a state of feeling such little contact with the environment that they feel numb. Laing accepted that there were insane people but was quick to point out that there were also lots of people called sane, even if their minds were possibly unsound, or who truly were a danger to themselves and others, but society did not regard them as psychotic. Moreover, "the cracked mind of the schizophrenic may let *in* [sic] light which does not enter the intact mind of many sane people."[86] This judgment was a harbinger of Laing's eventual turning away from psychiatry, although at the time this was barely recognized, and he continued to get grants from the mainstream Foundations' Fund for Research in Psychiatry.[87]

Laing demonstrated that Kraepelin, in a now famous interview of a schizophrenic patient, made no attempt to understand the patient and believed that what the patient said was incomprehensible.[88] Laing then showed that the patient's remarks were understandable.[89] He went further and advocated that the therapist should draw on his or her own "psychotic possibilities." Only in that way could he or she comprehend the patient's "existential position:" not the patient's psychopathology but his "distinctiveness, and differentness, his separateness and loneliness and despair."[90] Laing's existential viewpoint was that psychiatrists had to be able to recognize and give credence to the patient's world, accept his or her feelings, and understand what the patient said and meant, but without psychiatrists going mad themselves.

Four years after *The Divided Self* was published, Laing, together with Aaron Esterson (1923–1999), also a psychiatrist and existential psychoanalyst, published a study of the families of schizophrenic patients that they had been working on for six years, entitled *Sanity, Madness, and the Family*.[91] In the interval from his first book, Laing's concerns had broadened, and his outlook on schizophrenia had shifted. He listed his interests as not only schizophrenia and families but also as "varieties of experience including mind-expanding drugs." He now maintained, repeatedly throughout this study and in another book three years later (1967, see below), that "to regard [schizophrenia] as fact is unequivocally false."[92] Echoing Szasz, whose book he cited, he insisted that one could not say a person is suffering from a disease if its etiology was unknown. "We reiterate," Laing added, "that we ourselves are not using the term 'schizophrenia' to denote any identifiable condition that we believe exists 'in' one person."[93]

After *The Divided Self*, Laing visited the United States and met not only with psychiatrists involved in treating schizophrenic patients and their families but also with Goffman and with Gregory Bateson, an anthropologist with a theory of the familial origins of schizophrenia (see below). Based on the views of his American contacts and his and Esterson's study, Laing argued for the social origins of schizophrenia. Laing and Esterson contended that the experience and behavior of "schizophrenics" are "socially intelligible" in light of family interactions and contexts. They concluded that their work and discoveries constituted a historical breakthrough as significant as the "shift from a demonological to a clinical viewpoint three hundred years ago."[94]

As Laing developed his views about the social origins of schizophrenia and considered the relationship between sanity and madness, he became widely known as an authority on the alienation of the modern human being. Alienation in Western society was a topic of considerable concern to the counterculture. For the hippies and the flower children, for example, there was a strong pull to create a communal society that could overcome the alienation they felt in industrialized and urban society; but these sentiments had a sympathetic ear outside the counterculture as well. Therefore, Laing's next work, *The Politics of Experience* (1967), was eagerly read and went into several printings.[95] He said his message was that there was no "normal man" anymore because "society clamps a straitjacket of conformity on every child who is born. In the process man's potentialities are devastated and the terms 'sanity' and 'madness' become ambiguous. The schizophrenic may simply be someone who has been unable to suppress his normal instincts to conform to an abnormal society."[96] How had Laing arrived at this conclusion?

With his family studies, Laing had begun to question whether schizophrenia should be considered an illness since it had social origins or, later, whether schizophrenia existed at all. At this point he had left the medical model and the world of medicine. In *The Politics of Experience*, moreover, Laing's tone had changed. It was more dramatic, and his diction was at times not readily understandable.[97] His intended audience had also broadened and he was widely read. Parts of his new book were published in *Peace News*, *The New Left Review*, and the *Psychedelic Review*.

Laing announced his book to be a discourse on alienation and its inevitable results: To begin with, "we are born into a world where alienation awaits us," which means we are always violating our very selves. We are all "murderers and prostitutes."[98] Furthermore, because of our alienation, we can never know how we each experience each other. Therefore, Laing proposed a new field, "social phenomenology," whose task it was to relate one's experience of the other's behavior to the other's experience of our own behavior. While psychoanalysis had its merits, he argued, it dealt only with the intrapersonal. Laing echoed Szasz's contention that psychoanalysis should be concerned with "man's relationship to his fellow men." Laing also used the notion of games to describe human behavior, another link with Szasz. This then was the substructure that formed the basis of Laing's new conception and understanding of schizophrenia and his reaction to previous investigations of it.

First of all, Laing declared, it should be realized that schizophrenia is neither a condition nor an illness. It is a label, he asserted, referring to two works of Scheff.[99] Yet even though a label, "the label is a social fact and the social fact a *political event*."[100] It was therefore necessary to appreciate that so-called mad behavior may not be mad at all when viewed in its context. Laing gave two examples. The first drew from Kraepelin, who, in the course of the examination of a schizophrenic patient, employed certain physical tests.[101] From Kraepelin's point of view this was rational; after all, it was the patient who was insane. But when Laing examined Kraepelin's tests—all of which were physically intrusive—from the viewpoint of the patient, they became bizarre. The second example Lang took from Goffman's *Asylums*, where Goffman argued that a patient's behavior, diagnosed as "regression" or "deterioration," made perfect sense when viewed in the context of the patient being in isolation or on a back ward.[102] Now Laing had set the stage for his ultimate conclusions.

If one studied the interpersonal environments of schizophrenics, one readily saw, Laing maintained, that their families were disturbed. He turned to the "double-bind" hypothesis of the anthropologist Gregory Bateson (1904–1980), a theory enjoying wide usage in psychiatry in the 1960s. Bateson had contended that the children in these disturbed families were consistently placed in no-win situations to which they had to respond. So, Laing asserted, "When one person comes to be regarded as schizophrenic, it seems to us that *without exception* the experience and behavior that gets labeled schizophrenic is a special strategy that *a person invents* in order to live in an unlivable situation."[103] Extrapolating broadly from this, Laing declared that schizophrenia is a "social adaptation to a dysfunctional society."[104] Although Laing regarded the process as self-evident, he noted that, nevertheless, society persists in stigmatizing the schizophrenic. Once the label of "schizophrenic" is affixed, there is a tendency that the labeled individual will always be regarded as "schizophrenic." This is significant because it involves the "*political* order...the ways persons exercise control and power over one another."[105] Thus did Laing portray the stigma attached to certain psychiatric diagnoses.

Laing wanted to negate the possibility of stigma and, therefore, to look upon schizophrenia as a state where the affected person finds her- or himself in "inner space and time." The person has embarked on a journey, experienced "as going back through one's personal life, in and back and through and beyond into the experience of all mankind...and perhaps even further into the beings of animals, vegetables, and minerals. [Then there is] a return voyage from inner to outer, from death to life...from a cosmic fertilization to an existential rebirth."[106]

Perhaps, Laing wrote, all of us would profit from such a journey because "our sanity is not 'true' sanity." The madness of our patients "is not 'true' madness [but] is an artifact of the destruction wreaked on them by us and by them on themselves."[107] Since "normal" is a product of repression and denial, Laing argued, it makes no sense to talk about supposed schizoid, schizophrenic, and hysterical "mechanisms." With "normal" behavior, "we are going to exterminate ourselves."[108] He predicted that "future men...will see that what we call 'schizophrenia' was one of the forms in which...the light began to break through the cracks in our all-too-closed minds."[109]

How does one account for the widespread appeal of Laing's remarkable ideas about schizophrenia? One explanation is that in the 1960s, knowledge about the etiology of schizophrenia was so scant that even outlandish ideas about the "functional psychoses" were being considered. Some of the non-Laingian theories of the familial origins of schizophrenia by quite mainstream psychoanalysts now seem fairly odd in retrospect.[110] But the appeal of Laing and other antipsychiatrists went beyond wrestling with the causes of schizophrenia. The ethos of their era must be factored in, and we will turn to this shortly.

RADICAL PSYCHIATRISTS

But first, the epic of the antipsychiatry movement would be incomplete without introducing the radical psychiatrists, a psychiatric group who wanted fundamental change in American society. Along with other social and political activists, they staged demonstrations and disruptions at the annual meetings of the American Psychiatric Association starting in 1968. Like Scheff and Goffman, they advocated a social model of mental illness, although unlike them, they had a political and economic agenda. They published a journal called *Radical Therapist* for two years (1970–1972), from which it is possible to extract their beliefs and goals.[111]

The radical psychiatrists attacked what they saw as the intentions of traditional psychiatry: maintaining power in society and pursuing prestige, economic well-being, and control over others. Psychiatrists did this, they said, by employing the medical model. Using this model, psychiatrists could maintain dominant power in the mental health field; everyone else had to occupy a subsidiary role. They also had domination over their patients who were kept in sick and dependent positions. Psychiatrists guarded the practice of psychotherapy as a skill that supposedly only they could do, but actually it was not a medical act "but an area of common humanistic endeavor drawing on biology, behavioral and social science, education, philosophy, psycholinguistics, communication theory, general systems theory, mathematics, literature, theology, and common horse sense."[112] Therefore, all who desired training as mental health workers should be afforded this opportunity via community instruction.

Expanding on Scheff and Goffman's position, radical therapists claimed that American psychiatrists had overstressed intrapsychic determinants of mental illness at the expense of social, economic, cultural, and political factors. In one article after another, the radical therapists posited an enormously wide range of causative agents of mental disorder, in essence issuing an indictment of American society. They listed "racism, sexism, overpopulation, unlivable cities, bureaucracy, technological growth, pollution and ecological imbalance, the war in Vietnam, militarism and imperialism, capitalism, the consumer economy and lack of meaningful work, and such faulty institutions as monogamous marriage, contemporary child rearing, and American schooling."[113] They asserted that traditional psychotherapy based on psychological understanding only compounded social ills by supporting the status quo through encouraging patients to adapt to an oppressive, imperialist, racist, sexist, and materialistic society.

To meet the needs of underserved populations—the homeless, drug users, the poor, and minority groups—community mental health centers, which had existed since 1965, should offer twenty-four-hour crisis intervention and emergency care. The radical psychiatrists were angry that community psychiatry had not responded to the special needs of the underserved but had instead offered traditional talk therapy to the middle class. (This was quite an accurate observation.) Each day, clinics should provide every type of helpful service ranging from traditional counseling to political organizing. All mental health services should be under community control.[114]

Agreeing with Laing, the radical psychiatrists took the position that "insanity is social and cultural, rather than medical...and a very appropriate solution to an insane world."[115] They argued especially for the rectification of Freudian psychiatrists' subjugation of women and against prejudice toward homosexuals. Moreover, articles in the *Radical Therapist* repeatedly criticized most available therapies, including the use of medication, shock therapies such as electrconvulsive therapy (ECT), behavior modification, and traditional psychoanalysis.

The radical psychiatrists undertook organizing and then protesting during an era when there were strong challenges to the Establishment in racial, social, and political matters. Once organized, they contributed to the furthering of the antiauthority climate by attacking the structures that underlay their own profession. While the radical therapists did not change the mindset of most psychiatrists, they prodded a minority into examining themselves and their motives. John A. Talbott, a prominent mainstream psychiatrist, for example, was moved to investigate the radicals' positions. He pointed out that their indictment of American society and of psychiatric practice held a lot of truth and, if ignored, would cost the profession in the end. In certain respects, Talbott was prescient.

Everywhere in the antipsychiatry movement the medical model was under assault. One of the bedrock arguments for this was that psychiatrists had no studies to prove the etiologies of mental illness. Therefore, it was asserted, psychiatrists falsely used the language of sickness to create the appearance of illness where it did not exist. Yet one must note that the leading figures of the antipsychiatry movement, aside from Laing and the radical psychiatrists, ignored the issue of human suffering. Whether these men talked in terms of "odd behavior," residual deviance," or "career contingencies," they leapt over evidence of the toll of auditory hallucinations, overwhelming anxiety, and fearful isolation to the suffering individual. Even Laing eventually turned a blind eye to the suffering caused by schizophrenia, seeing the illness as a positive journey. The antipsychiatrists' siege against the idea that psychiatry was a part of medicine was undermined by their failure to acknowledge the personal misery induced by the symptoms of mental disorder.

AN AMERICAN ZEITGEIST

The popularity of Laing and other antipsychiatrists was considerable and quite influential in the 1960s and 1970s because it reflected the mood of the era. Antiestablishment thinking was strong, especially hardened by the racial tensions of the time and the opposition of many to the Vietnam War. With his condemnation of a society that turned individuals sick, Laing developed a strong following. Moreover, the counterculture was not limited to hippie communes but could be found on many college campuses among students and faculty, including junior and senior professors. Also, as regards Laing specifically, the use of "mind-expanding drugs," which he had openly stated as one of his "research" interests, endeared him to a wide audience.

Furthermore, the antipsychiatry movement in general enjoyed wide political support, with the coming together of both ends of the political spectrum. The right wing took the position that people exhibiting strange behavior ought not to be supported by tax dollars but should take responsibility for their own lives. The Right also wished to undo the medicalization of social issues. Among the libertarians on the right, there was animus toward the role of the courts in enabling commitment procedures. A good example of this would be the stance of Thomas Szasz, who argued that the only time an individual should be incarcerated is when the person committed a crime and a jury found him or her guilty. There should be no commitment to state mental hospitals based on behavior that was noncriminal, even if it might be strange.

The left wing, meanwhile, was fighting for the civil rights of individuals whose family or physicians had petitioned the court for their commitment. The Left demanded that judges be scrupulous in respecting citizens' liberties. Not "locking up" people had a good antiestablishment resonance, as did arguing for their release from enforced hospitalization. The Left also argued that intrapsychic explanations for mental illness were less valid than social, cultural, and political ones, so confining people was less important than attending to issues of racism, poverty, slums, and unemployment. It should also be noted that the Left engendered sympathy from a number of liberal and social psychiatrists who were receptive to the issues of civil rights and social justice.

By the start of the 1970s, efforts on behalf of the rights of the mentally ill had reached a crescendo. Civil rights advocates often had the backing of the legal profession. In 1961, the American Bar Association had published the results of a lengthy study of the rights of the mentally disabled. Its conclusion indicated a shift from the traditional focus on professional needs to one on patients' rights. Around the same time (1960) a lawyer and a physician, Morton Birnbaum (1926–2005), had written an article for the *American Bar Association Journal,* arguing that patients had a constitutional right to treatment. He asserted: "An institution that involuntarily institutionalizes the mentally ill without giving them adequate medical treatment for their mental illness is a mental prison and not a mental hospital."[116] Five years later, Judge David Bazalon (1909–1993) adopted Birnbaum's argument on the constitutional right to treatment. In a decision in *Rouse v. Cameron,* 1966, Bazalon talked about rights under the Eigthth Amendment (from cruel and unusual punishment) and the Fourteenthth Amendment (the right to due process and equal protection of the laws). Similar decisions were made in lower federal and state courts.

In 1972, a civil liberties lawyer, Bruce J. Ennis (1940–2000), published a book with the arresting title, *Prisoners of Psychiatry.* Ennis charged that "[most] persons with severe mental disorders [will be] ignored, left to fend for themselves in the cheerless corridors and barren back wards of the massive steel and concrete warehouse we—but not they—call hospitals....The central problem...is the enterprise itself....They are put away not because they are, in fact, dangerous, but because they are useless, unproductive, 'odd,' or 'different.'"[117] The year after Ennis' book appeared, the Board of Trustees of the APA called a special meeting to consider what to do about their public image, and one of their resolutions was to call for a new *Diagnostic and Statistical Manual of Mental Disorders (DSM)* that would portray psychiatry as a more medical and scientific field. But the legal momentum did not slacken. In 1975, Ennis got the support of the U.S. Supreme Court, which, in a unanimous decision, upheld the rights of the nonviolent mental patient. Thus, in many states of the U.S., a resolute lawyer or judge could often prevent the civil commitment of even gravely mentally ill individuals unless they attacked someone. Beyond that, however, some civil rights activists used reasonable judicial decisions, such as the one that found prefrontal lobotomy a violation of First Amendment rights because it interfered with mentation, to campaign against all forms of psychiatric treatment.[118] This legal activity served only to increase emotions on both the right and left wings of the political spectrum.

Moreover, flushed with the headiness of 1960s activism, and sharing some of the goals of the New Left in American society, many social psychiatrists—still within organized psychiatry—wanted to use their medical expertise to advance liberal causes.[119] As psychiatrists they argued against the war in Vietnam and against school segregation. They defended themselves against challenges that they had inappropriately moved into political debates and were making social value judgments on the basis of their medical degrees. Believing that social stresses and dysfunctions were causes of mental illness, they rallied against injustices in American society: poverty, racism, unemployment, misogyny, and homophobia, including some of the varied indictments made by the radical psychiatrists.

PSYCHIATRY'S DIFFICULTIES MOUNT

The social psychiatrists were criticized within the wider profession on the grounds that they had made mental illness appear to be infinitely elastic. Alan Stone, the president of the APA in 1976, pointed out that "as each new community mental health center opened, more troubled people came forward to be treated." There was a growing and dismayed faction in the APA who felt that "social psychiatry and social activism, carrying psychiatrists on a mission to change the world, had brought the profession to the edge of extinction."[120] E. Fuller Torrey (b. 1937), a psychiatrist believing in the biological, not social, origins of schizophrenia, attacked social psychiatry, and to some extent all of psychiatry, in a widely quoted book, *The Death of Psychiatry*.[121] Conservative and activist psychiatrists battled. Meanwhile, the general animus against psychiatry grew broader. Competing mental health professionals such as clinical psychologists and psychiatric social workers, using divisions among psychiatrists, continued to push their own expertise. The unpopularity of state mental hospitals grew. Federal policy-makers preferred local community-based mental health care to large, often distant institutions. This long-wished-for reform was to produce new difficulties.

Once Medicare and Medicaid were in place in 1965, with assured federal funding, "deinstitutionalization" appeared a realistic goal. The program had also been sped along by the revolutionary introduction of psychotropic medications in the 1950s and 1960s, starting with Thorazine (chlorpromazine), an effective antipsychotic for the overpowering auditory and visual hallucinations of schizophrenia. Tofranil (imipramine) and Elavil (amitriptyline) were early tricyclic antidepressants for the often debilitating effects of depression. Eskalith and Lithobid (lithium carbonate) were used to deal with the afflictions of mania. Finally, three tranquilizers, Miltown and Equanil (meprobamate), Valium (diazepam), and Librium (chlordiazepoxide), which could soothe crippling anxiety, rounded out the new psychiatric drug treatments at the mid-twentieth century.

Discharges of state hospital patients proceeded apace. From a peak of 550,000 residents in state hospitals in 1955, the census plunged to 370,000 in 1969, and by 1994 was at 80,000.[122] Some of the released patients, who were elderly or physically ill, immediately clambered aboard buses that took them straight to nursing homes. But a significant percentage was discharged to be followed up by the community mental health centers. This became a problem because with inadequate funding, never near enough CMHCs were opened, only 500 out of a projected 1500, and even the ones opened were beset by monetary quandaries. There were thousands of severely mentally ill patients who had nowhere to go and became homeless, lacking necessary social services and often medication. Not only was this a profound failure of mental care, but the homeless on the streets frightened people in their neighborhoods. Another embarrassment was now laid at the door of the psychiatrists.

Psychoanalysts in particular were shown to be unready to deal with serious and debilitating mental illness. In 1962, the APA had responded to this situation by convening a four-day conference together with the Canadian Psychiatric Association on graduate psychiatric training. It was concluded that the teaching of the epidemiology and physiology of the major psychiatric diseases was being neglected.[123] Yet, a decade later, little had changed, as reported in a 1975 study conducted by the APA and NIMH and written up by a prominent analyst, Judd Marmor (1993–2003).[124] Perhaps the findings were not surprising, but they were authoritative. Psychiatrists with private-office practice treated well-to-do professional and business people and not individuals with severe mental illness. This was one more reproach aimed at the dominant—although beginning to wane—psychodynamic establishment.

Added to psychiatry's worries was the fact that research and treatment dollars were shrinking; from 1963 through 1972, there was a seventeen percent reduction in the number of research grants awarded by the NIMH.[125] And there were other disquieting situations, tellingly documented by the psychiatrist Mitchell Wilson. Soon after coming into office, President Jimmy Carter established a Commission on Mental Health, which made its report in 1978.[126] The report expressed the perplexity of the Commission's members: "Documenting the total number of people who have mental health problems...is difficult not only because opinions vary on how mental health and mental illness should be defined, but also because the available data are often inadequate or misleading."[127]

Even earlier, insurance companies had begun to voice concerns. In the 1960s, federal government employees were reimbursed for treatment of psychiatric illness by Aetna and Blue Cross, their insurance carriers, on a par with coverage for other medical illnesses. These good mental health benefits drew people to the Washington, DC, area to work for the government. (The word at the time was that there were more psychiatrists practicing in suburban Maryland than in New York City, the proverbial home of American psychoanalysts.) But in 1975, the APA's *Psychiatric News* splashed across page 1 of an issue: "Blue Cross VP Says MH Prospects Cloudy." It quoted Robert J. Laur, a vice-president of Blue Cross:

> Compared to other types of [medical] services there is less clarity and uniformity of terminology concerning mental diagnoses, treatment modalities, and types of facilities providing care....One dimension of this problem arises from the latent or private nature of many services; only the patient and therapist have direct knowledge of what services were provided and why.[128]

Recall the psychoanalytic position on diagnosis: Diagnosis was not necessary because all psychopathology stemmed from the same basic unconscious conflicts. This belief had come to affect adversely the legitimacy of psychiatry from the viewpoints of what constituted a mental disorder and professional accountability for treatment.

An influential senator was perturbed: "Unfortunately, I share a congressional consensus that our existing mental care delivery system does not provide clear lines of clinical accountability."[129] Already, three months earlier, Aetna had acted decisively and cut back mental health coverage to twenty outpatient visits and forty inpatient hospital days per year.[130]

Chronicle III: "Schizophrenia in Remission" and "Sexual Deviations"

"ON BEING SANE IN INSANE PLACES"

The dwindling fortunes of American psychiatry were depleted even further by two highly public events of 1973. The year started with a sensational—albeit scholarly—exposé in the staid and prestigious columns of *Science*. Following the articles "Earliest Radiocarbon Dates for Domesticated Animals," "Maternally Acquired Runt Disease," and "Gene Flow and Population Differentiation" came the attention-grabbing title "On Being Sane in Insane Places."[131] The author was David L. Rosenhan (1929–2012), at that time a little-known Stanford psychologist and lawyer with an expertise in abnormal psychology.[132] After the *Science* article was published, he was catapulted to instant fame.

In the heated climate of the antipsychiatry movement, Rosenhan's first sentence was arresting: "If sanity and insanity exist, how shall we know them?"[133] He began to answer his question by citing the evidence showing how psychiatrists disagree on diagnoses. He concluded that it is "a simple matter" to distinguish the sane from the insane if one can only demonstrate whether the characteristics leading to a diagnosis are within the patients themselves or in their environments. Rosenhan referred to the work of Goffman, Laing, Szasz, and Scheff, who asserted "that psychological categorization of mental illness is useless at best and downright harmful, misleading, and pejorative at worst."[134]

Rosenhan proposed an experiment. Suppose one got normal people with no history of psychiatric disorders admitted to a mental hospital and then determined "whether they were discovered to be sane and, if so, how." To do this, he engineered the secret admission of eight sane people to twelve different mental hospitals in five separate states on the East and West coasts, unbeknownst to the hospital staffs. The "pseudo-patients" were varied in age and occupation and employed pseudonyms. They telephoned ahead for appointments, and when they arrived, complained of hearing voices, specifically the words "empty," "hollow," and "thud." "Beyond alleging the symptoms and falsifying names, vocations, and employment, no further alteration of person, history, or circumstances were made...None of their histories or current behaviors were seriously pathological in any way."[135] Once the pseudopatients reached the psychiatry wards, they stopped hearing voices, had no symptoms of any kind, and acted their usual selves. Their behavior on the wards, as recorded by nurses, was that they were "friendly," "cooperative," and "exhibited no abnormal indications."

The pseudopatients were never detected. They had been admitted with the diagnosis of "schizophrenia" (one was called "manic depressive") and when discharged were determined to have "schizophrenia in remission." The quality of the hospitals was never an issue. The length of the hospitalizations varied from seven to fifty-two days with an average of nineteen days. Quite a number of their fellow patients concluded that the pseudopatients were not ill at all but were either journalists or professors. (The pseudopatients were taking notes.) Yet, Rosenhan scornfully announced, no one on the staff ever raised the issue of their sanity. The reaction of psychiatrists was to criticize Rosenhan's indictment of the profession. They said that when a person presents him- or herself at an admissions office and complains of hearing voices, there is no reason not to trust the legitimacy of the individual and the legitimacy of the symptoms. If the psychiatrists did not accept at face value what they had been told, they would be endangering the health of many.

In his discussion, Rosenhan pointed out that being diagnosed with a psychotic illness was no small matter; a psychiatric diagnosis carried with it "personal, legal, and social stigmas." So it was important to see if the diagnostic process could go the other way. Could the hospital staff spot pseudopatients if the staff knew in advance that some were going to be admitted?

> An experiment was arranged at a research and teaching hospital whose staff had heard [about Rosenhan's] findings but doubted that such an error could occur in their hospital. The staff was informed that at some time during the following 3 months, one or more pseudopatients would attempt to be admitted into the psychiatric hospital. Each staff member was asked to rate each patient who presented himself at admissions or on the ward according to the likelihood that the patient was a pseudopatient.[136]

The staff rendered decisions on 193 patients, and a substantial minority was adjudged to be pseudopatients. Then Rosenhan revealed that no pseudopatient had come to the hospital in the past three months. He delivered a verdict. "One thing is certain: any diagnostic process that lends itself so readily to massive errors of this sort cannot be a very reliable one."[137] Regardless of the psychiatrists' critiques of Rosenhan's original experiment, at this point they found it very difficult to defend their diagnostic procedures.

Rosenhan had dropped a bomb. Just three pages into his article, no matter what he wrote afterward, readers were already staggered. The remainder of Rosenhan's article, by which he sought to cement his judgment on psychiatric diagnosis, was almost anticlimactic. He examined the issues of psychiatric "labeling" and of staff responses to patient-initiated contact, as well as what he called "depersonalization," by which he meant the origins and consequences of dehumanizing the patient.

The discussion of labeling showed Rosenhan's indebtedness to Scheff and Goffman, whose work had been around for over a decade. Rosenhan believed he had proved that once a person had a psychiatric diagnosis, he or she was stuck with the label. Once on a psychiatry ward, even normal behavior was disregarded or misinterpreted. A psychiatric diagnosis was dependent on the environment and context rather than the patient's health, he argued, and he presented some persuasive examples of a diagnosis overcoming reality.

First, a pseudopatient's ordinary-sounding history of his relationships with his parents was entered on his chart as "a long history of considerable ambivalence [where] affective stability is absent." Rosenhan deduced this to be a judgment evocative of the current psychiatric theory of the "schizophrenigenic" family.[138] The second example Rosenhan gave stemmed from the fact that all the pseudopatients took notes while on the ward. While other patients frequently commented on this, no one on the staff ever approached a pseudopatient to ask about it. Only afterward, one patient's chart was seen to contain a nurse's note of pathology: "Patient engages in writing behavior."

Rosenhan declared that the professional conclusion was that if "the patient is in the hospital, he must be psychologically disturbed."[139]

Rosenhan also contended that, according to notes kept by the pseudopatients, if a patient was mistreated by an attendant and went "berserk," his behavior was always laid at the door of his pathology, never connected with the staff–patient interaction. Finally, Rosenhan maintained, labels led to self-fulfilling prophecies. Both mental health workers *and* the patient assumed that the latter's behavior should be termed "schizophrenic," and the patient acted accordingly. There was psychiatric evidence to support some of Rosenhan's observations. When he wrote in the early 1970s, schizophrenia was being overdiagnosed in the United States, a fact recently acknowledged as a result of an important study.[140]

Rosenhan next considered staff response to patients who had initiated contact once on the ward. He reported that the staff's response to a question was usually minimal. "By far, [the staff's] most common response consisted of either a brief response to the question, offered while they were 'on the move' and with head averted, or no response at all."[141] Little eye contact and little verbal contact diminished the human status of the patient; the patient had undergone "depersonalization."[142] Moreover, Rosenhan argued that institutional treatment of patients emphasized their dehumanization and powerlessness in repeated ways. He offered his records of patients who were beaten when they tried to talk to an attendant, then he enumerated patients' loss of agency when they were committed: shorn of many legal rights, credibility gone, movement restricted, unable to initiate contact with the staff, privacy minimal (including many bathroom stalls without doors), and everyone—even volunteers—having access to the patient's chart.

Rosenhan held that the fundamental origins of depersonalization in a psychiatric hospital were threefold. There were the "fear, distrust, and horrible expectations" of the mentally ill, leading to avoidance. There was little contact with patients, especially by physicians whose "behavior inspires the rest of the staff." Yes, Rosenhan admitted, there were staff shortages owing to monetary constraints, but patient contact was one of the very first things to go. Finally, there was the heavy reliance on psychotropic medications, which convinced the staff they had done all they needed to do by way of treatment. One of the consequences of depersonalization, Rosenhan declared, was that there were sane people locked away, unrecognized as such, because they were responding to a "bizarre setting," what Goffman called "mortification," or socialization to life in a psychiatric hospital.

It was Rosenhan's closing judgment that one could not tell the sane from the insane in a psychiatric hospital because the environment itself led to false interpretation of behavior. Not only the patients but also the staff were controlled by the environment. There was a need, therefore, to change the environment to a "benign" one without "global diagnosis." This could be achieved, he urged, by discharging patients to community mental health centers, relying on the human potential movement, and turning to behavior therapies that eschewed psychiatric labels.[143] We now know his proffered solutions were naively rosy.

The year 1973 turned out to be a calamitous one for the public perception of American psychiatry. The first disaster was the Rosenhan study. The second riveting episode revolved around how the APA came to remove the designation of homo-sexuality as a mental illness from its *Diagnostic and Statistical Manual of Mental Disorders*.[144]

HOMOSEXUALITY AS A DIAGNOSIS OF PATHOLOGY BY THE APA

In the late 1960s, heavily influenced by civil rights activism—rallies, marches, picket lines, and sit-ins—various gay groups decided to attack directly long-established cul-tural, social, and even political prejudices against homosexuality. In particular, gay groups focused their attention on psychiatrists whose manual declared them ill. They were partly buoyed by Szasz's assertion of the medicalization of social behavior.

A newly formed, radical gay group, the Gay Liberation Front, drew sustenance from protests against American imperialism (war in Vietnam), racism (black segregation), and male domination (women's subordination). First, gay men began to talk publicly about their painful experiences while in psychotherapy, which they declared had had the effect of sharpening their sense of being unworthy in the wider society. Then they mounted "Gay Pride" demonstrations, drawing from the black declaration of "Black is Beautiful," and demanded an end to sodomy laws that made a private act a public crime. Gay groups organized pickets, demonstrations, and sit-ins targeting not only psychiatrists who gave public lectures on the "disease" of homosexuality but also the Catholic Church and the mass media. They also began staging disruptions based on the model of anti-war protests.

At the height of the antipsychiatry movement, "antagonism toward psychiatry could be transformed into a focused assault upon the psychiatric profession."[145] The APA became the target of homosexual attack in 1970 when gay activists in San Francisco decided to disrupt sessions of the APA's annual convention. The activists, joined by other protestors who had a more general antipsychiatry stance, formed a human chain around the convention center to prevent psychiatrists from entering the meeting.[146] Indoors, shouting matches and derisive laughter greeted a psychiatric expert on homosexuality, Irving Bieber (1908–1991), at a session on transsexual-ism and homosexuality. One protester called Bieber a "motherfucker." At another panel on "Issues of Sexuality," demonstrators loudly disrupted and demanded to be heard, whereupon the meeting was declared adjourned. Pandemonium broke out. The psychiatrists at the session began denouncing the activists. When "a protestor attempted to read a list of gay demands, he was denounced as a 'maniac.' A feminist who spoke out was called a 'bitch' .... One physician called for the police to shoot protestors."[147]

At this point, because of the risk that the entirety of the next year's APA meeting would be under siege, the program chair agreed to have a panel at which gay men and lesbians could present their views. Nevertheless, when May 1971 came around, gay activists, joined by anti-war demonstrators, still waged disruptions. In meetings throughout the country, psychiatrists began to divide on the issue of how to regard homosexuality.

A triggering event for gay demands to take homosexuality out of the DSM occurred in 1972 when the New York Gay Alliance decided to "zap" a meeting of behavior therapists, to call for the end of the use of aversion techniques on homosexuals in an effort to change their sexual orientation. At this meeting, a psychiatrist at the New York State Psychiatric Institute at Columbia University, Robert Spitzer, came into contact for the first time with homosexuals demanding an end to the official APA stance on homosexuality. Spitzer was impressed by what he heard, and he did two vital things. As a member of the APA's Committee on Nomenclature, which oversaw the DSM, he arranged for the gay men and women to present their arguments to the Committee. He also said he would sponsor a panel at the APA's 1973 meeting on whether homosexuality should be a diagnosis in the DSM. Both scientific evidence and civil rights would be discussed at the panel. After the gay participants had met with the Committee on Nomenclature in February 1973, Spitzer was resolved to push the issue forward.

By the time the full APA met in May 1973, Spitzer had become increasingly convinced that there were many homosexuals who led perfectly "normal" lives and functioned successfully in society. Why, then, should they be considered to have a "psychiatric disorder"? As to the promised panel specifically, he arranged a debate between psychiatrists who were convinced that gay individuals had had a flawed upbringing on the one side, and psychiatrists who believed that there was no tenable scientific evidence to support designating homosexuality as a mental illness on the other. One psychiatrist took the Szaszian position that it was not the job of psychiatrists to be social "watchdogs." A gay activist, Ronald Gold, also spoke. The panel drew an audience of 1,000 and was heavily covered by the press.[148] The tide seemed to be shifting in favor of changing the DSM.

To top things off, Gold brought Spitzer to a secret meeting of gay psychiatrists who were members of the APA. They were initially outraged at Spitzer's unexpected presence because of the risk to their jobs and to their family relationships if their homosexuality were revealed. Alix Spiegel, granddaughter of the 1973 president-elect of the APA, John P. Spiegel (1911–1991), reports that there were closeted gay chairmen of psychiatry departments at the meeting. Her grandfather, also in the closet, "came out" to his family eight years later.[149] Gold convinced the gay psychiatrists to take this historic occasion to speak to Spitzer. They did, and Spitzer was persuaded "that being homosexual had little to do with one's capacity to function at a high level."[150]

Spitzer thereupon drew up a compromise proposal: to delete the word "homosexuality" from DSM-II, where it was the first diagnosis under "Sexual deviations," and replace it with "sexual orientation disturbance," which would apply only to homosexuals who were unhappy with their lives as gay individuals and who sought psychiatric help. Simultaneously, the Committee on Nomenclature unanimously approved a statement on the civil rights of homosexuals; on the issue of whether homosexuality represents psychopathology they were divided. But when the issue reached the APA Council on Research and Development, a body devoted to scientific matters, the Council voted "unanimously to approve the deletion of homosexuality from DSM-II," the then current edition of the diagnostic manual. After approval by the Council, the proposal went to the Assembly of the District Branches of the APA, which reflected patient treatment concerns. "The overwhelming majority voiced approval."[151] At each step of the deliberative process, tensions mounted. Next in the chain was another APA body, the Reference Committee, composed of the chairs of all the various APA councils and the president-elect. This group also endorsed Spitzer's nomenclature proposal. With everyone now expecting the APA Board of Trustees to give final approval, gay activists pushed for the decision to be announced at a press conference. First, though, the Board heard from psychiatrists opposing the change, although this was a pro forma gesture. Then it discussed the issue, with a majority accepting "the distinction drawn by Spitzer between sexual behavior that was not normal and that which ought to be termed a psychiatric disorder."[152] On December 15, 1973, the Board accepted the recommendation from the Reference Committee to change the homosexuality classification in DSM-II to "sexual orientation disturbance" and also overwhelmingly approved Spitzer's civil rights proposal. Across the country, newspapers vividly described the APA's decision.

Privately, however, many psychiatrists expressed displeasure and bitterness at their association's decision. Among opponents of the new position, the main criticism was that psychiatry had abandoned its scientific posture. An Ad Hoc Committee Against the Deletion of Homosexuality from DSM-II was immediately formed. The committee drew up a petition to demand a referendum of the APA's entire membership and quickly got the requisite 200 signatures from those attending the winter meeting of the American Psychoanalytic Association. Observers were astonished. Psychiatric disorders would be decided by a democratic vote? And the same psychiatrists who had denounced the APA's Board's "capitulation to political pressure" should now be calling for a referendum? Nevertheless, the APA duly sent out ballots in the mail, and America's psychiatrists thereupon formally asserted in 1974 that homosexuality should be removed from DSM-II. The press had a field day, and psychiatry's reputation as a scientific field sank even further.

The 1960s and 1970s were wrenching years for American psychiatry. The profession faced a widespread and determined activism that challenged its very legitimacy, a situation made tangible by the dispiriting decision of insurance companies to reduce payment for treatment of psychiatric disorders. Struggling to maintain its dignity with the public, the profession was rocked by David Rosenhan's provocative hospital experiments and the APA's infelicitous balloting of its members to ascertain whether homosexuality was psychopathology. Yet, though realized by only a very few, a revolution was beginning to take shape that would lead psychiatry not simply to a new era but to eventual seeming repute, even though the new approach was hotly debated within the profession.

2

EMIL KRAEPELIN:
BIRTH OF MODERN DESCRIPTIVE
PSYCHIATRY

To look insightfully at the theoretical position that American psychiatry began to assume in the last quarter of the twentieth century, it is useful to locate this stance in the context of the cyclical nature of much of Western psychiatry in the last two centuries. This contextualization will also help to situate psychiatry in the nineteenth-century traditions from which Emil Kraepelin, the influential German psychiatrist, emerged. In this discussion, the term " neo-Kraepelinian"—used to characterize the psychiatry that succeeded in trumping antipsychiatry—will become meaningful. The neo-Kraepelinians espoused a descriptive and biological approach to psychiatry in ways very similar to that which guided Kraepelin and in somewhat analogous circumstances. DSM-III reflected the Kraepelinian and neo-Kraepelinian mode of thought. Moreover, in certain respects, the problems of psychiatry that preceded both Kraepelin's and Robert Spitzer's revolutionary contributions are also comparable; Spitzer can be ranked as the most influential psychiatrist in the late twentieth century, as significant as Kraepelin was in the early part of the century.

In 1856, Kraepelin was born into a Germany that stressed—indeed sometimes worshiped—realism, materialism, and positivism in politics and science. In politics it was a time of German unification through the vehicles of nationalistic—some might say ruthless—wars, which cast into sharp disrepute the earlier failure of Germany to unify under liberal and intellectual auspices. Arms brought what ideas could not do. In science it was a time of the increasingly triumphal development of basic science and medicine in which Germany captured the leadership of the Western world.

The materialistic emphasis of German science was in part a response to nonmaterialistic ways of thinking that had been dominant in the first thirty or forty years of the 1800s; these ideas have been subsumed under the rubric of the Romantic era. Set in this earlier science was *Naturphilosophie*, a structure of beliefs in the interconnectedness of all nature, in an energy source that was common to all life—the idea known as vitalism—and in a preoccupation with self-consciousness and the unconscious. Hypnotism was valued and regarded as perhaps a key to the understanding of all phenomena. Knowledge based on intuition was accorded respect, as seen in the "speculative physics" of the philosopher Friedrich W. J. von Schelling (1775–1854). Fundamental questions were raised concerning the relationship of human beings to the universe and to what purposes nature functioned as it did.

In psychiatry, a fledgling discipline, the human being was seen as a psychobiological entity. Moreover, as George Mora has pointed out, Romantic psychiatry "focused on the individual and on his unique response…to an individual [medical] approach."[1] The psychiatrist—or alienist, as he was then called—did not usually draw sharp lines between sickness and health. The height of sophisticated Romantic thought found expression in an 1845 textbook of the physician, poet, and philosopher Ernst von Feuchtersleben (1806–1849), *Lehrbuch der ärztlichen Seelenkunde*, almost immediately translated into English, as *Principles of Medical Psychology*. The demand for Feuchtersleben's book became so intense that the publisher recalled copies given gratis to the trade so that they could be given to booksellers.[2] Feuchtersleben declared that "all branches of human research and knowledge are naturally blended with each other." He could not give a "complete view" of any science without discussing what "other departments" had to say about it. He believed philosophers and physicians had things to say to each other, and in considering what the mind was, physicians should investigate the views of the philosophers Spinoza, Kant, Fichte, Schelling, and Hegel. He decided that "the notion, *mental disease*, must therefore be deduced, neither from the mind, nor from the body, but from the relation of each to the other."[3]

Feuchtersleben and others took a sophisticated interest in emotional, irrational, and hidden forces in human nature. He in particular introduced a differentiation between psychoses and neurosis. Yet it must be said that the understanding of such matters and of the principles governing human relationships were subjectively divined and not put to experimental confirmation. And even though asylums for the mad existed by then, physicians neglected what could be learned from clinical experience in favor of a priori constructions.[4]

REACTION AGAINST NONMATERIAL THINKING

After more than a generation of preoccupation with universal concerns, scientists and physicians concluded that this approach to scientific knowledge had netted them precious little. They condemned, often in harsh tones, the philosophical, especially teleological, concerns of the Romanticists. A nineteenth-century German historian of medicine, Theodor Puschmann (1844–1899), accused them of "los[ing] touch completely with practical life" as they plunged "into the mystico-transcendental realms of speculation." (We shall hear an echo of these words in reference to psychoanalysis from the neo-Kraepelinians in the next century.) Puschmann dismissed as fanciful the Romanticists' psychobiological orientation. German psychiatry, he warned, should never return to "the question of the essential nature and ultimate foundation of things."[5]

A cohort of often brilliant physiologists, physicists, pathologists, and embryologists arose to displace *Naturphilosophie*. Such men as Emil du Bois-Reymond (1818–1896), Ernst Brücke (1819–1892), Hermann von Helmholtz (1821–1894), Rudolf von Kölliker (1817–1905), Carl Ludwig (1816–1895), and Rudolf Virchow (1821–1902)—all born within four years of each other—put Germany in the forefront of science and medicine. With the exception of Kölliker and Virchow, these men have been identified as "the school of Helmholtz" or, perhaps more accurately, the "biophysics movement of 1847."[6] Scientifically and philosophically, their approach to medicine had three aspects.

First, there was a belief in the materialism and tangibility of all matter. In 1842, du Bois-Reymond wrote:

> Brücke and I pledged a solemn oath to put into effect this truth: "No other forces than the common physical-chemical ones are active within the organism. In those cases which cannot at the time be explained by these forces one has either to find the specific way or form of their action by means of the physical-mathematical method or to assume new forces equal in dignity to the chemical-physical forces inherent in matter, reducible to the force of attraction and repulsion."[7]

Second, they agreed that the only way the scientist learned about these forces was through experimentation and observation.

And finally, the Helmholtzians found no evidence of any teleological force in nature. In 1858, Virchow showed that disease develops when severe stimuli disturb the life processes of the cells. Any vitalist notion that invisible, ethereal substances were at work was ruled out; all cells came from other cells. It could now be shown that a causality completely intelligible to ordinary perception could explain nature's processes. Nothing seemed to stand in the way of solving all the mysteries of life, organic and psychological, through the new materialistic scientific methods. When Brücke published his *Lectures on Physiology* in 1874, he proclaimed that there were "no spirits, essences or entelechies, no superior plans or ultimate purposes" in the evolution of life."[8]

We should note that the Helmholtzian school's dedication to the use of observation and experiment, to the reduction of nature to physics and chemistry, and to antiteleological beliefs were also emotional commitments. Du Bois-Reymond had declared fervently, "Brücke and I pledged a solemn oath to put into effect this *truth*." Their world view was based on a repugnance for and violent reaction against the goals of the old *Naturphilosophie*. Rather than try to address ultimate questions regarding human existence, du Bois-Reymond, in influential lectures in 1872 and 1880, avowed a philosophy of *ignoramus et ignorabimus*—we do not know and we shall never know.[9]

At the end of the nineteenth century, Puschmann, looking back at the past fifty years, lauded the "positivism" of German science, which had "rediscovered the lost path." "The civilization of the present day has been established on the abundance of *newly-discovered facts* which have enriched the natural sciences [and] have rendered possible a simplified view of the life of nature." And again: The "*positive knowledge of scientific facts* must be presupposed as a self-evident requisite for any intellectual activity [that might] prove fruitful or could hope to win any serious regard" (italics added).[10] The new psychiatrists also saw themselves as an integral part of a scientific medicine, just as would the neo-Kraepelinians. The reverence for "facts" of the late nineteenth and early twentieth centuries was akin to the reverence for "data" and "evidence" of the late twentieth century.

It is relevant to note that the same year that Feuchtersleben published his textbook declaring that physicians should pay attention to the great philosophers and that "mental disease must...be deduced...from mind and body," another psychiatrist, Wilhelm Griesinger (1817–1868), published the antithetical *Mental Pathology and Therapeutics*.[11] This book was dedicated to the idea that all psychiatric disease is brain disease, although Griesinger admitted that it had not yet been possible to discover any specific brain damage that corresponded to individual mental disorders. Yet, he said, it was important that psychiatry move away from poetic speculations about insanity and study it only from the medical point of view. All nonmedical, "particularly all poetical and ideal conceptions of insanity [are] of the smallest value."[12] A whole school of brain psychiatry came into being. Especially with the advances in microscopy, an enormous literature began to develop in anatomy and pathology. Physicians became hopeful that they had found the key to mental illness, and many theories about alleged brain pathology were formulated.[13] In the tradition of Helmholtzian science, the brain psychiatrists were convinced that only material changes could produce mental changes. But they made no real discoveries to sustain their beliefs. Contemporaries derided the classification of mental diseases based on the theory of localization of pathology in the brain. The neuropsychiatrist Hans Gruhle (1880–1958) called it "brain mythology" and Emil Kraepelin, "speculative anatomy."[14] Though intensive brain research vaulted many a physician into a professorship, it yielded few practical results for psychiatry and was largely worthless to clinicians.

Clinicians dealing with patients clearly saw that there was a large group of individuals with severe mental disorders in which no positive postmortem findings could be detected. These psychaitrists began to feel that the most useful method to follow was a strict empiricism that refrained from causal speculations, limited itself to minute observation of the patient, followed each stage of the disease carefully, and described its total course. Perhaps on these grounds they could erect a classification that might help them in patient management. Continually searching for a way to order the piles of clinical material, German psychiatrists proffered one short-lived classification after another. Their efforts were so noticeable that the composer Berlioz remarked that upon completion of schooling, a rhetorician writes a tragedy, and a psychiatrist a classification.[15] The busy classifiers and energetic brain researchers characterized psychiatry in the closing decades of the nineteenth century.

THE CONTRIBUTIONS OF EMIL KRAEPELIN

It is on this scene that Kraepelin thrust a way forward (Fig. 2.1, Pictorial Essay). He proposed a resolution that would divide the "functional"—or cause unknown—psychotic disorders into three large groups: dementia praecox, manic-depressive illness, and paranoia. The first two categories, in spite of being severely criticized at the outset,[16] became part of psychiatric tradition, although they acquired new names in the twentieth century, schizophrenia and bipolar disorder, respectively. It should be recalled that schizophrenia, while similar to dementia praecox in many ways, is somewhat different, even though Bleuler entitled his book *Dementia Praecox or the Group of Schizophrenias*. Not only did Bleuler talk about the group of schizophrenias, he also did not believe, as Kraepelin did, that the disorder always led to deterioration. Bleuler also had a more symptom-oriented approach, whereas Kraepelin emphasized the course of the disorder.[17]

When the majority of Western psychiatrists eventually accepted Kraepelin's new categories, it had the unintended consequence of creating a common language for them with regard to the psychoses.[18] Kraepelin's categories were somewhat helpful to the efforts of creating a useful classification, but in the United States, because of the hegemony of psychoanalysis, the goal of a common language and a classification was not a high priority. We will see that these were goals for the neo-Kraepelinians— including the psychiatrists and psychologists who were on the Task Force that created DSM-III—because to them, accurate communication among psychiatrists would go a long way toward assuring reliability in diagnosis. The problem still in the late twentieth century was that two or more psychiatrists seeing the same patients often did not agree on the same diagnosis.

A common language was not actually Kraepelin's goal when he first hastily (over the 1883 spring hiatus between semesters) put together a compendium of psychiatry based on his culling of current thought, diagnoses, and classifications in the German-speaking world. But he was appalled by the array of differences in terminology and conceptions that confronted him, and he thus tried to bring some order to his observations, at least enough to organize a small book. Like other contemporary psychiatrists and neurologists, Kraepelin was bewildered by the phenomena he saw or that were reported by peers. In subsequent editions of his textbook, which evolved from his compendium, he was able to group certain behaviors into various categories; these categories developed slowly during the 1880s and 1890s.

Kraepelin eventually postulated that the functional psychoses could be divided into three groups, although most of the attention was focused on two: dementia praecox and manic-depressive insanity. To give the reader a sense of what Kraepelin faced in trying to make order out of a host of symptoms, following are descriptions of the psychopathology that confronted physicians in an era almost totally devoid of psychopharmaceutical aids. Some of the psychopathology that Kraepelin described is no longer seen today. We have a fortunate guide in Kraepelin because he excelled at descriptive prose, partly by paying deliberate attention to his writing.[19] His composite portraits, based on numerous patients he had seen, became a pedagogical device, creating at least three generations of European and English psychiatrists devoted to observation and phenomenology—the study of signs and symptoms in psychiatric illness. It would be hard to find any psychiatrist who has described the symptoms of dementia praecox and manic-depressive illness with the vividness and thoroughness of his clinical pictures.

To read Kraepelin's early chapter, "Psychic Symptoms," in the section of his textbook on dementia praecox, is an intense experience.[20] In rapid fire, tumbling out on one another, are descriptions of fifty-three symptoms in sixty-eight pages.[21] In agitated dementia praecox, Kraepelin vividly describes the frequent hallucinations:

> The patients...see mice, ants, the hound of hell, scythes, and axes. They hear cocks crowing, shooting, birds chirping, spirits knockings, bees humming, murmurings, screaming, scolding, voices from the cellar....The voices say "filthy things," "all conceivable confused stuff, just fancy pictures"; they speak about what the patient does....They say: "That man must be beheaded, hanged," "Swine, wicked wretch, you will be done for."[22]
>
> Delusions...are developed with extraordinary frequency....The feeling of disease takes on insane forms; the brain is burned, shrunken, as if completely gone to jelly, full of water, the mind is "drawn like rags from the brain."...The tongue is made of iron, the lungs are dried up, blood is in the spinal marrow,...the flesh is loosened from the bones....The patient is not a human being any longer....
>
> These delusions are frequently accompanied by ideas of sin. The patient has by a sinful life destroyed his health of body and mind, he is...the greatest sinner, has confessed unworthily...has denied God....God has forsaken him, he is eternally lost, he...is going to hell.
>
> In connection with these ideas of sin ideas of persecution are invariably developed....The patient notices that he is looked at in a peculiar way, laughed at, scoffed at, that people are jeering at him....People spy on him; Jews, anarchists, spiritualists, persecute him, poison the atmosphere with poisonous powder, the beer with prussic acid.[23]

Moving to manic-depressive psychosis, Kraepelin points out that in "simple" depression

> the performance of actions is here made difficult, even impossible....Activity...which after much hesitation is at last begun, comes to a stop every moment, as the energy of vigourous decision is lacking. The patient no longer finishes anything, does everything the wrong way....[H]e is weighed down in gloom. A female patient said that she had dressed early intending to go out, and in the afternoon she was still at home.[24] The patient lacks spirit and will-power....The smallest bit of work costs him an unheard-of effort; even the most everyday arrangements, household work, getting up in the morning, dressing, washing, are only accomplished with the greatest difficulty and in the end indeed are left undone.
>
> The fundamental mood...is most frequently a somber and gloomy hopelessness. The patient's...heart is like stone; he has no pleasure in anything....[There is

a] decrease of emotional interest, the loss of inner sympathy with the surroundings and with the events of life, which the patient usually feels most bitterly. Within [the sufferers] all is empty and vain, everything is indifferent to them, is no concern of theirs, seems "so stupid" to them; music "sounds strange."…They cannot weep any more; they experience neither hunger nor satisfaction, neither weariness nor refreshment after sleep, no longer any bodily desire; God has taken away from them all feeling.

[T]orment…which is nearly unbearable, according to the perpetually recurring statements by the patients, engenders…weariness of life, [and] only too frequently also a great desire to put an end to life at any price.…The patients, therefore, often try to starve themselves, to hang themselves, to cut their arteries.…In carrying out injuries on themselves, they are often quite indifferent to bodily pain. One of my patients struck his neck so often on the edge of a chisel fixed on the ground that all the soft parts were cut through to the vertebrae.[25]

In manic states, Kraepelin goes on,

increased busyness is the most striking feature. The patient feels the need to get out of himself, to be on more intimate terms with his surroundings, to play a part. As he is a stranger to fatigue, his activity goes on day and night; work becomes very easy to him; ideas flow to him. He cannot stay long in bed.

His pressure of activity causes the patient to change about his furniture, to visit distant acquaintances, to take himself up with all possible things and circumstances, which formerly he never thought about. Politics, the universal language, aeronautics, the women's question, public affairs of all kinds and their need for improvement, gives him employment.…The patient…builds all kinds of castles in the air.…He has 16,000 picture post-cards of his little village printed.…At the same time the real capacity for work invariably suffers a considerable loss.

In the talk of the patients the flight of ideas and the pressure of speech are both at the same time conspicuous. He cannot be silent for long; he talks and screams in a loud vice, makes a noise, bellows, howls, whistles…strings together disconnected sentences, words, syllable, mixes up different languages…or suddenly com[es] to an end in unrestrained laughter.

We invariably meet with a very much exaggerated opinion of *self*. The patient boasts about his aristocratic acquaintance, his prospects of marriage, gives himself out as a count,…speaks of inheritances which he may expect, has visiting cards printed with a crown on them,…boasts of his performances and capabilities; he understands everything best,…he can take the place of many a professor or diplomatist.

The restriction of his freedom he regards as…the perverse ongoings of his relatives.…Those, not he, are mentally afflicted, who did not know how to appreciate his intellectual superiority and his gifts.…

Mood is predominantly exalted....On the other hand there often exists a great emotional irritability....When he comes up against opposition to his wishes and inclinations trifling external occasions may bring about violent outbursts of rage. In his fury he thrashes his wife and children, threatens to smash everything to smithereens, to run amuck, to set the house on fire.

In more severe excitement a state of genuine mania is developed by degrees. Impulses crowd one upon the other and the coherence of activity is gradually lost. [Finally] the patient sings, chatters, dances, romps about, does gymnastics, beats time, claps his hands, scolds, threatens, and makes a disturbance, throws everything down on the floor, undresses, decorates himself in a wonderful way.[26]

Yet Kraepelin's legacy is not just his virtuostic emphasis on observation and description. His other contributions are that the course of an illness must be studied because it is vital to the making of a diagnosis; there are two major groupings of functional psychoses; and scientific knowledge comes only through empirical research. This broad summary only partly covers his views; it says nothing about his sophisticated classificatory statements and his frank confessions regarding his alleged accomplishments. So first let us examine his familiar legacy, and then turn to the more obscure parts.

PICTORIAL ESSAY

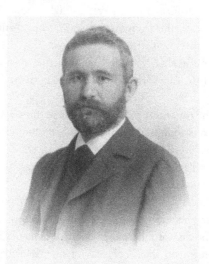

FIG. 2.1 Emil Kraepelin (1856–1926) at age 39, shortly before he published his textbook that included the separation of the psychotic disorders into two main groups: dementia praecox and manic-depressive illness (with some alterations, modern schizophrenia and bipolar disorder, respectively). The various volumes and editions of the textbook became authoritative and were remarkable contributions to descriptive psychiatry. From Max-Planck-Institute of Psychiatry, Munich, Historical Archives.

PSYCHIATRIE.

EIN LEHRBUCH

FÜR

STUDIRENDE UND AERZTE

VON

Dr. EMIL KRAEPELIN,

PROFESSOR AN DER UNIVERSITÄT HEIDELBERG.

SECHSTE, VOLLSTÄNDIG UMGEARBEITETE AUFLAGE.

II. BAND.

KLINISCHE PSYCHIATRIE.

MIT 6 TAFELN IN AUTOTYPIE, 3 TAFELN IN PHOTOGRAPHIE, 16 CURVEN,
3 DIAGRAMMEN UND 13 SCHRIFTPROBEN.

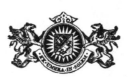

LEIPZIG,

VERLAG VON JOHANN AMBROSIUS BARTH.

1899.

FIG. 2.2 The title page of the sixth edition of Kraepelin's famous textbook, *Psychiatry: A Textbook for Students and Physicians* (1899). The book was published by J. A. Barth, a German scientific publishing house founded in 1780. Volume II, "Clinical Psychiatry" contained the chapter about "Dementia praecox" and "manisch-depressives Irresinn." Later in life Kraepelin wondered if there really was such a clear-cut division between the two psychoses. From Max-Planck-Institute of Psychiatry, Munich, Historical Archives.

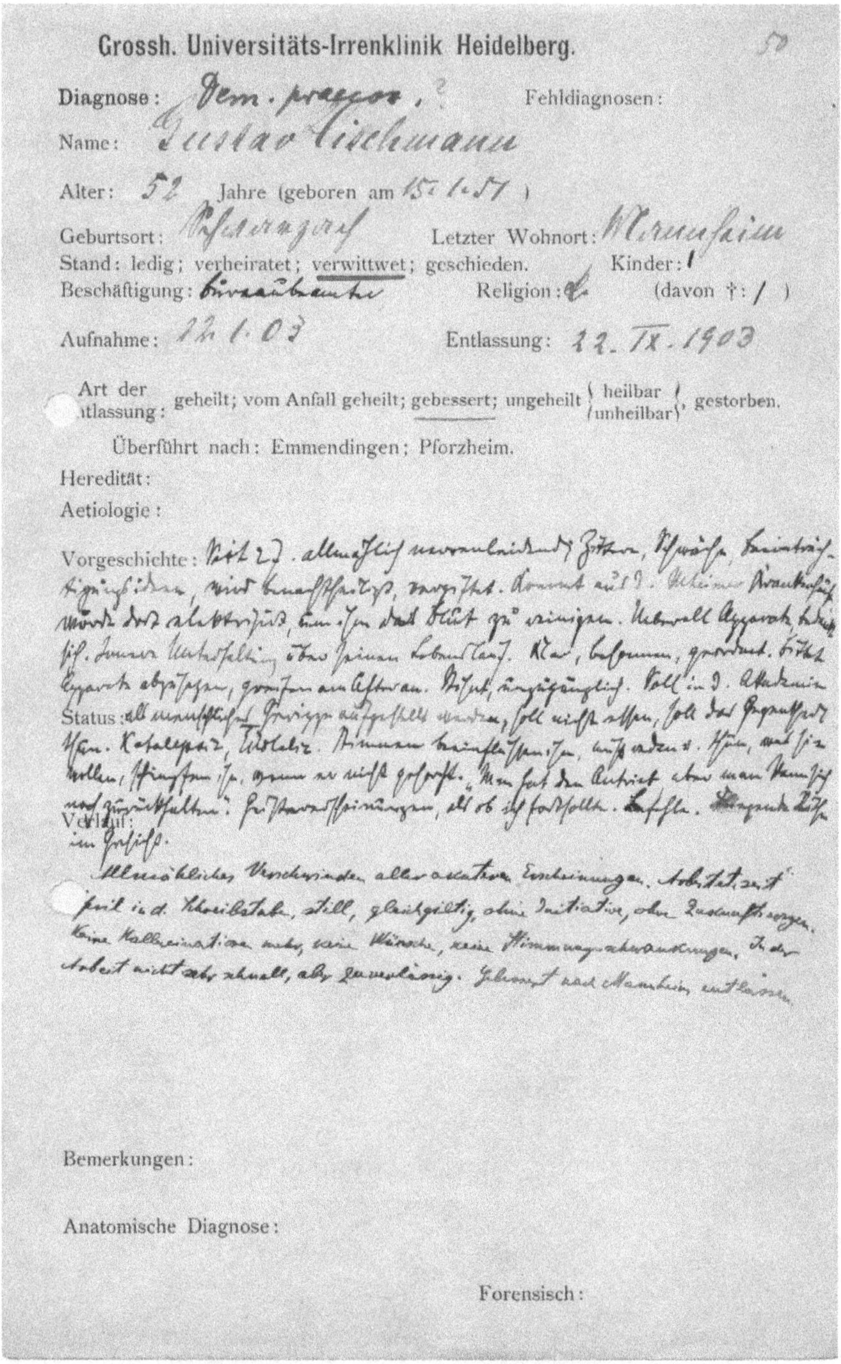
Grossh. Universitäts-Irrenklinik Heidelberg.

Diagnose: Dem. praecox. ?   Fehldiagnosen:

Name:

Alter: 52 Jahre (geboren am 15. 1. 51)

Geburtsort: Letzter Wohnort:

Stand: ledig; verheiratet; verwittwet; geschieden.   Kinder: 1

Beschäftigung: Religion: (davon †: /)

Aufnahme: Entlassung: 22. IX. 1903

Art der Entlassung: geheilt; vom Anfall geheilt; gebessert; ungeheilt {heilbar / unheilbar}, gestorben.

Überführt nach: Emmendingen; Pforzheim.

Hereditat:

Aetiologie:

Vorgeschichte:

Status:

Verlauf:

Bemerkungen:

Anatomische Diagnose:

Forensisch:

FIG. 2.3 A patient index card (Zaehlkarte), one of thousands Kraepelin compiled, this one written in 1903 at the Heidelberg Clinic. The 52-year-old patient described here has a diagnosis of dementia praecox with thoughts that he is being controlled and discriminated against. From Max-Planck-Institute of Psychiatry, Munich, Historical Archives.

CREATING DIAGNOSES

As the years passed, and as Kraepelin's initial compendium grew into a textbook, each edition larger than the previous one, he slowly worked on developing diagnoses. He did most of this work while director of the Psychiatric Clinic at Heidelberg University from 1891 to 1903. He has left us a description of how he and his colleagues sought to discover and define discrete nosological categories through the use of a "diagnosis box." (We can bear this in mind when we later see how Robert Spitzer and his Task Force created and described diagnoses.)

> After the first thorough examination of a new patient, each of us had to throw in a note with his diagnosis written on it. After a while, the notes were taken out of the box, the diagnoses were listed and when the case was closed, the final interpretation of the disease was added to the original diagnosis. In this way, we were able to see what kind of mistakes had been made and were able to follow up the reasons for the wrong original diagnosis.[27]

Clearly, through this procedure, Kraepelin and his staff were constantly revising their diagnostic criteria so as to make a reliable diagnosis. Vital to this enterprise was the "follow-up," returning after an interval to find out if the original diagnosis had been correct. This was another important part of arriving at a diagnosis and, as we shall see, one which dominated the thinking of the neo-Kraepelinians. Nevertheless, as Kraepelin came to admit, the follow-up was difficult to achieve.

In the fourth edition (1893) he introduced the term "dementia praecox" as a diagnostic entity. In the Preface of his fifth edition (1896) he announced his work as a "decisive step from a symptomatic to a clinical view of insanity....The importance of external clinical signs has...been subordinated to consideration of the *conditions of origin*, the *course*, and the *terminus* which result from individual disorders. Thus, all purely symptomatic categories have disappeared from the nosology."[28] This was a most significant step because the same symptoms, for example, hallucinations, can appear in different diseases. It was just this fact that had contributed to the chaos of attempts at classification and had slowed progress in formulating diagnoses. As the neo-Kraepelinians from Washington University in St. Louis later proclaimed, "classification in medicine is called diagnosis."[29] In Kraepelin's sixth edition (1899) (Fig. 2.2, Pictorial Essay) there was a clear dichotomy of endogenous psychoses, the separation of dementia praecox from a newly named entity, manic-depressive insanity. Kraepelin asserted that dementia praecox was usually characterized by mental deterioration, whereas manic-depressive insanity had a much more favorable prognosis. Moreover, in studying manic-depressive disease, family history was important because the disease appeared to run in families.

Another aspect of Kraepelin's legacy is his legendary devotion to empirical research. Two examples will suffice here. Very early in his career, he came under the tutelage of Wilhelm Wundt (1832–1920), the father of experimental psychology. Then, while in his first professorship at Dorpat (Tartu) in Estonia, at that time under Russian rule, Kraepelin set up his own equipment for the measurement of mental reactions to stimuli as well as the mental effects of drugs, caffeine, tea, and fatigue. He wanted to apply Wundt's methods to psychiatry in order to construct separate disease categories.[30] Over the years, he carried out this work himself or tried to hire staff who were skilled in experimental psychology. Much later, when he held the chair of psychiatry at Munich, he presided over the opening of the German Institute for Psychiatric Research (1917), an institution that was copied throughout the Western world. He sought out the most talented scientists he could find to work on pathological anatomy, histology of the cerebral cortex, brain localization, genetics, serology, metabolism, and experimental psychology.[31]

At the Institute, there was no room for psychoanalysis; Kraepelin found it totally unscientific:

> We meet everywhere the characteristic fundamental features of the Freudian trend of investigation, the representation of arbitrary assumptions and conjectures as assured facts, which are used without hesitation for the building up of always new castles in the air ever towering higher, and the tendency to generalization beyond measure from single observations.... As I am accustomed to walk on the sure foundation of direct experience, my Philistine conscience of natural science stumbles at every step on objections, considerations, and doubts, over which the likely soaring tower of imagination of Freud's disciples carries them without difficulty.[32]

Kraepelin's sarcasm and disdain would later be echoed by the neo-Kraepelinians at Washington University in St. Louis.

TOWARD AN EVALUATION OF KRAEPELIN

We now turn to less known aspects of Kraepelin's thought, some of which actully contradict the ideas for which he is famous.

Kraepelin taught that psychiatrists should shy away from postulating etiologies to make a diagnosis and instead observe the course of the illness, attend to its final state, and do follow-up studies, where possible. He insisted to his students that they not interpret what they saw, but only describe it.[33] But he did not take his own advice. In the fifth edition of his textbook, he talked about considering "the conditions of origin." For the etiology of dementia praecox he posited a "disease process in the brain, involving the cortical neurones [and brought about] by an autointoxication...as a result of a disorder of metabolism."[34] On the origins of hysteria Kraepelin talked about "morbid" constitution, "defective heredity," and certain environmental conditions. He considered the possibility of uterine disturbances but said the role played by "the female sexual organs...is not clear."[35] In the eighth edition of his textbook (1909–1915) he devoted seventy pages to considering the origins of paranoia: was it an outgrowth of "the hard blows life delivers to everyone," or was it due to innate degeneracy where "morbid germs…were already present in the disposition" as in a genetic disease like Huntington's chorea?[36] Kraepelin opted for degeneracy.

The Kraepelinian legacy to modern psychiatry includes his distinction between dementia praecox and manic-depressive illness and his separating sharply the mentally healthy from the mentally ill. This division was often buttressed by a belief in the overriding role of genetic predisposition in illness. But often overlooked is the fact that he reconsidered these conclusions. Toward the end of his life he regularly said that there was nothing holy about his nosology: "What we have formulated here is only a first sketch, which the advance of our science will often have occasion to change and to enlarge in its details, and perhaps even in its principal lines."[37] He even wondered whether his differentiation of the two psychoses was right. In 1920 he wrote, "We must, then, accustom ourselves to the idea that the phenomena of illness which we have hitherto used are not sufficient to enable us to distinguish reliably between manic-depressive illness and schizophrenia in all cases."[38] This problem has continued to vex psychiatrists and has preoccupied the makers of DSM-5.

In addition, Kraepelin relinquished his insistence on there being a fixed line between the healthy and the ill, when he argued that "there are no fixed, but only blurred borders between mental health and mental illness,"[39] thus opening up the possibility of a continuum. There seems to be no evidence to suggest that the neo-Kraepelinians took any notice of Kraepelin's shifting insights as the years passed. But again, the developers of DSM-5 have sought to address this issue, conceptualizing some disorders as occurring in a continuum, in "dimensions." This actually brings them closer to the psychoanalytic belief in this regard, which the neo-Kraepelinians dismissed.

Finally, Kraepelin openly confessed his shortcomings. Adolf Meyer (1866–1950), often called the dean of American psychiatry in the first half of the twentieth century, and others critiqued Kraepelin's formulation because he did not publish a monograph with a literature review and comments on others' work.[40] Kraepelin took time to reply to this criticism in his *Memoirs*, in essence admitting the truth of Meyer's criticism. He acknowledged his failure to compare his work with others. He said he had presented his ideas as "the current state of knowledge" and then went on to note, "[I] simply could not spare the time to substantiate my opinions."[41] Moreover, although he stressed the importance of follow-up studies in making diagnoses, he found it more and more difficult to pursue this avenue. "I was soon forced to admit that this work became increasingly impossible with the continuously growing amount of patients."[42]

Kraepelin also cut a corner in another way, casting doubt on the scientific nature of his classification. During the very years he was developing his separation of dementia praecox and manic depressive illness through observation and diagnosis of thousands of patients, he began to severely limit the period of observation. This practice directly affected the prognoses he assigned—that is, slow deterioration for dementia patients and recovery for manic-depressive patients.[43] This is important because prognosis was "perhaps the most fundamental criterion that Kraepelin employed in his clinical research to differentiate dementia praecox from manic depressive illness."[44] When he first came to Heidelberg to head the psychiatric clinic there, he required of himself and his co-workers that a diagnosis and prognosis be made within the first four weeks after [the patient's acute] admission. Then, after the patient was discharged to [a state] asylum, his or her prognosis was to be monitored in regular and systematic examinations. In this way, it was hoped, conclusions could be drawn and corrections made in the original diagnosis. However after [two years] and in conjunction with the...pressures of overcrowding, Kraepelin required that patients' prognoses be made not after four weeks, but rather immediately following their first examination in the clinic.[45]

The question inevitably arises: How much of Kraepelin's classifications came from rigorous observation and how much from preconceived notions? Furthermore, an argument has also been made that the index cards (*Zählkarten*) (Fig. 2.3, Pictorial Essay) that Kraepelin kept on patients, which he used in his classificatory scheme, were brief and general and sadly lacking in detail. Of a large group of cards studied by Matthias Weber and Eric Engstrom, half of them contained no diagnosis, and more than half said nothing about the course of the illness.[46]

While assessment of Kraepelin's work and influence is a complex issue, some of his accomplishments are clear and indisputable. He proposed the useful idea that, since the etiology of almost all mental illness was unknown, physicians should devote themselves to identifying an illness on the bases of describing it, noting its course, and predicting its prognosis. His own descriptions of the psychopathology of his hospitalized patients were brilliant and without parallel. This achievement and his characteristic conscientiousness made him a master teacher. He even said that one of the reasons for developing a correct classification was that it enabled him to teach. In addition to his teaching in lectures and on rounds, he prepared a highly readable book of his clinical lectures and several editions of textbooks for students and physicians. His division of the "endogenous" psychoses into dementia praecox and manic-depressive illness allowed physicians, if they assessed the patients correctly, to offer prognoses for the future. This was very useful to all concerned, in an era where there were essentially no effective treatments beyond custodial care. Furthermore, Kraepelin's founding of an institute for psychiatric research in Munich provided an outstanding path to the scientific study of mental illnesses.[47] Finally, as the years went on, Kraepelin began to realize that the dichotomies he had made so sharply throughout most of his career might not actually be so clear-cut. Having divided the psychoses into two main groups, he concluded in his *Lectures on Clinical Psychiatry* that his verdict might be only a "first sketch." The originally unambiguous line between mental illness and mental health began to appear somewhat blurry.

One aspect of Kraepelin's work that was necessary often had unfortunate consequences. In the effort to construct a classification that would lead to a diagnosis, Kraepelin was interested in what patients had in common. To arrive at a reliable diagnosis, in addition to following the course, he had to define the components—the signs and symptoms, the "criteria"—that would enable him to sure-footedly make the correct diagnosis when seeing a patient. To this scientific end, he had to weed out from consideration the unique factors of the patient that defined him or her as an individual. For the practice of good medicine, however, these are factors that must be considered when the physician interacts with or treats the patient. As seen in the earlier descriptive examples, what emerged in Kraepelin's textbooks were composite portraits rather than individual ones—clinical pictures that exemplified the disease as a whole. This often led to a mentally ill person being regarded as just a collection of symptoms. Combined with factors discussed below, a psychiatry devoid of humaneness appeared. Yet what complicates the picture is that, in Kraepelin's treatment of hospitalized mentally ill patients, he saw to it that their *physical* needs were carefully attended to. Such concern was not necessarily the case among other psychiatrists, whose disregard for their patients' physical well-being only added to their ignoring of their patients' uniqueness.

There were other negative aspects to Kraepelin's pursuit of a scientific psychiatry. He had a fixed notion of what was scientific and what was not. A scientific study of psychiatry was to focus on lab research and clinical description, negating other approaches. This methodological emphasis had the effect of making patients' complaints secondary. The line of attack was often to study one organ and not the whole person. This rested on the assumptions that the researcher could study a particular structure or function isolated from the rest of the body, and that the accuracy of the findings was not affected by this isolation. This type of science commonly led to a materialistic and sometimes mechanistic outlook. One might talk here of the tyranny of empirical data. Moreover, Kraepelin's desire to integrate psychiatry into medicine often led to the view that all mental disease is physiologically based and strongly hereditary in origin, thus ignoring personal and social factors.[48]

Indeed, psychiatric medicine had changed by Kraepelin's day. The moral treatment of the early nineteenth century, involving personal contact of the patient with the physician, various forms of psychotherapy, and "milieu" therapy (adjusting the hospital environment for therapeutic purposes) had been by and large discarded. This shift owed much to changed concepts of mental illness and treatment and the intervention of the state, via large asylums, in the care of the seriously mentally ill. Since Kraepelin and his colleagues concentrated on what they could observe and the making of diagnoses, there was no special concern for the role of a therapeutic relationship. It should be noted, however, that the word "psychotherapy" was somewhat in vogue at the end of the nineteenth century, and there were eminent psychiatrists who practiced it, though they were in a decided minority.[49]

At first, Kraepelin's classification was welcomed and was stimulating, because it enabled psychiatrists to make some sense of the multiplicity of psychiatric symptoms they encountered. But soon psychiatrists became pessimistic as they realized that what they could do therapeutically was extremely limited. Neither brain psychiatry nor clinical psychiatry could propel them forward. Karl Jaspers (1883–1969), the psychiatrist turned existentialist philosopher, in recalling the mood of the time, wrote:

> The realization that scientific investigation and therapy were in a state of stagnation was widespread in German psychiatric clinics.... The large institutions for the mentally ill were built constantly more hygienic and more magnificent [but]

the best that was possible consisted in shaping...the lives of the unfortunate inmates...as naturally as possible as, for example, by successful work therapy. In therapeutics we were basically without hope.[50]

Kraepelin himself, at the opening of the German Institute of Psychiatric Research (1917), reminded his audience that

along with our knowledge has come a lack of confidence in the efficacy of our medical practices. We know now that the fate of our patients is determined mainly by the development of the disease.... [W]e can rarely alter the course of the disease.... [O]ur ability frequently to predict what will happen keeps us from falsely assuming...that our treatment will appreciably influence the outcome of the disease....We must openly admit that the vast majority of the patients placed in our institutions...are forever lost.[51]

THE CYCLICAL NATURE OF PSYCHIATRY: FROM THE ROMANTIC ERA TO DSM-III

The optimism of the laboratory scientists had not borne fruit. It is at this juncture that the challenging ideas of Sigmund Freud—born the same year as Kraepelin—begin to intrude, and the cyclical pattern of psychiatric history showed itself once more.

We began this chapter with an account of the early nineteenth-century Romantic emphasis on finding the source of all mental illness, coupled with spiritual, religious, and intangible concerns. The roles of emotion and intuition were important. Unconscious ideation was recognized. This was accompanied by a belief in the fundamental relationship of all human beings to each other. An optimistic "moral" (psychological and environmental) treatment accompanied this phase of psychiatry.[52]

There followed a severe reaction to the early nineteenth-century ignoring of the empirical and factual. A new generation turned to studying basic sciences. They attempted to formulate laws based on laboratory findings, looked for answers to the enigma of mental illness in the brain, and wondered about a little-understood hereditary degenerative process to account for many otherwise unknown etiologies. In clinical psychiatry there was a helpful development when Emil Kraepelin formulated a new diagnostic system for serious mental illness. But this was insufficient to affect treatment. It was the time of a custodial system of care in large institutions where it was thought little could be done for patients with unknown genetic illnesses.

Onto this scene burst the provocative ideas of psychoanalysis, positing a common psychosexual development for all human beings and explaining mental illness in terms of universal unconscious conflicts. This was akin to Romantic psychiatry, with its emphasis on the inner life and stress on the universality of human development. In psychoanalytic thought, a strict empiricism was no longer necessary. With such beliefs, diagnosis and classification were not terribly important. There was much disdain for the "shallow" psychiatry limited to descriptions and lacking explanations. Psychoanalysis optimistically offered a lengthy course of psychotherapeutic treatment at the end of which there was supposed to be psychological health, since unconscious conflicts, the theory went, had become conscious and could be resolved. (Although Freud had only offered to change "hysterical misery into common unhappiness,"[53] the analytic epigone offered more.) The unconscious, dreams, and fantasies—intangibles—now mattered very much. One historical cycle—Romantic-intuitive (early nineteenth century) to empirical-scientific (late nineteenth century) to unconscious-developmental (early twentieth century)—was now complete.

The next swing began a half-century later in St. Louis among a very small group of men who were to be given the name "neo-Kraepelinians." We will next turn our attention to these psychiatrists. They were antagonistic to psychoanalytic "speculation" and believed that valid diagnoses and classifications were of essential importance. They recognized that they did not know the etiology of most mental illnesses, thus all they could rely on were accurate descriptions, family history, and patient follow-up. Yet they were optimistic where Kraepelin had been pessimistic. Laboratory tests for etiology, they were sure, would some day be discovered. Meanwhile, other empirical knowledge was the route to psychiatric progress that they believed they could bring about. Their ideas became the basis of DSM-III, and a new cycle in modern psychiatric history was launched.

3

KRAEPELIN'S PROGENY:
THE "NEO-KRAEPELINIANS"

DSM-III made an intellectual journey of half a century before it finally emerged in finished form in 1980. Fascinatingly, we can trace its roots to 1927, from a physicist at Harvard who enunciated a method of gaining scientific knowledge that he named "operational analysis." Psychiatrists at Harvard, interested in making their work "scientific," used the idea in the 1940s and 1950s. From Harvard it was transferred in the 1950s and 1960s to psychiatrists at Washington University in St. Louis who employed the notion increasingly in research and teaching. It was ultimately developed under Robert Spitzer at Columbia in the 1970s, in an extended manual for the entire American psychiatric profession, clinicians as well as researchers.

In this chapter we will trace the story of the evolving creation of DSM-III from its psychiatric origins at Harvard and examine the lives of its principal pioneers at Washington University. This is not to write a Whig history of ever-upward progress but to narrate the circumstances of another turn in the two-hundred-year cycle of modern psychiatry. We will follow the determined assault on the then-dominant psychoanalytic paradigm by a group of distinctly confident and dedicated researchers. They sought to displace an explanatory etiological model based on the universality of unconscious conflict with a model based on empirically observable phenomena with few explanatory etiologies. These researchers were akin to the Helmholtzians one hundred years before them. They triumphed because of the concurrent crisis in American psychiatry and because Spitzer made their work one of the bases of DSM-III.

THE KRAEPELINIAN TRADITION

In the 1950s and 1960s a small band of psychiatrists—Eli Robins, Samuel Guze, and George Winokur—at Washington University in St. Louis, labored in relative obscurity. They were dissatisfied with and critical of the state of American psychiatry. As they saw it, the psychiatry then being practiced dealt with nonpsychiatric pursuits, eschewed for the most part the medical model, did not value classification and diagnosis, and rejected necessary distinctions between mental illness and mental health. Many in psychiatry also seemed unbothered by the abysmally low scores of inter-rater reliability—two or more psychiatrists coming to the same conclusion about the diagnosis of a patient they had both interviewed. The Washington University psychiatrists and their few sympathizers believed that only empirical psychiatric research with a strong focus on biology held any hope for the treatment and betterment of the mentally ill. The domination of American psychiatry by psychoanalytic and psychodynamic thinking, they felt, was responsible for its unscientific character. What they believed was needed was a psychiatry that limited itself to the description of the mentally ill and avoided speculation about etiology, particularly psychoanalytic theories, because they felt etiology was unknown for almost all psychiatric diseases. As one Washington University author announced in a textbook, he and his colleagues were going to avoid "meaningless" explanations such as "functional," "psychogenic," and "situational reaction."[1] Thus, in addition to description, they urged that the course of illness be observed and that case follow-up and family histories play significant roles in diagnosis. Descriptive psychiatry would lead to better communication among all psychiatrists, which would be the first step toward accurate research, the only path to progress, they insisted self-assuredly.

The "Wash. U." psychiatrists were greatly buoyed in their theoretical stance and professional goals by a psychiatric textbook, *Clinical Psychiatry*, which first appeared in 1954. The book stood prominently apart from the psychoanalytic literature that dominated the 1950s, and the "neo-Kraepelinians," as they were eventually called, repeatedly referred to it. The text was written by three British psychiatrists, the senior author being Willy Mayer-Gross (1889–1961) (Fig. 3.1, Pictorial Essay).[2] Mayer-Gross had lived and practiced in Germany until 1933, and his longest affiliation (1918–1933) had been with the psychiatric clinic at the University of Heidelberg, the same clinic that Kraepelin directed from 1891 to 1903. During Mayer-Gross's years at Heidelberg, the Department of Psychiatry there was well known for searching out "diagnostic criteria" by the "exact observation" of psychiatric patients and "precise description" of their symptoms. This approach "supplied a logical complement to the work of the Kraepelinian school in sorting out forms of mental disorder by long-term follow-up."[3]

In his textbook, Mayer-Gross attacked psychoanalysis unmercifully, agreeing only with the notion that unconscious ideation exists. Other than that, psychoanalysis had halted the advance of science because of its "flight into the air" (p. 2). Mayer-Gross rejected the psychoanalytic conceptualization that every psychiatric illness is unique to the individual (p. 5). Excessive preoccupation with individuals was counterproductive, he argued, because with that approach one could not construct data on which to progress. Rather, the psychiatrist needed diagnosis to build on past knowledge. Treating a patient only with psychotherapy was the same as "universal purging and bleeding" (p. 6).[4] Psychoanalysis was a form of "faith-healing" (p. 17) based on a "mechanistic mythology" (p. 11), Mayer-Gross' tirade continued. The data that might bring understanding to the role of sociological factors in psychiatric illness simply did not exist. So psychiatry needed to be defined neither as the study of human behavior nor as the study of interpersonal relationships. Rather, psychiatry was a part of medicine because there was an "immense body of evidence showing that in the major psychiatric disorders the specific factors in causation are those of a constitutional and physiopathologic kind" (p. 4). Psychiatry, concluded Mayer-Gross, needed experimentation, clinical observation, and follow-up and had to aim for diagnoses, even though, quite mistakenly, that pursuit had become unpopular. Here he was referring to the popularity of psychoanalysis.

The Wash. U. psychiatrists' work was carried on in the traditions established by Kraepelin and Mayer-Gross. But sensitive to the claims of psychoanalytic "humaneness," as opposed to the "coldness" of biological research, the Wash. U. physicians felt the need to argue that scientific research had humane ends. In a 1969 paper, published in 1970, one of these physicians, Samuel Guze, argued for the "Need for Toughmindedness in Psychiatric Thinking."[5] The paper touted biological psychiatry and was antipsychoanalytic. In concluding, he asserted the following:

> It is argued that because it is difficult to measure psychologic phenomena and to characterize psychiatric disturbances…too much should not be expected.…But to abdicate the role of constructive critic is to abandon the field to the tender-minded. The difficulties of the field seem to require just the opposite: a commitment to toughmindedness.…
>
> Paradoxically, such toughmindedness is sometimes attacked in the name of humanitiarianism. It is asserted, or implied, that a critic who demands "data," who asks about controls, who insists that the burden of proof is on the affirmative, reveals thereby that he is not interested in people.…
>
> But scientific skepticism is in no way incompatible with compassion for the sick or disabled. In fact, it is the desire to help patients that causes one to be frustrated by the lack of definite knowledge about what really helps and what does not.[6]

PSYCHIATRY AT WASHINGTON UNIVERSITY IN ST. LOUIS

The foremost leaders of the Wash. U. group were all of the same generation, born within four years of each other: Robins in 1921, Guze in 1924, and Winokur in 1925. Their backgrounds were similar, all coming from eastern European Jewish families that had recently immigrated. They shared science and socializing. For years they ate lunch together every day, brainstorming, sounding out ideas, each drawing from the others the emotional conviction that they were on the right track. Robins' wife, Lee Nelken Robins (1922–2009), a Harvard-trained sociologist, provided much to the breadth and depth of their work with her ground-breaking studies in psychiatric epidemiology.[7] At night there were legendary parties, usually given by the Robinses. Their isolation in the 1950s from the many voluntary psychoanalytic faculty members in the department drew them ever closer. They were reminded of their outcast status when the NIMH, into the 1950s and up to the late 1960s, refused to fund their grants for clinical studies. They were only funded, said Guze, if their application was for doing "basic pharmacology or biochemistry."[8] One way of combating their isolation was to maintain links with British and European psychiatrists who did research in the model of Kraepelinian psychiatry, and there were visiting professorships back and forth.[9]

In their residency program, the Wash. U. psychiatrists trained embryonic psychiatrists in descriptive psychiatry and imbued them with their—the professors'—fervor. All of the residents were required to do original research, either on their own or working with a member of the faculty.[10] In so doing, one of the residents, John Feighner (1937–2006), later wrote:

> It became painfully clear to me that the state of the art of psychiatric diagnoses was frankly in a mess. Trying to draw conclusions from the scientific literature with regards to virtually any area of the major psychiatric disorders was extremely difficult. Patients that were described in one article as having acute schizophrenia, showing a very positive response to electroconvulsive therapy (ECT), seemed quite different from patients described in other articles as having a similar disorder and responding poorly to ECT but positively to neuroleptics. Also, with the progressive use of lithium and other more specific pharmacological treatments at that time, it seemed imperative to me that we refine our diagnostic criteria to assist us in selecting specific treatments for specific patients and to improve communication between research centers.[11]

Feighner found that in his contacts with his teachers, particularly Robins with his "no-nonsense data oriented approach," it was apparent that something should—and even better—could be done. So in his third year as a resident, Feighner began to develop diagnostic criteria for the affective disorders, specifically depression and mania, and discussed with Robins, Guze, and Winokur the possibility of expanding the criteria to include other psychiatric disorders. During Feighner's fourth year he began to do this and, with the Wash. U. triumvirate, particularly Robins, a committee was set up to carry out this task. The committee had six members, the four already mentioned, plus a junior faculty member (Robert Woodruff) and another resident (Rodrigo Munoz). All six men attended every meeting.[12] Feighner reviewed close to a thousand articles and from these data proposed criteria for a variety of disorders. The criteria were gone over by the committee, which met every week or two over a period of nine months. They met in Robins' office, and "he was clearly in charge."[13]

Feighner, although a resident, was a very active and questioning member. He completed a paper, after everyone had reviewed his drafts, that was published in the research-oriented *Archives of General Psychiatry*.[14] Although the co-authors of the article included Robins, Guze, and Winokur, the diagnostic criteria become immortalized as the "Feighner criteria." Feighner et al.'s paper became the most cited paper ever published in a psychiatric journal.[15] "From 1972 through 1980, there were 1,157 citations to this article in the *Science Citation Index*. This was an average of 144.6 citations per year. In contrast, the average article published in the *Archives of General Psychiatry* received only 2.1 citations per year."[16] Robins himself said it was one of the two most important papers he had ever written.

Robins' other pivotal paper was on how to achieve a valid diagnosis in psychiatry, written two years earlier with Guze and foreshadowing the Feigner article.[17] This earlier paper did not spell out diagnostic criteria for specific psychiatric disorders but did lay out five steps that Robins and Guze thought necessary to develop a valid (i.e., useful because correct) classification: (1) description of the clinical picture (signs and symptoms); (2) laboratory studies (which they admitted did not exist for "the more common psychiatric disorders"); (3) exclusion criteria to weed out patients with other illnesses; (4) follow-up studies; and (5) family studies.[18] Robins and Guze tried to show briefly how the five steps would apply to schizophrenia. The paper included the memorable phrase: "classification is diagnosis."[19]

The Feighner paper echoed the argument about the necessary five steps and announced that their "communication is meant to provide common ground for different research groups so that diagnostic definitions can be emended constructively.... The use of formal diagnostic criteria by a number of groups should expedite psychiatric investigation."[20] Note here that at this juncture, Feighner and colleagues were talking only about research, not clinical work. The Feighner authors also took a jab at the current *Diagnostic and Statistical Manual* of the American Psychiatric Association (*DSM-II*), which was heavily influenced by psychoanalytic thought.[21] They proclaimed that in contrast to DSM-II, "in which the diagnostic classification is based upon the 'best clinical judgment and experience' of a committee and its consultants, i.e., opinions and theories, [their (Feighner et al.'s)] communication [would] present a diagnostic classification validated primarily by follow-up and family studies,"[22] in other words, data-based evidence.

Follow-up studies especially were deemed crucial by the Wash. U. psychiatrists. They reiterated tirelessly the message that these studies were necessary in the making of a reliable diagnosis. Two examples (out of many) are a 1969 paper on obsessional neurosis and a 1970 one on hysteria.[23] Furthermore, when Robins and Guze published a paper suggesting a new classification of affective disorders, they relied on a variety of follow-up studies—"data," as they would say. Because of their method, they asserted, their new classification—which also avoided "etiological implications"—would "bring order out of relative chaos."[24] Kraepelin had strenuously advocated following patients after their initial hospitalization, although, as we have seen, he often fell short of his goal. Later in the same century, the Wash. U. physicians argued that precisely because the causes of most psychiatric illnesses were unknown, the psychiatrist needed studies that would

> determine whether or not the original patients are suffering from some other defined disorder that could account for the original clinical picture. If they are suffering from another such illness, this finding suggests that the original patients did not comprise a homogeneous group and that it is necessary to modify the diagnostic criteria.... Until we know more about the fundamental nature of the common psychiatric illnesses, marked differences in outcome should be regarded as a challenge to the validity of the original diagnosis.[25]

The need to study a "homogeneous group," an oft-repeated mantra of the Wash. U. group, meant an intense stress on using diagnostic criteria. Another necessity was the follow-up. Twice Donald W. Goodwin (1942–1999), a junior colleague of Guze and Robins, quoted the words of Peter D. Scott (1914–1977), a well-known British forensic psychiatrist: "The follow-up is the great exposer of truth, the rock on which many fine theories are wrecked and upon which better ones can be built; it is to the psychiatrist what the post-mortem is to the physician."[26]

It must also be noted that the Feighner group were diagnostic purists; they took a very radical view of just how many psychiatric illnesses could be reliably diagnosed. This is why they limited their diagnostic criteria to sixteen psychiatric illnesses. The Feighner criteria inspired Robert Spitzer, the eventual head of the task force that produced DSM-III. But first Spitzer created the Research Diagnostic Criteria (RDC), which numbered twenty-five diagnoses (discussed in detail in Chapter 7). He then turned to develop DSM-III, which was meant to be used by both researchers *and* clinicians. DSM-III was a very large book, with 265 diagnoses.

At the same time that work on DSM-III started, in 1974, a new textbook by the Wash. U. psychiatrists, *Psychiatric Diagnosis*, was published; it was limited to just twelve psychiatric illnesses.[27] The authors—Robert Woodruff, Donald Goodwin, and Guze—said they were going to write only about "valid" diagnoses. In the Introduction, one of the authors wrote that "there are many diagnostic categories in psychiatry, but few are based on a clinical literature where the conditions are defined by explicit criteria, and follow-up studies provide a guide to prognosis....Not every patient can be diagnosed by using the categories in this book. For them, 'undiagnosed' is, we feel, more appropriate than a label incorrectly implying more knowledge than exists."[28] Examples they gave of diagnoses that lacked studies were "passive-aggressive personality" and "emotionally unstable personality," personality disorders being common diagnoses made by psychoanalysts.[29]

Guze attempted to bring the makers of DSM-III, the Task Force, around to this way of thinking. He recalled that in an early meeting on DSM-III, he proposed

> that perhaps we should urge [the APA] that, until there had been at least two long-term follow-up studies from different institutions with similar results, we shouldn't give the entity a status in DSM-III. The alternative was to have a lot of undiagnosed cases. We could have a way of subcategorizing undiagnosed patients in which the label would indicate what the diagnostic problem was. That would put us on a stronger scientific basis and it would constantly remind psychiatrists of our ignorance and what kinds of questions needed to be studied.
>
> I couldn't [Guze continued] get that group to vote in favor of my suggestions. The answer that I was given was that they said we have enough trouble getting the legitimacy of psychiatric problems accepted by our colleagues, insurance companies and other agencies. "If we do what you are proposing, which makes sense to us scientifically, we think that not only will we weaken what we are trying to do but we will give the insurance companies an excuse not to pay us."[30]

Now, keeping in mind the Wash. U. stand on diagnostic "legitimacy," which revolved around follow-up studies, avoiding etiological "speculations," and having a category of "undiagnosed," let us examine the Feighner diagnostic criteria for schizophrenia as an example of their overall proposal. If, as Robins and Guze declared, "classification is diagnosis," then the building blocks of diagnosis, the diagnostic criteria, would be vital. The psychiatrist's diagnosing of his or her patients would rest on the correct, that is, valid, criteria.

Schizophrenia.—For a diagnosis of schizophrenia A through C are required. [For comparison, "schizophrenia" in DSM-II (1968) was dealt with in a series of descriptive paragraphs over three pages and in DSM-III (1980) was dealt with both by descriptive paragraphs and diagnostic criteria totaling over thirteen pages.]

A. Both of the following are necessary: (1) A chronic illness with at least six months of symptoms prior to the index evaluation without return to the premorbid level of psychosocial adjustment. (2) Absence of a period of depressive or manic symptoms sufficient to qualify for affective disorder or probable affective disorder.

B. The patient must have at least one of the following: (1) Delusions or hallucinations without significant perplexity or disorientation associated with them. (2) Verbal production that makes communication difficult because of a lack of logical or understandable organization. (In the presence of muteness the diagnostic decision must be deferred.)

C. At least three of the following manifestations must be present for a diagnosis of "definite" schizophrenia, and two for a diagnosis of "probable" schizophrenia. (1) Single. (2) Poor premorbid social adjustment or work history. (3) Family history of schizophrenia. (4) Absence of alcoholism or drug abuse within one year of onset of psychosis. (5) Onset of illness prior to age 40.[31]

Critics made inevitable fun of the diagnostic criteria, calling them the "Chinese menu" approach. Guze's response was that it was another neo-Kraepelinian who used that terminology. "It did resemble a Chinese menu approach to things, but coming from [a like-minded colleague], we didn't take offence at it."[32]

Feighner et al.'s paper concluded with the message that their diagnoses rested on a "synthesis of existing information, a synthesis based on data rather than opinion or tradition."[33] But it is clear from the detailed remembrances of Rodrigo Munoz, at that time a resident on the Feighner committee, that the sixteen diagnostic criteria borrowed heavily from already-published literature that was not always based on empirical studies.[34] Moreover, the originality of the neo-Kraepelinians lay not in the invention of diagnostic criteria, which had been used in several individual studies (see Chapter 6), but in the novel idea that one could use diagnostic criteria to develop an entire classification. This appeared to the Wash. U. group, and later to Spitzer, as a way out of the scientific impasse that so many—even if not most psychoanalysts—felt psychiatry had reached.

GERALD L. KLERMAN—A GIFTED PSYCHIATRIC LEADER

The Wash. U. physicians and others who shared their philosophy and goals were given the name "neo-Kraepelinians" in 1978 by a Harvard psychiatrist, Gerald L. Klerman (1928–1992) (Fig. 3.2, Pictorial Essay).[35] Klerman, born in New York City, went to college at Cornell University and medical school at New York University (NYU). He did a residency in psychiatry at Harvard followed by a two-year stint at the NIMH. He entered psychoanalytic training but never received his psychoanalytic certification "because he was too much of a maverick, and continued to question the dogma," a junior colleague has maintained. "The leaders [felt they] could never trust him, so they wouldn't let him graduate."[36] He shifted from a psychoanalytic orientation to a descriptive stance, although many years later he developed "interpersonal psychotherapy." This was a therapy specifically designed for people who had the DSM diagnosis for depression; it was a psychotherapy that was tailor-made for a specific illness.[37] Klerman had a talent for phrasemaking. He once entitled an article "Psychotropic Hedonism vs. Pharmacological Calvinism."[38]

The fact that Klerman publicized the work of the neo-Kraepelinians was of great benefit to them because he was an influential thinker. He was very creative, had a fertile mind, and was known for his ability as a synthesizer, historian, and philosopher of psychiatry. In the course of his life he held many high-level positions because of his impressive intellect, originality of thought, and restless energy. Toward the end of his life, while on kidney dialysis, he traveled the world to meetings and in response to the many invitations he received to lecture.[39]

Klerman reported that a Kraepelinian revival was occurring among researchers and academicians while there was a Meyerian (a reference to the "psychobiosocial" thought of Adolf Meyer) and a Freudian decline. One proof of Klerman's observation of the Kraepelinian revival was the publication of a book, *Manic Depressive Illness*, written by three Wash. U. psychiatrists, George Winokur, Paula J. Clayton, and Theodore Reich.[40] At every turn, it harkened back to Kraepelin's descriptive and theoretical work on manic-depressive illness and concluded that there was no "hard evidence in favor of the psychologic and social approaches" to the disease.[41] Yet the Wash. U. people disliked being labeled neo-Kraepelinian. "We would never have used the term ourselves [Guze recalled]. I think we were afraid it would seem too old-fashioned an idea, even though we insisted that all our residents read Kraepelin's monographs and emphasized his work with the medical students. But we were worried that the label didn't point in the right direction."[42]

Nevertheless, having coined the term, Klerman took the opportunity to create a nine-point "credo" of the neo-Kraepelinians, six of which (points 4 through 9) incisively challenged psychoanalytic positions.

1. Psychiatry is a branch of medicine.
2. Psychiatry should utilize modern scientific methodologies and base its practice on scientific knowledge.
3. Psychiatry treats people who are sick and who require treatment for mental illnesses.
4. There is a boundary between the normal and the sick.
5. There are discreet mental illnesses. Mental illnesses are not myths [an obvious reference to Szasz's *Myth of Mental Illness*.] There is [sic] not one but many mental illnesses. It is the task of scientific psychiatry, as a medical specialty, to investigate the causes, diagnosis, and treatment of these mental illnesses.
6. The focus of psychiatric physicians should be particularly on the biological aspects of mental illness.
7. There should be an explicit and intentional concern with diagnosis and classification.
8. Diagnostic criteria should be codified, and a legitimate and valued area of research should be to validate such criteria by various techniques. Further, departments of psychiatry in medical schools should teach these criteria and not deprecate them, as has been the case for many years.
9. In research efforts directed at improving the reliability and validity of diagnosis and classification, statistical techniques should be utilized.[43]

With Klerman's particular exposition of neo-Kraepelinian beliefs, let us now turn to examine the careers of the three pioneering Wash. U. psychiatrists, Robins, Guze, and Winokur, as well as their forefather, Mandel Cohen.

PICTORIAL ESSAY

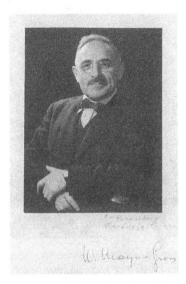

FIG. 3.1 Willy Mayer-Gross (1889–1961), a German-British psychiatrist who advocated the Kraepelinian approach to psychiatry: "exact observation" and "precise description" of patients. His 1954 textbook, much prized by the psychiatrists at Washington University in St. Louis ("Wash. U."), attacked the psychoanalytic emphasis on the uniqueness of psychiatric illness for each individual, arguing that such a belief impeded scientific progress. This was at a time when psychoanalysis was the dominant force in American psychiatry. From the Bethlem Art and History Collections Trust, UK.

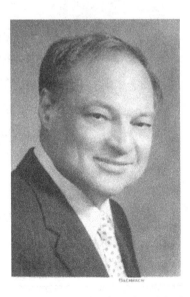

FIG. 3.2 Gerald L. Klerman (1928–1992), a much-admired psychiatrist with a wide array of skills and talents. Klerman coined the term "neo-Kraepelinians" to refer to Robins, Guze, and Winokur at Washington University and to others who shared their psychiatric approach. Courtesy Dr. Robert M. A. Hirschfeld.

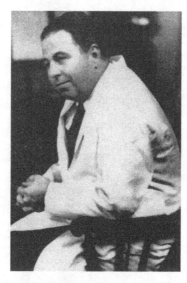

FIG. 3.3 Mandel E. Cohen (1907–2000) at Harvard in the 1940s when he was conducting research in clinical psychiatry that set him apart from his psychoanalytic colleagues, whose theories he openly derided. Eli Robins, a resident, was attracted to Cohen's argument that using "operational criteria" when making diagnoses would make psychiatry more scientific. Courtesy Dr. Anne Hamlen Cohen.

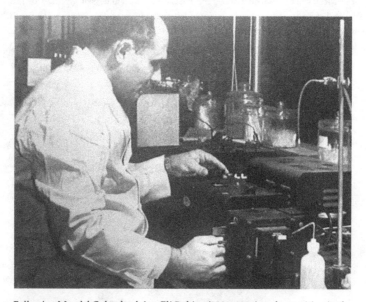

FIG. 3.4 Following Mandel Cohen's advice, Eli Robins (1921–1994) took a position in the Department of Psychiatry at Washington University in St. Louis, one of the few psychiatry departments in the United States that was biologically oriented. There he began educating others in the use of operational criteria for psychiatric diagnosis. Here is Robins c. 1960, working in one of the two laboratories he ran. Copyrighted by *Missouri Medicine,* Vol. 90, No. 6, 1993. Used with permission.

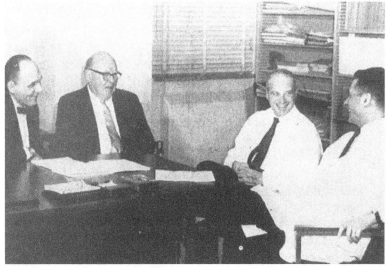

FIG. 3.5 Robins (left) and his intimate colleagues, George Winokur (1925–1996) (in the corner) and Samuel Guze (1924–2000) (far right), meeting in the early 1960s with Edwin Gildea (1898–1977), chair of the Psychiatry Department, who agreed to the plan that the three take responsibility for various Washington University psychiatric programs and services. The three men hoped to make a "dent" in American psychiatry. Robins became chair of the department in 1963. Copyrighted by *Missouri Medicine*, 1993. Used with permission.

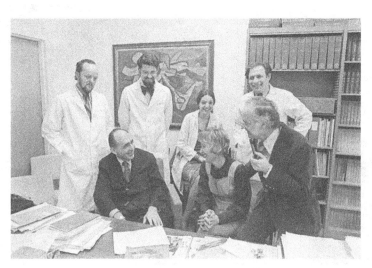

FIG. 3.6 Eli Robins and Psychiatry Department colleagues at Washington University in 1974. From left to right in the rear: Robert Woodruff (DSM-III Task Force), Robert Cloninger (eventual Wash. U. Psychiatry chair), Ann Mazur (chief resident), and Theodore Reich (expert in psychiatric genetics). In front: Robins, Paula Clayton (DSM-III Task Force), and George E. Murphy (specialist in affective disorders). From Washington University Libraries, Department of Special Collections.

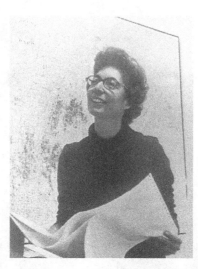

FIG. 3.7 Lee Nelken Robins (1922–2009), c. 1960. Robins was a sociologist who became a
psychiatric epidemiologist providing vital demographic data for the psychiatry research
projects at Washington University. She and Eli Robins were known for their parties and
hospitality, which were all the more important because at first, the Washington University
Psychiatry Department was professionally isolated. Copyrighted by *Missouri Medicine*, 1993.
Used with permission.

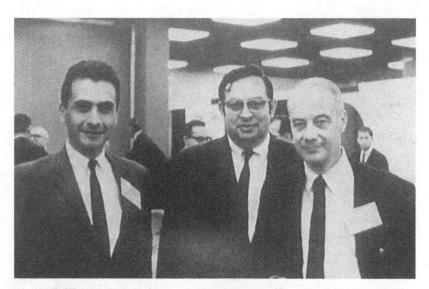

FIG. 3.8 Samuel Guze (left), dedicated teacher and intent on making psychiatry fully a part of
medicine, and George Winokur (right), prolific researcher in affective disorders and genetics,
also the department's impertinent wit. William McKnelly, Jr., is in the middle. (Photo from the
early 1960s.) Copyrighted by *Missouri Medicine*, 1993. Used with permission.

ELI ROBINS (1921–1994) AND MANDEL COHEN (1907–2000)

Eli Robins was born in a small Texas town, just south of Houston. He attended Rice University (then Institute) in Houston and graduated at age nineteen. He completed the first two years of medical school at the University of Texas Medical Branch in Galveston. He then finished up at Harvard when he was twenty-two and had residencies in both psychiatry and neurology there.[44] He also underwent a year of personal analysis with Helene Deutsch (1884–1982), one of the well-known émigré psychoanalysts from Europe, but psychoanalysis appeared to him to be "silly,"[45] and he never applied for psychoanalytic training, unusual for a Harvard psychiatrist at that time.[46] "It is [also] possible that Robins held a special grudge against analysis. A close relative who developed severe depression was treated with analytic therapy at McLean Hospital [a Harvard-affiliated private hospital], where he died after jumping from an upper storey [sic]."[47]

Much more influential than anything else was Robins' training with a Harvard psychiatrist fourteen years his elder, Mandel E. Cohen (Fig. 3.3, Pictorial Essay), at Massachusetts General Hospital (Mass. General, or MGH). When Robins was in the Army and en route from Texas to Germany, he developed bad pain in his left shoulder. He went to an Army hospital in Waltham, MA, where he was diagnosed with hysteria. Cohen, who worked in the neurology department at Mass. General, was called in as a consultant and found some weakness in Robins' shoulder and ordered a lumbar puncture. The test showed an increase in lymphocytes, and Cohen diagnosed Robins with polio, since there was then an epidemic of polio in Texas.[48] Having been treated by Cohen and appreciating his nonpsychoanalytic approach to his shoulder pain, Robins turned to train under him.[49]

Cohen had a data-intensive approach to psychiatry, evident in the title to an article he wrote in 1959 with two other physicians: "The Electrocardiogram in Neurocirculatory Asthenia (Anxiety Neurosis or Neurasthenia): A Study of 203 Neurocirculatory Asthenia Patients and 757 Healthy Controls in the Framingham Study."[50] That Cohen would take psychiatric diagnoses (anxiety neurosis, neurasthenia) and try to study their cardiovascular components and rename the disorders "neurocirculatory" also illustrates his biological psychiatric interests.

While Cohen had postgraduate training at Harvard, he was "persona non grata" to his psychoanalytic colleagues, who "maligned him unmercifully."[51] The feelings were mutual, as he waged a continuous war with them, making liberal use of sarcasm and put-downs. He annoyed them continuously by always asking, "But where are your data?"[52] He could have a wicked tongue, referring to a female visiting analyst as "a witch who commuted on her broomstick."[53] He had been analyzed by the European émigré Hanns Sachs (1881–1947) from 1939 to 1941, and he called the analysis "a terrible waste of time."[54] He began referring to analysts as "Freudists and Stalinoids." When arguing a point of view with colleagues, Cohen preferred a quick, direct thrust rather than "long-winded…civil discussion."[55] A younger colleague referred to his "stiletto-in-the-heart questions." He was so much "on the out with the analysts, who back in the 1940s and 1950s ran the Department of Psychiatry at Mass. General," that he did not have an appointment in the Department of Psychiatry. "Basically, he was too biological for them and they cut their relationship with him," says David Sheehan, who had a residency at Mass. General in the 1970s. Cohen "had an appointment in the neurology department, even though he was a psychiatrist."[56]

According to Sheehan, "[a] long time back, in the 1930s and 1940s, Cohen said diseases of the mind have to be studied like any disease—you have to define your diagnostic criteria precisely and apply them consistently."[57] The physicist and mathematician, Percy Williams Bridgman (1882–1961), a Harvard colleague, probably influenced Cohen in this regard.[58] In 1927, Bridgman published a small volume, *The Logic of Modern Physics*, in which he introduced the concept of "operational analysis."[59] He proposed that any concept be defined in terms of the "operations" that had been carried out to determine its existence. He asserted "that we shall no longer permit ourselves to use as tools in our thinking concepts of which we cannot give an adequate account in terms of operations.... The attitude of the physicist must therefore [be] one of pure empiricism. He recognizes no *a priori* principles."[60] Bridgman's idea was widely hailed in the 1930s and 1940s, including by Harvard scholars, as an advance in science, and was adopted especially by psychologists and sociologists whose urge was to make their fields "scientific." Harry Stack Sullivan (1892–1949), the well-known psychiatrist and psychoanalyst, even tried to apply Bridgman's suggestions to psychiatry in the 1940s. Bridgman's star waned thereafter, but the widespread use of the term "operational" in a variety of fields has persisted.

In the late 1930s and 1940s, Cohen was formulating the concept of "operational criteria," and it seems unlikely that he, also being at Harvard, would not have heard about Bridgman's much talked-about propositions. When David Healy, the psychiatrist, interviewed Cohen shortly before he died, he asked him about the origins of operational criteria. Cohen replied, "I just thought that we were doing studies and we should try to be scientific. If you have a disease that had eight different names, particularly when you wanted to do a family study—we showed that it ran in families—you would need criteria."[61]

Cohen, a cardiologist before he became a psychiatrist, insisted on the medical model and published in major medical—although not psychiatric—journals. Gradually, he attracted a coterie of devoted followers. With these students and residents he was on social as well as professional terms, inviting them to his home and attending their weddings.[62] He was very loyal to these individuals, supporting them for jobs and memberships, and keeping in touch with them. But even in the 1980s, when the psychiatry department was no longer fundamentally psychoanalytic, it still denied him an appointment. He was nonetheless a major force behind one of the biggest shifts in American psychiatry because of his profound influence on Eli Robins.

Sheehan recounts that he (Sheehan) was involved in the early 1980s in the planning of a conference on anxiety disorders at the psychiatry department at Mass. General that was to bring together the world's leading experts on the topic. Sheehan wanted to invite Mandel Cohen because he knew the history of Cohen's career at Mass. General. But, as Sheehan recalled:

> You cannot imagine the level of resistance that I ran into at the Mass. General in getting them to allow me to invite him...to speak at the meeting [even though] he was an entire generation ahead of his time....I put him first on the agenda because of the interesting historical background, but also as a way of letting the assembled

demi-gods know that...here was this guy who an entire generation earlier had anticipated almost everything they had done....I remember a lot of people were saying, "Who is this man? Who is Mandell (sic) Cohen?" And this little old man gets up and proceeds to give his talk. [The experts sitting in the audience were completely] bowled over. He stole the show on everyone....This guy had anticipated almost everything we had done [re operational criteria] and understood very clearly where the field was going to be. [He was] a seminal figure in American psychiatry without people knowing about it..[63]

While still a resident at Harvard, Eli Robins along with Cohen and another physician published a paper on hysteria in *JAMA* in 1951. This is probably the first neo-Kraepelinian paper, which, of course, is very important historically.[64] Cohen's influence was evident. The authors announced their intention to "provide factual data that might be useful to the clinician in the diagnosis of hysteria"[65] and closed by saying that they could not provide any knowledge of the cause of hysteria or about the mechanisms of its symptoms. Cause and mechanisms

will be discovered by scientific investigation, rather than by the use of nonscientific methods such as pure discussion, speculation, further reasoning from the dictums of "authorities," or "schools of psychology" or the use of such pretentious undefined words such as "unconscious," "depth psychology," "psychodynamics," and "Oedipus complex."...Fundamental investigation must rest on a firm clinical basis.[66]

Cohen's importance to Robins never diminished. When, thirty years later, Robins authored a key work on suicide, he dedicated his book to Mandel Cohen.[67]

Cohen recommended that Robins (Fig. 3.4, Pictorial Essay) take a position at Washington University because the chair of the psychiatry department there, Edwin F. Gildea (1898–1977), was biologically oriented—the "great hope for American psychiatry," as Cohen put it. Gildea's research centered on attempts to correlate levels and metabolism of blood lipids and thyroid function with mental disorders.[68] Robins then introduced Cohen's idea of operational criteria to Samuel Guze and George Winokur. (Fig. 3.5, Pictorial Essay). Recalls Guze: "George and I were immediately persuaded that this was the way to go....So these ideas were there from the early 1950s and, once Eli persuaded us of their validity, we began to use them [in our research]."[69] A psychiatrist who had his medical school and psychiatry residence at Washington University remembers that his teachers in the psychiatry department spoke "reverently" of Cohen, and that he was required to read his papers. Cohen was held up as an icon to follow.[70]

With Cohen as a model, Robins greatly influenced many. Guze spoke for himself and others when he said, "I owe to Eli opening up to me [the] whole field of [research] literature. No one had taught me about that literature; Eli was the one."[71] Everyone was agreed on Robins' warmth and leadership. "It was because of Eli," said Guze, a brilliant and resourceful man himself, "that I decided to devote my life as a psychiatrist to psychiatric research."[72] Moreover, in 1975 Winokur helped found the American

Academy of Clinical Psychiatrists (AACP) for like-minded psychiatrists, and in 1988 the Academy began publishing a journal, *Annals of Clinical Psychiatry*. Cohen was a strong supporter.

Eli Robins brought much to the psychiatry department at Washington University. (Fig. 3.6, Pictorial Essay). He was an intellectual and a voracious reader and had enormous energy, running two laboratories at the same time that he was carrying on clinical studies. This entailed working late and on weekends, but he was always very lively and exuberant.[73] Robert Spitzer, who stayed at Robins' house several times, remembers him as warm and friendly and that he had "wonderful times" with Robins and his wife Lee (Fig. 3.7, Pictorial Essay).[74] As catalyst, mentor, and a man of great charisma, Robins fulfilled the role of an exemplary department chair and was the main force behind the department's extensive development of laboratories. He had an interesting quirk, though. In the early years none of the department's laboratories was dedicated to drug research because of Robins' disbelief in the efficacy of new psychotropic medications. He particularly distrusted the antidepressants and did not prescribe them.[75] But he authored over 175 publications and in almost all of them was the consummate biological psychiatrist. He achieved all of this in spite of the fact that for a large part of his life he suffered from ever-more debilitating multiple sclerosis, from which he died in 1994 at the age of 73. By the age of 50, at the time he was working on the Feighner criteria paper, he was already having difficulty with speaking and moving.

Robins arrived at Washington University in 1949 at 28 years of age. He worked both as an NIMH pharmacology fellow—under Oliver Lowry (1910–1996), an internationally famous pharmacologist and biochemist—and as a clinical investigator and teacher in the Department of Psychiatry. Beginning in the 1950s, he published throughout his life in the fields of brain neurochemistry and histology, concentrating in the areas of suicide, depression, schizophrenia, and alcoholism. In the 1960s he developed an interest in the problem of vague descriptions of psychiatric disorders, a highly significant topic, which culminated in the 1970 paper that he and Guze published on the establishment of diagnostic validity in psychiatric illness. Recall that it was this paper that formed the foundation on which Feighner et al. two years later based their use of diagnostic criteria.

One example of Robins' work that demonstrated early his basic philosophy and efforts before Feighner, was a book chapter on antisocial personality. This was an attempt to establish diagnostic criteria in a personality disorder, a field that had long been considered the purview of the psychoanalysts.[76] Other instances of pre-Feighner work were papers on male and female sexuality that were based on studies supported by NIMH grants, which showed that by 1969, the NIMH was willing to fund Wash. U. clinical studies. Not surprisingly, the papers were highly descriptive and eschewed any thoughts on etiology. Yet, remarkably for the Wash. U. group, the paper on lesbians reported that "psychological responses are crucial to the classification of female homosexuals." The study on male homosexuals challenged psychoanalytic beliefs, presciently pointing out that the subjects had infrequent psychotherapy and seemed to be "able to make the necessary adjustments and compromises on their own." Eighty-four percent, the authors said, had no disability, "psychiatric or social" to any significant degree.

Lastly, Robins spent years studying suicidal behavior and in 1981 published a book on his work, *The Final Months*. This was the book dedicated to Mandel Cohen.[77]

In 1974, Robert Spitzer, Jean Endicott, and Robins and colleagues presented a paper on their new Research Diagnostic Criteria at the First CNS Symposium of The Squibb Institute For Medical Research,[78] officially allying Robins with Spitzer and Endicott who were at the New York State Psychiatric Institute. Endicott remains there.[79] Robins and Spitzer first came into contact, according to Spitzer, under the auspices of Martin M. Katz, Ph.D., at the NIMH, who brought them together in 1971 to work on an NIMH study of the psychobiology of depression—a large project still going on today.[80]

Guze reported that after Robins' and Spitzer's initial meeting, Spitzer came to Washington University to give a talk and stayed a while, and the Wash. U. people saw that Spitzer shared their "foundational" views 100%, though they differed slightly in other matters.[81] Spitzer points out that Robins was initially surprised to find that he "would be interested in or know something about psychiatric diagnosis [coming] from Columbia and the psychoanalytic center there." He recalls coming to St. Louis with Endicott around six times in 1972–74 to develop with Robins an extension of the Feighner criteria, the Research Diagnostic Criteria,(RDC) which was being sponsored by the NIMH.[82] The RDC was a vital prelude to Spitzer's work as head of the DSM-III Task Force. Paula Clayton, later on the Task Force, was in the early 1970s an assistant professor at Washington University. She says Spitzer came to the university with Jean Endicott to virtually "sit at the feet" of Eli Robins to learn the Wash. U. "approach."[83] It is clear that Robins had a career-changing influence on Spitzer who, up to that time, had been engaged in developing rating scales and structured interviews and only tangentially working with diagnostic criteria.

From Robins we move to Samuel Guze.

SAMUEL B. GUZE (1924–2000)—PSYCHIATRY IS A PART OF MEDICINE

Samuel B. Guze was born in New York City and graduated from high school at age fifteen. He then attended college for two years at City College of New York (CCNY). He transferred to Washington University because he was told at CCNY that it would be hard for him, as a Jew, to be accepted to a medical school from there. He did his medical school, internship, and residency at Washington University. As early as medical school, from which he graduated at age twenty-one, he thought psychoanalysis was "baloney."[84]

Guze began a residency in medicine at Wash. U. but did not enjoy his work, so he was allowed to take some time off one of his medical rotations to work under a psychiatrist, George Saslow (1907–2006). Saslow had come to Washington University to develop links between medicine and psychiatry via a psychosomatic medicine division. He was strongly antipsychoanalytic, having been influenced by Mandel Cohen, and was eventually appointed to the task force for DSM-III. Guze was very impressed with Saslow, who was a charismatic teacher, and with his skill as an interviewer.[85] Despite his ambivalence about medicine, Guze did a third year of medical residency at the VA

Hospital affiliated with Yale University. He returned to Washington University in 1950 to work as a fellow under Saslow, who had a grant from the Commonwealth Fund. The Fund "was very interested in medical education and in trying to inculcate an awareness of social and personal factors in health and illness."[86] Guze remembered it as a "wonderful" year. It was then also that he met Robins and George Winokur. It is paradoxical that Saslow and Guze, both antianalytic and biologically oriented, were being funded to teach medical students and residents about "social and personal factors in health and illness."

Guze next took a residency in psychiatry at Washington University and ended up a faculty member with a joint appointment in medicine and psychiatry. A psychiatric resident at the time remembers him as "intense, highly organized [and] a dedicated educator."[87] Throughout his professional career, Guze was unwavering in advancing the idea that psychiatry must be regarded as a part of medicine.

In the 1950s, when there were a lot of psychiatrists who were psychoanalytically oriented, Guze said, "you had to know [their] language. Even [when I was] most critical, [I] always told the residents you had to know the language in order to be critical [of psychoanalysis]."[88] Guze gave lectures to the medical students and residents and one introductory lecture concerning psychoanalysis. The lecture had an accompanying handout that had sixty defined psychoanalytic terms on it. Guze remembers saying to students "that if you understand these terms, what they mean and how to use them, there's no reason why you can't hold your own in any context."[89] An indication of the influence that the Wash. U. troika had in the department is that Guze, who had no use for psychoanalysis, taught it.

Guze remembered that he, Robins, and Winokur decided to teach their residents how to pass their board exams as the three knew there would be psychoanalytically oriented examiners. They did very careful, detailed coaching and encouraged residents to approach the exams with a "covert, hostile, competitive attitude. It had to be covert, but [they were] there to beat the examiner....Those who failed almost always did so because they didn't take our advice and got into arguments. They forgot the insistence on being covert.'"[90]

After a while, in 1955, Guze thought of going into an internal medicine practice, but then he was offered a leading position in the psychiatry department. As he later recalled, "Winokur, Robins and I suddenly realized [by the late 1950s] we were now in a position to try to shape the department in the direction we thought it should go. We didn't want a psychoanalytic department, we wanted a broad research effort, and we wanted to put tremendous emphasis on improving the diagnostic system in psychiatry."[91] So they went to the department chair, still Edward Gildea—a man permissive by nature—[92] with a plan that presented what they would do in each year with the medical students and each year of the residency training, which would include cultivation of research. Gildea was taken aback by this ambitious plan, its comprehensiveness, and its totally nonpsychoanalytic nature, but he welcomed its orientation and said he would back them; he continued to do so even though he received many criticisms and complaints.

Ultimately, Robins, Guze, and Winokur divided up the main responsibilities in running the department. Robins directed medical-student teaching; Guze became director of the psychiatric outpatient clinic and consultation-liaison service, an outgrowth of the psychosomatic division under Saslow; and Winokur assumed direction of the inpatient service and residency training.[93] In every way research was encouraged not only in clinical psychiatry but also in neurochemistry, pharmacology, genetics, and epidemiology. In the 1950s and 1960s it was rare to see such a program at a medical school or residency.

Guze asserted that another factor that helped them to achieve their goals was that most of the psychoanalysts in St. Louis went into full-time private practice rather than full-time academia after World War II. Washington University had a strict rule that all full-time people had to turn in their private-patient earnings to the department. The psychoanalysts preferred not to do this. "So," as Guze recalled, "we didn't have to cope with full-time and therefore influential psychoanalysts." Nevertheless, when the analysts opened the St. Louis Psychoanalytic Institute, Guze remembered, "it was clear that there was going to be a long, protracted 'war' with our department."[94] Perhaps it was at this time, or after they had pushed the analysts out of the department when Robins became chair in 1963, that they hung a picture of Freud over the urinal in the men's room.[95] (It might have been the brainchild of the irreverent and caustic Winokur.) In any event, as Guze, Robins, and Winokur discussed things over lunch, they were imbued with the notion that they "could really make a dent in American psychiatry."[96]

Before we return to Guze's career, this is a good moment to note that his and his colleagues' hope for influencing psychiatry coincided with significant changes coming from several directions. The psychoanalytic hegemony was on the wane. The introduction of psychopharmacological agents offered a new area for research. The professional climate concerning the need for description of psychopathology and for diagnosis was shifting. Recognizing a need for a new approach, for example, "in 1965, the Psychopharmacology Research Branch of the NIMH sponsored a conference on classification in psychiatry." Their view was that there had been significant technological and methodological changes. High-speed computers were now available, making it possible to manage large-scale data sets and complex statistical operations. Rating scales and other psychometric techniques could quantify and assess symptoms, behavior, and personality.[97] Structured diagnostic interviews such as Spitzer and Endicott's Schedule for Affective Disorders and Schizophrenia (SADS) were becoming prominent.[98]

Moreover, there was a growing interest in genetics. This in particular attracted all three of the Wash. U. pioneers. Guze became one of the first Americans to use studies of twins as a means of identifying the role of heredity in psychiatric illness. And Winokur, as we shall see, began to investigate the role of genetics in affective disorders (Fig. 3.8, Pictorial Essay). Family members of patients with such disorders were found frequently to have the same difficulties. (Kraepelin, it will be remembered, believed that for psychiatric research to go forward, he had to include a geneticist among the scientists at his Munich Institute.)

Furthermore, the Wash. U. psychiatrists began to realize, Guze recalled, that "there were people around the country who felt that they wanted something different and were looking for some place to take the lead. For many years that was a big advantage to us when it came to recruitment. Residents who were looking for something other than psychoanalytic training were always told to go out to St. Louis. We got a lot of interesting residents."[99]

Finally, there is also a strong possibility that some of the people who either sought biologically oriented residencies from the start or turned away from Freudian approaches at other stages of their careers had had an earlier negative experience with psychoanalysis, like Robins with his relative at McLean. Another more definitive example of this phenomenon comes from the experience of psychopharmacologist and eventual member of the DSM-III Task Force, Donald Klein (b. 1928), who was in training at the New York Psychoanalytic Institute, at that time a prominent and highly regarded (and very traditional) program. Klein wanted to do research, which his analyst interpreted as a sadistic wish that they would have to work through.[100] This was a defining moment for Klein in his journey away from psychoanalysis and in his eventual denigration of it. There was also a generation of well-known, analytically trained psychiatrists, Spitzer among them, whose commitment to psychoanalysis lessened or faded, with varying amounts of new allegiance to descriptive or biological psychiatry.[101]

To return to Washington University: Guze's organizational skills brought him appointments as Vice Chancellor for Medical Affairs and President of the Washington University Medical Center, from 1971 to 1989. He also was head of the Department of Psychiatry from 1975 to 1989 and again from 1993 to 1997 after Robins had to step down because of his deteriorating health. This row of administrative positions placed Guze in an ideal position to support the research and biological work of the psychiatry department and perhaps boost the exposure of his own work.[102] In 1979, he was elected to the National Academy of Science's Institute of Medicine, one of the highest recognitions a physician can achieve in the United States.

Guze made two very influential contributions to American psychiatry. One was his dedicated, skillful teaching and mentoring of almost two generations of medical students, residents, and junior colleagues. Among other achievements, he recommended Paula Clayton, a professor in the Washington University psychiatry department, for the position of head of the psychiatry department at the University of Minnesota.[103] In 1980, Clayton was the first woman in the United States ever to hold such a job.

Guze's other major contribution was his long-term commitment to remedicalize psychiatry. In the service of this goal, to give just one example, he wrote or co-authored five papers on hysteria, all in a true Kraepelinian mode. He argued strongly against the traditional psychoanalytic interpretations of this illness. Instead, he asserted, psychiatrists did not know enough to explain the etiology of hysteria and needed instead to stick to describing the clinical course, do follow-up studies to see if the original diagnosis had been correct, and study family history, which could help confirm the patient's diagnosis. Guze established diagnostic criteria for hysteria and stated that diagnosis was vital because there could be no research on the disorder without a valid classification. However, if a diagnosis was not clear, the answer was to declare that there was no diagnosis.[104]

Many years later, when "hysteria" as a main diagnosis was out of the DSM and "somatoform disorders" and "dissociative disorders" took its place, Guze co-authored a book chapter that discussed the validity of four separate subdiagnoses under "soma-toform disorders." Although a quarter of a century had passed since Guze's first paper on hysteria, in his own estimation little had changed from the medical point of view: "Establishing whether particular criteria define a valid disease entity remains...prob-lematic, since independent correlates of validity, such as laboratory tests or biopsies, do not yet exist. [Therefore] much research is required before we can accept the validity of the four DSM disorders." He did, however, give a grudging nod to the DSM-III criteria; they provided "a framework for the needed studies."[105]

Guze continued in this mode throughout his career. He repeatedly lionized Kraepelin as the psychiatrist who represented the history of descriptive psychiatry and who had blazed the path whereby "symptoms, signs, and course are paramount in understand-ing and classifying psychiatric illness."[106] In 1992 he published *Why Psychiatry Is a Part of Medicine*, a culmination of the key positions he had enunciated for many decades.[107] If the book had any major weakness, it was Guze's playing down of the role of psy-chological events in mental illness, although because of his fellowship with Saslow in psychosomatic medicine, he accepted that "psychological significant events...can affect the body's physiological state," but added that we do not know why. Yet, regard-less of where the reader stood on this mind–body issue, the book is an impressive work by an uncommonly intelligent and thoughtful man who brought historical, biological, and philosophical depth to his subject. Guze included a chapter entitled "Philosophical Issues," in which he spelled out the implications for a psychiatry that adhered to the medical model. He dealt with the issues of causality, teleology, the relationship between the mind and the brain, reductionism, free will, consciousness, the meaning of illness, and ethical decisions.[108] He also had a chapter on psychotherapy where he continued to assail psychoanalysis because it insisted on causal linkages and etiology. He offered a replacement, "rehabilitative psychotherapy," which encompassed cognitive-behavioral therapy and Klerman's nonanalytic interpersonal therapy, because they were compat-ible with the medical model, "requiring no assumptions concerning etiology."[109]

When all was said and done, despite Guze's continued criticism of the unsatisfac-tory rate of psychiatric progress toward the Wash. U. goals, in 1995 he was willing to admit that there had been a "neo-Kraepelinian revolution in psychiatric diagnosis."[110] Yes, he declared, diagnosis, disease specificity, and the study of brain physiology had been missing from American psychiatry for half a century, but now the new DSM-IV (1994) gave evidence that they were no longer banished.[111] Psychiatry, he declared, had returned to its Kraepelinian roots.

GEORGE WINOKUR (1925–1996): LONG-TERM FOLLOW-UP AND AFFECTIVE DISORDERS

The third of the Wash. U. triumvirate was George Winokur, who was born in Baltimore, received his bachelor's degree from Johns Hopkins, and then his medical degree three years later from the University of Maryland.[112] He came to St. Louis from Baltimore in 1951 for a last year of residency training, wanting to learn something about what was going on at Washington University. He quickly became involved with Robins and Guze and ended up not going back to Baltimore to have psychoanalytic training, as he had planned. He joined the Department of Psychiatry faculty in 1954 at age twenty-nine. Eighteen years later, he was one of the authors of the Feighner et al. article.

As Guze later noted, "[o]ne of...Winokur's most outstanding characteristics was his ability to attract people into research and to encourage them to pursue their careers in this area."[113] He was also known for his phenomenal memory. His very ready humor appears to have been quite pointed, sometimes even causing embarrassment. But Guze in his obituary for Winokur observed that "very few individuals could get away with being as candid and open as [he, but] somehow, people recognized that he was not being mean."[114] Richard Hudgens, a psychiatrist who worked with Winokur, believes that the antipsychoanalytic reputation of the department "owed much to the drum-fire of mockery which Winokur rained down on its proponents." Winokur freely said that the "only worthwhile attacks on psychoanalysis were *ad hominem* attacks" because there were no substantive issues since the analysts had no real data in support of their positions.[115]

Hudgens remembers Winokur as "an outspoken and stimulating teacher" who had an unusually close day-to-day influence on first-year residents. Later on, as chair of a psychiatry department, he was equally involved with his faculty. Moreover, as a committed and creative researcher, he had an ongoing interest in studies involving large numbers of patients, which he used to his great advantage. Continuing the Wash. U. emphasis on follow-up studies, Winokur took part in the Iowa 500 Research Project, which involved the long-term (30–40 years) follow-up of patients originally diagnosed with schizophrenia, depression, and bipolar illness in the 1930s and 1940s.[116] He also published prolifically throughout his career.

Winokur remained at Washington University for twenty years, until 1971, when he accepted a chair and the chairmanship of the psychiatry department at the University of Iowa College of Medicine.[117] In this way, the Wash. U. "approach," as Guze termed it, was carried to other medical schools and gave birth to additional influential neo-Kraepelinians.[118] Iowa spawned the future editor of the *American Journal of Psychiatry*, Nancy Andreasen, and Ming Tsuang, a biological researcher who later moved to the Massachusetts Mental Health Center at Harvard. Donald W. Goodwin moved from Washington University to Kansas City, where he became chair of the Department of Psychiatry at the University of Missouri. Paula Clayton, who served her residency and then became a full-time faculty member in the Washington University psychiatry department, was heavily influenced by Winokur to become an expert on affective disorders.[119] She then moved to the University of Minnesota as chair. (Andreasen, Goodwin, and Clayton were all on the Task Force that developed DSM-III.) Paul H. Wender had a year of residency at a Wash. U.–affiliated hospital and went on to have a distinguished career, known especially for his work on attention deficit hyperactivity disorder (ADHD). Wender's contribution is discussed further in Chapter 12.

Early in his career, Winokur began to focus on affective disorders—depression and mania—and was one of the first psychiatrists in the United States to use lithium on patients with mania. He and his junior colleague Paula Clayton were pioneers in defining and conceptualizing affective disorders.[120] Winokur also wrote a landmark monograph on manic-depressive illness with Clayton and another member of the department at Washington University. This book provides yet another piece of evidence connecting Wash. U. psychiatrists with Kraepelin.[121]

Winokur ultimately published over four hundred articles and individual book chapters as well as a dozen textbooks and monographs. Beginning in 1963, Winokur and co-authors started publishing a series of papers on various aspects of affective disorders.[122] At this time, he also wrote on chronic anxiety neurosis and on depression among medically ill patients.[123] Meanwhile, in 1964–1965, supported by NIMH grants, he and Clayton studied 426 patients with the diagnosis of primary affective disorder, including data from and about close family members. Winokur and Clayton then reported their findings in a 1967 seminal paper, which established that there existed separately unipolar (depression alone) and bipolar (depression and mania) diseases; they based their conclusion on family history, age of onset, and disease course.[124] Simultaneously, on the basis of the same study, Winokur and Clayton wrote on sex differences in primary affective illness. Since Winokur's special interest was in bipolar illness, using their 1964–1965 data set, he and Clayton followed mania patients and their families longitudinally (going forward) in a landmark book, *Manic Depressive Illness* (1969). Their study was deeply rooted in Kraepelin's observations and conclusions.

Not resting on his laurels, Winokur continued to investigate genetic factors in manic-depressive disease.[125] He also published an important review of the literature on the various types of affective disorders. This article included his proposal of a classification of the affective disorders and diagnostic criteria for mania and primary depression.[126]

In the early 1970s, ever exploring, Winokur shifted his main focus from manic-depressive illness (bipolar disorder) to depressive disease (unipolar disorder).[127] Over a five-year period, from 1971 to 1976, we can trace how his thinking developed. On the strength of this work, he decided that unipolar depression could be subdivided into depression spectrum disease, a depressive condition in which a first-degree family member has alcoholism and/or antisocial personality disorder, and pure depressive disease. He found that the course of illness was different in the two groups and posited that the depression spectrum disease might be linked to certain specific genetic markers.[128] Winokur's conception of the possibility of spectrum disorders was a generation ahead of his time.

Winokur's papers always had about them the upbeat tone of a dedicated and imaginative researcher who had great confidence in the use of diagnostic criteria and in the underlying foundation of the work he was doing. So it comes as a surprise to learn that Winokur decided that there were significant weaknesses in depending on diagnostic criteria.[129] After all, the diagnostic criteria system had been touted as a vital achievement of reliability because it would mean that psychiatrists everywhere would be in agreement on exactly what they meant by a certain diagnosis. But now he wrote about important shortcomings of the system in the *Archives of General Psychiatry*, eighteen years after DSM-III had come into existence.

In his article, Winokur challenged the assumption of reliability. Working with two others in the psychiatry department at Iowa, he conducted an experiment in diagnosing—both originally and in follow-ups—98 patients. It turned out that there were serious discordances among the diagnoses of the three co-workers. Winokur also read diagnostic studies from other institutions and discovered flaws in their methods and decisions. On the basis of his experiment and literature review, he came to four significant conclusions:

1. It was a fiction that the data could speak for themselves (this from a data-driven researcher.)
2. It is impossible to eliminate clinical judgment in making diagnoses.[130]
3. Carelessness in following a set of criteria occurred. ("We hope," wrote Winokur, "it is a rare event.")
4. There was an "insidious problem [among different institutions] of…inconsistencies in criteria interpretation and application."[131]

The Wash. U. authors of the Feighner criteria (who included Winokur), Spitzer et al. with their NIMH-sponsored Research Diagnostic Criteria, and the DSM-III Task Force had all presented their diagnostic systems as giant leaps toward achieving diagnostic reliability. Winokur was now shaken. Referring to the song lines, "Jesus loves me, this I know, 'cause the Bible tells me so," he concluded, "The Bible may tell us so, but the criteria don't. They are better than we had, but they are still a long way from perfect."[132]

However, as far as Winokur's career is concerned, we should not end on a negative note. True, he had published a warning of great importance that contained welcome insight because it came from a Wash. U. pioneer. Nevertheless, it must be stressed that Winokur made seminal discoveries in the conceptualizing and diagnosing of affective disorders that stand to this day. Like Guze's emphasis on psychiatry being a part of medicine, Winokur's great interest in genetics provides another link to Kraepelin.

One cannot but conclude that Robins, Guze, and Winokur formed a remarkable trio. Their bonding together over the years is noteworthy in itself because of the great differences in temperament: Robins, warm and inviting, yet clearly the strong leader in spite of his MS; Guze, organized and "intense," driven by his desire to unite psychiatry and medicine; Winokur, outgoing and mocking, unflaggingly imparting his research ethos to residents and junior faculty. But they had much to keep them together. There was the sense of being beleaguered, surrounded as they were by the sea of psychoanalytic dominance. So they clung together tightly, impelled by the vision that they could bring about a change in American psychiatry. They adamantly persisted, addressing ongoing scientific concerns over the lunchtime they shared each day, and then were socially buoyed by the legendary parties that Eli and Lee Robins unfailingly hosted. Like the generation of Helmholtz in the mid-nineteenth century, they rebelled against a non-material approach to knowledge, insisting on an empirical psychiatry. Bequeathing to us both the progress we can praise and the problems we now struggle with, their empiricism prevailed. That they transformed modern psychiatry, as seen in the theoretical and clinical challenges inherited by the DSM-5 Task Force, is indisputable.

Yet the Wash. U. ideas might not have received their wide dissemination and broad influence without the coming together of Eli Robins and Robert Spitzer. Spitzer was a psychiatrist, originally trained as a psychoanalyst, working in the Biometrics Unit at New York State Psychiatric Institute at Columbia University. He was an individual of penetrating intellect, open to new ideas, possessed of astonishing energy, politically adept, and intently set on achieving his goals. We now turn to learn about this remarkable man.

SECTION II

The People

4

ROBERT L. SPITZER,
PSYCHIATRIC REVOLUTIONARY

In 1969, the NIMH convened a landmark conference organized by both Martin M. Katz, a research psychologist who was Director of the Clinical Research Branch of the NIMH, and Gerald Klerman, the formulator of the neo-Kraepelinian "credo," to consider new ideas about depression and its treatment. They believed that depression had become a significant public health problem. Since there had been important developments during the 1950s and 1960s regarding conceptions of the nature and etiology of affective disorders, the implications of those changes now needed to be addressed. Specifically, Katz and Klerman concluded that research advances meant "that we were on the verge of linking physiology, psychosocial factors, and behavior in [affective] disorders, which would...make possible the development of a coherent and valid psychobiologic theory of depression."[1]

The NIMH invited to the conference a group of research scientists and clinical investigators from all over the country who were "asked to analyze the state of the field and to develop a recommendation to guide further research in the affective disorders."[2] The conferees addressed both of their assigned tasks and issued three major recommendations:

1. There were technical obstacles to comparing results from one study to another. Especially vital was the need to establish "consensus on and reliability of the measurement of the...symptomatic and behavioral facets of [each] affective disorder." Therefore, it was crucial to develop interview methods that would be reliable in different clinical settings.
2. It was necessary to determine the reliability of new classifications that were being devised, by comparing traditional nosologies with the new ones. Therefore, there had to be research to resolve "the issues underlying the uncertainty of nosology" in affective disorders.
3. Finally, the conferees concluded that since there were already influential genetic and biochemical findings, there had to be a means of conducting studies to confirm or disconfirm the new information that had arisen from the research.

The conferees decided that no single institution could provide the multiple resources needed to implement their recommendations or "conduct replicative studies in the biological sphere." Hence, there had to be "collaboration across disciplines, laboratories, and clinical settings."[3]

Responding to this comprehensive advice, Katz decided to form an advisory group on collaborative research on the psychobiology of depression. He already knew Robert Spitzer from meetings of the American College of Neuropsychopharmacology (ACNP) and felt that Spitzer would be a logical member of the new advisory group, which was to include Eli Robins as well. Katz wanted the two men to meet. It is under these circumstances that Eli Robins and Robert Spitzer came together in 1971.[4]

Robins, aged fifty, was on the verge of publishing the propitious nosology that would shortly appear as the "Feighner criteria." Spitzer, aged thirty-nine and trained as a psychoanalyst but soon to quit practicing as one, was doing research on structured interviews, which could be used to improve and facilitate research. A structured interview is an interview format worked out in advance so as to ask exactly the same questions of a group of selected patients, to achieve greater reliability in diagnosis. Spitzer, together with the Columbia psychologist Jean Endicott, had already formulated DIAGNO, a computer program for psychiatric diagnosis, Spitzer having studied Fortran IV at IBM.[5] In the coming years, he and Endicott would develop other interviewing formats, including the Global Assessment Scale (GAS), to measure the severity of psychiatric disturbance, and the Schedule of Affective Disorders and Schizophrenia (SADS.)[6]

Following the recommendations of the advisory group on collaborative research on the psychobiology of depression, the NIMH designated five centers in the United States, plus the NIMH itself, in Rockville, MD, to form a clinical studies group, separate from a coexisting biological studies group. The five clinical studies centers were the Massachusetts General Hospital and the Harvard Medical School in Boston; Rush-Presbyterian-St. Luke's Medical Center in Chicago; the University of Iowa in Iowa City; the New York State Psychiatric Institute in New York City; and the Washington University School of Medicine in St. Louis. Through this mechanism, Spitzer, at the Psychiatric Institute in New York, and Robins, at Washington University in St. Louis, maintained contact for a number of years.[7] We should also remember that after meeting Robins at the NIMH, Spitzer went to St. Louis to learn from him what the Wash. U. psychiatrists were doing.

ROBERT SPITZER: LEADER AND REBEL
FACING A CRISIS IN PSYCHIATRY

Spitzer, as always, displayed his characteristic energy, his openness to new ideas, and his enterprising nature. Shortly after meeting with Robins and becoming intrigued by Robins' system of diagnostic criteria, he brokered the effort to remove homosexuality as a diagnosis in DSM-II. Simultaneously, he was angling for the job of leading the Task Force that would construct DSM-III. Since DSM-III is a prodigious achievement—whether one is sympathetic to it or not—and represents a historic change of direction in American psychiatry, we must search out the person who produced this radical revision of DSM-II. Spitzer replaced a 134-page booklet with a 494-page tome and formally terminated the entrenched, albeit faltering, psychoanalytic domination of American psychiatry.

Let us begin with historical theory. Thomas Kuhn has argued that a radical development in science, a "paradigm shift," often occurs following a state of crisis in a field.[8] To Kuhn's model, we should add the phenomenon of the remarkable leader who often emerges at the time of the crisis and effects change. In Chapter 1 we explored the crisis in American psychiatry—the antipsychiatry movement, the effects of deinstitutionalization, the legal challenges, the APA vote on homosexuality, and the "pseudopatient" fiasco in mental hospitals. All of this occurred immediately before Spitzer became head of the APA Task Force charged with revising the diagnostic manual. This model of crisis and the emergence of a leader can be accurate for nonscientific situations as well. We are used to seeing such a pattern in history on a larger scale. An illustration of this occurred in the sixteenth century when a crisis in the Roman Catholic Church was taken in hand by an ardently devoted and charismatic monk and theologian, Martin Luther. The Protestant Reformation resulted. This is not at all to compare Spitzer to Luther nor DSM-III to the Protestant Reformation, but the *pattern* of a crisis and a dynamic leader coming together to effect major change holds true.

The combination of a crisis and new leadership occurred in psychiatry over a century ago. Psychiatry in the late nineteenth century was in a state of paralysis, unable to advance, and the impasse was addressed by both Emil Kraepelin and Sigmund Freud (the two men were born in the same year). In one instance, as we have seen, the historic division of psychosis into dementia praecox and manic-depressive illness pushed the conceptualization and prognosis of psychotic illness forward. In Freud's case, his development of psychoanalysis allowed for the conceptualization and treatment of "neurotic" conditions like hysteria, anxiety, and obsessions, as well as character pathology. This offered a way out of the pessimistic gloom of therapeutics documented so tellingly by both Kraepelin and Karl Jaspers. With the division of psychosis and the treatment of neurosis, Kraepelin and Freud, men of unusual strength and determination—and in Freud's case an outright rebel as well—responded to the predicament that encased their field.

There were similar circumstances in the late twentieth century. Robert Spitzer, a leader and a rebel from his early days, faced with the plummeting of regard for his field, became determined to halt it and redirect psychiatry. Whether or not one agrees with his solution and its consequences, still, as the creative, energetic, and resolute head of the DSM-III Task Force, Spitzer ended up turning American psychiatry in a new direction via a drastically revised nosology. He himself moved down a startlingly new path, away from the psychoanalysis in which he had been trained. Feeling increasingly dissatisfied by his work as a psychotherapist, he rebelled against psychoanalytic thinking, turning away decisively from the men who had supervised and analyzed him. Although there were losses as well as gains, Spitzer ended up bringing psychiatry into a new dimension. Because Spitzer's achievement was so influential, this chapter will explore the first half of his life, up to the publication of DSM-III in 1980.

We have an unusual opportunity to see Spitzer's development into a leader and rebel by exploring his home and school life from an early age, as we have access to some of Spitzer's childhood records from the school he attended, Walden School, a progressive Manhattan private school (pre-K–12). We also have the transcript of a revealing interview he gave when he was fifteen and a sophomore at Walden high school. Spitzer was part of a study by the famous sociologist David Riesman (1909–2002), author of the much-lauded *The Lonely Crowd* (1950), an examination of post–World War II conformity and suburban anomie.[9] In the 1940s, Riesman and his younger colleague, sociologist Nathan Glazer (b. 1924), conducted interviews of students at Walden as part of a study of the way "people expressed political attitudes or their absence." In this study, Spitzer appears as "Henry Friend," a student at "San Guardino," a private school supposedly on the outskirts of Los Angeles.[10] As part of the study, Riesman had access to Spitzer's entire school records, from which it becomes obvious that Spitzer had been a rebel every since his kindergarten days.

According to Spitzer's own later account, he enjoyed controversy and troublemaking.[11] Rebelliousness by itself, however, is insufficient for leadership. In fact, many childhood rebels end up as criminals or increasingly alienated. But a leader who brings forth a successful paradigm shift perforce remains within the Establishment. Spitzer obviously met this necessity. He also brought to bear considerable intelligence, a driving ambition, and an avowed comfort with being "ruthless" on occasion, exhibiting these qualities as early as adolescence. Combined with these traits was a palpable exuberance and enthusiasm.

SPITZER'S CHILDHOOD AND ADOLESCENCE

Robert L. Spitzer was born in White Plains, New York, on May 22, 1932. His middle initial is for Leopold, a name his father bestowed on him in celebration of a Hungarian king.[12] His family soon moved to another New York City suburb, Scarsdale. In the 1930s and 1940s Jewish families, or even nonobservant families of Jewish background, did not usually choose these two wealthy and conservative suburbs, which often had anti-Semitic restrictive clauses for residence. Shortly thereafter the Spitzers moved again, this time to West 83rd Street in Manhattan, the Upper West Side, which was quite diversified and had a substantial and often liberal Jewish population. (The move may have been occasioned by the death of the family's oldest child.) Although Spitzer was born when the United States was deeply in the grip of the Great Depression, the Spitzer family was not severely touched by it because Spitzer's father "did not believe in the Stock Market" and had invested none of his money there.[13]

Robert Spitzer was the last-born child of Benjamin Spitzer and Esther Pfeffer. Spitzer's father was born in Hungary and had come to the United States at a young age, and his mother was born in New York City, although all her older siblings were born in Europe, probably in Poland. Benjamin's and Esther's families were Jewish. At birth, Spitzer had two older sisters—Elaine, six, and Louise, four. When Spitzer was two, Elaine died of meningitis, this being before the days of antibiotics. It was a disaster for the family. Apparently, Spitzer's mother became depressed, and she began seeking psychoanalytic treatment.

Spitzer's father was an engineer who designed the first X-ray machine for use by dentists. He worked for General Electric and then developed models of teeth that dental students worked on. According to Spitzer he was a successful businessman.[14] Spitzer also remembers that in his early adolescence his father told him that "if he had to do it all over again, he would have become an internist and specialized in diagnosis." If true, this is a startling statement in light of both Spitzer's future defiance of his father and his ultimate career choice. Benjamin Spitzer was a quiet, even "withdrawn" man, according to Louise Albert, Spitzer's older sister.[15] After dinner he would go into the bedroom to read the newspaper. He had few friends, except for those who shared his pro-Stalinist politics. He did belong to the New York Ethical Culture Society and there initiated a group, the "Workers' Fellowship," to discuss Communist politics.[16]

Spitzer remembers Benjamin as being not very demonstrative; previous commentators on Spitzer have concluded that his father was "cold." But this is not the full story. The relationship was far more complex as it evolved over the years. Robert Spitzer's school record from the age of six states: "He is completely identified with his father—talks about him endlessly." Yet Spitzer himself recalls very little interaction between the two of them, aside from a few instances. His father encouraged him in science and gave him[17] the gift of a microscope when he was ten,[18] for Spitzer a "pleasant memory." And we know from the Riesman interview with Spitzer that once when his father invited him to go for a walk he declined and felt guilty afterward. It was also during Robert's adolescence that he and his father began to argue over left-wing politics.[19] His father was passionate in his support of Stalinist Russia, during the late 1940s, and Robert began to dissent. His pulling away started in 1948, when the Communist ruler of Yugoslavia, Josip Broz Tito (1892–1980), broke with Stalin.[20] Father and son argued politics obdurately. The antagonism became so bad that at times they stopped speaking to each other. The two had not been close for many years, and teenage rebellion now entered the picture.

The Spitzer house was staunchly Stalinist until Nikita Khrushchev (1874–1971), General Secretary of the Communist party of the Soviet Union, destroyed the cult of Stalin after Stalin died in 1953. Challenging the household loyalty to Stalinist Russia was the perfect subject on which to disagree because Robert was very conversant with the prime issues of left-wing politics. He could not have picked a more perfect matter to rebel against. As part of his interview at fifteen, in response to a question about his politics, he replied:

> I used to consider myself a real Communist—but now I feel closer to Wallace [left-wing presidential candidate], less dogmatic. The Communists are clear on economic matters but not on social laws, and they don't understand why people act as they do. Most middle-class Communists are not mentally healthy; they are sex-negative, authoritarian. I have similar doubts on Russia—we must change not only economic conditions but also human structure. This is [my] change of the last few months—reading *The Sexual Revolution* and being analyzed by a Reichian.[21]

Spitzer's belittling of "middle-class Communists" obviously was meant to include his parents (his mother was actually a member of the Party, his father was not).[22]

One subject that Spitzer always remained true to was his father's atheism, and he has remained an atheist throughout his life. Political and religious rebellion was ensconced in the Spitzer family.

Esther and Benjamin's politics appears to be one of the few things that united them. Spitzer's mother was a piano teacher, but what Spitzer recalls especially is that she was an unhappy woman who cried a lot and was in psychoanalytic treatment much of the time. Spitzer's sister concurs on the unhappiness and the continual analyses—"3/4 of her life," but remembers her as always angry.[23] She says their mother was an aggressive woman, interfering with and critical of her children and consequently hard to get along with. When Spitzer was in high school, he talked to the interviewer about hating how his mother needled him. He described her as "the boss" at home and his father as not paying "much attention."[24] In contrast to her husband's frequent silence, Esther was a "compulsive talker." Louise Albert has lamented, "It was a marriage made in hell."[25] And it was a marriage from which the children did not emerge unscathed. Albert has acidly typified their family life as "lousy," filled with "conflict and pain" for both children. She comments that Robert had "a hard time" growing up. The consequence was that the two children had a very close relationship, having "a common enemy" in their parents. Albert remembers that they were a big help to one another.[26] This childhood misery had to leave its imprint, something we must not forget as we learn about Spitzer's professional life and relationships. Yet it is worth noting the obvious: Spitzer and his sister also inherited and absorbed strengths. Both of these unhappy children achieved success in school and college and in their chosen fields. Louise is an author and a teacher.

Perhaps Esther Spitzer's greatest misery came from the sudden death of her oldest child, a time of "real trauma." She became "overwhelmed with grief" and withdrew from her baby—Robert—who was not even two, Albert asserts. It was then that she turned to psychotherapy, especially with either Karen Horney or one of her disciples. Esther Spitzer herself became a Jungian therapist later in her life.[27] Albert recounts that after her mother died, she gave a eulogy at a memorial service, and much to her surprise her brother—a man reported by colleagues as not given to showing his feelings—started to sob, testifying to some deep emotion.[28] We know that whatever Spitzer's negative feelings were about his mother, he took from her his love for playing and performing on musical instruments.

SCHOOL YEARS

At three years of age, Spitzer's parents enrolled him in the nursery school program at the Walden School, a not surprising choice for his parents. Riesman reported that Walden was thought of as "experimental" and "radical."[29] Spitzer remained at Walden through grade school and high school. Soon after his entrance, a note appeared in his school records: "Defies routine demands by pretending not to hear," though this is matched by a cooperative side: lets "other children play with toys he brings to school."[30] At age five he was "a perfect five-year old [who is] happy all the time [and] a leader." At age six, the teacher noted, he was not only intelligent but he strove to do things "way beyond" his capabilities. That same year he questioned the right of another child's "right of leadership in the 'gang.'" At age seven the rebelliousness and leadership continued to assert themselves: "Looked up to as leader—shows no fear of physical contact [he had had the previous year]. Defiant. Resents authority. Says 'You can't make me.'" An example is given: the other children wrote letters to their parents and ended them with "Love." Spitzer refused to do this.[31]

At eight years it was noted that he daydreamed but then sometimes went on rampages, jumping over desks, knocking down chairs, leading the class singing at the top of their voices. Walden seems to have accepted his behavior as "clowning antics." He was called "big boss" by the children when he raised "hell." But his position was challenged at the end of the year.[32] "He was miserable and insecure at losing his position. Children decided to take turns in leadership. He tried to influence the invitations other children extended for parties by threatening not to attend himself." The school notes go on: "He is disturbing to whatever group he is in…needs a class all by himself." All of this was followed the next year by Spitzer being unable to reassert his leadership, despite many attempts. The year after that, at age ten, he was always alone but did not seem unhappy; the notes read, "[he] enjoys dancing and is popular with girls," and later that year, "he is very popular in the group now. Has a great need to be the 'best.'"[33] Spitzer displayed this quality again in Riesman's own study and, not surprisingly, at various times in his adult life.

Significantly, we have from Spitzer himself two revealing self-reports of his preadolescence. At age eleven or twelve, Spitzer was given a school assignment to write about himself, which he did in the third person. The result is remarkable and at times unusually sophisticated. Riesman, who analyzed many high school interviews, said it was "unusual for its frankness and insight."[34] Here are Spitzer's own words in response to the assignment:

> Likes to have power…flirts with girls…only works on something very interested in, i.e., math and science. Likes to be frank with people. Likes to be with the underdog. Talks about people's faults to other people. Is very irresponsible and knows it. Will talk about his faults to his friends. Has an inferiority complex. Good sense of humor. Can do a good job if he really wants to. Likes to get attention. Is very frank with himself. Used to go to a psychoanalyst.[35]

The second self-report is Spitzer's remembrance at age seventy-four. It is notable because his recollection is predictive of his later career bent. As Spitzer tells it,

> When I was—I don't know—10, 11, or 12, I went to summer camp, and my bed was against the wall. And on the wall, I made a graph of my feelings towards five or six ladies and it, over time, went up and down.…That's a strange thing for somebody to do, but that's the kind of person, I guess, that ends up doing what I did; in other words, translating feelings into some kind of a system.[36]

In a National Public Radio (NPR) profile, a journalist, Alix Spiegel, commented, "You see, the little boy who graphed his passions onto cabin walls grew up to be the man who revolutionized the *Diagnostic and Statistical Manual*, the American Psychiatric Association's official listing of mental disease."

Spitzer also recalled a noteworthy incident from early adolescence, when his mother dragged him to an optometrist against his will, and he struck her in the face. One of the ways his mother dealt with this episode was to arrange for him to see a psychotherapist.[37]

At this point our information about Spitzer jumps to age fifteen, when he was a subject of Riesman's study. Riesman and Glazer constructed a written public-opinion poll and a set of wide-ranging interview questions and hired university students to administer the poll and conduct the interviews. These were relatively brief encounters, squeezed into 40 to 50 minutes, the length of a class period. The interviewers put their questions to three boys, all in the same class at Walden. In addition to the opinion poll and the interview, Riesman and Glazer asked the interviewers to prepare a "personality sketch" of each boy. The student who interviewed Spitzer painted a particularly appealing picture:

> Henry Friend is an engaging youth of fifteen. He has great charm, an attractive smile, unusual vivacity. In the interview he appeared quite secure and reflective— not unduly talkative; he was scrappy but with a smile. He is freckled and looks like the all-American boy, lithe and quick, but the warmth and liveliness of his manner were quite unusual and stood out in a day of interviews.[38]

Riesman observed that the three boys who were polled and interviewed were more "radical, more prominent, more politically involved, [more] extreme" than their classmates. Still, Henry Friend stood out. Riesman prefaced his assessment by declaring that he had beeen "struck, on analyzing these three, [that] Henry Friend is already the young rebel leader, astonishingly energetic, ambitious, and charismatic; he is definitely 'going places.'" He is in possession of "an exceptional maturity."[39] Riesman also added that from the vantage point of "mode of adaptation: autonomy, adjustment, or anomie," Friend "seems almost arrogant in his belief in his own autonomy."[40]

On what grounds did Riesman make these extraordinary statements, which turned out to be so prescient of Spitzer as an adult? Perhaps we should preface any answer to this question by noting what Riesman nowhere states—that adolescence is a time for rebellion. We must therefore keep in mind another question: on balance, what about Spitzer at fifteen was "normal" teen-age rebellion, and what of Spitzer's rebelliousness was an essential part of his personality? There is yet another complicating factor: Riesman overlooked the facts that Spitzer came from a politically rebellious family and the school he attended fostered politically rebellious attitudes. What from the outside might look like rebellion may actually have been a kind of conformity. Nevertheless, Riesman was correct to focus on the subject of Spitzer's rebellious nature, which was readily evident and indeed a life-long trait.

In the same year that Spitzer was involved in Riesman's study, he demonstrated his rebelliousness by decisively defying his parents. As a sophomore, Spitzer had a substitute English teacher, Robert Kronomeyer, who taught less about English and more about sex, emphasizing how society causes harm to people by not recognizing the importance of sexual expression. Intrigued, Spitzer went to speak to the English teacher and learned that he was a psychotherapist. Kronomeyer offered to help Spitzer be more liberated emotionally and sexually, but said that he would have to get the permission of his parents. Spitzer went to his parents and asked for their permission and, not surprisingly, they said no.

Undeterred, Spitzer started seeing Kronomeyer once a week and paying him $5.00 per session. His therapist turned out to be a student of Wilhelm Reich (1897–1957), an Austrian-born psychoanalyst who, in his later years, claimed to have discovered a new form of energy, "orgone energy," and built "orgone accumulators"—telephone booth–like structures in which to sit and absorb orgone energy. (At the end of his life, Reich became delusional and ran afoul of the law.) Spitzer became enamored of Reich's book, *The Function of the Orgasm*.[41] "That was his basic stuff which I later decided was nonsense," Spitzer proclaimed many years after. Spitzer's therapy consisted of some talking and a lot of yelling and pounding of pillows, the therapy Reich had developed. Spitzer went to Kronomeyer for about two years and gradually came to the conclusion that he was not being helped.[42] (For future reference, we should note that Spitzer once quipped to a colleague at the New York State Psychiatric Institute that "it was one of the many attempts—unsuccessful attempts at psychotherapy.")[43] It is true that Spitzer underwent many different types of psychotherapy in his life. Simultaneously with his Reichian therapy, Spitzer was seeing a conventional psychiatrist that his mother had arranged for, feeling her son was having problems socially and relating to his family. Spitzer resented this latter arrangement.[44] One can't but wonder if Spitzer's seeing Kronomeyer had an additional rebellious fillip, a counter to his parents' decision to seek treatment for their son on their terms.

RIESMAN ON HENRY FRIEND'S POLITICS AND POTENTIAL IN LIFE

Henry Friend's rebellious political positions—what Riesman called his "dauntless radicalism"—were directly connected with his capabilities as a leader. Friend had an impressive amount of political experience for a person of his age, and he spoke convincingly on a number of issues. He unabashedly declared that he took the lead in discussions in school, and Riesman pointed out that the other students trusted his political opinions. For example, since 1948 was a presidential election year, Friend took part in the election by organizing a Young Citizens for Wallace club in his area. Henry Wallace (1888–1965) had been vice-president under President Franklin D. Roosevelt from 1941 to 1945 and in 1948 was running for the presidency under a third party, the Progressive Party, with many left-wing views. Leftists, including Communist sympathizers, supported him. This was not Friend's first foray into politics. In 1944, at the age of twelve, he worked in the Roosevelt campaign. For the Wallace Campaign, Friend circulated many petitions and talked about political issues and current events at Wallace meetings with informed views on war, the draft, revolutionary events in Czechoslovakia, and what it meant to have the burden of working for a living.[45]

For a political rebel like Friend, the Establishment was the enemy. Friend declared that the National Association of Manufacturers, the Republicans, and the Democrats were "lined up against him.... The press is controlled against the interests of the man in the street."[46] His teachers were not exempted. Friend characterized his behavior in class in the following words: " I squawk—yes I do, as any. The teachers are afraid of me—I'm sometimes too ruthless."[47] He cast more light on this statement when he declared, "I always have a tough time with the teachers on whom I spilled resentments against my family."[48] (Was this statement something that a psychotherapist had told Spitzer?) The school psychologist found Friend "an aggressive and argumentative youngster," yet in a private school like Walden, the teachers were tolerant. One stated that it is "hard to convince him that his teachers are well meaning and try to be fair. If Henry could over-come his distrust of the adult world he would be more relaxed."[49] The teachers liked his intelligence, humor, and charm; if only he would overcome his mistrust of them. Riesman observed that his "aggressive and rebellious drives bring him at every point into conflict with his environment. [Yet he] is a successful leader who is not intimi-dated by the hostility he arouses in some. He seems from the record to manage his daily life not too badly, and he impresses his fellows....At every point Friend's resonance with others—peers, parents, teachers—is evident."[50] As we shall see, in the making of DSM-III, Spitzer was an impressive leader and formidable opponent.

Perhaps Friend's rebelliousness was so tolerated because it was accompanied by an obvious exuberance for life, what Riesman described as his "high spirits [and] his enthusiastic desire to explore all the resources of self." Friend declared that a person should "live with gusto."[51] When asked what he would do if he had only six months to live, he proclaimed that he would stop going to school, find a girl, sleep with her, play the guitar, travel "—boy what a time I'd have!"—make as many friends as pos-sible, and write a Kinsey Report on the sex lives of his teachers.[52] Riesman noted his "high affect...hardly another subject [in the study] uses so often phrases such as 'I like,' 'I want,' 'I hope.'"[53] If one looks closer, it can also be argued that Friend's energy had a certain driven quality. He wanted to be up-to-date in sex and politics and was eager not to miss any experiences "the others" were having. When asked to comment on six possible "paths of life," his response to one possibility was that "enjoyment *is* hectic; not warm and comfortable—one has got to be hurried; driving ambition is good." Indeed, Friend commented that he was one of the more ambitious students at Walden.[54] But ambition is not necessarily a negative quality. As Riesman put it, Friend was "going places."

Riesman also emphasized Friend's maturity. He had as evidence Friend's self-assessment at age twelve, in which he had examined himself; he had been reflec-tive and frank, Riesman found. Friend's political knowledge and leadership and the "consistency with which he support[ed] his position" were also impressive. Riesman noted that "the maturity of his language which is so much greater than many [and] his occasional flashes of insight go far beyond the norm of even very gifted and venture-some adolescents."[55]

Riesman pondered what the future held for Henry Friend. One possibility was that his extremism, activity, and spontaneity, which worked for him at the present, might not outlast his student days. "His credo which today adds piquancy to his relationships with parents and teachers will, if he clings to it as an adult, alienate him from all but a few extremists. Having…a tendency to ruthlessness, he might harden still more, and his charm failing become still more ruthless in a vicious circle." Or "Friend may continue to live in situations which are stabilizing for him, situations where his views and behavior receive attention and approval….In his energies and gifts Henry Friend has more to offer than most."[56] Riesman's second scenario turned out to be more correct than his first one, although one or two elements from the first remained. Much of his positive predictions were quite prescient.

One thing up to this point seems certain: Walden School had provided nurturance for Spitzer and his sister, Louise Albert, who also attended the school. At age fifteen, when asked, Spitzer agreeably found his school to be a democratic institution.[57] Albert recollected it as a "wonderful" place where the two Spitzer children had an "emotional home." Other children were glad when the summer came and they got out of school. With Spitzer and Albert it was the opposite. They were unhappy when the summer came and glad when school started again.[58]

Spitzer had an additional source of emotional sustenance when he was in high school. He recalls: "Someone [sic] who psychologically was very important to me were actually two brothers, Cuban brothers, who taught me classical guitar when I was fifteen. That was very important to me because I was not close to my father and these two guys, I had lessons twice a week for several years. That meant a tremendous amount to me emotionally. I used to often eat there, wonderful Cuban food."[59]

COLLEGE, MEDICAL SCHOOL, RESIDENCY, AND PSYCHOANALYTIC TRAINING

Robert Spitzer graduated from the Walden School in 1949 and went to Cornell University in Ithaca, New York, the same university from which his older sister had graduated. He was premed with a major in psychology and was inducted into the National Psychology Honorary Society and the National Premedical Honorary Society. He graduated from Cornell with honors in 1953. In his sophomore year, Spitzer married a fellow student at Cornell. Early marriages among college students were not at all unusual in the 1950s.

In his senior year, a remarkable incident occurred. Its inception had actually been a few years earlier when Spitzer began to believe that his therapy with the Reichian analyst, Robert Kronomeyer, was not helping him. Gradually, he began to question Reichian therapy and Reich's claims about orgone energy and the orgone accumulator, which Spitzer asserted he had sat in "a bit" during college.[60] Reich had argued that not only was orgone energy good for neurotic problems but it could also cure cancer and explain phenomena such as the origin of life. At the start of his last year at Cornell, Spitzer devised eight experiments to study Reich's claims about the existence of orgone energy, which Reich had presented in his book, *The Cancer Biopathy*.[61] For some of the experiments, Spitzer enlisted other students to serve as subjects. Other experiments he carried out by himself. After testing Reich's claims, Spitzer concluded "that careful examination of the data in no way proves or even hints at the existence of orgone energy." Never one to hide his light under a bushel, the young scientist sent off his paper to the *American Journal of Psychiatry*, which promptly rejected it.[62]

This was not the end of the episode, however. One day, before he had graduated, Spitzer was visited by someone from the Food and Drug Administration (FDA), who explained that the agency was attempting to stop Reich from distributing orgone accumulators. The agency had gotten Spitzer's name from the American Psychiatric Association—which publishes the *American Journal of Psychiatry*—because the FDA was looking for an expert witness to testify against Reich, and Spitzer seemed to meet their criteria. A year and a half later, the FDA filed for an injunction to prevent Reich from distributing orgone accumulators through interstate commerce for treating or preventing diseases. Reich refused to be judged by a court on the grounds that he was a scientist and a court could not make a scientific determination. He refused to appear and was jailed for contempt, so Spitzer was never called to testify. Reich, who in his early years had been an important psychoanalyst, came to a sad end. Embittered and psychotic, he died in prison of a heart attack a year later.

After graduating from Cornell, Spitzer returned to New York City for his medical training at the New York University School of Medicine (NYU). While there, he, with co-authors, published three papers in the *American Journal of Pediatrics*, one of which challenged the work of a very well-known child psychiatrist at NYU, Lauretta Bender (1897–1987). Bender posited that childhood schizophrenia could be caused partially by the failure of the nervous system to develop. This failure, she argued, could be demonstrated in schizophrenic children by a "primitive reflex," so that if one twisted their heads slightly the children would keep on turning, all the way around. It occurred to Spitzer to try the same maneuver with normal children and, to his delight, they did the same thing. Here was the opportunity for another paper. Unfazed by the fact that Bender was on the faculty of the Department of Psychiatry at his medical school, Spitzer openly disputed her conclusion.[63] Later on, when Spitzer applied for residency training at the Columbia Department of Psychiatry, the chairman of the department there, Lawrence Kolb, was impressed by the fact that he had written a paper in medical school. At NYU, Spitzer became a member of Alpha Omega Alpha, the prestigious National Medical Honorary Society, and upon graduation in 1957 received the Bernard Wortis Prize for Excellence in Psychiatry, Medicine, and Neurology.

Spitzer took an internship at Montefiore Hospital in the Bronx in 1957–1958. He had wanted this internship specifically because it had a six-week elective that could be done anywhere. He chose to spend his elective rotation at the New York State Psychiatric Institute (Columbia) and was assigned to a biological unit that was testing the effects of LSD. Spitzer himself took some. In the 1950s, Spitzer recalls, "there was no [such thing as] 'informed consent,' we just did it. It was a very interesting experience." While an intern, Spitzer interviewed for psychiatric residencies, one of which was at Columbia, where he was accepted.

On the personal side, Spitzer remembers one specific moment of this interview because Lawrence Kolb asked him how his marriage was going, and he said "fine." One month later he and his wife of six years separated; there were no children. Shortly thereafter, he married a physician, who also went on to become a psychiatrist, and the couple had two children.

Spitzer began his residency in 1958 and, wasting no time, conducted an experiment on the effects of monosodium glutamate (MSG) on elderly psychotic men living in a state hospital. Again, like at NYU, he attacked the presumed wisdom of past studies. This time Spitzer challenged a series of experiments that had shown MSG to be helpful to their subjects. In Spitzer's study, the patients had not benefitted at all. This time the *American Journal of Psychiatry* published his paper.[64] Spitzer's goals upon entering his residency were to combine seeing patients and doing research. In the latter sphere he was interested in the problem of how to evaluate treatment. "That was what really turned me on," he later recounted.[65] Since early life, carrying out measurements had been an interest of his.

In Spitzer's second year of residency, he began psychoanalytic training at the Columbia Psychoanalytic Institute. Psychoanalytic training in the late 1950s was the path to pursue if a psychiatrist wanted to be where the action was. Many of the psychiatrists whose stories we will follow were in psychoanalytic training mainly for that reason. Spitzer immediately had an important decision to make: Whom should he choose to be his training analyst? He decided that if he was going to be able to truly understand himself and have his analysis help him, he had to have a very experienced analyst. So he chose Abram Kardiner (1891–1981) who was an anthropologist as well as a psychoanalyst and was well known for having applied Freudian theory to anthropology. In 1959, Kardiner was 68 years old. He had been analyzed by Freud, but came to believe that Freud's model of the psyche was too ethnocentric and so had developed a form of psychoanalysis that he believed could be used in various cultures.

As it turned out, Kardiner was a "classical" analyst, one of whose characteristics was to sit quietly behind the analysand and say very little. Sitting behind the patient was likely a carryover from Freud's earliest days when he sat behind patients while hypnotizing them, often pressing their foreheads and urging them to remember events he said they were blocking from consciousness. But this physical relationship, leaving the analyst unobservable, had achieved a later theoretical justification. The analyst's being out of sight and his or her silence were said by analysts to be necessary for the treatment. The justification ran as follows: A central path to a successful analysis lay in analyzing the transference. The analysand would project onto the silent and invisible analyst all the thoughts and feelings the analysand had about significant figures in his or her past. Then the analyst could point to the existence of these feelings as dominating the patient's present-day relationships, usually to his or her detriment. The transference could best occur and be explained if the analyst remained an unknown figure.[66] However, Spitzer grew increasingly uncomfortable with Kardiner's continual silence and, after a few months at most, switched analysts.[67] "Also," Spitzer adds, "I think I was having trouble with some analytic supervisors, so that was another reason I thought I ought to switch."[68]

The man Spitzer picked to replace Kardiner was Arnold M. Cooper (1923–2011). At that time Cooper was one of psychoanalysis's rising stars. He had been supervising Spitzer on a case, and Spitzer was "enthralled" with him.[69] "I realized that his approach to treating patients and understanding patients was totally different from everybody else," Spitzer later related. Cooper was influenced by Edmund Bergler (1899–1962), a Viennese psychoanalyst who had fled to the United States. "Bergler," explains Spitzer, "had this idea that there is really one neurosis—psychic masochism—and it had the answer to everything. And I liked a system that had the answer to everything, but then I moved on. So, that worked for a few years. I thought that explained everything. . . . So, I read Bergler most of the time that I was in analysis with Cooper. The theory behind it was Bergler's stuff. It didn't work, but it had a big influence on me at the time."[70] Cooper himself went on to establish an outstanding reputation with his work on the interrelationship of narcissism and masochism.

At Columbia, Spitzer also found himself drawn to Willard Gaylin (b. 1925), another training and supervising analyst. He had no official relationship with Gaylin but found him to be a friendly faculty member, "quite nice . . . very cordial."[71] Gaylin was interested in fields that spilled over from psychiatry into other disciplines, such as law and theology. He was soon to cofound The Hastings Center, a bioethics research institute for examining ethical issues relating to health, medicine, and the environment. Gaylin has received near-universal acclimation for his writing, teaching, and lecturing.

But in spite of positive connections, Spitzer's career as a neophyte-analyst was not fulfilling. About these years at the Columbia Psychoanalytic Institute he has said, "I was always unsure that I was being helpful, and I was uncomfortable listening and empathizing." Basically, he concludes, "I just didn't know what the hell to do."[72] We will see that the discomfort in empathizing did not stop here and would play a role as Spitzer's career unfolded. Also, he had become disenchanted with his own analysis.[73] Still, his professional training was moving along on schedule. In 1961 he finished his psychiatry residency, and in 1966 he graduated from the Psychoanalytic Institute, though just "barely."[74] "I ran into some difficulties there," he says, "so they were not too happy with me, but I graduated."[75] In the midst of so much else, wanting greater computer literacy, he also took courses in the Data Processing Division of IBM in data processing, general computer programming, and the computer languages, FORTRAN II and IV, which opened up for him the world of algorithms. As a result, Spitzer's technical skills were strong.

ENTERING PROFESSIONAL LIFE

Upon finishing his residency, Spitzer went to work at the New York State Psychiatric Institute (PI), affiliated with Columbia University, beginning a life-long connection from which he never moved and did not retire until 2010. He became an instructor in psychiatry and a research fellow in the Biometrics Unit under a psychologist, Joseph Zubin (1900–1990),[76] who played a "critical" role in Spitzer's career. Zubin had "a department which encouraged me to do the kind of work I did," Spitzer has declared. Zubin "created [for me] an atmosphere. Also he had the motto, kind of, in his department [that] anything that is worth studying has to be quantitative. If you can't count it or measure it, we are not interested. . . . In other words, [there should be] an attempt to systematize, make subjective things objective."[77] Clearly this is a key statement as one views Spitzer's lifework in perspective. In Zubin's department Spitzer turned to devising rating scales and standardized interview schedules, subjects that also suited him temperamentally.[78] Zubin helped bring Spitzer into the research community, introducing him at the annual meetings of the American Psychopathological Association (APPA) and the American College of Neuropsychopathology (ACNP). Spitzer sums up: "They are both kind of the elite in psychiatric research [so] that was very important."

At PI, Spitzer embarked on fulfilling his goals: doing research and seeing patients. In the 1960s, together with others, he developed instruments for the evaluation of patients—the Mental Status Schedule, the Psychiatric Evaluation Form—and proposed a path to measure change in psychotherapy.[79] He began to receive grants and to publish regularly and then prolifically. (Over the years, Spitzer has found he often does his best work when he writes together with a colleague. He says they start with the title and then compose the rest.) In the 1960s and early 1970s, together with Jean Endicott, a research psychologist also at PI, he devised DIAGNO, a computer program for psychiatric diagnosis, and began to evaluate the automation of psychiatric case records.[80] He climbed the academic ladder and received research promotions. He taught in the psychiatry department and analyzed patients. An outsider might look with admiration on this busy and seemingly successful academic psychiatrist and clinician. Yet Spitzer did not feel he had a satisfying career, nor did he believe he was making a distinctive contribution. Clearly, this must be seen in the light of his self-professed ambitious drives.

Still, academic life had its perks. Lunch at PI, for example, could be a leisurely break when people from various units within the department discussed their work while eating in a pleasant dining room replete with table linen and waitresses. In this atmosphere Spitzer made friends. At one lunchtime a senior colleague said, "Bob, I'm chairing this DSM-II committee and we're almost finished [but] I need somebody to take notes, do a little editing. Would you be interested?" Spitzer asked if there was any kind of remuneration. The answer was "no." Spitzer quickly decided that that was not important and joined the committee. The chair of the DSM-II committee (officially the Committee on Nomenclature and Statistics of the American Psychiatric Association) was Ernest Gruenberg (1915–1991), a psychiatrist and epidemiologist.[81]

DSM-II appeared in May 1968 and was reprinted in October 1968, this time with a guide for using the new nomenclature that Spitzer co-authored.[82] There had been no such guide in DSM-I, but it was Spitzer's style to be innovative and expansive where he deemed necessary. Gruenberg thanked him in the foreword for his important contributions "to the articulation of Committee consensus as it proceeded from one draft formulation to the next."

But DSM II did not attract much interest. While there was some new language and emphases in it that distinguished it from its predecessor, fundamentally it was little different from DSM-I (1952). And even though DSM-II supported a psychoanalytic viewpoint, it was given hardly any attention by the analysts themselves, who did not care much about diagnosis because, as they saw it, all neurosis was caused by remarkably similar unconscious conflicts. Recall that just five years earlier the analyst Karl

Menninger had written: "There is only one class of mental illness—namely mental illness. [Therefore] current nosologies and diagnostic nomenclature are not only useless but restrictive and obstructive."[83]

Spitzer remained on the APA Committee on Nomenclature and Statistics, and it was partly in connection with this position that he became involved with the crisis over the existence of the diagnosis of homosexuality in DSM-II. Thus, even before becoming involved with DSM-III, he began to think about diagnosis and the definition of a mental disorder.

Spitzer's role in brokering a solution to the challenging circumstances created by gay activism against the APA thrust Spitzer into the limelight before the Association's leadership. He defused an issue that had been a source of great challenge to Establishment psychiatry in the heyday of the antipsychiatry and civil rights movements in the early 1970s (see Chapter 1). Moreover, it must be noted that the situation was dealt with throughout in a characteristic "Spitzerian" style of decisiveness and thoroughness.

CHAIR OF THE DSM-III TASK FORCE

Spitzer's membership on the Committee for Nomenclature made him sensitive to the whole matter of classification, and he became aware that the current World Health Organization's (WHO) International Classification of Diseases, ICD-8, was being revised. That meant the DSM, according to an international treaty that the United States had signed, needed to be updated to be compatible with ICD-9, due out in 1979. The APA Board of Trustees was aware of this and even before Spitzer was chosen to lead the revision, they had decided that this as well as other situations called for a new DSM. Becoming head of the Task Force to create a new DSM appealed to Spitzer, and he had backing in the APA.[85] There was no competition for the job because no one paid much attention to the DSM. Past statistical and diagnostic manuals had existed primarily to document numbers, diseases, and deaths of state hospital patients, but American psychiatry was now at a time when state hospital psychiatry was a relatively small part of the field as a whole. Yet Spitzer wanted the job. He was at loose ends. One aspect of his career was at a standstill; he had become disappointed with his own analysis and frustrated with doing psychoanalyses, as we have seen. He recalls, "I learned that ICD-9 was being developed so it occurred to me this was an opportunity for DSM-III. So, I spoke to Mel Sabshin, who was the medical director at the APA and I said: 'With this ICD-9 coming out, we ought to have a DSM-III, and I would love to head that thing.'"[86]

A subsidiary element to the story of the APA's decision to produce a revised DSM is the testimony of a psychologist, Theodore Millon (b. 1928), who later served on the DSM-III Task Force. Millon has asserted that he played a role in getting the APA to authorize work on a "forward-seeking, contextually oriented and empirically-grounded DSM-III."[87] In 1971, he occupied a position as head psychologist at the Neuropsychiatric Institute (NPI) of the University of Illinois Medical Center. His chief was the psychiatrist

Melvin Sabshin (1925–2011), who was then also chair of the particular APA Council that oversaw the Task Force on Nomenclature and Statistics. Millon has written that he sent a memorandum to his chief in his—Sabshin's—role as the chair of that APA Council, urging him "to bring fresh perspectives to our archaic taxonomy [since there had been a] total lack of creative innovation in the DSM-II." Millon suggested that Sabshin form a committee "to review research data and coordinate theoretical proposals for the next DSM."[88] Sabshin did appoint an ad hoc committee to evaluate models of classification, especially since the update of WHO's ICD was expected soon, but no policy decisions were ever made. Then, in 1974, when Sabshin became Medical Director of the APA, Millon recalls that he again urged Sabshin to re-evaluate the APA's official classification and to schedule a meeting that would ensure the updating of a new DSM. (As we shall see, Sabshin needed little prompting since his stated goal as the new Medical Director was to take steps to move psychiatry away from "ideologies" and make it more "scientific.") As Millon recollects, he, Sabshin, and Robert Spitzer met and agreed that "new blood was needed in the Task Force" and decided to ask the incoming president of the APA to appoint "a substantially reconstituted Task Force," which indeed was carried out.[89]

However, Donald Klein, a psychiatrist who served at PI with Spitzer and also became a member of the DSM-III Task Force, stresses Spitzer's version of events: "When Bob was appointed to the DSM-III, the job was of no consequence. In fact, one of the reasons Bob got the job was that it wasn't considered that important. The vast majority of psychiatrists, or for that matter the APA, didn't expect anything to come from it." The psychoanalysts certainly didn't use the DSM—this was the day before health insurance companies demanded DSM diagnoses—and couldn't see any value in mere description. Klein adds: "Psychoanalysts dismiss symptoms as being unimportant, and they say that the real thing is the internal conflicts. So to be interested in descriptive diagnosis was to be superficial and a little bit stupid."[90]

Thus, Spitzer's interest in taking on the job of shepherding the next DSM was welcomed by officials at the APA—except there was a problem. The Task Force that would undertake the revisions—the Committee on Nomenclature and Statistics—already had a chairman, Henry Brill (1907–1990), a distinguished state hospital psychiatrist and administrator, and the APA had no intention of dismissing him. But now there occurred a *deus ex machina*: Brill resigned, and Spitzer was appointed the new chair and hence the leader of the Task Force on DSM-III (Fig. 4.1). Spitzer has said: "It was a job that I asked for. They didn't come and say, gee, we need somebody for DSM-III. Maybe Bob Spitzer will do it. That was not the way it happened."[91] Today, the job of head of the Task Force to revise a DSM is highly sought after, which is a measure of what the DSM became under Spitzer's leadership. The present Chair and Vice-Chair of the DSM-5 Task Force, David Kupfer and Darrell Regier, respectively, even have high visibility among the general public. Spitzer adds an important recollection: The Wash. U. people "were delighted that I got the job because [they] were totally outside of the mainstream. They were just absolutely delighted that I...was getting to use the diagnostic criteria."[92]

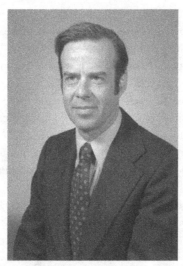

FIG. 4.1 Robert L. Spitzer, 1978, 46 years of age, head of the DSM-III Task Force. Courtesy New York State Psychiatric Institute.

The first thing Spitzer did was to begin appointing people to the Task Force. He was in a good position to do this because no one was paying attention. As he tells it, it was "totally under my control. I didn't have to clear it with anybody. So about half of them, you would say would be neo-Kraepelinian."[93] Another thing he kept in mind was the work that had been coming out of St. Louis. Recall that after he met Eli Robins at the NIMH conference, he and Jean Endicott, the research psychologist at PI, went to St. Louis to soak in the knowledge coming out of Washington University. Spitzer became very interested in Robins' and Guze's proposal on how to establish diagnostic validity in psychiatric illness and was fascinated by the idea of employing diagnostic criteria to establish reliability in psychiatric illness, as Feighner et al. had attempted.[94] He was for a time also intrigued by the Wash. U. position that "there were [only] 16 [diagnoses] that were valid, so as far as they were concerned, almost all of DSM-II was a lot of nonsense."[95] Spitzer was absorbing it all intently.

THE RESEARCH DIAGNOSTIC CRITERIA AS GATEWAY TO DSM-III

As Spitzer began work on the new manual, he was simultaneously engaged in a related project. Actually, he had begun this project even before he was appointed head of the DSM-III Task Force. The Clinical Branch of the NIMH had suggested to Spitzer and Robins that they work together to enlarge the Feighner criteria of 1972 and produce a document that researchers would find useful in their studies. The two men assented to the plan, and Spitzer turned to this enterprise with great enthusiasm, bringing Jean Endicott into the venture. It received the name "Research Diagnostic Criteria" (RDC). While it had a life of its own precisely for the audience for which it was designed, it became in Spitzer's hands the prelude to DSM-III. When he began leading the construction of DSM-III in 1974, he brought over much that had already been formulated for the RDC. In Chapter 7 we will investigate the relationship between the RDC and DSM-III in some detail because of the significant overlap of the NIMH project with the APA's revision of DSM-II. Moreover, when Spitzer started to publicize his work on DSM-III, he was often drawing on what had been accomplished in the RDC.

THE PASSIONATE EMBRACE OF DSM-III

As Spitzer worked on the RDC, he quickly exercised his leadership as Chair of the Committee on Nomenclature and Statistics. In addition to the Task Force being filled with research-oriented people, he eventually created fourteen advisory committees, each dedicated to a different group of psychiatric disorders, for example, the Advisory Committee on Organic Mental Disorders or Advisory Committee on Substance Abuse Disorders. He appointed himself to eleven of the committees so he could take an active part in the work of each one. The only three committees he did not sit on were Infancy, Childhood, and Adolescent Disorders; Eating Disorders; and Psychosomatic Disorders. A full discussion of the people who were appointed to the Task Force and advisory groups will appear in Chapter 5.

Spitzer became a man possessed. "I mean, I was married, I had kids, but I was working, you know, 12, 16 hours a day," he has said. He would awaken his wife at night, asking for her opinion on a point. He answered every letter the committee received, no matter how trivial the issue. He responded to every critical article about DSM-III no matter how obscure the journal in which it had appeared. Sometimes he even telephoned in response to a letter.[96] Jean Endicott, the psychologist who worked closely with him for many years, remembers, "He would come in on Mondays having clearly worked on [the DSM revision] all weekend....If you sat by him on the plane going to a meeting, there was no question what you were going to be talking about."[97] His intense focus was not always appreciated. "He was famous for walking down a crowded hallway and not looking left or right or saying anything to anyone," another colleague remembers. "He would never say hello. You could stand right next to him and be talking to him and he wouldn't even hear you. He didn't seem to recognize that anyone was there."[98]

But Spitzer's work compulsion was more than that. It was linked to more general personality traits. "Despite [his] genius at describing the particulars of emotional behavior, he didn't seem to grasp other people very well....He got very involved with issues, with ideas, and with questions. At times he was unaware of how people were responding to him or to the issue," Endicott explains. "He was surprised when he learned that someone was annoyed. He'd say, 'Why was he annoyed? What did I do?'" Eventually Spitzer came to confront this aspect of his persona, one he says he still wrestles with. He told Alix Spiegel, "I find it hard to give presents....I never know what to give. A lot of people, they can see something and say, 'Oh, that person would like that.' But that just doesn't happen to me."[99] When interviewing Spitzer, I experienced this first-hand. When asked to describe the personalities of some people he worked with, he struggled with this and then said he couldn't, and that he knew that was odd because this is what a psychiatrist is supposed to be able to do.[100] Today, Spitzer has reached the point where he can make jokes about this personality characteristic. When giving Grand Rounds at PI in 2006, his talk was entitled "DSM and Psychiatric Institute: A (Very) Personal History." Why "Personal," he asked the audience and then answered his own question: Janet, his wife, had advised, "[Since] some people don't think you're very human...if there are a lot of personal things, you'll come off better." The audience laughed.[101]

Working on the manual seventy, eighty hours a week, Spitzer began to neglect his family and eventually fell in love with the woman he had hired as a text editor, Janet Williams, a social worker (Figs. 4.2 and 4.3, Pictorial Essay). He and his wife separated in 1979, and he married Williams several years later (Fig. 4.4, Pictorial Essay). He has two children, a son and a daughter, by his second marriage, and he and Williams have three sons (Fig. 4.5, Pictorial Essay). Williams went on to become Project Coordinator for the NIMH field trials of DSM-III and to receive a doctoral degree in social work. She was on the faculty of the psychiatry department at Columbia and worked at PI for many years.

PICTORIAL ESSAY

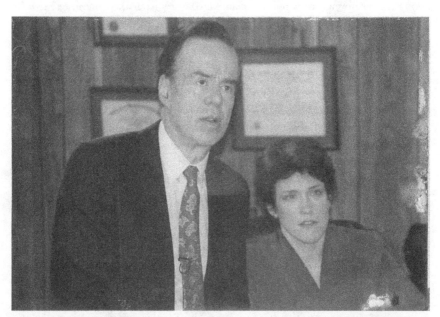

FIG. 4.2 Robert Spitzer and Janet B. W. Williams at work, 1982. During the making of DSM-III, Williams became its Text Editor, Coordinator of Field Trials, and Spitzer's colleague in many other matters. Eventually, Spitzer and Williams married. Courtesy Drs. Spitzer and Williams.

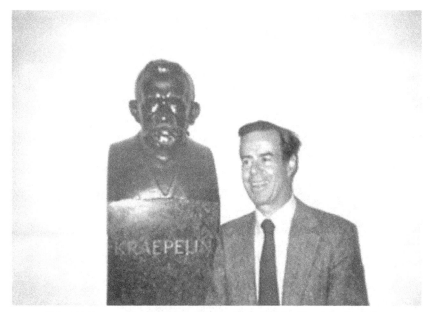

FIG. 4.3 Robert Spitzer next to a bust of Emil Kraepelin in the Max-Planck-Institute for Psychiatry in Munich. Courtesy Dr. Janet B. W. Williams.

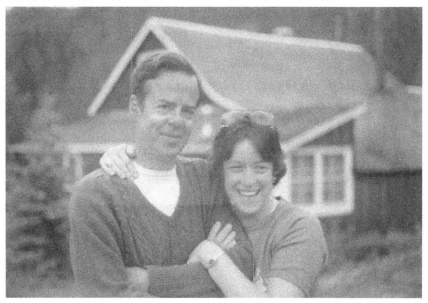

FIG. 4.4 Spitzer and Williams relaxing in Colorado the year after DSM-III was published. Courtesy Dr. Janet B. W. Williams.

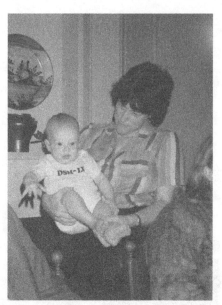

FIG. 4.5 Janet Williams and baby Noah Spitzer-Williams wearing a "DSM-IX" t-shirt, 1984. Courtesy Dr. Janet B. W. Williams.

The making of DSM-III took five years, two more than originally planned. One preliminary working document and two full drafts were circulated for opinions, and eventually field trials were held, Spitzer receiving an NIMH grant of $93,286 to conduct the trials.[102] The vicissitudes of the lengthy process of producing the revolutionary manual are addressed in Chapters 7 through 13. The APA Assembly of Delegates accepted the final version of DSM-III at a dramatic session at the annual APA meeting in May 1979, and the manual appeared in 1980. After its appearance, Spitzer and Williams were invited to speak throughout the world, which was a personally exciting time for them as they were often lionized "like rock stars," Williams says[103], and the speaking tour was also lucrative.[104] In the United States, evaluations and critiques of DSM-III poured in, stimulating journal articles, debates at professional societies, panels at APA meetings, and large conferences with published proceedings. Also available were casebooks relating to DSM-III and videos of how to conduct a diagnostic procedure according to the new manual. Though originally unanticipated, Spitzer's royalties were considerable. Within a short while, recognizing the many critiques, Spitzer decided that DSM-III needed some reworking. A revision process took place starting in 1983, and in 1987 it yielded DSM-III-R.

During the period leading up to the publication of DSM-III, Spitzer was promoted to the positions that he held until his retirement from PI in December 2010. He replaced Joseph Zubin as Chief of Psychiatric Research, Biometrics Research Department, at PI in 1976, achieving the same year the high grade of Research Scientist VIII at the New York State Department of Mental Hygiene. Three years later, Columbia University promoted him to full Professor of Psychiatry, replacing his former title of Professor of Clinical Psychiatry. His position as head of the

APA Task Force working on DSM-III earned him a place on the working committee preparing reports for the President's Commission on Mental Health in 1977. PI and Columbia University honored him in 1979 with the Van Gieson Award for Distinguished Achievements in Psychiatry. And the WHO invited him to join their Psychiatric Nomenclature Project, 1978–1980. He continued to be recognized for the work he had done on computer applications and rating scales.[105] Understandably, of course, he was now approached to write on his most recent expertise, nosology, and he submitted articles designed to acquaint readers with the Research Diagnostic Criteria (RDC), since this system was the model for the new DSM that was being worked on.[106]

Throughout the five-year gestation period of DSM-III, Spitzer found time to both edit and co-edit a number of books and to publish numerous articles.[107] He struck up a constant drum roll of articles and book chapters on the development of DSM-III and on the issues aroused by the classification of a variety of psychiatric disorders. These publications are too numerous to specify, but it is clear that he wanted the widest possible publicity about the coming DSM in order to prepare American psychiatrists for new classifications and the use of diagnostic criteria. In 1978 alone there were twelve articles or book chapters, in addition to numerous in-house drafts and memoranda, oral presentations, and letters. In one memorable letter, he vigorously protested against being labeled a neo-Kraepelinian.[108]

Furthermore, Spitzer published a closely argued rejoinder to David Rosenhan's famous *Science* article, "On Being Sane in Insane Places," which had raised the issue of whether a psychiatric diagnosis is actually the result of the environment of the patient rather than an intrinsic disorder of that individual. Rosenhan, it will be recalled, argued that sane people are only insane because they have been diagnosed as insane and not because of an inherent illness. The pseudopatients, he also argued, should have been given the diagnosis of "hallucinations," not schizophrenia.[109] He thus challenged both the reliability and validity of psychiatric diagnoses, which were, in 1973, acknowledged weaknesses of psychiatry. Spitzer went on the attack at a symposium called in order to debate the merits of Rosenhan's article, and the papers of the participants were later published in an issue of the *Journal of Abnormal Psychology*.[110] About his presentation he boasts, "The paper I am most proud of is the critique of Rosenhan's study. That is the best thing I have ever written."[111]

Spitzer criticized the logic of Rosenhan's experiment, tearing at his propositions and conclusions point by point, including arguing for the validity of the diagnosis of schizophrenia for the pseudopatients. Moreover, by the time Spitzer wrote this rejoinder, he had been thinking for some time about issues surrounding psychiatric diagnosis and could challenge Rosenhan knowledgeably. He laid out the case for the significance and usefulness of psychiatric diagnosis, although admitting that there were problems with reliability and validity. But he pointed to the positive changes that had already taken place with the Feighner criteria and the reliability already shown by using the RDC. He predicted that the next edition of the DSM would probably have similar diagnostic criteria. Rosenhan, Spitzer asserted, did not know enough about psychiatry to speak intelligently.[112]

The appearance of DSM-III did not halt Spitzer's attempt to publicize and to educate about using his new methods to diagnose psychopathology. Articles and book chapters continued to flow rapidly. After DSM-III appeared in 1980, Spitzer also devoted much time to developing and testing additional structured interviews.

At this point, let us shift our central gaze from Spitzer to the men and women he appointed to the DSM-III Task Force. The original eight members of the Task Force bonded as a group from the very start and were determined to construct an empirically based manual. As the years of developing the manual progressed, these two women and six men—with some later additions—turned out to be very influential in charting Spitzer's course on several issues and played a pivotal role in his negotiations with the psychoanalysts. Let us now meet the Task Force.

5

THE DSM-III TASK FORCE AND PSYCHIATRIC EMPIRICISM

As soon as he was appointed Chair of the APA's Committee on Nomenclature and Statistics, Spitzer began recruiting members of the Task Force that would create DSM-III. Having carte blanche to choose this committee, he assembled a small, research-oriented group, although he did ask two psychoanalysts to join, both of whom turned him down. The analysts' initial lack of interest in a diagnostic manual would cost them dearly in terms of their later problems in influencing the development of DSM-III. This issue will be specifically addressed in Chapters 11 and 13.

Some of the members of the new Task Force were stars in their fields, and there were some with strong personalities who exerted influence on the final shape of DSM-III. There was also one decided "comer," Nancy C. Andreasen (b. 1938), whose career has been meteoric since the 1970s. None of the group had a psychoanalytic orientation, and some of them took an openly anti-analytic stance. Psychoanalysis, they firmly believed, had gone "too far." It had de-emphasized diagnosis and classification, choosing instead to stress "the nature and source of intrapsychic conflicts." It had, moreover, according to Andreasen, "led to a significant de-emphasis on careful observation of signs and symptoms [teaching that] the patient's self-report of both symptoms and other internal experiences should be discounted. [Instead the analyst was expected to] dig beneath self-report to reach the real truth."[1] The evaluation of overt psychopathology had sadly dwindled, she concluded.

PHENOMENOLOGY AND PSYCHOANALYSIS

Before meeting the individual members of the Task Force, it is pertinent to spell out, albeit briefly, the differences that separated them and the psychoanalysts. The empirically minded Task Force members were phenomenologists—descriptive psychiatrists—who followed the Helmholtzians' and Kraepelin's material emphases. The psychoanalysts and psychodynamically oriented psychiatrists trod in the footsteps of the early nineteenth-century non-material Romantic psychiatrists, those who believed in "moral treatment," and later, of course, Freud. In 1974, when the Task Force began meeting, the analysts still occupied many powerful positions in American psychiatry, though an alert observer might have noticed signs of this dominance lessening.

The phenomenologists did not accept psychoanalytic explanations of mental disorders because they believed the analysts had no scientific proof—as the phenomenologists defined scientific proof—of the etiologies the analysts thought to be true. Phenomenologists believed that psychiatrists actually did not know the etiologies of many mental disorders; they argued that the first step toward knowledge was to make a diagnosis. Still, before they could even make a diagnosis, they had to gather information. In their widely cited 1970 paper on validity in psychiatric diagnosis, Eli Robins and Samuel Guze, two phenomenologists, outlined what was necessary to make a valid diagnosis and used schizophrenia as a model of how to go about it. What was needed was (1) full clinical observation; (2) laboratory studies, which they admitted they did not have; (3) delimitation from other disorders in order to obtain a homogeneous group to study; (4) family studies; and (5) follow-up studies. To achieve reliability in diagnosis, the descriptive psychiatrists argued for the use of diagnostic criteria, based on observable symptoms. Phenomenologists believed most mental disorders were sharply divided from each other and separate from normality.

Psychoanalysts and psychodynamically oriented psychiatrists looked down on what the phenomenologists believed was necessary. The analysts thought that making lists of diagnostic criteria and publishing tables of findings based purely on close observation were shallow and superficial activities and did not enable psychiatrists to treat suffering people. The analysts felt they appreciated each individual as unique and capable of being understood deeply through an exploration of that person's mind and unconscious mental processes. They believed that at the root of most psychopathology were intrapsychic conflicts. The anxiety generated by these conflicts led to various types of neurosis. To resolve the neurosis, analysts and psychodynamically oriented psychiatrists treated people with psychoanalysis and psychodynamically oriented psychotherapy.

These clinicians published numerous articles and books based on the analyses of their patients that contained theoretical discussions built on their findings. They presented clinical evidence of the many ways they had been able to bring about change in a given patient's workaday life and relationships. Sometimes a psychoanalytic article was about the psychoanalysis of just one patient and the knowledge that had been gained. When this was criticized, the analysts took the position that one case might actually be quite significant and yield important new information.[2] The analysts and psychodynamically oriented psychiatrists thus pointed to numerous successes in helping people ease their suffering and live more satisfying lives. Their field was sometimes called "depth psychology" because of the "deep" analyses they conducted over the course of several years and the seemingly profound knowledge that the patient and analyst discovered arising from lengthy examination of the patient's unconscious mind. Analysts asserted that psychopathology could be fluid and that it existed within a spectrum (on a continuum) going from seriously disordered to normal.

The phenomenonolgists were scornful of all this. A study that neatly illustrates the contempt with which many phenomenologists viewed the psychoanalysts is a 1951 paper by James J. Purtell, Eli Robins, and Mandel E. Cohen, entitled "Observations on Clinical Aspects of Hysteria: A Quantitative Study of 50 Hysteria Patients and 156 Control Subjects."[3] It is a study that gathers facts, is purposely inconclusive as to any deeper meaning at that present time, and is devoid of suggestions for therapy—exactly the kind of study that the analysts derided as empty of any real significance. It is, however, the precise, limited, observational type of study that the phenomenologists believed is the only road to knowledge. It is also a condemnation by the phenomenologists of the psychoanalysts' allegedly "nonscientific speculations." This paper has been briefly discussed in Chapter 3, but merits further attention here.

Purtell, Robins, and Cohen touted the importance of careful observation and description, which would be used to achieve their three circumscribed goals: (1) determine whether the past clinical impression of hysteria was accurate; (2) provide factual data that could be used to diagnose hysteria; and (3) "provide a sound clinical basis for further research in hysteria." Hysteria, of course, was the original disorder that Freud set out to cure, and the analysts were sure they knew what it was and how to treat it. Of what possible benefit, they thought, would be the facts from a study based on observation and recording? But in their conclusion, Purtell and colleagues rejected any legitimacy of the analysts' approach to diagnosis. (The forthright phraseology, no doubt, owed much to Mandel Cohen's predilection for bluntness.)

> Some clinicians rely on finding that the patient has a worry, problem or conflict. In our opinion this is so nonspecific that it is grossly unreliable. Other writers emphasize specific psychological "mechanisms" such as "conversion" or specific "complexes" as important in the diagnosis of hysteria. These approaches have arisen largely from limited, uncontrolled observations on isolated cases, from speculation or from attempts to apply unproved theories and are not based on facts.[4]

Thus, mutual disparagement characterized the relationship of the phenomenologists and psychoanalysts. Concrete examples of this relationship were the wars between Mandel Cohen and the psychoanalytically oriented Department of Psychiatry at Harvard, as well as the two opposing psychiatric camps in St. Louis: Eli Robins' Department of Psychiatry at Washington University and the St. Louis Psychoanalytic Institute and Society.

THE DSM-III TASK FORCE CONVENES

The original Task Force of eight members began meeting in the fall of 1974. The group consisted of five psychiatrists, two psychologists, and a specialist in biometrics. The psychiatrists were Nancy Andreasen, M.D., Ph.D., Donald F. Klein, M.D., Henry Pinsker, M.D., George Saslow, M.D., Ph.D., and Robert A. Woodruff, M.D. The psychologists were Jean Endicott, Ph.D., and Theodore Millon, Ph.D., and the biometrician was Morton Kramer, Sc.D. We will also consider briefly two later members because of the roles they played: Paula J. Clayton, M.D. and Dennis P. Cantwell, M.D., a child psychiatrist, both of whom had trained at Washington University, as had Woodruff. The Wash. U. influence in the Task Force is obvious. Saslow had been on the faculty at Washington University, and Andreasen had been a resident under Winokur at Iowa.

The night before the first meeting, they wondered what was in store for them, according to reports by Andreasen. She and Robert Woodruff found themselves talking about wanting more reliability using diagnostic criteria—what she calls the "mid-Western idea" with roots in Washington University and the University of Iowa. Yet there was a "sense of apprehension" since she and Woodruff thought of diagnostic criteria as "avant-garde." But everyone in the room the next day agreed: there should be "more objective, reliable and criterion-based diagnosing." There was a feeling, Andreasen recalls, that we were creating a "small revolution."[5]

We have from Andreasen a memorable description of that first meeting. Each individual knew in advance that they were expected to contribute large amounts of time and energy to developing a new DSM that "would help improve the rather sorry state of the diagnostic process in psychiatry," she recorded.[6]

Spitzer began the first meeting by asking each of the members to describe his or her background and what he or she was hoping to accomplish—what changes they would like to see in DSM-III. One person immediately began talking about the imprecision of diagnosis in DSM-II and his hope for more objective definitions. Another wanted the new manual to be based on research data instead of opinion. Someone proposed that all the illnesses should have specific criteria for diagnosis. One member asserted critically that DSM-II was "an embarrassment to the profession." Andreasen recalled:

> When all the members of the task force had finished speaking, they were clearly astonished at the extent to which they agreed with one another. Each had come expecting to represent a minority point of view and to argue for increased objectivity and precision. Instead, each of the members was part of a unanimous majority. The members confronted their new task with an attitude that one called "dust bowl empiricism." [Another judged that] an era of opulent theorizing was passing into history.[7]

In a mood of "joy and excitement,"[8] there was a universal consensus that DSM-II should be totally revised, and that DSM-III "should be evidence based, use diagnostic criteria instead of general descriptions [like DSM-II had], and strive for maximal reliability."[9] This would mean returning to the scientific method "to know...about the world through observation, testing, and empirical truth," Andreasen has written. She noted that Philippe Pinel (1745–1826), one of the founders of modern psychiatry had written of his resolution

> to notice successively every fact, without any other object than that of collecting materials for future use; and to endeavor, as far as possible, to divest myself of the influence, both of my own prepossessions and the authority of others.[10]

In this spirit, the Task Force now articulated a group of "lofty goals:" to improve communication between clinicians; to provide reliable diagnoses that would be useful in research; to train psychiatry students in differential diagnosis; and to realign American psychiatry with that of Great Britain and Europe and with ICD-9—the World Health Organization's (WHO) International Classification of Diseases.

And so they set to work, a "small and close-knit group."[11] Five of them are still alive: the psychiatrists Nancy Andreasen, Donald Klein, and Henry Pinsker and the psychologists Jean Endicott and Theodore Millon. Ten more appointments to the Task Force were made over the next few years of the life of the panel. Two years after the original Task Force had begun meeting it had increased to fifteen members, eleven of whom were psychiatrists.[12] The central place for Task Force meetings was in New York City at the New York State Psychiatric Institute at West 168th Street in the Columbia University medical complex. Occasionally, the group might meet in another city. Sometimes Task Force meetings were called for two or three days at a time. Those not in the New York area—Andreasen, Kramer, Millon, Saslow, and Woodruff—nevertheless traveled long distances to attend these meetings, leaving their usual work, with no payment, except that the APA covered their air travel, room, and meals.[13] Spitzer also received no remuneration from the APA, drawing only his usual salary from PI. After the first year, the full Task Force did not meet frequently. A lot of work was done via phone calls and memorandums.

As work proceeded in the early years, a small core group in the Task Force became the main shapers of the new manual, along with Spitzer.[14] This group included Jean Endicott, Donald Klein, Nancy Andreasen, and Robert Woodruff, joined later by the child psychiatrist Dennis Cantwell. They were a "bunch of idealists," remembers Andreasen.[15] They often clustered around Spitzer, all of them talking as he banged out text on his typewriter. There were no computers, and revisions were made by manual cutting and pasting.[16] Millon and Pinsker also took part, but to a lesser extent. The least influential members were Saslow and Kramer.

The Advisory Committees, or even small subsections of each of the committees, did the actual writing of most of the manual. Spitzer was a member of many of the committees, and from time to time was involved in writing specific parts of the manual. Occasionally, Spitzer would choose someone whom he wanted to work with for a particular portion, and the two of them would compose it together. There were occasions when Spitzer very much wanted the input of a particular specialist who was not on an Advisory Committee, usually someone who was in a different city. Spitzer launched a correspondence requesting information, to which some experts responded readily and others only grudgingly. In the latter situation, Spitzer kept writing letters anyway, pushing for a reply in his determined attempt to solve a particular conundrum. Sometimes, Spitzer would write up the diagnostic description on his own, but this was rare. The Task Force was the ultimate arbiter where there was conflict or disagreement.

The original group met often over the first year of its existence and by the end had hammered out some basic principles from which they and Spitzer never departed.

Each disorder would be systematically and comprehensively described; each would have its group of diagnostic criteria, there would be a multiaxial format that would put psychotic and affective disorders on Axis I and personality disorders on Axis II; and in mid-course of the DSM revision there would be extensive and formal field trials. Spitzer received a special grant from the NIMH to cover the costs of some of the field trials. The Task Force and Spitzer were also committed to a policy of "syndromal inclusiveness," so that the DSM would incorporate all conditions that clinicians were called on to deal with.[17] A joke made the rounds that Spitzer had proclaimed, "I never saw a diagnosis that I didn't like."

Of course, inclusiveness works against validity. Recall that the Wash. U. psychiatrists were very limited in their naming of diagnoses because they believed that, beyond several unambiguous diagnoses, they could not assure validity, psychiatry lacking the necessary diagnostic tools. They preferred in doubtful situations to give a label of "psychiatric disorder without diagnosis." Robins and Guze's 1970 paper on how to achieve psychiatric validity became a classic. We will see, therefore, that there were times when the Wash. U. people objected to the inclusiveness.

Now let us turn to the professional lives of the original DSM-III Task Force. All of them had decidedly significant, some even high-powered, careers.

PICTORIAL ESSAY

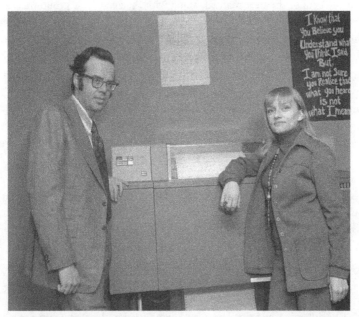

FIG. 5.1   Robert Spitzer and Jean Endicott, a research psychologist, were close colleagues on the DSM-III Task Force and collaborated on numerous research projects and publications for many years. Here, they are in the computer room at the New York State Psychiatric Institute in 1974. Courtesy of New York State Psychiatric Institute.

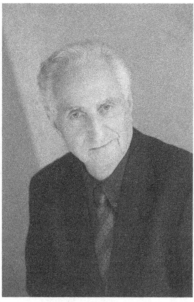

FIG. 5.2 Donald F. Klein in a recent photograph. Klein, a biological psychiatrist, was a very influential member of the DSM-III Task Force, Spitzer's close colleague, and clearly antipsychoanalytic in his views. Klein has made important contributions to the field of psychopharmacology. Courtesy of Child Mind Institute, New York, NY.

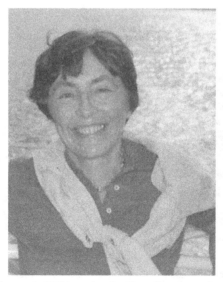

FIG. 5.3 Nancy C. Andreasen in 1978 in a relaxed setting after a research meeting. Simultaneous to and sometimes informing the creation of the DSM-III was the NIMH Collaborative Study of the Psychobiology of Depression. Spitzer, Jean Endicott, Andreasen, and psychiatrists from Washington University were all involved in the study. At their meetings, the group often held informal parties. Courtesy Dr. Nancy C. Andreasen.

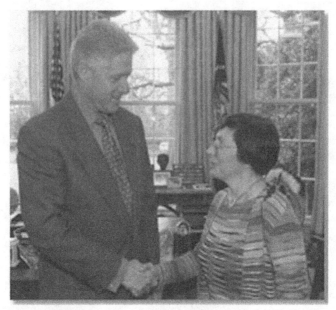

FIG. 5.4   Nancy C. Andreasen receiving the National Medal of Science from President Bill Clinton in 2000. After serving on the DSM-III Task Force, Andreasen went on to have an illustrious career as an expert in the fields of both schizophrenia and creativity. She was Editor-in-Chief of the *American Journal of Psychiatry* for 13 years. Courtesy Dr. Nancy C. Andreasen.

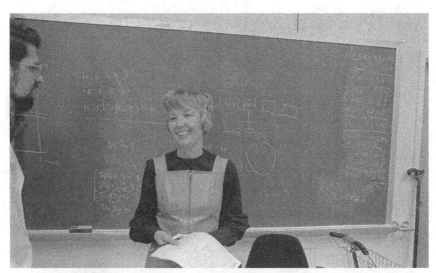

FIG. 5.5   Paula J. Clayton, 1974, DSM-III Task Force member who replaced Robert Woodruff, in front of genetics diagrams at Washington University with Robert Cloninger, at left. Eli Robins' motorized chair and cane can be seen in lower right. In 1980, Clayton became the first woman chair of a department of psychiatry in the United States. From Washington University Libraries, Department of Special Collections.

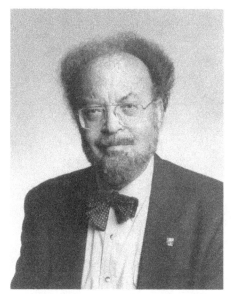

FIG. 5.6   Theodore Millon in 1978, a psychologist on the original DSM-III Task Force, and a specialist in psychopathology and personality disorders. He has had a prolific career in creating psychological assessment instruments. Courtesy Dr. Theodore Millon.

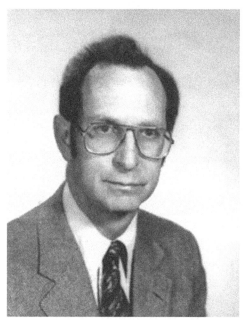

FIG. 5.7   Henry Pinsker, c. 1980. Pinsker represented the concerns of the clinician on the Task Force. He was also a teacher and administrator and had an interest in the diagnosis of psychopathology, especially that of hospitalized patients. His diagnostic interests were not shared by his psychodynamically oriented colleagues dominant in the 1960s and 1970s. Courtesy Dr. Henry Pinsker.

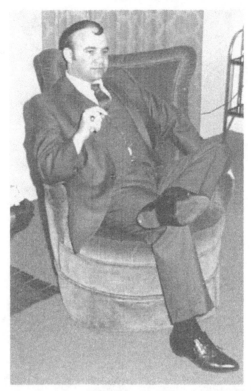

FIG. 5.8   Dennis P. Cantwell, c. 1972. Although Cantwell (1939–1997) was not one of the original eight members of the DSM-III Task Force, after he joined it he was very active. He had been both a medical student and resident in psychiatry at Washington University. In 1972, he joined the faculty of the UCLA Neuropsychiatric Institute, where he had a brilliant career until his untimely death from chronic heart disease at age 58. Courtesy Dr. Susan Cantwell-Selby.

JEAN ENDICOTT

One of the first recruits was Jean Endicott (b. 1936), who was Spitzer's research and writing partner for many years (Fig. 5.1, Pictorial Essay). There are some notable working relationships in the making of DSM-III, and the Spitzer-Endicott coupling is one. They were a "dream team," synchronous in their interests and ways of thinking. Endicott is a research psychologist with a specialty in psychometrics and an impressive record of publications and honors. Theodore Millon, the other psychologist on the Task Force, called her "a conceptualizer and research implementer of the first rank."[18]

Endicott was doing her psychology internship at PI the year after Spitzer had completed his residency, and they met at a party at the home of a mutual friend. Spitzer inquired as to her plans after graduation, and Endicott replied that she wanted to do full-time research, not have a clinical practice. When Spitzer learned the details of the kind of work Endicott wanted to do, he told her he had a new grant and invited her to meet with him so he could tell her about his project and see if she might have a role in it. As Endicott recalls, "It just fit perfectly with my background, the courses I had taken, and it was a project developing a measure for a psychiatric status schedule." She began working for Spitzer as a research assistant, but "it moved into a collegial relationship fairly quickly because I had had the courses in psychometrics, and when it came time to develop scoring systems and issues about reliability studies and validity studies, I had had some special training in that, and we both had an interest in doing whatever we could to make that a real good procedure." Endicott remained in Spitzer's department from 1964, working on a variety of projects, until 1980, the year DSM-III was published.[19]

In 1974, Spitzer appointed Endicott not only to the Task Force but also to three of the advisory groups: Schizophrenia, Paranoia, and Affective Disorders; Anxiety and Dissociative Disorders; and Multiaxial Diagnosis. The atmosphere on the Task Force pleased Endicott:

> The people on the DSM-III Task Force were all what I call DOPS—"data oriented people." What is the evidence? Has it been studied? Has anyone looked at this or looked at that? So that when we would be working on diagnostic criteria, or we would be working on what is the evidence that this is a different disorder from something else, everyone had what I would call a scholarly attitude—is there any evidence, has anyone done any studies? ... It was an intellectually stimulating learning and also [had] the feeling that this could be an important advance.[20]

Endicott went on to a distinguished research and publishing career at PI, and the width and depth of her work is remarkable. She is the author of many rating scales and has served on several editorial boards. She became an Honorary Fellow of the American Psychiatric Association and President of the American Psychosomatic Society. Endicott remains an active researcher.

DONALD KLEIN

Another early appointee to the Task Force was Donald F. Klein (b. 1928) (Fig. 5.2, Pictorial Essay), who had become interested in diagnosis in the 1960s. He and Spitzer had inevitably met at professional meetings. They found that they shared similar points of view and became friends. Spitzer appreciated his analytic mind and so appointed him to the Task Force.[21] He played an important role in shaping some decisions because of his outspokenness and directness. In the view of Allen Frances, a member of the DSM-III Personality Disorders Advisory Group (and later the head of the DSM-IV Task Force), Klein was perhaps the most influential person on the DSM-III Task Force because of his very authoritative way of speaking. Spitzer looked up to him a lot, says Frances, and his judgment was valued.[22] Spitzer and Klein shared the experience of training to be psychoanalysts and having rejected that path. Evidence of their familiar relationship is that during the time Klein was on the Task Force he and Spitzer published two books together.[23]

Everyone had strong feelings about Klein, ranging from distaste to wildly positive. In interviews those who did not like him shied away from saying anything on the record, often communicating their opinions with significant nods and looks. Those who respected him held him in high regard. Henry Pinsker belonged to this group. Elaborating, he declared that Klein was "erudite" and "impressive," speaking authoritatively on any number of subjects. After he had studied a large number of of of patients, Pinsker pointed out, Klein was able to formulate the new diagnosis of Panic Disorder. Klein, he thought, was the most creative of the Task Force members. Pinsker referred to one of Klein's recent papers as "very philosophical."[24] To see this proclivity, the reader might turn to his paper "A Proposed Definition of Mental Illness," which Klein delivered in 1977 at a meeting of the elite American Psychopathological Association (APPA), one of the organizations to which he and Spitzer belonged.[25] But not everyone viewed Klein in this way. In historical-autobiographical accounts of the DSM-III process, Theodore Millon, the other psychologist on the Task Force, quoted at length Klein's memos to show Klein's blunt and sometimes sarcastic language.[26] Nevertheless, Millon found him to be "a brilliant and inventive adversary."[27]

Klein was a psychopharmacologist who separated out Panic Disorder as a discreet diagnosis under Anxiety States. He had originally embarked on psychoanalytic training, but for an unusual reason. In college he had come across Freud and was at first taken by his focus on sex. Yet, though he found Freud very interesting, he was skeptical. "I never bought it," is how he puts it. He thought to himself he would like to test these ideas and devised the notion of becoming a research psychoanalyst. He then went to medical school, because to become a widely respected psychoanalyst in the United States—a member of the American Psychoanalytic Association—one needed an M.D. degree.[28] He was accepted to the prestigious New York Psychoanalytic Institute in 1957, but left in his fourth year, having become disillusioned with both of his training analysts. Klein locked horns with the first one over his desire to do research via drug studies on human beings, the analyst telling him this plan was a sadistic wish that would have to be worked through.[29] In regard to his second analysis, Klein did not report any one incident that finally soured him on psychoanalysis but labeled the analyst a "dishonest fool," and he stayed with him for only five months.[30]

Klein was influenced by two incidents that took place before his psychoanalytic training. In his first year of residency at Creedmoor (NY) State Hospital, in 1953, before any effective antipsychotic medication was available, he dealt with untreated psychotic patients and grew doubtful about psychoanalysis. "It was very difficult to see how it applied to these people."[31] Then, in the U.S. Public Health Service (USPHS) Hospital in Lexington, KY, in 1956, he treated some backward psychotic men—some of them mute for years—with chlorpromazine (Thorazine), and they began to speak rationally. "That was an honest to God miracle," Klein remembered. After abandoning psychoanalysis in 1961, Klein pursued a prominent research career, for many years at Hillside Hospital (Queens, NY), becoming Director of Psychiatric Research. He became Director, Department of Therapeutics at PI in 1976, while he was on the DSM-III Task Force.

As well as being on the Task Force, Klein was on three of the advisory groups: Anxiety and Dissociative Disorders, Personality Disorders, and Impulse Control Disorders. He found the meetings of the Task Force lively, with a group of Young Turks who were interested in descriptive psychiatry and wanting to get away from psychoanalysis. He recalled:

> It was a very high IQ bunch. We had a lot of interesting discussions in which we had to thrash out principles that we just hadn't faced before. Bob was very much the Chairman. He very much was sitting there with the typewriter...and worked very close with Jean Endicott. And essentially, we would bring up issues and Bob would type it down and then we would come back to it....It was a very animated discussion.[32]

NANCY ANDREASEN

Nancy C. Andreasen (b. 1938) (Fig. 5.3, Pictorial Essay) was also part of the early core group. The details of her career and accomplishments are a fascinating story. Andreasen was a rising star as early as college, where she had a triple major in English, history, and philosophy, and graduated summa cum laude. Before receiving her Ph.D. in English Renaissance literature, she was a Woodrow Wilson scholar at Harvard and a Fulbright fellow at Oxford. After receiving her doctorate, she immediately became an assistant professor and began teaching English literature. Then a life-changing event occurred. Becoming severely ill after the birth of her first child, her interest was piqued by medical illness, and she decided to go to medical school and take a residency in psychiatry. Her medical career was as meteoric as her literature career—she even combined the two at times—and she has become world-renowned as an expert in schizophrenia, neuroscience, and neuroimaging. She has also done research into the connection between creativity and mental illness. Andreasen brilliantly served three terms—13 years—as editor-in-chief of the *American Journal of Psychiatry*, the APA's main professional journal, increasing its stature greatly. She has written four books for the lay public, three of them a series on the brain, and one of them was nominated for a National Book Award.[33] In 2000, President Bill Clinton awarded her the National Medal in Science (Fig. 5.4, Pictorial Essay).[34]

Andreasen came to the Task Force with the blessing of George Winokur at Iowa, where Andreasen served her residency in psychiatry and immediately became an assistant professor. This was the year before work started on DSM-III; while on the Task Force she was promoted to associate professor. Beginning as a resident, she built up a notable record of publishing. Since she worked under Winokur, a specialist in affective disorders, some of her early research centered on mood disorders, especially those involving thought, language, and communication. Under this emphasis, she gradually began research into schizophrenia and while on the Task Force, her strengths were clearly recognized. She served on three advisory groups: Schizophrenic, Paranoid, and Affective Disorders; Reactive Disorders; and Glossary of Technical Terms, a glossary being one of Spitzer's innovations for DSM-III. Moreover, when the Task Force agreed on a new diagnosis that had become clear as a result of the Vietnam War, Post-Traumatic Stress Disorder (PTSD), Andreasen wrote the description, thus laying the foundation for the study of stress disorders that has become so significant in our own time.[35]

ROBERT WOODRUFF

Only a little can be said about Robert A. Woodruff, Jr., because he committed suicide midway in the development of DSM-III.[36] He was in his early forties, at the beginning of a very auspicious career. Woodruff was born in Michigan and attended Harvard as an undergraduate. He came to Washington University for his medical training and stayed on as a resident (he became chief resident) and then became a member of the faculty. He was attracted to the Washington University psychiatry department because of its reputation as a place of "scientific rigor" that was "quantitative and data-oriented."[37]

Woodruff was the principal investigator on a major grant to study and then follow up 500 psychiatric outpatients. He thus had access to a wide range of data that he subsequently used in articles on various subjects, although he wrote on affective disorders more than on any other topic. He therefore served on the Schizophrenic, Paranoid, and Affective Disorders Advisory Group. However, he also published papers on hysteria, ECT (electroconvulsive therapy), structured interviews, psychiatric diagnosis, and alcoholism, all of which appeared from 1967 to 1979—forty-two articles and one co-authored book in all. Eight papers alone were published in 1971. He was the lead author of the minimalist textbook *Psychiatric Diagnosis*, which was limited to twelve "valid" diagnoses. He and Eli Robins were part of the original discussions about DSM-III with Robert Spitzer and Jean Endicott, but since Robins could not travel to New York to be on the Task Force because of his MS, he appointed Woodruff in his stead. Robins' action alone speaks to Woodruff's outstanding capacities, and he became intimately involved with the development of the new manual.

Paula Clayton, a fellow medical student and resident, characterized him as a man with very broad interests, well read, intellectual, and quite charming. He was very bright, understood complex things easily, and was meticulous with his clinical duties— a person of great promise, she said. Woodruff had been having marital problems and was depressed over them; Clayton was treating him for depression.[38] But both she and Andreasen agree that when he committed suicide they, and indeed all his colleagues, were shocked—no one had thought he was anywhere near such an action.[39] [40] He had not appeared to be brooding, had not been reclusive, and his intense involvement in the revision of the manual had not slackened.[41]

PAULA CLAYTON

Woodruff's place was taken by Clayton (b. 1934) (Fig. 5.5, Pictorial Essay), his friend and colleague at Washington University. We have already met Clayton in Chapter 3, where we learned of her work in affective disorders as junior colleague to George Winokur.

Clayton was one of four women to earn a medical degree from the Washington University School of Medicine in 1960, where she also took her residency in psychiatry. In 1964, she became the chief resident, and the following year took her place on the faculty, becoming a full professor in 1974. In 1967, she and Winokur had become the first Americans to describe the separation of mood disorders into unipolar and bipolar illnesses. Clayton went on to become an expert on bereavement. It was her specialty in this area that influenced Spitzer to exclude simple bereavement from the diagnosis of major depression. This exclusion lasted through DSM-IV, but its inclusion in DSM-5 has led to considerable controversy over the issue of whether normal grief was being wrongly medicalized.

Clayton went on to have a distinguished career. In 1980, she became Chair of the Department of Psychiatry at the University of Minnesota School of Medicine, the first woman to chair a department of psychiatry in the United States and the first woman to head any department at the university's medical school. She later served as President of the American Psychopathological Association and the Society of Biological Psychiatry. After retiring from Minnesota, she became a professor of psychiatry at the New Mexico School of Medicine. Currently she is Medical Director of the American Society for Suicide Prevention.

THEODORE MILLON

Theodore Millon (Fig. 5.6, Pictorial Essay), the psychologist and an expert in personality disorders, was another early appointee.[42] Millon (b. 1928) is voluble in style and unusually prolific in publication and in designing clinical testing instruments. His "Millon Clinical Multiaxial Inventory" is only one of a host of tests and assessments he has created.[43] Henry Pinsker, who was friendly with Millon, remembered he had a lot to say. He was "an important person [who brought] a different perspective." Pinsker found him "warm [and] likable."[44] Although personality disorders were given a separate axis in DSM-III (Axis II), Millon was the only expert in this field invited to be on the Task Force. Millon also felt he represented psychology in Task Force proceedings.[45]

Millon, being strongly empirical, found psychoanalysis to have "questionable tenets and conceptual presumptions that are unsupportable by usual empirical or clinical criteria."[46] As described in Chapter 4, Millon maintains that he played a "central role" in getting the APA to authorize work on a "forward-seeking, contextually oriented and empirically-grounded DSM-III."

Millon served on the Personality Disorders Advisory Group. He saw personality disorders as arising from damaged interpersonal relationships that reflect "particular features of social and familial behavior" which influence the individual. This is based on an "external social system," which Millon says is a different construct from that of another expert in the field of personality disorders, the psychoanalyst Otto Kernberg (b. 1928). Kernberg gives primary attention to the capacity of the person's ego, an internal structure, says Millon. However, he is willing to accept that there is "a rationale for utilizing both intrapsychic and external dynamics."[47] Originally, personality disorders had been the bailiwick of psychoanalysts, but Millon stressed an empirical approach to all psychological conditions, making him quite welcome on the Task Force. He also maintained a long-standing interest in classification in psychopathology. In 1990 he introduced the Millon evolution theory, in which he attempted to ground his theories of personality styles and disorders in the wider theory of evolution.[48] Currently, Millon is Dean of the Institute for Advanced Studies in Personology and Psychopathology, with whose activities he has been involved since 1994.

Millon has written at length on the major issues with which the DSM-III Task Force had to deal and has penned an impassioned defense of the Task Force and its proceedings. In all of his several writings about the making of DSM-III, he has been one of its staunchest promoters. During the course of the Task Force's deliberations, Millon recalls, it had to contend with wild rumors and bizarre stories that swirled around them:

> Philosophical and conceptual positions were ascribed to the DSM-III Task Force as if the committee were composed of clones that rubber stamped some higher authority, rather than being a highly diverse collection of outspoken and independently thinking professionals with clearly disparate views. Troublesome also were the questionable, if not malicious, motives attributed to the committee....Little of what I heard or read corresponded to either the process of the DSM-III's evolution or the product that finally emerged.[49]

Millon insists that what materialized as DSM-III came from "a strongly shared committee consensus [owing to] the open and equalitarian spirit that prevailed in the task force's early deliberations." Millon proceeds:

> Not that there was a paucity of vigorous disagreement from both internal and external quarters or that impassioned polemics were invariably resolved, but these divergences and spirited controversies resulted in neither group discord, traditional academic schisms, nor professional power struggles....However wrongheaded or deficient the manual may be, it was, in fact, an outgrowth of scholarly debate and empirical test [sic], and not of any real or imagined ventures of psychiatric imperialism.[50]

We should note here Millon's emphasis on the "equalitarian" spirit and lack of "psychiatric imperialism." These words were written for an audience of psychologists, who often felt that psychiatrists treated them as second-class citizens. Of course, there exists a turf war between psychiatrists and psychologists. Psychologists are aware that they usually get paid less than psychiatrists for similar psychotherapeutic work. Psychiatrists insist on the importance and relevance of their medical expertise and fight legislative attempts to allow psychologists to prescribe medication. One of the central issues that engaged the Task Force was how to define mental disorders, in light of Spitzer's desires to call them a subset of medical disorders. When the American Psychological Association learned of this in 1976, it fought successfully against such a definition. Chapter 8 recounts Spitzer's battle with the Association, one of a very few he lost. The phrase "medical disorders" never found a home in DSM-III.

HENRY PINSKER

Millon became especially friendly with Henry Pinsker (b. 1928) (Fig. 5.7, Pictorial Essay), a psychiatrist with a great interest in psychopathology, especially that of the hospitalized severely ill. Before going further into the career of Pinsker, however, we should recognize that, with regard to the original eight-member Task Force, an age cohort can be found. We have seen that such a cohort existed among Robins, Guze, and Winokur. In the case of the Task Force, Millon, Pinsker, and Klein were all born in 1928, and in total, five of the original eight members were born in the decade 1928–1938—six out of nine, if we add Spitzer (born 1932). The many shared experiences of this group—all "DOPS"—and the commonality of their abundant memories of the past in general, could not but help them to bond and work well with each other, as happened with the three Wash. U. pioneers.

Pinsker, as he describes himself, was primarily a clinician, teacher, and administrator, a "user" of psychiatry, as he puts it. When teaching residents, he would direct their attention to overt behavior and its meaning, "not psychoanalytic psychotherapy." Millon calls him "a compassionate clinician whose feet are planted firmly on the ground."[51] Allen Frances, of DSM-IV fame, was an intern when Pinsker was a young attending physician and remembers Pinsker fondly as one of his first teachers, a man who was "wise, funny, and wry [and] a brilliant clinician. He could do a great five minute interview." Frances, who served with Pinsker on the Personality Disorders Advisory Group, says Pinsker was not the type of person who would exert influence directly—he was "too modest to force his opinion"—but he brought leavening and perspective to a group discussion. He was also a physician who saw things more historically than most. He read the writings of the great French psychiatrist Pierre Janet (1859–1947)—recognized today as one of the pioneers in the understanding of trauma and dissociation—before it was popular to do so. Pinsker is currently reading century-old texts on psychiatric treatment.[52]

About his fellows on the original Task Force, Pinsker says there were many "heavy weights" on the committee. With reference to himself, he self-deprecatingly says, "I'm a lightweight, not a scholar, not a researcher. I represent the clinician,"[53] even though he has published many papers and book chapters. Pinsker was also active in APA affairs. Because he was engrossed with the study of psychopathology, he was interested in diagnosis and thus unhappy with DSM-I (1952), where all disorders were labeled "reactions."[54] Spitzer was attracted by his outlook and by how Pinsker combined these views with his career as a hospital psychiatrist. In a 1967 paper, Pinsker found the then-current DSM-I at times useless for the general patient population he dealt with every day in a community-based general hospital. His words would have been music to Spitzer's ears:

> The diagnostic system we are required to use is without utility and is irrelevant to contemporary psychiatric practice....The emphasis on an underlying illness, just as much as the sometime preoccupation with the events of childhood, leads to a

loss of interest in the phenomena of mental illness and a lack of curiosity about psychopathology....A solution to the problem of inadequate and unsuitable nosology is possible within the medical tradition, by use of standardized, operational, descriptive terms.[55]

Yet Pinsker modestly maintains that he was chosen only because Spitzer did not know many people in the country, and not many people wanted to sit on the DSM-III Task Force.[56] While this claim echoes the view of Donald Klein as to why Spitzer got the job as Chair of the Task Force, it is immediately challenged by the high caliber of the researchers Spitzer was able to recruit. Actually, this point is worth a minute of contemplation. Spitzer says he got the job as chair because no one wanted it. Nonetheless, he could attract a superior group to serve under him. True, he appointed people he knew personally, and some were recommended by the Wash. U. psychiatrists. Yet did Spitzer have some charismatic qualities to win over outstanding psychiatrists and psychologists? At Walden School he had been repeatedly tagged as a leader by teachers, psychologists, and even his classmates.

Once on the Task Force, Pinsker found that he and the others were busy with a lot of material to read and comment on. About the discussions, he has only good to say: "Stimulating, intriguing, enjoyable"—with one big exception. Spitzer was absorbed with the issue of how to define "mental disorder" and spent months considering it. This made Pinsker impatient because he didn't see the need. Other physicians just treated patients without worrying about how to define a medical illness, he stated. Today, Pinsker states, general practitioners and internists, without pondering definitions, go ahead and treat erectile dysfunction. But, he asks, is that a disease?

Pinsker remains voluble about his disgruntlement with the psychodynamically oriented psychiatrists with whom he had to deal on the wards and at meetings:

> In the golden years of psychoanalytic influence, nothing mattered but understanding the patient. Discussing diagnosis at a case conference was seen as a sterile pursuit, comparable to chasing butterflies; it implied deficiency of zeal for understanding patients, and possibly lack of aptitude for the profession. Since the treatment was the same for all conditions, it didn't really matter that diagnosis was ignored. Diagnosis didn't matter [in the mental hospitals] because almost everyone was diagnosed schizophrenia (sic). When Thorazine arrived, around 1956, almost everyone got it.

Although Pinsker's views were not synchronous with his psychoanalytic surroundings, this did not retard his academic and hospital career. Before he reduced his work schedule in the 1990s, he held the rank of Professor of Clinical Psychiatry at the Mount Sinai School of Medicine (1987–1991) and Associate Director, Department of Psychiatry at the Beth Israel Medical Center in New York (1973–1992). His publications span an unusually broad variety of topics, suggesting a wide intellectual curiosity. While on the Task Force, he and Spitzer collaborated on a book chapter on the classification of mental disorders in DSM-III.[57] In recent years, Pinsker has published two books on supportive psychotherapy.[58]

GEORGE SASLOW

It is not surprising that George Saslow (1907–2006), an unusual and eminent psychiatrist and physiologist who had been at Washington University from 1943 to 1955 and had been Samuel Guze's mentor, was on the Task Force. Millon described him as "a gentleman, a scholar, and intellectual's intellectual."[59] This praise was apt because Saslow had trained in four medical fields and was a voracious reader in many areas.

Saslow had a very long and fertile career. He held a Ph.D. in physiology (NYU) and an M.D. from Harvard, and he completed residencies in neurology-neurosurgery at Boston City Hospital and in psychiatry at Worcester State Hospital (MA) and Massachusetts General Hospital (MGH). He also had a year of psychoanalysis with Hanns Sachs, one of Freud's close colleagues. Saslow reported that Sachs had told him after a year that he needed no further psychoanalysis. Still, Saslow developed an antipathy to psychoanalysis because of what he regarded as its unscientific character, there being no attempt to test rival hypotheses in the field to see which was correct.[60] Also, he was influenced by Mandel Cohen's anti-analytic bias while he was a resident at MGH. Right after his residency Saslow went to Washington University to start a psychosomatic division, the area in which Guze struggled to find his niche in either internal medicine or psychiatry. Like so many other residents who worked under Saslow throughout the years, Guze found him to be a charismatic teacher and a masterful interviewer.[61] It is very probable that Saslow was recommended to Spitzer by Robins or Guze and, of course, found himself at home with the ethos of the Task Force.

Saslow had a rich diversity of academic and research fields. In addition to his study of psychosomatic illness, he was interested in PTSD, the biological basis of mental illness, refining the technique of the psychiatric interview, and developing brief psychotherapeutic interventions. While on the Task Force he served on the Anxiety and Dissociative Disorders Advisory Group. His greatest love was teaching residents how to conduct interviews and do psychotherapy. His primary insistence was that they should above all listen to the patient, a skill he reported he found less and less as the years passed. After leaving Washington University, Saslow taught briefly at the Harvard Medical School and then went to Portland to become the first full-time chairman of the Department of Psychiatry at Oregon Health and Science University (OHSU), a position he left in 1973 only because of mandatory retirement. He then became Professor of Psychiatry at UCLA and Chief of Mental Health and Behavioral Science at the VA Hospital in Sepulveda, CA, before returning to OHSU to teach and to see patients. It was during his work in Portland and Sepulveda that he was a member of the Task Force.

Saslow had an interesting past relative to his expertise on the role of stress and his skill at interviewing. While he was a resident, there was a calamitous fire in Boston at the Coconut Grove Night Club; 492 people died and hundreds more were injured. Saslow's interviews of the survivors contributed to the early development of grief theory and the understanding of post-traumatic stress. Then, while at Washington University, he became a psychiatric consultant to the Manhattan Project at Los Alamos, NM, where the first atomic bombs were developed, and at the Los Alamos Medical Center, subsequently under the control of the Atomic Energy Commission (AEC) from 1947 on. For over twenty years, while first in St. Louis and then in Portland, he studied work-related stress for the AEC. In his interview with Roland Atkinson at OHSU, he described vividly the kind of psychiatric emergencies he was called on to deal with at the Manhattan Project where the scientists lived closeted, pressurized lives without their families. He was an amazing Renaissance man in both psychiatry and medicine.

MORTON KRAMER

We have now learned about seven of the eight members of the original Task Force. The group also had an official biometrician, Morton Kramer (1914–1998), who had served on the panels that formulated DSM-I (1952) and DSM-II (1968). Kramer was a highly skilled statistician and epidemiologist who had been Director of the Biometrics Branch of the NIMH since 1949. At this point one should recall Robert Felix, the ebullient and politically connected psychiatrist who created the NIMH and was its first chief, in the heady days after World War II. Far-seeing and expansive, Felix realized that the mental health program he was trying to implement needed a strong biostatistical arm, and he hired Kramer. At first Kramer protested that he knew little about mental health. But Felix persuasively replied: "Who knows anything about it at this point? Join me, and we'll show the world what we can do."[62]

Early in his tenure at the NIMH, Kramer had been invited by the APA Committee on Nomenclature and Statistics to join it, as they wanted to revise and consolidate the competing classifications then in use by American psychiatrists. The committee required a statistician. The reporting of annual statistics by state mental hospitals needed to be standardized and a diagnostic scheme devised for presenting tabulations of mental disorders that would be coherent with the new nomenclature of the revised classification. Kramer performed these jobs for both DSM-I and DSM-II. For DSM-II, he wrote a special introduction on the historical background of ICD-8, which had been approved by WHO in 1966 and was scheduled to become effective in 1968.[63] Henry Pinsker, a clinician who valued his close contact with patients, remembers Kramer as a very serious man who stuck determinedly to his role as statistician: "The realities of sick people were not part of the equation," Pinsker reports.[64] Kramer was indeed an epidemiologist who made conclusions based on data about masses of patients, not individual ones.

Kramer gained renown in psychiatric statistical and epidemiological circles, working at an early date (1952) on the problem of reliability by getting state mental hospitals to agree on some basic definitions for terms used in their reports on patients in their hospitals. Kramer was also involved in the U.S./U.K. study on differences in diagnosis between the two countries. He produced data showing that the rate of admission into hospitals in England for manic-depressive disorders was ten times that in the United States.[65] For its part, the United States had lopsidedly large admissions of patients with schizophrenia. Kramer went on to develop a standardized diagnostic instrument that was used in mental hospitals in both Great Britain and the United States. On the weight of this instrument, he saw that the differences between the U.K. and U.S. patient populations could be attributed to differences in training of psychiatrists in the two countries.[66] Spitzer was very interested in this because of his concern with how DSM-III could help solve the problem in reliability of diagnosis. In an interview, Kramer recalled about his diagnostic instrument: "This work had a considerable impact on the recognition of the need to develop good diagnostic criteria for mental disorders that could be used both nationally and internationally."[67]

Kramer came to be called "the father of mental health statistics." He received the Distinguished Service Award from the U.S. Public Health Service and was elected to the prestigious Institute of Medicine of the National Academy of Sciences. WHO honored him with a medal, and the APA made him an Honorary Fellow. In 1976, Kramer became a Professor of Biostatistics at the School of Hygiene and Public Health at John Hopkins University, where he had received his Sc.D.

DENNIS P. CANTWELL

Some note should also be made of Dennis P. Cantwell (1939–1997) (Fig. 5.8, Pictorial Essay), although he was not one of the original eight members. Cantwell was a famous child psychiatrist. Like Andreasen, he was just at the start of his illustrious career when he served on the DSM-III Task Force, where he contributed considerably.[68]

Cantwell graduated with highest honors from Notre Dame University and was both a medical student and resident at Washington University, where he came especially under the influence of Samuel Guze. He completed his training in child psychiatry at the Neuropsychiatric Institute at UCLA and joined the faculty there in 1972. After only eight years he received a chaired professorship. He remained at UCLA for the rest of his life, though often wooed by other institutions. He probably received every available research award for a child psychiatrist. Cantwell made his name as a researcher and teacher about children with handicaps, particularly those with speech and language disorders, autism, and ADHD (Attentionn Deficit Hyperactivity Disorder). He published over 200 papers and authored or edited five books before he met a premature death at age 58 from chronic heart disease. At UCLA, he was renowned for his brilliance as a teacher and innovator in psychiatric education. Residents flocked to study with him.[69]

Cantwell was interested in evidence-based psychiatry and so was an especially good fit on the empirically minded Task Force. His presence there, along with Woodruff, Andreasen, and Saslow and eventually Paula Clayton—all five exceptionally talented—reminds us of the important continued influence of the Wash. U. psychiatrists in the history of the development of DSM-III.

"A SMALL REVOLUTION"

The Task Force expanded over the years, ultimately growing to 18 members, to some extent because Spitzer added individuals with whom he found it useful and congenial to work. Others were added to please certain psychiatric constituencies. But the tone and goals of the Task Force had been set early on, and from these there was no deviation. To expand on the point made early in this chapter, something unintended seemed to be happening. Nancy Andreasen has emphasized, "As the writing evolved, Task Force members began to comment to one another that they were writing a new textbook of psychiatry [with] a variety of new principles and innovations." The Task Force believed that they were producing a volume that was "atheoretical about etiology" since, upholding the Wash. U. psychiatrists, etiology was unknown (a direct repudiation of psychoanalysis.) Within the first year, it had been decided that there would be diagnostic criteria for each disorder, which should help communication, reliability, and research; there would be a glossary to define the terms used in the criteria; the term *neurosis* would be dropped (since it was based on "speculative" principles); and there would be a "multiaxial approach to classification in order to incorporate medical and psychosocial components of a clinical evaluation." The authors of DSM-III knew, concludes Andreasen, "that they were creating a small revolution in American psychiatry."[70]

We know now that the revolution turned out to be a large one that would affect the whole field of psychiatry and influence American society in ways that no one could have accurately predicted. The next section of this book lays bare the creation of DSM-III and we learn about the forces—conceptual, scientific, economic, and political—that were at play. We will also meet additional individuals who had a major influence in determining the structure of the new manual. The five-year saga of the actual construction is preceded by two subjects: a description of nineteenth- and twentieth-century interests in the development of psychiatric classifications, and a recounting of a major problem in twentieth-century psychiatry—achieving reliability in diagnosis from one psychiatrist to the next. This troublesome issue exists in part because much of psychiatry lacks definitive biological tests to establish the etiology of a given disorder.

SECTION III
The Making

6

A BRIEF HISTORY OF MODERN
CLASSIFICATION AND PROBLEMS
WITH RELIABILITY IN DIAGNOSIS

Two matters must be briefly considered before we join Spitzer and his Task Force of eight empiricists around the table in the fall of 1974. One subject is the history of classification in the nineteenth and twentieth centuries, and the other is the challenge of achieving reliability in diagnosis. We might remember again at this point that Robins and Guze took the view that "classification is diagnosis."

The DSM-III Task Force was convened to write a new classification that would be a radical departure from what had come before. Revised diagnostic descriptions would hinge on that classification. Ideally, the goal of a diagnosis would be to lead to an accurate etiology, prognosis, or therapy. If the Task Force decided that these were largely unknown, their goal would be instead to describe groupings of disorders that appear related to each other.

In addition to defining the basic rationale of their classification, the DSM-III Task Force was informed that they had to solve another problem, that of achieving reliability in psychiatric diagnosis. Generally speaking, reliability means that (1) two separate (or more) interviewers are in agreement on the diagnosis after they have interviewed a patient, and further, when the interviewers discuss the diagnosis of a patient they have interviewed, they mean the same thing when they settle on a diagnosis; and (2) the initial diagnosis remains the same in a subsequent interview. This last is exactly what the Wash. U. psychiatrists meant when they talked about the importance of the follow-up.[1]

Spitzer himself had actually been working on the issue of reliability through developing structured interviews of patients long before he was appointed to chair the writing of a new manual. Then, at Washington University, he was influenced to construct a more reliable manual through the use of diagnostic criteria.

We will turn first to a pertinent history of classification and then move to consider the conundrum of reliability.

CLASSIFICATION IN PSYCHIATRY: AN OVERVIEW

Classification is a necessary endeavor that human beings automatically carry out from early infancy on in order to comprehend the world they live in. Thus, for example, infants separate out pain from pleasure or mother from father, with the distinguishing attributes of each.[2] Yet, developing a reliable classification is no simple feat, because there is always the danger of creating artificial divisions and categories where none exist. A child may decide that a flower and a kite are interchangeable because they are both red, until later knowledge shows the error of that judgment. The challenge psychiatrists always face when writing a classification is to develop "real"—valid— categories that will stand the test of time. But that inevitably means that as new knowledge enters the field, classifications must be periodically revised.

With the aim that it can ultimately help in treatment, a classification is desirable— first, to bring about accurate and meaningful diagnoses that are valid, and second, to enable communication of knowledge among researchers and practitioners that is reliable. Validity is the accuracy of a diagnosis. The more validity, the more likely that useful treatment will emerge.

It has been argued that the urge to classify and diagnose had different roots and goals in the European world and in the United States in the nineteenth century. In Europe the desire to construct a classification—a nosology—that would make sense of the diz- zying array of symptoms confronting psychiatrists was strong. Therefore, psychiatrists strove for accurate groupings. In the United States, the emphasis on the uniqueness of each affected individual, which had begun with moral (psychological and environ- mental) treatment, made grouping seem less necessary for a while. Thus, while the idea of a classification based on symptoms ignited a quest among European alienists for a nosology, in the United States, alienists were put off by the notion of basing a classifica- tion on a multitude of confusing symptoms. In the United States, where pragmatism often prevailed, classifying was at first prompted by the desire of the federal Bureau of the Census to collect statistics on the number of patients in mental hospitals; the demographic characteristics of patients; admission and discharge rates; the disorders they were suffering from; and, finally, death rates.[3] It was not until the end of the nine- teenth century that psychiatrists in the United States took an intellectual interest in the course of an illness and its outcome, although even then, Kraepelin's classification was still not immediately accepted. Eventually, however, American psychiatrists joined their European counterparts and developed parallel concerns. Therefore, let us first come to understand nineteenth-century developments in Europe.

THE MODERN TRADITION OF CLASSIFICATION

In Europe in the nineteenth century, there were several medical and psychiatric cir- cumstances that spurred desire for and smoothed the road toward the construction of a psychiatric nosology. First, there was the general impetus to classify that existed throughout the whole of medicine at that time because of rapid scientific advances. Second, in psychiatry in particular, there was pressure to classify because of the widely acknowledged confusion in understanding mental illness and failure to develop effec- tive treatments. Third, there was the influence of faculty psychology—the belief that the mind is divided up into separate "faculties" designed to perform certain mental tasks. Franz Joseph Gall's (1758–1828) phrenology—the belief that one can chart personality traits by measuring particular bumps on the head—was an expression of faculty psychology. Although the Catholic Church and establishment science condemned Gall's theories, they were popular in Paris salons and later in the United States. Fourth, after 1857, Benedict Augustin Morel's (1809–1873) theory of degeneration affected first French psychiatric classification and later that of other countries as well.[4] His thesis was that mental illness afflicting one generation would afflict the next one, with ever-worsening deterioration. In each generation, the physical signs of degeneration were different, thereby creating a new clinical picture. Morel's impact was widespread. Thomas Mann (1875–1955) won the 1929 Nobel Prize in literature for his novel *Buddenbrooks* (1901), which traces the declining fortunes of a bourgeois family over four generations.

Finally, under the influence of Kraepelin, in most of Europe and the United Kingdom, it was seen that in order to make a differential diagnosis between dementia praecox and a major affective disorder (manic-depressive illness in Kraepelin's terminology), it would be useful to accumulate homogeneous patient groups to study pathology. Moreover, being able to diagnose the one disorder as distinct from the other would allow for a more accurate prognosis.[5]

The pressure to classify also arose from the inadequacy of pre-nineteenth-century concepts of insanity. Madness then was considered a state of existence which, once having occurred, was unending. This made it hard to understand why remissions took place. So the notion of "lucid interval" was created to account for periodic normal behavior in order to maintain the view that the affected person remained mad in some fundamental way. But clearly, the state of madness was a topic that beckoned further consideration.

Thus, in the nineteenth century, there came about a new understanding of insanity as existing in time and, therefore, fluctuating. Karl Kahlbaum (1828–1899) and Emil Kraepelin (1856–1926) used this temporal quality of mental disease to launch the concept of a disease course, and postulated that the pathology was located in the brain or occurred as the result of a faulty metabolic process. The notion of disease having a specific course had a nosological effect of reducing the number of disorders described in a classification and was eventually used by Kraepelin to create the two overarching diagnoses, dementia praecox and manic-depressive illness. These two categories have lasted more than a century, although terminology and conceptualization have been modified, and there has been ongoing intermittent questioning of the dichotomy that Kraepelin had created. The psychiatrists planning DSM-5 have struggled with the issue of the relationship and division of the two disorders. Indeed, late in his life, Kraepelin himself began to have doubts whether his division was valid.[6]

Classificatory clarity was hard to achieve—and remains so—because psychiatrists could find only a limited etiological base for their nosology and thus were usually limited to describing symptoms. True, most had distanced themselves from the earlier notion that sin and God's punishment accounted for mental derangement. Psychiatrists embarked on a secular scientific approach. For example, one result of Kraepelin and his colleagues' work was establishment of the idea that theories of insanity could not be only theoretical but had to be based on observation.

But psychiatry in the nineteenth century had run into roadblocks with regard to treatment, creating a void that psychoanalysis tried to fill. Freud, although certainly aware of symptomatic differences among his patients, did not feel the need to create a taxonomy since he believed he had discovered the universal underlying etiology of mental illness, which was psychological rather than physical. He thought a descriptive psychiatry led to a superficial understanding of mental illness. (Although one could argue that Freud, without deliberately planning it, created a descriptive classification of outpatient "neurotic" conditions, for example, "anxiety neurosis.") Psychoanalytic understanding, by contrast, was "deep" because he and his followers believed that it could disclose more about a given individual than could a psychiatric diagnosis, that is, the patient's being assigned to a category. Psychoanalysis shared with moral treatment the belief in the uniqueness of each individual.

The Wash. U. psychiatrists rejected psychoanalytic etiology and believed the etiologies of most mental illnesses had not been discovered at all. To them, as we have seen, even description had its limits, and they created only a restricted number of diagnoses that they considered valid.

Spitzer accepted the Washington University system based on diagnostic criteria and used it to create the Research Diagnostic Criteria (RDC) and DSM-III. But for the new DSM he came to believe that there was little limitation on the diagnoses he could include, as long as he used a descriptive psychiatry, accompanied by diagnostic criteria, that clinicians and researchers found useful for their goals. For Spitzer, reliability trumped validity.

CLASSIFICATION IN THE UNITED STATES

Moving now from a European and more general overview of classification, let us consider developments in the United States specifically. The road to DSM-III had been a long one, stretching back almost a century and a half in American psychiatric history. Recognizing the growth of asylums in the early nineteenth century, the U.S. government decided to count and diagnose asylum patients in the 1840 Census. However, all patients were listed under one diagnosis. "idiocy/insanity," the Census officials making no distinction between what might appear to us to be mental retardation as separate from mental illness. No further description appeared until 1880, when the Census listed seven diagnoses: mania, melancholia, monomania, paresis, dementia, dipsomania, and epilepsy. This was a testament to the burgeoning of ever-larger asylums, as well as the growth of psychiatry as a distinct medical discipline. While Census officials continued to use the 1880 classification for a while, various asylums became dissatisfied with the U.S. government's delineation and grouping and began composing and publishing their own nosologies, creating an ever-bewildering diversity.

In recognition of this unscientific situation, the American Medico-Psychological Association (later to become the American Psychiatric Association), together with the National Commission on Mental Hygiene, developed in 1917 a classification of twenty-two diagnoses to be used nationwide, and the Bureau of the Census adopted it for its own collections of statistics. This was used until 1935, when it was revised and became a part of the American Medical Association's (AMA) *Standard Classified Nomenclature of Diseases*. This was the situation when the United States entered World War II in 1941.

Within a short while, Army psychiatrists saw that this system, designed for diagnosing chronic inpatients with severe disorders, was almost totally unsuited for most of the many psychiatrically sick soldiers whom they were seeing; up to ten percent of all discharges were for psychiatric reasons. By the end of the war there were four separate classification entities, although there was some overlap: the AMA's *Standard Classification*, a U.S. Army classification, a U.S. Navy classification, and a Veterans Administration (VA) classification. Some of these classifications were also being used by post-war psychiatrists who tended increasingly to be psychodynamic in their outlook and saw private patients in their offices. To complicate this picture, in 1948 the World Health Organization (WHO) took responsibility for producing a sixth edition of the *International Causes of Death* and renamed it the *International Classification of Diseases, Injuries, and Causes of Death* (ICD-6); this contained its own system of classification of mental disorders, but U.S. psychiatrists did not find it useful for them.

Thus, the American Psychiatric Association decided to publish its own classification, which was to be a revision of the ICD-6 classification and would meet the needs of its members. The APA's Committee on Nomenclature and Statistics devised a document that was also based on the VA's system that actually had been developed by the psychoanalyst William Menninger (1899–1966). Their effort appeared in 1952 as the 132-page *Diagnostic and Statistical Manual of Mental Disorders (DSM-I)*, which contained a discussion of diagnostic categories ("Definition of Terms"), their exact format shaped by the idea of mental disorders as "reactions." This schema reflected both what psychiatrists had observed in soldiers during the war and the psychobiosocial views of Adolf Meyer (1866–1950), the so-called dean of American psychiatry. Meyer had taught that mental disorders represented the reactions of the affected person to psychological, biological, and social factors. DSM-II (134 pp.) came into being sixteen years later (1968), dropping the idea of reactions and often reflecting the psychoanalytic orientation of many American psychiatrists at the time. DSM-II was based on the ICD-8 classification but with definitions useful to the Americans, ICD-8 having no glossary until 1972.

The decision of the APA in the 1970s to produce a new DSM was an effort not only to improve psychiatry's image but also to coordinate the DSM with the upcoming ICD-9.

THE CHALLENGE OF ACHIEVING
RELIABILITY IN DIAGNOSIS

Yet, even after the APA had begun publishing nationwide classifications after World War II, psychiatrists and psychologists became increasingly aware that the concordance of diagnoses was seriously flawed, thus raising questions on how good the classifications were. The diagnoses in use did not mean the same from one occasion to another, from one hospital to another, and from one psychiatrist to another. Especially if categories were to be used in research—keeping in mind the ultimate goal of effective treatment—it was necessary to create homogeneous groups of patients for study, all of whom had been declared to have the same illness. But how could this be accomplished if psychiatrists could not agree on what to call the illness? The problem of reliability was recognized long before either the Wash. U. psychiatrists or Spitzer came on the scene.

We can view the issue of reliability in psychiatric diagnosis in two stages. In the first, psychiatrists bewailed the state of diagnostic unreliability but offered little to directly attack the issue. In the second stage, they attempted to remedy the situation by the use of informative specific factors—"criteria"—to make a diagnosis. It will be remembered that Mandel Cohen had introduced the concept of "operational criteria" in the 1930s and 1940s, but psychiatrists, aside from his acolytes such as Eli Robins, ignored his work at that time.

What follows are a few examples of early studies in which the factor of unreliability in diagnosis was emphasized. In 1927, Dr. E. B. Wilson addressed the APA about studies he had been conducting at the Boston Psychopathic Hospital,[7] where he observed the great variability of reports among psychiatrists dealing with the same material. He inspired an assistant professor of statistics at the Harvard School of Public Health to conduct experiments (also at Boston Psychopathic) of "a single observer repeating his results on given material and...of different observers working on the same material."[8] The experiments revealed large areas of disagreement. A discussant of these results underlined "how far from reliable some unusually carefully prepared classifications were."[9]

Outside the United States, a well-known British psychiatrist and geneticist, Eliot Slater (1904–1983), also addressed the problem of reliability. In 1936, in attempting to portray the genetics of manic-depressive illness, Slater found that in the materials with which he was working, there was a great deal of confusion of schizophrenia and manic-depressive illness, which hampered his investigation.[10]

Two years later, in 1938, two Chicago psychoanalysts, Jules H. Masserman (1905–1994) and Hugh T. Carmichael, reported on a comprehensive and detailed study of one hundred patients admitted to the Psychiatric Division of the University of Chicago Clinics. The mean stay of the patients was twenty-four days. On their discharge the patients were diagnosed according to the nomenclature of the National Committee for Mental Hygiene *Statistical Manual*, newly published by the Utica (New York) Hospital Press. The patients had been treated with various forms of psychotherapy, and the chief aim of the study was to see whether one year later they had maintained the progress they had achieved while in the hospital. While the main goal of the study was not to evaluate reliability of diagnoses, the report incidentally provided such information. First, at follow-up, forty percent of the original diagnoses had to be revised. Then, the investigators tried to see if the diagnoses of their patients were comparable to those of similar hospitalized patients at the Maudsley Hospital in London. They found almost no correspondence and concluded that the "wide differences of classification illustrates...the looseness and inadequacies of the psychiatric nosological concepts at present in use."[11]

The final early study of the reliability of diagnosis, in 1949, was that by a psychologist, Philip Ash (1917–2002), which was based on a study of psychiatric interviews of fifty-two white males. Ash described the categories of the particular diagnostic system he used but not its formal name. In his experiment three psychiatrists interviewed thirty-five patients together but wrote up their evaluations separately. Then two psychiatrists interviewed the remaining seventeen patients with a similar procedure. There was wide disparity of agreement in both groups. The three psychiatrists agreed on a specific diagnosis (e.g., schizophrenia) only twenty percent of the time and on a general category (e.g., psychotic disorders) only forty-six percent of the time. The two psychiatrists agreed on a specific diagnosis thirty-one to forty-four percent of the time and a general category fifty-eight to sixty-seven percent of the time. Ash concluded, "The extremity and frequency of disagreement make it quite legitimate to raise the question of the reliability of the diagnostic system."[12]

After Ash's study, interest in the subject of reliability continued sporadically, partly held in check by the influence of psychoanalysis, with its disdain for diagnosis. An analyst, Kenneth Mark Colby, for example, published *An Introduction to Psychoanalytic Research*, in which he lamented the system of classifying patients, arguing against diagnosing anyone as schizophrenic.[13] Those few psychiatrists who bothered to write on the issue came to the predictable conclusion that "psychiatric diagnosis at present is so unreliable as to merit very serious question when classifying, studying, and treating patients' behavior and outcomes."[14] During the 1950s, psychologists appeared to be more interested in the subject than psychiatrists.[15]

Perhaps psychiatrists started to take a sharper notice of their diagnostic imbroglio after 1962, when Aaron T. Beck (b. 1921), the future founder of cognitive therapy for depression and eventually cognitive behavioral therapy (CBT), published two articles on the unreliability of diagnosis. The first was influential because it was a review of the literature of studies reporting on the poor reliability of psychiatric diagnosis.[16] The second was important because Beck and his colleagues conducted their own study with the aim of ensuring the highest possible percentage of agreement. Their psychiatric interviewers were strictly prepared by the researchers' attention to "the nomenclature used by each psychiatrist, the minimum level of training and experience of each psychiatrist, and the type of diagnostic procedures to be employed." Yet the results showed only a fifty-four percent level of concordance, which Beck et al. declared was not sufficient for research and treatment. They also made the telling point that most studies of reliability were unrealistically high because they included the diagnosis of organic brain syndromes (OBS), which tended to be eighty to ninety percent concordant and thus compensated for the poor results for other types of psychiatric diagnoses. Beck and his co-workers strove for a less skewed evaluation and excluded OBS from their study.[17]

Simultaneously, Beck, a psychoanalyst, began to establish himself as a psychiatric thinker in the field of depression. Part of Beck's interest in reliability had been prompted by his inability to get fellow psychoanalysts to agree on what constituted depression.[18] He then developed criteria for depression and, in 1961, created what came to be known as the Beck Depression Inventory (BDI), a twenty-one-question, multiple-choice, patient-reported questionnaire designed to provide a quantitative assessment of the severity of the patient's depression over the past week.[19] The BDI represented a theoretical shift from a Freudian, psychodynamic view of depression to one focused on the patient's own self-defeating thoughts or "negative cognitions."

Deciding that the time had come to deal seriously with the issue of diagnosis, the American Psychiatric Association and the NIMH convened a conference in November 1965 to discuss classification in psychiatry and psychopathology. The Wash. U. axiom, "classification is diagnosis," received formal acknowledgement. Participants at the meeting included Joseph Zubin, Spitzer's chief at New York State Psychiatric Institute (PI) (Biometrics Unit), and Seymour Kety (1915–2000), a highly respected researcher at the NIMH. The tone of the conference demonstrated appreciation of phenomenology—descriptive psychiatry—and the attendees' concluded that the subject of etiology of psychopathology not be considered closed, which was a slap in the face of psychoanalysis. The primary editor of the *Proceedings* was Martin Katz, the NIMH research psychologist who just a few years later would decide that Spitzer and Robins had to meet. The *Proceedings* of the conference appeared in 1967.[20] With this publication, reliability of diagnosis had become a visible professional concern of American psychiatry.

In the same year as the *Proceedings*, a study tackled the issue of why, from one study to the next, the percentage of diagnostic reliability reported was always different. The lead author was none other than Robert Spitzer, this being seven years before he began creating DSM-III. Working on a grant from the NIMH, while still in the midst of psychoanalytic training, Spitzer evinced his interest in measurement. Spitzer and his colleagues described "several defects in current procedures used to assess diagnostic agreement" and offered a mathematical solution based on a statistically derived method. In the article, they also reported on a study of computerized diagnosis for which Spitzer had written a computer program using the training he had received at IBM on FORTRAN IV.[21]

ATTEMPTS TO ESTABLISH RELIABILITY IN SCHIZOPHRENIA STUDIES

An attempt to remedy diagnostic unreliability came first in the field of schizophrenia studies. A burning diagnostic question in the 1960s was that of prognosis in cases of schizophrenia. Psychiatrists in the United States had decided that there were two kinds of schizophrenia—good prognosis (remitting) or poor prognosis (deteriorating.) But they could not predict in advance which kind any given patient might have. They did not receive much help from the widespread use of Eugen Bleuler's diagnostic criteria, the four "A's": disturbance of affect, loosening of associations, ambivalence, and autism.[22] It is true that Bleuler had a much more optimistic view of schizophrenia than did Kraepelin. Bleuler knew that it did not inevitably lead to deterioration. But Bleuler had no predictive criteria. Psychiatrists' diagnostic dilemma about prognosis, we now know, came from their lack of ability, when dealing with a patient, to distinguish schizophrenia from an affective disorder. American psychiatrists also tended to overdiagnose schizophrenia in the 1960s. The very important "U.S.—U.K. study" showed that when it came to major psychiatric illnesses, by the late 1960s, U.S. psychiatrists were heavily diagnosing schizophrenia while U.K. doctors favored the affective disorders.[23] The study had a great impact on psychiatric sensibilities.

Some workers in schizophrenia studies were engaged in a debate over what signs and symptoms would indicate "true" schizophrenia, meaning the deteriorating kind. In 1960, Gabriel Langfeldt (1895–1983) of Oslo, a well-known researcher since the 1930s, tried to bring order into the disarray. Based on many studies and a lifetime of experience, he set forth four diagnostic criteria by which he felt true schizophrenia could be recognized: "(1) A break up in the development of a personality. (2) Catatonic stupor or excitement. (3) Symptoms of depersonalization and derealization. (4) Primary delusions as seen in paranoid cases."[24] However, these four criteria were weighted on the side of observation and judgment, which meant that empirical researchers did not set much store by Langfeldt's proposal.

Moreover, Langfeldt's criteria excited little attention in the United States, psychiatrists here having moved away from European traditions of descriptive psychiatry because of their interest in psychoanalysis. Still, a Harvard psychoanalyst, George E. Vaillant (b. 1934), read Langfeldt's work as well as that of six other researchers from 1927 to 1956 and immediately plunged into the debate on predicting outcome in schizophrenia. The question, he pointed out, in 1962, was whether a patient with a good outcome had been correctly diagnosed to start with. On the basis of his reading of others' studies,[25] Vaillant compiled a list of six diagnostic criteria that seemed to presage recovery in schizophrenia and designed a study to see if these criteria held true. The criteria held up in a number that was statistically significant. (Vaillant's six criteria were acute onset, precipitating factors, depression, non-schizoid premorbid adjustment, confusion, and heredity positive for affective psychosis.) Vaillant became optimistic: "Perhaps it is possible to adapt a group of objective criteria to prognosis, much as [T. Duckett] Jones [d. 1954] devised his criteria for the diagnosis of rheumatic fever."[26] (Valiant, we now realize, had some success because his recovering patients had a family background of an affective disorder and most likely suffered from an affective disorder, and not schizophrenia.)

In spite of positive results, Vaillant wanted to go beyond his first study, and he evaluated three additional studies by others. He then designed a prognostic study with seven criteria for predicting a remitting—"good"—schizophrenia. To his six criteria in the previous study he added concern with death. His seven criteria were based on clinical observation and judgment, follow-up, and a consideration of heredity (family study). Schizophrenia studies were beginning to move toward the criteria that were soon to be adopted by Robins and Guze.[27] (Thus, note that the attempt at formulating diagnostic criteria for schizophrenia had not started with the Feighner criteria.) In terms of follow-up, Vaillant declared, "Prognosis must depend upon longitudinal factors and cannot be evaluated by paying attention only to the admission picture." As to reliability, he commented, "The prognostic scale was more accurate than clinical judgment [alone]....Despite deliberate use of evaluation by inexperienced clinicians [first year residents], subsequent clinical course was correctly predicted in 82% of cases."[28]

Yet another list of diagnostic criteria for schizophrenia was that presented by John S. Strauss and colleagues in 1974.[29]

SPITZER'S WORK ON RELIABILITY BEFORE DSM-III

Still, unreliability in diagnosis continued as a galling problem. Long before his involvement with revising the DSM, Spitzer was actively considering two solutions: the structured interview and psychiatric evaluation through the use of a computerized program. He turned to the first of these just three years out of his residency and not even finished with psychoanalytic training. In 1964, he published his Mental Status Schedule (MSS), informing his readers, "Until now, a standardized interview to assess the major dimensions of mental status, in which the content and order of questions are fixed, seems never to have been reported."[30] A fixed interview held great appeal for him. Measuring and evaluating had been his research goal for many years. Being in Joseph Zubin's Biometrics Research Department nurtured this activity. But, more than this, precision and quantification had attracted him since an early age. Now, many years later, professional enjoyment of the unstructured psychoanalytic relationship did not bring as much satisfaction as did an attempt at empirical research. Accordingly, Spitzer brought to bear the full weight of his intelligence to the mapping out of a structured interview as a vehicle to deal with the challenging issue of diagnostic unreliability.

Since the MSS was Spitzer's first foray into the world of structured interviews, some details about it are warranted. Spitzer was senior author with the support of three other members of the Biometrics Research Department. Spitzer introduced the instrument as

> an easily learned technique for simultaneously examining, recording, and evaluating the mental status of a psychiatric patient....The evaluation focuses on current behavior and therefore can be repeated to assess changes in patients after treatment.[31] Properly administered, the interview has the feel of a clinical evaluation. However, unlike the usual clinical interview, the use of a specific schedule of questions, a fixed order of presentation, and uniform coverage of the same areas of psychopathology with every patient make it more likely that differences observed among patients will reflect basic differences rather than differences due to variations in interviewing procedures.

Spitzer reported in the article that the interview would take twenty to fifty minutes. He then discussed the methods by which the schedule had been developed, the fact that it was based on observable behavior without reference to unconscious processes,[32] that it used diagnostic criteria (without calling them that), how it was possible for the examiner to "speak in a natural manner," the methods of scoring, and the reliability and validity that had been achieved using the instrument in various studies. He addressed at length the reluctance that some experienced psychiatrists would have to use a standardized interview because they believed it would interfere with the patient–doctor relationship. In sum, the article was carefully crafted.

After introducing the MSS in 1964, Spitzer continued to publish regularly reports of his research employing structured interviews. He also introduced new instruments that have been widely used since. Four of the more prominent ones should be mentioned here. The first is the Schedule for Affective Disorders and Schizophrenia (SADS), initially published in 1978.[33] The second is the Structured Clinical Interview for DSM-III-R and, later, DSM-IV (SCID I for Axis I disorders [psychotic disorders] and SCID-II for Axis II disorders [personality disorders]).[34] The third is the PRIME-MD, a short procedure for the diagnosing of mental disorders by primary care physicians.[35] Finally, there is the Global Assessment of Functioning (GAF) Scale for overall psychosocial functioning (Axis V in DSM-IV).[36]

At the same time that he was introducing and assessing standardized interviews, Spitzer, again working with associates, began to publish frequently on quantitative psychiatric research.[37] Then, in the area of computerized evaluation, Spitzer and Endicott introduced DIAGNO in 1968 and DIAGNO II the next year.[38] However, after developing DIAGNO III, they began to see the limitations of computer diagnostics. One study compared the degree to which DIAGNO III agreed with a pair of experts. The result was that the experts agreed with each other more than the computer program did. It was especially noticeable that DIAGNO diagnosed affective psychosis poorly. Routinely made human clinical diagnoses were superior to the diagnoses made by a particular computer system.

Spitzer and Endicott asserted in 1974—just as the Task Force was about to begin its work—that the major constraint to computerized diagnosis was the traditional diagnostic system itself as embodied in DSM-II, and that the Feighner criteria had shown a far more superior way to diagnose. Moreover, it was argued that the collaborative studies on the psychobiology of depression being directed through the NIMH would change "the diagnostic system itself with emphasis on simplification, explicit criteria, and limiting the categories [of psychiatric illness] to those conditions for which valid evidence exists." Spitzer and Endicott pointed out that the NIMH program had already led to the development of the RDC, which had shown that clinicians using its criteria for diagnosis had a "far superior reliability than that obtained on the same cases when clinicians use the vague criteria of DSM-II."[39]

In concluding this section on attempts to lessen diagnostic unreliability before the publication of DSM-III, it is important to note the paper published by Spitzer and Joseph Fleiss, a biostatistician in Spitzer's department, also in 1974. Although by this time Spitzer had introduced a structured interview (the MSS), a computer program, and the RDC in an attempt to ameliorate diagnostic unreliability, his and Fleiss' review of the field showed that little had changed since Beck had published his pessimistic findings in 1962. Beck had found fair to very poor agreement, with the exception of diagnosing organic brain syndrome, mental deficiency, and alcoholism. Yet Spitzer was optimistic. He declared that psychiatrists did not agree well when technical terms were used (i.e., "depression") because these terms meant different things to different psychiatrists. He argued for alternate language, asserting that psychiatrists have more reliability when specific behaviors are rated (i.e. "stays in bed most of the day.") He referred again to the Feighner criteria of the Wash. U. psychiatrists as a model for using diagnostic criteria to deal with unreliability. Spitzer concluded firmly, "These two approaches, structuring the interview and specifying diagnostic criteria are being merged in a series of collaborative studies...sponsored by the N.I.M.H. We are confident that this merging will result not only in improved reliability but in improved validity which is, after all our ultimate goal."[40]

The strong leadership, frequent tactical brilliance, sheer energy, total dedication to his task, and even ruthlessness[41] that Spitzer demonstrated as Chair of the Task Force will now be recounted in the next several chapters. He was a man on a mission who threw himself into the plethora of situations he encountered with zest, only occasionally distressed about the process or outcome of positions he had maintained.

7

THE REVOLUTION BEGINS, 1973–1976

The APA's Board of Trustees had made the decision to revise DSM-II even before Spitzer was appointed to the position of Chair of the Committee on Nomenclature and Statistics. The Trustees stipulated that the chair, whoever that might be, would report to the APA's Council on Research and Development (R&D). The decision to create a new edition of the DSM was made by the Trustees in an atmosphere of crisis. From February 1 to 3, 1973, the Trustees convened at a "Special Policy Meeting" in Atlanta.[1] This meeting occurred right after David Rosenhan's startling article about the admission of "pseudopatients" appeared in *Science*. The year previously, Bruce Ennis, the civil liberties lawyer, had indicted the entire "enterprise" of the psychiatric care of mental hospital patients in his accusatory book, *Prisoners of Psychiatry*.

At their special meeting, the Trustees tackled two difficult topics. One was to address internal organizational chaos in the APA created by an alarming multiplication of APA councils, task forces, committees, commissions, and boards, as well as their relationship to each other. The second was to confront the problems that had arisen for American psychiatry externally: the "rampant criticisms;" the lack of a strong public conception of psychiatry as a medical specialty, coupled with the failure to recognize the psychiatrist's special competence in mental health care; the increasing attempts by the insurance industry and government agencies to regulate psychiatric treatment; and recent court cases in which the psychiatrist's medical judgment had been overruled.

The Trustees drafted or recommended a number of decisions that were intended to reverse the perturbing recent events and public perception of psychiatry. One step was the decision to revise DSM-II, which had been in effect only five years. (DSM-I was in effect sixteen years before a revision was published.) With a sense of urgency, the Board urged that "the task be completed within two years."[2] They also specifically directed that the new classification relate to "the problem-oriented-record-system approach." This was a recent concept of record-keeping in American medicine requiring that all findings and necessary information about a patient be listed, that the major problems needing attention be outlined, and that there be a plan for treatment of each problem by "all the health care personnel directly involved in the care of the patient."[3] It was anticipated that this aspect of the revised manual would tie psychiatry more closely to medicine. The Trustees also directed that, since the present DSM-II Task Force was helping to revise the psychiatry section of ICD-9 for American clinical usage, the new task force should have "close working ties" with the old one. (This does not seem to have come about.) The Trustees advocated in addition "that whatever classification is ultimately adopted should contain provision for designating the *degree* of functional disability that accompanies a diagnostic category" and for expressing the disability in percentages. Finally, "the Trustees recommended the formation of a new Task Force to Define Mental Illness and What is a Psychiatrist.... It was the Trustees wish that the definitions that this Task Force develops be used as a preamble to the new DSM-III."[4] Clearly, the Trustees were hoping that DSM-III could be a tool to strengthen the medical aspects of psychiatry and reorient its image.

SPITZER'S OWN PLAN TO REVISE THE DSM

Along with the Trustees, and many members of the APA, Spitzer shared the desire to bolster and make visible a psychiatry that he believed was clearly part of the medical establishment. What the Trustees were probably not aware of when they appointed Spitzer, however, is that he already had in mind exact plans for how to create a new DSM and what to put in it.

There exists a remarkable document, "DSM-II: A Reply," prepared as a result of a meeting called to evaluate DSM-II very soon after its publication in 1968. Spitzer's statements at that time were four years before his appointment as head of the DSM-III Task Force.[5] In replying to a host of comments at a meeting on the new DSM, he and a colleague, Paul Wilson, suggested ways in which the making of the eventual DSM-III could be improved, anticipating in precise detail what actually came about. Their first suggestion was that the small central committee engaged in producing DSM-II, the Task Force, be aided in their work by a collection of subcommittees of experts on the various kinds of psychiatric disorders—these, of course, were the expert Advisory Committees that Spitzer ultimately appointed upon assuming leadership of the Task Force. Spitzer and Wilson next recommended that before its final publication the draft version of DSM-III be sent to a large number of psychiatrists for their review. The actual Task Force did just that. Then Spitzer and Wilson urged that after the drafts were reviewed, they should be given clinical trials in various appropriate settings (something that had not happened for DSM-I and DSM-II.) Indeed, Spitzer later saw to it that there were field trials of the draft versions of DSM-III. Finally, Spitzer and Wilson proposed that some of the problematic diagnostic issues raised by DSM-II could be at least partly resolved by "a multidimensional approach to diagnosis ...a system under which individuals are described in terms of more than one clinical dimension."[6] Advisory Committees, large professional review of the draft versions of DSM-III, field trials, and the multiaxial diagnostic system were already decided on years before any actual work took place.[7] A similar type of organization has lasted down through DSM-IV-TR (2000).

SPITZER AT THE STARTING POINT

Soon after the Task Force started meeting in 1974, Spitzer began to send the Chair of the Council on R&D updates on its progress, so we have a paper trail of Spitzer's early decisions and the initial activities of the Task Force.[8] Spitzer and the Task Force plunged into their assignment and showed early on an impressive array of accomplishments.

We see here the first evidence of the energy Spitzer was to bring to all his endeavors to produce DSM-III as well as the speed at which he moved, often outpacing any of the opposition he might encounter.

After just one meeting of the Task Force, Spitzer reported that possible innovations for the new manual would include, among others, a "definition of mental disorder and a defense of the medical model as applied to psychiatric problems, operational criteria for the diagnostic categories, ...provision for an undiagnosed psychiatric disorder category for patients who do not meet the criteria in the specified diagnostic groups, a bibliography of standard references justifying the diagnostic categories as valid entities, [and] a glossary of critical psychiatric terms." Spitzer assured the Council that the innovations planned for DSM-III would be compatible with the mental illness section of ICD-9 then being developed by the World Health Organization (WHO). It was also "agreed [by the Task Force] that etiology should be [the] classificatory principle only when it is clearly known," as with organic brain conditions. (This was the initial indication that psychoanalytic etiological explanations were imperiled; the phrase "clearly known" could carry various meanings.) Approaches to multiaxial diagnostic systems were also discussed by the Task Force. Spitzer reported that Advisory Committees now existed for the areas of disorders in sexual activities, psychosis, personality, and childhood and adolescence, and he attached lists of their members. "All of the [advisory] committees will have had their first meeting by mid November," he added.

Spitzer promised that the membership of the APA would be continually apprised of the deliberations of the Task Force: there would be a special session at the next APA meeting (May 1975) in which a progress report on DSM-III would be given, and *Psychiatric News* (the APA's news magazine) would be contacted to run an article about the Task Force's work and "invite interested members to send in suggestions for the DSM-III."[9] Throughout his tenure, Spitzer kept soliciting feedback from the psychiatric profession via personal letters, reports, and publications. The Chair of the Council on R&D was impressed by Spitzer's accounting and reported to the APA membership that the Task Force was "working vigorously," that the final draft was scheduled for 1977, and that the new manual would be published in 1978.[10]

THE RESEARCH DIAGNOSTIC CRITERIA: ELABORATION OF THE FEIGHNER CRITERIA AND LINK TO DSM-III

It is vital to our story to pay particular attention to the creation and development of the Research Diagnostic Criteria (RDC), for two reasons. The first is that the RDC and DSM-III were so intricately intertwined that Spitzer's public presentations of the work on the RDC provide an invaluable guide to where his thinking was focused in the early months of the development of DSM-III. The issue of reliability was uppermost in his mind as he sought to elaborate on the necessity for diagnostic reform. Moreover, in his talks and publications on the RDC, we can see the forthright declarations he was providing on what to expect from DSM-III, given, of course, that American psychiatrists were paying any attention. One could even say that as Spitzer sought to publicize DSM-III in its earliest days, he was actually presenting what work had already been done on the RDC.

The second significance of the RDC is that it is the vital bridge that connects what Spitzer had learned from Robins, his use of it, and, his making widely known the work that had come out of Washington University. Those with historical awareness of what the men in St. Louis had taught their medical students and residents in the 1950s and 1960s,[11] leading up to the publication of the Feigner criteria in 1972, often ponder: What was Robins' contribution to the creation of DSM-III? How do we titrate the Robins–Spitzer balance? What is recounted below will help answer these questions.

The Clinical Research Branch of the NIMH, it will be remembered, had brought Robins and Spitzer together in connection with its ambitious undertaking to study the psychobiology of depression. (Endicott says that much of the early work done for DSM-III was really done for the NIMH collaborative study of depression in which she took part.)[12] In addition to the collaborative study, the NIMH now sponsored an attempt to extend the use of diagnostic criteria as "an elaboration and expansion" of the Feigner criteria. It was planned that Robins and Spitzer would work together on this expansion. Spitzer was enthusiastic about the proposal and quickly applied himself to it, bringing in Endicott. Robins, restricted by the impediments from his multiple sclerosis from full participation, nevertheless contributed his ideas. Thus was born the Research Diagnostic Criteria. All this is also a reminder that over the years, the NIMH and the APA have shared ideas and personnel, and the NIMH has supported some of the APA's projects.

There were sixteen diagnoses in the Feigner criteria, and twenty-five were developed for the RDC.[13] As Spitzer and Endicott worked on it, they joked about there being the Feigner criteria and now the "finest criteria," that is, the RDC.[14] Spitzer adds: "We also enjoyed that the RDC kind of replaced the Feigner criteria." Of course, they were only too aware of the great sensation the Feigner criteria had made after they were published.

When asked if he knew exactly what he was going to do when appointed to head the DSM-III Task Force Spitzer has responded, "No, [except] the Feigner criteria, the Research Diagnostic Criteria—we've got to do that for all the mental disorders. And that's about as much as I thought through."[15] But that was not totally accurate. While working on the RDC, he was also actively making crucial recruiting decsions for the overall Task Force and for the novel advisory groups. And as far back as 1969, he had considered the multiaxial system of diagnoses that he put in place in DSM-III and was thinking about having field trials to test its draft version.[16] Thus Spitzer had more in mind about constructing DSM-III than he was later willing to admit.

The Feigner criteria had first appeared in January 1972. Within two and a half years of that date, the twenty-five diagnoses and diagnostic criteria of the RDC were developed and tested for their reliability by studying records of psychiatric cases.[17] In June 1974, just a few months before the DSM-III Task Force began its work, the initial draft of the RDC was presented at a conference sponsored by the Squibb pharmaceutical company. Spitzer and Endicott, lead authors of the paper (Robins was third author), opened their presentation with a short discussion of the long-standing problem of diagnostic reliability in psychiatry. "This sad state of affairs," they argued, "is responsible in part for the low regard with which psychiatric diagnosis is often held both within psychiatry and the general field of medicine." Rosenhan's sensational article in *Science* of just a year before, asserting that psychiatrists could not tell the difference between sane and insane patients, still weighed heavily on Spitzer's mind, and he had made up his mind to rebut it.[18] But first, at the Squibb conference, he presented his solution to the problem of unreliable diagnoses.

Studies had shown that the main source of unreliability was the variation among clinicians in the methods they used to make diagnoses, Spitzer declared. (Note that with the use of the word "clinician," Spitzer and his co-authors were now significantly extending the scope of the RDC to psychiatrists who treat patients, no longer limiting it to researchers who conduct studies.) DSM-II was not helping the problem, Spitzer asserted, because "the paucity of specific criteria in this manual forces the clinician to rely heavily on his own concepts of diagnostic categories …based on his particular training, experience, and interests." Spitzer and his colleagues proposed a solution whereby diagnostic criteria could be standardized. This innovation would be "the development of specific inclusion and exclusion criteria for each diagnosis that the clinician is required to use, regardless of his own personal concept of the disorder." With this approach, the clinician's task was twofold: to determine the presence or absence of specific clinical phenomena, and then to apply the comprehensive rules provided for making the diagnoses.[19] Because of Robins' influence, it was proposed that there be a category of "other psychiatric disorder," since "some patients with obvious psychiatric disturbance will not meet the criteria for any of the specific categories."[20] This precise option was later dropped from DSM-III.[21] (DSM-III had categories for diagnoses that were "Atypical," "Residual," or "Nowhere Else Classified," but not "Other Psychiatric Disorder.")

Within a year of the Squibb conference the wider psychiatric community was apprised of Spitzer's plan to include specified diagnostic criteria in DSM-III, via a 1975 article in the *American Journal of Psychiatry*, the official journal of the APA. Spitzer's goal was to "improve the reliability and validity of routine psychiatric diagnosis." But mindful of the fact that the diagnostic criteria had been developed for research only, Spitzer initially announced that "the criteria that may be listed in DSM-III would be 'suggested' only, and any clinician would be free to use them or ignore them as he saw fit."[22] Yet when Spitzer's plan was called to his attention in an interview several years ago, he seemed genuinely surprised. He had no memory of ever having written it.[23] In any event, there is a clear disjunction between Spitzer's 1974 paper at the Squibb conference (there would be "specific inclusion and exclusion criteria that the clinician is required to use, regardless of his own personal concept of the disorder") and his 1975 paper ("any clinician would be free to use them or ignore them as he saw fit"). It is evident with this clash of intentions that when Spitzer first began to work on DSM-III, he was still not sure how his revision of DSM-II would be received.

But Spitzer was certain of one thing: he had decided that the main method of curing unreliability in psychiatry was to nail down specific criteria for each mental disorder. At the Squibb conference he made his belief explicit: "Our main point is that most studies have shown that the major source of unreliability still is the criteria and not the perception and not even the interaction with the patient."[24] Previous DSMs had failed to produce reliability, and now Spitzer argued that he had the answer. He skewered DSM-II. "The DSM-II definition of schizophrenia …is just a general statement and it doesn't tell you how to make the diagnosis, what to do in borderline cases, etc.…DSM-II was written to offend as few people as possible." But, Spitzer promised, "if you use the RDC criteria, you will really be giving a much more comprehensive description of what criteria were applied than if you merely said we used the DSM-II categories."[25] Users could rest assured that many of the RDC criteria had research evidence supporting their validity, although, Spitzer admitted, some were only "an initial attempt to operationalize concepts whose importance for diagnosis is based on a considerable amount of clinical wisdom," that is, without research evidence. Still, he stressed, the RDC would at last allow accurate communication among psychiatrists.

Although it is likely that only a few paid attention at this juncture, Spitzer gave clear notice of what American psychiatrists should expect in DSM-III:

> We [will] have to give examples for many of the concepts that are in the RDC, such as the phrase "obvious overt thought disorder." We have to define that, because there is such a tremendous disparity on what is considered thought disorder. [The same goes for] the concept of bizarre or fantastic delusions.…This thing kind of gets a momentum of its own.… [W]e want to avoid making up a whole glossary of psychiatric terms although we know we have to do some of that. *Many of the new terms and criteria used in the RDC are likely to be part of the revised nomenclature of the American Psychiatric Association, DSM-III* [Italics added].[26]

How this would emerge Spitzer made abundantly plain in a comparison of the DSM-II category of "manic-depressive illness, depressed type" with the RDC category of a new diagnosis, "major depressive disorder," which included psychotic depressive reaction, involutional melancholia, and severe forms of neurotic depression. The DSM-II entry was twenty-one lines, and the RDC entry was seventy-one lines.[27]

Spitzer argued that there was yet another advantage to the use of "specified criteria:" they would improve the training of psychiatric residents and psychology interns because the employment of these criteria would "sharpen and focus many discussions of differential diagnosis."[28] This was predicted almost forty years ago, but from our present vantage point the use of the DSMs, which developed out of the RDC, has had some drawbacks. It has often led residents to think that all that is necessary when meeting a new patient is to check off the criteria and then make a diagnosis instead of listening to the patient for more than one visit and getting to know him or her. Consider now the language in Spitzer's 1974 Squibb proposal. Once given "specific inclusion and exclusion criteria for each diagnosis …the clinician's task is twofold: to determine the presence or absence of specific clinical phenomena, and then to apply the comprehensive rules provided for making the diagnosis." The physician's "own personal concept of the disorder" is to be swept aside.

To the neophyte this plan of action might appear to be a godsend. The warning that appeared in the Introduction to DSM-III, that treating a patient requires more than a DSM-III diagnosis, has frequently been overlooked.[29] All too often, unsure psychiatric trainees have grabbed on to the criteria like a drowning person to a life preserver. Diagnosis is reduced to going down a symptom checklist of "present" or "absent," a procedure some new psychiatrists come to rely on throughout their professional lives.[30] With the shortening of psychiatric sessions, as fewer and fewer psychiatrists do psychotherapy or only engage in a truncated form of it, they limit themselves to the prescribing of medications. This not infrequently results in the 15-minute "med checks" so beloved by managed care. Psychotherapy is carried out by psychologists or social workers, who are paid less for their time than physicians. The DSMs were never meant to be textbooks,[31] never meant to teach about psychiatric care, but this is a role they have often assumed, made even more convenient because there is a pocket edition of the DSM, handy for ready reference to names of diagnoses and their codes. Should we ask at this point: can the use of research criteria be applied to an everyday clinical situation?

But to return to the history of the RDC: even while Spitzer and Endicott were working on and publishing about the development of DSM-III (as well as after DSM-III was published), the RDC had a life of its own. It had been developed as a research instrument and continued to be useful for research because in some cases it had certain subtypes for making diagnoses that the same DSM-III diagnoses lacked. Major depressive disorder in the RDC, for example, had eleven subdivisions, allowing for more precise delineations. In 1978, Spitzer, Endicott, and Robins published a follow-up to their 1975 preliminary report on the RDC, discussing usages of the document in three studies of newly admitted psychiatric inpatients.[32] By this time, a second edition of the RDC was in use, and further revisions appeared into the 1980s. In many respects, this 1978 paper was also publicity for DSM-III, spelling out Spitzer's plans. We should emphasize the frequent interchangeability of information in papers on the RDC and DSM-III. Spitzer took every opportunity to write about the progress of the DSM-III Task Force.

The main aims of Spitzer and his colleagues at this juncture were to highlight the attempts to achieve reliability and to explain the diagnostic concepts that underlay the RDC, the "rationale" behind its development. The RDC had been repeatedly revised "until it appeared that further revisions would not increase reliability without a loss of validity."[33] The results of three studies undertaken had indicated that the reliability of the RDC categories was "very high....With only a few exceptions, the reliabilities reported ...[were] higher than [those] reported in other research studies." (It must be remarked, however, that reliability was better in the studies at New York State Psychiatric Institute than in the studies at Washington University.) Much thought, Spitzer et al. said, had also gone into the determination of diagnostic categories to include in the RDC. The decision had been made to emphasize the affective disorders and schizophrenia, broadly defined. The bulk of the 1978 article was devoted to explaining the diagnostic criteria that had been chosen in each case. For example, Spitzer and his co-authors had considered the minimum period of time that a disorder had to exist before schizophrenia could be diagnosed. The article concluded buoyantly, "The use of operational criteria for psychiatric diagnosis is an idea whose time has come!"[34]

In conjunction with further development of the RDC, Endicott and Spitzer conceived of a structured interview, the Schedule for Affective Disorders and Schizophrenia

(SADS). After evaluating the instrument in two field trials, they reported that it had considerably increased the reliability of the RDC and, hence, its diagnostic validity. Part I of the SADS was designed to describe the current episode of illness at its most severe, and Part II was primarily designed for describing past psychiatric disturbances. In their report, they gave examples of the SADS that were being used to evaluate a manic syndrome. As in the 1978 article on the RDC, the publication of the SADS was also meant to showcase DSM-III, whose diagnostic categories would "be virtually identical with or slight modifications of those contained in the RDC."[35][36]

EARLY EVENTS: PUBLICIZING DSM-III, IMMEDIATE CRITICISMS, AND INTRA-APA DIALOGUES

Publicity for DSM-III started early. For example, Spitzer reported on the DSM-III Task Force's activity in the fall of 1974 at a Payne Whitney Clinic (New York Hospital) meeting. At this early date, the Task Force had actually not done very much work on the manual although it had determined much of its direction. But Spitzer was anticipating that the work he and Endicott had done on the RDC would find its way into DSM-III. Thus, many at Payne Whitney were startled at Spitzer's presentation.[37] As one in the audience wrote: "I had been informed last year that there would soon be a 'Revised DSM-II'....Now I hear that what is in store for the profession is a totally reworked classification, to be designated officially as 'DSM-III.' I am not the only one concerned to be caught so surprised."[38]

We will see that each time Spitzer made a public presentation or published an update in *Psychiatric News*, he encountered criticisms. At first these were few, but as more and more was revealed about DSM-III, the critiques mounted. After a "DSM-III in Midstream" meeting in June 1976, which attracted wide notice, Spitzer's job became hectic. The constituencies that entered the fray and the ways in which Spitzer contended with these challenges form the bulk of our story.

However, in the first few months of his leadership of the Task Force, Spitzer had first to tackle several issues raised by the Chair of the APA's Council on R&D. There had been some concern in the Council and within the APA Reference Committee, a high-level group concerned with scientific matters, about the "relative absence of minority members on the task force." Spitzer assumed this referred to women and argued that "no additional action is necessary," taking the position that the two women on the Task Force plus the one on "the subcommittee on sex" were sufficient. And three weeks earlier, in response to the Committee of Black Psychiatrists, who had asked about representation on the Task Force, he responded with the same explanation: "I applied what I had regarded as the principles of affirmative action in considering minority group members who had ...expertise in problems of classification....In so doing several women are members or consultants to the Task Force."[39] (Both episodes are quite unsettling today.) In his correspondence with the Chair of the Council on R&D, Spitzer also put in a plea for augmentation of the money budgeted for his Task Force.[40]

The Advisory Committees began their work shortly after the Task Force plunged into theirs. Within several months of the Advisory Committees' work, Spitzer had dramatic news. Writing on March 18, 1975, he stated that "initial drafts have been completed for well over half of the disorders that will be in DSM-III....In so far as possible, each disorder will be described under the following categories: essential clinical features, associated clinical features, course, age at onset, usual level of incapacity, differential diagnosis, premorbid personality, complications, prevalence, sex ratio, familial pattern and suggested operational criteria."[41] Spitzer also related that, as planned, the Task Force had organized a special session for the May 1975 APA meeting in Anaheim with a progress report on DSM-III. In addition to the APA panel, the ambitious "DSM-III in Midstream" meeting was being seriously discussed: this was the possibility (at that point) of a conference in 1976 to be sponsored jointly by the Task Force and the Missouri Institute of Psychiatry on the "problems of classification, standardized coding, and computer technology."

Spitzer closed his report to the Council on R&D with a request for additional funding to cover the expenses of bringing in special "one shot" consultants. Within a short while, the DSM-III Task Force's monetary needs had far exceeded that of any of the many other task forces reporting to the Council on R&D. Let us briefly examine this important budgetary issue.

The actual expenses of the Task Force on Nomenclature and Statistics were as follows:

1975–76	$13,858.
1976	$20,353.
1977	$54,252

For 1978 the authorized budget was $55,000, and Spitzer ended up asking for $60,000.[42] By comparison, the next highest budgetary expenses were for the Task Force on Electroconvulsive Therapy, which never spent more that $11,594 in one year, and the sums for all the other task forces reporting to the Council on R&D were paltry.[43] One chair of the Council, Louis Jolyon West, was called upon early on to justify the sums Spitzer had requested. West (known to his colleagues as "Jolly") forcefully wrote to Henry Work, the APA Deputy Medical Director for Professional Affairs, about Spitzer's need for funds to comply with the mandate of the Executive Committee "for the task force to go full speed ahead and accomplish as much as they can." West emphasized "this means numerous meetings, much travel, thorough reviews, and extensive consultation—all of which cost money. [Moreover DSM-III] is needed badly, and it is needed soon."[44] The feeling of urgency, connected to the hopes that a new DSM could restore the reputation of psychiatry in America, was palpable. And, West pointed out in his letter, "The Executive Committee took note of the fact that profits from the sale of DSM-III will repay the cost of preparing it many times over." This was a prediction that was more than fulfilled.

CONTENTIOUS ISSUES

After the progress report on DSM-III at Anaheim in May 1975 and an article the next month in *Psychiatric News*, Spitzer began receiving complaints about the Task Force's plans for DSM-III.[45] Much of it centered on the topic of sexual deviance. There were several points at issue. One was criticism of the way that Spitzer had proposed to deal with the issue of homosexuality, which the year before had been removed from the nomenclature and replaced with "sexual orientation disturbance." There were immediate objections to the Task Force's listing of "homosexual arousal" as a sexual object choice disorder, with fears that this would bring homosexuality back as a disorder in the nomenclature. One writer voiced specific fears that such a diagnosis would be tantamount to teaching impressionable psychiatric residents that the diagnosis was a "disease."[46] Moreover, within the year there was objection to keeping "sexual orientation disturbance" in DSM-III and criticism about changing the designation to "homodysphilia," Spitzer's suggested neologism.[47] Since a protracted and bitter fight over this and related issues mushroomed through much of 1977, going into 1978, these matters will be discussed at length in Chapter 10. The other aspect of diagnosing sexual deviance that quickly excited objections was Spitzer's proposal that in the new manual "subjective distress" was required for a diagnosis of sexual deviance. This will be discussed at the conclusion of this chapter within the larger problem of Spitzer's attempts to construct a definition of mental disorder.

Thus at this juncture let us turn to the protests Spitzer encountered that were other than those about sexual deviance. One writer was unhappy that the diagnosis of "borderline schizophrenia" was nowhere to be found. (Spitzer was trying to reduce the proven overuse of the schizophrenia diagnosis by American psychiatrists.) Another complainant launched a sarcastic critique of proposed new diagnoses such as "drug withdrawal syndrome of tobacco" and "amorous relationship maladjustment" Yet another psychiatrist believed that DSM-III was basically a "rehash of DSM-II," that "notoriously unreliable" classification. More than one writer was bewildered and appalled that DSM-III did not include traditional psychoanalytic explanations of the etiologies of mental disorders.[48] In the years that followed, psychoanalysts would often protest that the new manual was ignoring the years of knowledge and experience that they had accumulated.

The first indication that there was about to be a radical reordering of diagnosis came with psychodynamically oriented psychiatrists' awareness that "neurosis" was missing as a category in the new nosology.[49] (In DSM-II there were many different kinds of "neurosis." The term was used to denote a fundamental mechanism underlying the disorders that psychodynamic clinicians treat.) Should this lacuna have been a shock? One clue might have come with others' realization that Spitzer himself had stopped conducting psychoanalyses, although, of course, this was not widely known.

We also know that around the time the Task Force first began meeting, Spitzer asked Theodore Millon on the Task Force, who was not only a specialist in personality disorders but also had other wide-ranging interests, to prepare for him a brief history of the terms *neurosis* and *psychosis*.[50] Clearly, Spitzer had more than a passing interest in the meaning and use of these terms, but again, there is no way the psychoanalytic community could have known this.

Harbingers of the intent to challenge the psychoanalytic conception of mental disorder, although presented in a low key, could also be found in a long textbook chapter by Spitzer that had just appeared on classification in psychiatry.[51] This chapter seems to be the only published indication of Spitzer's views on the validity of psychoanalytic thought on the eve of his becoming head of the DSM-III Task Force. In an extensive critique of DSM-II, he declared that "some students of psychiatric classification have challenged the entity status of the neuroses, claiming that they are, in reality, nothing more than symptom complexes."[52] He went on to inveigh against psychoanalytic "tradition, training, and rhetoric" (p. 836) and rebutted the psychoanalytic interpretation of anxiety (pp. 841–842). The Wash. U. influence on Spitzer is evident (pp. 835–836.)[53] The chapter appeared at the same time that Spitzer began publicizing the work of the Task Force—hardly enough time for any outside conclusions to be drawn. Moreover, psychodynamically oriented psychiatrists would not have been interested in the subject of classification in psychiatry and unlikely to read a textbook chapter on the subject.

Spitzer began to present some of his thoughts on neurosis publicly after the Task Force had been working for about a year. John Talbott, the New York District Branch delegate to the APA Assembly, wrote to Spitzer, on behalf of some of his constituents, about the "eliminat[ion]of neurosis and psychosis" from the nosology.[54] Spitzer replied: "I am delighted that the District Branch is critically evaluating our work....We have eliminated neurosis and psychosis as a categorizing principle [although not] specific subtypes of neurosis and psychosis."[55] The controversy over Spitzer's decision about neurosis was to prompt a battle that continued right up to the moment of the APA Assembly of Delegates' vote on May 12, 1979, on whether or not to accept the new DSM-III.

THE MULTI-AXIAL DIAGNOSTIC SYSTEM

As we examine in detail the substantive work of Spitzer and the Task Force in the early years, we should note a truism of Spitzer's career as the architect of DSM-III: Spitzer had thought often about various stratagems of developing a new DSM, as well as what features the revised manual should contain, long before the APA named him head of the DSM-III Task Force. One of the aspects that preoccupied him for quite some time was the desirability of a diagnostic system that would present a multidimensional picture of the patient and his or her disorder, the totality of the individual's problems, as it were. Such a picture, he argued, could lead the psychiatrist to a more knowledgeable plan of treatment and to a realistic prognosis. Moreover, the multiaxial system that debuted in DSM-III was one of the innovations that pleased Spitzer the most. In an interview a few months after the APA hierarchy had approved DSM-III he was asked, "What do you think are the three biggest changes from DSM–II to DSM-III?" He began his answer by immediately naming the multiaxial patient evaluation system. (The other two changes were implementing diagnostic criteria and redefining schizophrenia.)[56]

Spitzer had a tradition to draw from; the multidimensional concept was far from original with him. The modern roots of the idea go back at least to the period right after World War II. Erik Essen-Möller, a Swedish psychiatrist, proposed a three-part evaluation system, but it was never widely accepted.[57] The notion of a multivariable diagnosis, however, did enter general medicine substantively in 1964 when the New York Heart Association drew up just this kind of system for the diagnosis of heart disease.[58]

Spitzer's thinking, again before he began to lead the DSM-III Task Force, was also strongly influenced by a study that WHO had sponsored, developing a multiaxial system for children.[59] Of two psychiatrists who reported on this WHO study, Spitzer appointed one as a special consultant (Michael Rutter) and another (David Shaffer) to the Multiaxial Advisory Committee. Spitzer talked about the inspiration of the WHO project to an interviewer. If a child had more than one disorder in the WHO study, Spitzer pointed out, "the idea was to put these different classes of information on different axes and ...have an axis for what they called the clinical psychiatric syndrome." DSM-III came to adopt the same term—the *clinical syndrome*—for disorders such as schizophrenia, affective disorder, or organic brain syndrome—and this category became Axis I. WHO had placed children's developmental disorders on a separate axis (Axis II), which is what DSM-III did for a portion of those disorders. The DSM also placed adult personality disorders on Axis II. Ultimately, Spitzer situated any relevant physical disorder of the patient on a separate axis—Axis III—thus emulating WHO's axis for physical disorder (although an early DSM-III draft in the fall of 1976 had "Intellectual Level" on the third axis.)[60]

When Spitzer first spoke to me about the multiaxial system, he said it was created to meet the concerns that psychoanalysts had expressed when they learned what the new DSM was going to look like.[61] But it is clear that the multiaxial system had been in his mind for a long time and was not constructed to please the psychoanalysts. He may have thought that he could assuage some of their concerns with this approach, but it was not his initial motivation.

A large (ultimately 13 members) Multiaxial Advisory Committee, on which Spitzer sat, carried out the development of the various axes. The committee began meeting either in late 1974 or early 1975. The basic issues to be decided were how many axes there would be and what they would cover. The committee debated the proposals of several different psychiatrists, including one of Spitzer's own suggestions. By the winter of 1975 or spring of 1976, the decision was to have five axes for both children and adults:[62] Axes I and II were in place in accordance with the WHO decisions, but Axes III through V were tentatively assigned: Axis III for intellectual level; Axis IV for relevant nonmental medical conditions; and Axis V for severity of concurrent psychosocial stressors. This last category was the trickiest. According to handwritten notes in the Archives, possibly Spitzer's, the problems were how to categorize psychosocial factors; how to code more than one stressor and which stressor should have priority; and, most difficult of all, how to rate severity.

However, by late 1976 or early 1977, "intellectual level" was dropped, the original Axis V (psychosocial stressors) became Axis IV, nonmental medical conditions became Axis III, and a new Axis V was added: highest level of adaptive functioning during the past year. Additionally, other axes were suggested, one for etiology and another for coping styles, although the Task Force did not accept these. The debates on these two axes were intertwined with the issue of whether DSM-III should contain information desired by psychoanalysts and are discussed in the context of the ongoing clashes between the Task Force and the psychoanalysts in Chapter 11.

While the Task Force and the Multiaxial Advisory Committee were in the midst of their labors, they were supported in their decision to adopt some sort of a multi-axial system by the published work of the psychiatrist John S. Strauss. Strauss was a professor of psychiatry at the University of Rochester Medical School with an interest in severe mental illness. He also held a continuum or dimensional conception of diag-nosis and proposed a "comprehensive" diagnostic system. He advocated the "routine evaluation" of five characteristics for every patient; these characteristics had both like-nesses and differences with the eventual DSM-III system. His proposal encompassed (1) symptoms, (2) circumstances associated with symptoms, (3) previous duration and course of symptoms, (4) quality of personal relationships, and (5) level of work function. Strauss made a strong case for the advantages of multivariable diagnosis: the patient would be seen as a "whole person;" the patient would not be forced into categories that either do not fit him or her or that are too broad to be meaningful; a multiaxial approach would provide greater information for determining prognosis and etiological factors; and more data for research would be gathered.[63] Spitzer later appointed Strauss to the Multiaxial Advisory Committee.

It is worth noting that everyone who spoke in favor of a multivariable system emphasized that such a system would be of great help in making a prognosis and planning treatment. WHO itself was so impressed by the value of using a multiaxial system for children that it evinced an interest in developing a multivariable approach for diagnosing adults.[64] Thus, a multiaxial design was part of the *Zeitgeist* of psychi-atric diagnosis. The APA's decision to adopt this approach to diagnosis was made in a supportive atmosphere. Also, in an era of a strong antipsychiatry movement, another influential force for a multiaxial diagnostic system was the belief of many psychia-trists that such a system, together with diagnostic criteria, would help their field to be thought of as both medical and scientific.[65] These broad factors cannot be separated from the central role played by Spitzer's fertile mind, energy, and determination in bringing about major changes. This confluence of the role of the individual and of the times in which he or she lives is a familiar pattern in history when momentous transformation takes place.

In any event, the DSM-III multiaxial evaluation system meant that every patient should be evaluated on five axes, but only the first three formed the "official diagnostic assessment." The following are examples of possible use of the five axes:

Axis I: Clinical syndrome, e.g., 296.6x, Bipolar Disorder, Mixed
Conditions not attributable to a mental disorder that are a focus of attention or treatment, e.g., V61.10 Marital Problem
Additional codes as specified at the end of the Classification[66]
Axis II: Personality disorders, e.g., 301.2 Schizoid Personality Disorder
Specific developmental disorders (mainly for children and adolescents), e.g., 315.00 Developmental Reading Disorder
Axis III: Physical disorders and conditions, e.g., congestive heart failure

Axis IV: Severity of psychosocial stressors, e.g., loss of job = Level 5, Severe

Axis V: Highest level of adaptive functioning during the past year: Levels 1–7, e.g.,
5 = Poor.

Nevertheless, Spitzer had trepidations about introducing the multiaxial system. He was aware that others had tried such a step, but their efforts had not met with much response. Spitzer had noticed that it was difficult to get agreement on what the axes should denote, and even after DSM-III had been approved, he was concerned that busy clinicians might not use such an elaborate course of diagnosis.[67] He pointed out that he himself had proposed in 1970 that "the standard nosology be supplemented by a multidimensional classification of each patient."[68] But in his 1975 textbook chapter on classification, he expressed very guarded optimism about the potential usefulness of this 1970 proposal, both in terms of its superiority and its adoption "except [in] special research studies."[69]

Over the years, the multiaxial diagnostic system has had a mixed reaction. Initially it looked complex, and at first many used only the first three axes; clinicians sometimes failed to use the last two or give them due weight. Often insurance reimbursement required only an Axis I or Axis II diagnosis, and the third—relevant medical conditions—was not too difficult to complete, especially as it often touched on treatment. But Axes IV and V, sometimes requiring much thought and getting to know the patient, were often slighted. (In DSM-IV-TR [2000] Axis V is called Global Assessment of Functioning and often is used because insurance payment may require it since it is a measure of just how ill a given patient is.) In any event, little use or disuse is a pattern Spitzer was worried about when he proposed such an ambitious plan.

THE DEFINITION OF A MENTAL DISORDER

In addition to a multiaxial system, another of Spitzer's goals that predated his appointment to Chair of the Task Force was his desire to produce a definition of mental disorder as a subset of medical disorders. This was long the dream of the Wash. U. camp, especially Samuel Guze. Now it also had become the desire of the Board of Trustees of the APA in order to combat the antipsychiatry movement. Moreover, Melvin Sabshin, the new Medical Director, had accepted the position with the express motive of moving psychiatry back into medicine. But Spitzer faced difficulties with achieving such a definition almost from the start, for two reasons. For one thing, many psychiatrists said they did not wish to be encumbered by a stated definition that might curtail their flexibility. For another, there were a number of psychiatrists who did not agree with the stance Spitzer had enunciated during the earlier homosexual controversy, that one criterion for a valid mental disorder had to be that the individual was experiencing "subjective distress." Thus, Spitzer had asserted, if a homosexual individual had no subjective distress and was socially effective, homosexuality should not be considered pathological. (But, said many psychoanalysts, who still saw homosexuality as pathological, then neither would a fetishist or exhibitionist, satisfied with his object choice or aim, merit a psychiatric diagnosis.)

While Spitzer eventually backed down on the issue of subjective distress, he did not let up on efforts to convince his colleagues about the importance of having a definition of mental disorder as a medical disorder. Not until the American Psychological Association officially balked at the notion did Spitzer abandon his position—after a two-year battle.

The story of constructing a definition begins in the early 1970s when Spitzer had begun thinking about what constitutes a mental disorder. At that time he became involved with the question of whether or not homosexuality is a mental disorder. One of his strong motivations for removing homosexuality from the nomenclature was that he wanted to show that psychiatry was a profession that defined very clearly what was and was not a disorder. He could then combat those critics who accused psychiatrists of medicalizing social behavior and demonstrate that psychiatrists were scientists who were owed lay and professional respect. After a session at the annual meeting of the APA in 1973, on the question "Should Homosexuality be in the APA Nomenclature?" Spitzer declared:

> By creating a new category, "sexual orientation disturbance" [and removing that of homosexuality] we will no longer insist on a label of sickness for individuals who insist that they are well [i.e., have no "subjective distress"] and who demonstrate no generalized impairment in social effectiveness. We will thus help to answer the charge of some members of our own profession who claim that mental illness is a myth and [claim] that by labeling individuals with psychiatric diagnoses, we are merely acting as agents of social control.[70]

Note that Spitzer incisively entitled the proposal from which these words are excerpted "Homosexuality as an Irregular Form of Sexual Behavior [i.e., not a disorder] and Sexual Orientation Disturbance [when a homosexual person is not happy with his or her orientation] as a Psychiatric Disorder."

Spitzer outlined his plans for a definition of a mental disorder to the Task Force at their very first meeting in 1974, but discord on this subject soon grew. While Spitzer later referred to the fact that not all on the Task Force agreed with him,[71] the DSM-III Archives provide only a specific description of objections by one member, Henry Pinsker. Pinsker was a New York clinician and Vice-Chair of the Department of Psychiatry at Beth Israel Hospital. After months of discussion, Pinsker summed up his general understanding of what had transpired, as well as his personal belief, in a June 1975 memo to the entire Task Force: "I think that the diversity of opinion about the definition of mental illness is so great that we are premature in hoping to bring about closure by propounding a new definition."[72]

However, Spitzer did not let the disagreement in the Task Force impede his strong desire to fashion a definition of mental disorder. He wrote to Pinsker in February 1976 about an encyclopedia article that Pinsker and he were writing: "I do think, that, with the exception of yourself, the committee intends to have a discussion of the definition of mental disorders in DSM-III, and since the profession expects this of us, there should be some reference in the [article]."[73] Spitzer here was overstating the case with regard to the unanimity of the Task Force and the expectations of American psychiatrists. But nevertheless, determined to win his point, he presented his definition and

views of a mental disorder before a special session at the APA annual meeting in Miami
in May 1976. Unfortunately, the Archives do not contain a copy of this 1976 definition,
but refer to the end notes to see Spitzer's 1975 and 1977 definitions of mental disorder (which were quite dissimilar from each other.)[74] The response of his colleagues in
Miami in 1976 surprised him:

> For the most part, to our chagrin, the reaction was negative. Some questioned the
> need and wisdom of having any definition. Many argued that the definition pro-
> posed was too restrictive, and if officially adopted, would have the potential for
> limiting the appropriate activities of our profession and would redefine the major
> educational activities of psychiatry; they also felt that it was out of keeping with
> trends in medicine that emphasize the continuity of health and illness. Furthermore,
> some questioned our claim that the definition that we proposed was actually help-
> ful in making decisions regarding the nomenclature. Rather, it was argued, deci-
> sions were made and then the definition tinkered with to justify them.
>
> It now seems unlikely [Spitzer continued] that any proposed definition will be
> found generally acceptable to the profession.... We also recognize that it is not pos-
> sible or useful to sharply define the boundaries between disorder and "normality,"
> as we had originally intended.[75]

(Defining sharp boundaries, of course, is what he ended up doing.)[76]

When Spitzer appointed the well-known family therapist and schizophrenia
researcher Lyman Wynne (1923–2007) to the Task Force in July 1976, he joked that
Wynne had "distinguished himself by being one of the few members of the psychiatric
profession to have found my attempt with Jean Endicott to define mental disorder,
useful."[77]

Yet despite the clear rejection at the Miami meeting, Spitzer reversed his initial acceptance of his colleagues' negative reactions. He decided to try again the next year before
a different psychiatric audience—one more attuned to research—with a reworked definition. This attempt will be discussed in a later chapter, as Spitzer mounted one more
presentation on the need for psychiatrists to situate their profession medically as a
means of counterattacking the antipsychiatry movement. Simultaneously, at that exact
time, he was doing battle with the psychologists over the question of whether a mental
disorder would be defined as a medical disorder. Spitzer did not surrender easily.

"SUBJECTIVE DISTRESS"

For the present, let us investigate the fate of the notion of "subjective distress." Spitzer's
changing positions about subjective distress constitute a major part of his focus during
the first year and a half of his chairmanship of the Task Force.

The topic of the necessity of subjective distress in the development of a definition
of a mental disorder first arose in connection with the question of whether homosexuality was a pathological disorder that should be listed under the "Paraphilias" (a term
that replaced "Sexual Deviations").[78] When Spitzer proffered to the APA in 1973 the

compromise diagnosis of "sexual orientation disturbance" to replace "homosexuality," he argued that as long as a homosexual individual experienced no distress about his or her homosexuality and functioned effectively in society, homosexuality could not be considered a disorder. If a homosexual individual *was* distressed about his or her sexuality, then the person could be given the diagnosis of sexual orientation disturbance, which was a disorder. This is a piece of Spitzer's continued attempt to show that psychiatrists went about defining a mental disorder scientifically and were not bent on social control of homosexuals, as some critics alleged.

Those psychiatrists who considered homosexuality to be a mental disorder argued against the notion that subjective distress should be considered a requisite for a psychiatric diagnosis. They pointed to the existence of many sexual deviations in which often the individual practicing them was not at all distressed but still these practices were considered pathological. (DSM-III listed as paraphilias fetishism, transvestism, zoophilia, pedophilia, exhibitionism, voyeurism, sexual masochism, and sexual sadism.)

Spitzer began his tenure as Chair of the Task Force on Nomenclature and Statistics adamantly refusing to designate as pathological a case of sexual deviance where there was no subjective distress. But gradually, over a span of about one and a half years, he shifted his position. He did this at first privately, until finally he made a pronouncement to a large number of individuals that the Task Force had never taken the stance that subjective distress was required for a diagnosis of pathology. We can see the evolution of his responses in his letters.

Even after the removal of the diagnosis of homosexuality in DSM-II in 1974, many psychiatrists continued to argue against the idea of requiring subjective distress in sexual deviance and wrote to Spitzer to protest. Some of them were energized to do so either by Spitzer's presentation at the May 1975 APA meeting or the June 4, 1975, article in *Psychiatric News*. For example, a psychiatrist who was also an analyst objected to Spitzer: "I learn that further changes are contemplated for DSM-III which remove from consideration as pathological behavior more categories of sexual behavior....You cannot make pathology go away by removing its label."[79] (Not at all atypical for him, Spitzer wrote him back two days later in a friendly tone: "Thank you for [your] candor....I hope that you will continue to critically examine our work and continue to make your views known.")[80] Another letter writer said he felt "ashamed for psychiatry; I am fearful we will be the laughing stock of our scientific colleagues."[81] But Spitzer clung to his position that sexual deviance was not pathological if there was no subjective distress.[82]

Spitzer let this decision guide him when he dealt concurrently with the issue of whether racism would be a diagnosis in DSM-III. On June 24, 1975, Charles B. Wilkinson, a prominent black psychiatrist in Kansas City, MO, wrote to Spitzer that he had learned about the revision of the DSM at a meeting of the Executive Committee of the APA and was "somewhat concerned [to learn that] no consideration [was being] given for an inclusion of racism in the diagnostic criteria."[83] Spitzer, although condemning racism in a warm and sympathetic letter, explained his decision. He asked Wilkinson to "understand our rationale [that] the racist is not necessarily in either distress or having difficulty with his general functioning, even though he makes others miserable....In DSM III we are using [such] a definition of mental disorder."[84] Six months later the Committee of Black Psychiatrists wrote to Spitzer about including racism as a mental disorder, and he had the same reply: "With our current working definition racism would not meet the criteria for a mental disorder since it is only in certain environments that it is associated with distress."[85]

Yet the same fall, after being approached by John A. Talbott, representing the New York APA District Branch, to answer a question on the definition of a mental disorder posed by one of the members, Spitzer informed Talbott confusingly:

> We have never [sic!] operated on the assumption that for a condition to be a mental disorder it must be accompanied by subjective distress. In the tentative definition of a mental disorder that I have proposed, subjective distress is merely one of the requirements for a condition to be considered a mental disorder. I recognize that the main problem here has to do with the classification of sexual disorders. Our committee is working in this area and expects to have a revised classification within the month..... I believe that this newer classification will be more acceptable than our previous attempts.[86]

Clearly, some members of the New York District Branch had questions about Spitzer's stance that there was no pathology if there was no subjective distress. But Spitzer's efforts to reassure them are very curious. As can be seen from the first two sentences in the above quotation, they completely contradict each other. The first is the *opposite* of his usual position of requiring subjective distress for a pathological diagnosis, and the second *is* his usual position that distress is "one of the requirements for a condition to be considered a mental disorder." This total confusion is difficult to understand unless we see it as an indication that Spitzer was beginning to bow to the continued pressure of the APA membership.

Soon after Talbott had written him, Spitzer received two letters from psychoanalytic organizations castigating him for his "unscientific" position, "unworthy of our profession." Requiring subjective distress as a measure of somatic disorders "would be ludicrous and/or harmful," opined one. Should we abolish the diagnoses of epilepsy or tuberculosis "unless the patient is willing to accept them as illnesses when applied to him," queried another.[87] Several weeks later (January 29, 1976), Spitzer replied to both letters in almost identical lengthy, conciliatory letters:

> For a relatively brief period of time, our position was that the sexual deviations were only to be considered mental disorders when associated with distress....This is no longer our position. We have added to our proposed criteria for a mental disorder the concept of disadvantage. If a condition, although not associated with distress or disability, is associated with disadvantage to the individual in coping with unavoidable aspects of the environment, then that condition is to be considered a mental disorder. A medical analogy would be color blindness.
>
> With this conception of a mental disorder, we do not believe that homosexuality per se meets the criteria for a mental disorder, but all of the remaining traditional sexual deviations do.

We hope that you will continue to critically evaluate [our work] so that we may further modify it to make it of maximum value to our profession.[88]

Then Spitzer cast in stone this private communication with a wider pronouncement in a "Progress Report" on the Task Force's work that was issued two months later in March 1976. Here he argued, not entirely accurately, that there had been "a widespread misunderstanding" of the "principles" by which the Task Force defined what constituted a mental disorder. "The most common misunderstanding is the assumption that the Task Force believes that acknowledged subjective distress is a requirement for a condition to be considered a mental disorder."[89]

A dramatic event occurring two months later was the denouement to the evolution of the applicability of "subjective distress." The charged incident was the highly negative response to Spitzer's proposed definition of a mental disorder at the 1976 Miami APA meeting, including formidable disagreement with his stance on subjective distress; both blows shook him powerfully. No sooner had he returned from Miami than he sent a memo to the members and consultants of the "Sex Subcommittee" (Advisory Committee on Psychosexual Disorders) with the subject "Implications of changed definition of mental disorder." The memo, along with two related memos, will be quoted almost verbatim because of their importance. The reader should consider the situation: Spitzer had maintained, just a few years earlier, that if a homosexual individual experienced no subjective distress or had no impairment in social effectiveness or functioning, that person did not have a pathological condition. This was the basis for the controversial removal of homosexuality as a disorder from the DSM, which had upset so many psychiatrists. Now—seemingly abruptly, although not actually so—Spitzer was about to definitively change his mind about sexual deviance with a new concept of "disadvantage," although still excluding homosexuality:

We have come to the conclusion [he informed the "Sex Subcommittee" on May 28, 1976] that we needlessly restricted the definition by requiring distress for the sexual dysfunctions.

One of the criteria that we have had for a long time [sic] has been the notion of disadvantage. [This concept] can be applied to any condition characterized by the inability to experience pleasure in situations that ordinarily are associated with pleasure.[90] With this formulation, the lack of sexual pleasure during sexual activity would meet the requirements for a mental disorder, whether or not it is associated with distress.

We are changing our position on this issue, not only because it is politically the wiser thing to do, but because we also believe that it makes sense. (Italics added.) This does not mean, of course, that every woman (or man) who derives no pleasure from sexual activity needs to be in treatment.

I hope that this revision, and its implications for defining the categories of sexual disorders, meets with your approval. Assuming that it does, this revision will have to be explained to the participants at the St. Louis [June 1976 Midstream] conference.[91]

Although at the Midstream Conference someone on the "Sex Subcommittee" referred to this memo and reported that "the issue of distress had been clarified immediately prior to the conference,"[92] the Committee did not in truth approve of Spitzer's change of heart. The month *after* the St. Louis conference Spitzer informed the Task Force and members of the Childhood and Adolescence Advisory Committee:

> As many of you know, our Sexual Disorders Subcommittee [Spitzer's underlining] has quite an independent spirit. I was so successful in convincing them that a sexual dysfunction was only a mental disorder when accompanied by subjective distress, that I am now unable to convince them otherwise, although my own views have changed. I believe that both for scientific and political reasons we are in a very bad position if we claim that lack of sexual pleasure of any kind is only a mental disorder when accompanied by distress. The capacity for sexual pleasure [Spitzer argued][93] is an orgasmic function, and its absence clearly represents a dysfunction which puts the individual at a disadvantage, compared to those individuals who do not have such a condition. I would like to be able to tell the Sexual Disorders Subcommittee that their own views on this matter must gracefully bow to the considered judgment of the Task Force [underlining in the original].
>
> Unless I hear from any of you to the contrary, I will assume that you support me in this decision [original underlining].[94]

Within the next eleven days, Spitzer cobbled together an agreement on this issue working with a member of the Sexual Disorders Subcommittee and a member of the Childhood and Adolescence Subcommittee. He recorded that "it was agreed that Sexual Orientation Disorder [original underlining] would remain a category only to be used for individuals who are distressed by their homosexual feelings." Spitzer and his colleagues also decided that individuals distressed by their homosexual feelings would not bear a diagnosis of "Sexual Orientation Disorder" but some other designation. The "Sex" Subcommittee and Task Force's decisions involving nondistressful homosexuality and the exact wording of a diagnosis for homosexuals with distress will be discussed in Chapter 10, since the relevant debate (actually a furor) took place mainly in 1977, after the key Midstream Conference.[95] Once the very open airing of the proposed DSM-III took place at this meeting, Spitzer and the Task Force were plunged into even greater activity.

This chapter has presented almost all of the issues occurring at the start of the DSM-III Task Force's work. As Spitzer and the Task Force began their assignment, there immediately cropped up a potpourri of situations that grabbed their attention as they organized themselves and launched into making decisions. Spitzer, in particular, assessed his mandate from the APA's Board of Trustees, planned a multiaxial diagnostic system, forecast the use of specific diagnostic criteria to improve reliability, and removed "neurosis" as a diagnostic category. He also attempted to define "mental disorder," which proved a rocky path, and the issue of subjective distress roughened it even further. Then he began to ponder a renaming of "sexual disturbance disorder" as a diagnosis for homosexuals unhappy with their sexual orientation. The issue of homosexuality in the nosology, supposedly settled, now raised its head again.

Whatever publicity there had been about Spitzer's objectives and about the decisions made by the Task Force in the early months of their work did provoke rejoinders, but they were basically isolated ones. The "DSM-III in Midstream" Conference, however, brought together about one hundred leaders in American and foreign psychiatry, psychoanalysis, and psychology, both researchers and clinicians. Here controversy erupted immediately, and organized reactions soon followed. Spitzer threw himself completely into the task of confronting the challenges to his revolutionary vision.

8

A SNAPSHOT IN TIME:
DSM-III IN MIDSTREAM, 1976

It is time to take a step back to examine what DSM-III looked like as it was developing and to learn about the major concerns of the psychiatric and related professions as they found out about its philosophy and contents. We will embark, so to speak, on a short voyage to chart a not yet fully discovered coastline and inland territories. After a year and a half of the Task Force's work on a new manual, what had been decided and achieved? What was still unsettled? What disorders had the Task Force focused on? What were the leaders in the field learning? What was the wider profession finding out? With regard to the latter, how was Spitzer trying to educate them and convert them to his ways of thinking? What impact was the new information having on its potential users?

Among Spitzer's plethora of goals, we know he had three overriding ones. He wanted to increase diagnostic precision—reliability—for two reasons: to enable researchers to go about their work with greater accuracy and to burnish the reputation of psychiatry among other physicians, many of whom regarded psychiatry with disdain. Diagnostic criteria and an empirically and descriptively based manual, he believed, would help accomplish those goals. A related aim was to combat the antipsychiatry movement by establishing firmly that mental disorders were medical disorders. The precisely right definition of a mental disorder, he hoped, would diminish the attacks—coming now from all quarters—on the psychiatric profession. Finally, he wanted to decrease the panoply of schizophrenia diagnoses, a runaway phenomenon in American psychiatry. The truth of this situation had been firmly established by the U.S.-U.K. study that showed that American psychiatrusts diagnosed an overwhelming number of patients as schizophrenic, while in the United Kingdom similar patients were largely diagnosed as manic-depressive or bipolar.

In 1976, Spitzer chose three ways to educate psychiatrists, psychoanalysts, and psychologists what he was about: the first was the Midstream Conference in June for leaders of these fields; the second for the wider psychiatric profession was an article in *Psychiatric Annals* (a continuing education journal) in September; and the third was a symposium for experts in November and its publication for a larger audience several months later. Spitzer wanted to educate broadly, in every possible venue.

The catalytic Midstream meeting in June was jointly sponsored by the University of Missouri Department of Psychiatry at the Missouri Institute of Psychiatry and the American Psychiatric Association through the Task Force on Nomenclature and

Statistics. The desire for the conference first arose with psychiatrists at the Missouri Institute of Psychiatry, who suggested early in the Task Force's existence that they and the Task Force have a meeting to discuss issues concerning the standardization of psychiatric concepts, a topic that concerned them both. Spitzer was agreeable, and after a while, he also wanted an effective way to publicize the work he and the Task Force were engaged in, "in order to obtain feedback from the psychiatric profession." He and the Missouri Institute came to agree "that there was a more immediate need to specifically discuss plans for DSM-III, which certainly would involve an attempt to standardize a very substantial segment of psychiatric concepts and descriptors."[1] Concrete planning for the meeting started in June 1975 in anticipation of a meeting a year later. The University of Missouri agreed to fund the conference.[2]

THE "PROGRESS REPORT" OF MARCH 1976: THE FIRST PUBLIC DRAFT OF DSM-III

As a prelude to the Midstream meeting, Spitzer and the Task Force issued in March 1976 a 325-page, double-spaced, typewritten manuscript "Progress Report on the Preparation of DSM-III," which was sent to all of the conference's ninety-one participants. They represented a wide variety of academic institutions, professional societies and groups, the NIMH, and some individuals preeminent in their fields. Those invited included at least seven psychoanalysts and at least seven psychodynamically oriented psychiatrists (fifteen percent total), although it is obvious that the majority of the attendees were predominantly interested in research. All participants were requested to prepare written comments, criticisms, and suggestions in response to the "Progress Report," which would then be circulated among them before the actual meeting.

The "Progress Report" had been put together by thirty-one contributors drawn from members of the Task Force, the Advisory Committees on particular areas, and special consultants. The report specified as contributors the current eleven members of the Task Force (eventually the Task Force numbered eighteen), the members of the six participating Advisory Committees (eventually there were fourteen of these committees), and sixteen Special Consultants. It was explained that the full Task Force had met only twice because many issues were resolved by telephone and mail, and that the bulk of the work was done by the Advisory Committees, which consisted of Task Force members and other experts, aided by special outside consultants.

Spitzer reported that he presided at all of the Advisory Committee meetings and added that he "spent considerable time personally answering letters from an assortment of friendly, irate, outraged, and supportive (a distinct minority) psychiatrists."[3] In addition, he reported on the "innovative features" of the manual: a definition of a mental disorder, very extensive descriptions of all the disorders, operational criteria for most of the disorders, a glossary defining all key diagnostic terms (e.g., "thought disorder"), and references from the research literature.

The report also contained the latest classification of DSM-III, discussions of the nosological issues in diagnosing each of fourteen main categories of disorders, and drafts of the actual texts and operational criteria included in DSM-III (which varied in completeness). The report concluded with a lengthy section, "Proposed Definition of Medical and Psychiatric Disorders," which included a twenty-seven-page "Rationale" and a two-page "Definition." Those invited to the St. Louis meeting were asked to address all of these various sections with their written critiques.

THE CONFERENCE CONVENES IN JUNE 1976: THE FIRST GENERAL SESSION

The Midstream meeting offers a revealing look at the vital issues, hotly held positions, and distinct, personal ways of strategy and behavior that became the concerns and challenges faced by Spitzer and the Task Force over the course of the next three years. A chronicling of the meeting also allows us to examine aspects of Spitzer's style of dealing with opposition.

A prestigious group of American psychiatrists, plus some from England and Canada, and a few research psychologists gathered in St. Louis at the Hilton Hotel, June 10–11, 1976.[4] After welcoming remarks from officials of the two sponsoring organizations, Spitzer extended greetings and declared that the Task Force had come to the conference to explain what they had accomplished to date and then to listen to and learn from the participants so that DSM-III would be a document of compromise "that would help unify the profession." He added that "there was no desire to force DSM-III onto the profession." The Task Force was there to help American psychiatrists "and this particularly included the practitioners." He discussed the matters of the definition of a mental disorder and the multiaxial system, the latter as a way "to bring back more psychosocial concepts into DSM-III." He stated also that the Task Force wanted to be conservative in not overstating knowledge concerning course and prevalence of a disorder if those areas lacked "adequate evidence."[5] Obviously, Spitzer recognized that he had to conciliate various constituencies.

Next on the agenda was a General Session where persons prominent in the field of diagnosis and classification and individuals representing professional organizations delivered brief talks summarizing their written responses to the "Progress Report." Several of the leading figures we have met in past chapters spoke on their well-known, habitual themes. Samuel Guze made a brief for one of the Wash. U. pet positions, that of giving many patients the diagnosis of "undiagnosed," since he maintained that many patients and illnesses could not be classified. This would result in greater acceptance of the diagnostic classification in DSM-III, Guze argued. He concluded by stating his "hesitan[cy] about deriving a general definition of disease."[6] Eli Robins even thought it a "fruitless task" to try to define a mental disorder but spoke in favor of "typology" (discrete categories) rather than "dimensions" (the concept of a continuum or spectrum) in classification and lauded the use of diagnostic criteria. John S. Strauss praised a multiaxial system as a way to bring more psychosocial concepts into DSM-III because the "Progress Report" had "tended to downgrade the psychodynamic schools." Nevertheless, he was concerned that some groups might not be ready for the multiaxial approach and advised putting it in an appendix for the time being. Joseph

Zubin, Spitzer's chief at the New York State Psychiatric Institute (PI), like others, "questioned the need" for a definition of mental illness. His main concern was improving the validity (the accuracy and veracity) of a diagnosis and thus wanted more studies to determine etiologies. We can round out the familiar names whose opinions were solicited for the General Session with the remarks of Gerald Klerman and Donald Klein. Klerman, insightful as usual, pointed out very clearly various problematic areas, so let us return to him when concluding this section. Klein made a sympathetic argument for the multiaxial approach, declaring it would allow for describing the patient's various aspects and make for better patient care. Yet he could not resist adding, in a sardonic vein, that he knew if he urged such an approach solely on the basis of arriving at a better diagnosis he would not be able to convert clinicians [7]

Toward the end of the General Session, new figures made their entrance, giving us a view into areas where they and Spitzer would lock horns right until the crucial moment when DSM-III was on the agenda for approval by the APA Assembly of Delegates. The psychoanalysts and their many dynamically oriented adherents spoke up, expressing their dissatisfaction and concerns with the path being taken by DSM-III. Two well-known analysts, Paul Chodoff (1914–2011), representing the American Academy of Psychoanalysis, and Silvano Arieti (1914–1981, editor of a famous textbook, *American Handbook of Psychiatry*), argued that psychiatrists did not only treat medical conditions.[8] Where was there provision for all the patients of psychoanalysts and psychotherapists, they asked? It seemed, they asserted, that the only category that could be used to diagnose these patients was "personality disorder—other." Psychiatry was about to return to a "predynamic era," the analysts prophesized. Psychoanalyst Everett Dulit (d. 2010) was "distressed" about what DSM-III meant for adolescent psychiatry, "where there are few hard edges," so that a "dynamic perception" was necessary. Repeatedly in the analysts' remarks was the charge that the Task Force was ignoring psychiatrists at large and the worry that third-party payers would no longer pay for some psychiatric diagnoses and treatments. A representative of the American Psychoanalytic Association called for "a liaison committee between the psychoanalytic groups and the Task Force."[9]

The analysts were not the only ones with fears. Spitzer's efforts to frame the definition of mental disorder as a medical disorder were challenged by the President of the American Psychological Association, Maurice Lorr (1922–1998). His argument was blunt: mental disorders "have psychological and social origins and...many other disorders have no known psysiological [sic] base." He was concerned that "since there is an implication that those disorders are diseases, social workers, psychologists, and educators lack the training and skills to diagnose, treat, or manage such disorders."[10] Spitzer also later recalled that Lorr had "expressed the view that mental disorders (as medical disorders) should be limited to those conditions for which a biological etiology or pathophysiology could be demonstrated."[11] Thus Spitzer, in his final remarks, assured Lorr that "the Task Force definition of medical includes all mental health workers."[12] Having in mind that he wished to establish that a mental disorder is a subset of a medical disorder, in order to fight the antipsychiatry movement, Spitzer was at pains not to antagonize the psychologists.

Gerald Klerman, who listened carefully, had a clear ear for professional worries of both the analysts and the psychologists. "Psychiatrists need to face the issue," he advised, "of whether or not to include categories which we may feel are real entities, but for which we have no data. We also need to face the issue that psychologists may feel we are preempting their field."[13]

The editors who later wrote the official "Summary of the Conference" sought to soothe fears. Their view was that there had been "considerable consensus" at the General Session on six points: (1) the purpose of DSM-III was to be of assistance to the profession, not just to facilitate academic research; (2) there should be compatibility with WHO's ICD-9 (then being drafted); (3) the classification systems had to be a product of many compromises; (4) there was no need "to define the broad concept of mental illness;" (5) there should be "adequate discussion and experimentation" before implementing DSM-III; and (6) the multiaxial approach should be eventually adopted "to include psychosocial variables."[14] This written summary was conciliatory. We might remember these six points as our story proceeds. To what extent did the Task Force end up implementing them?

Yet despite this "considerable consensus," Spitzer, Strauss, and others concluded at the end of the General Session that the subject of a multiaxial system needed further advocacy. Spitzer was already deeply committed to this system, so education of the conference participants was vital. Thus, a one-hour Ad Hoc Plenary Session on multiaxial concepts was scheduled for later in the afternoon. Strauss opened the session by pointing to the greater reliability and improved prognosis such a system would probably bring. John K. Wing, an English psychiatrist who had been a pioneer in devising structured interviews, discussed the possible aspects of the patient's life and illness that a multiaxial system could cover. An analyst, Dane G. Prugh (1918–1990), spoke from the floor. He praised "multiple axes" but reopened the topic of "the psychodynamic approach" and lambasted DSM-III's "discarding of the concepts of psychosis and neurosis." After hearing this, Spitzer quickly returned to the merits of the multiaxial approach, mentioning once more that the axes should include "a psychosocial axis so that social stresses could be given greater prominence."[15]

WORKSHOPS OF THE ADVISORY COMMITTEES

Over the two days of the conference, breakout workshops were hosted on six of the broad diagnostic categories being addressed by the DSM-III Advisory Committees: Schizophrenia, Personality Disorders, Childhood and Adolescent Disorders, Mood Disorders, Sexual Disorders, and Organic Mental Disorders. The members of these Advisory Committees had published very little based on the work going on in their meetings. Accordingly, these workshops provide both a conduit into the actual issues being debated at the on-going meetings of the committees as well as the concerns of other psychiatrists who were attending the workshops in St. Louis. Moreover, examination of the issues raised in the workshop discussions provides an excellent introduction to some of the basic conundrums of revising a classification and a nomenclature's impact on patient care. After the Midstream Conference, primed by their experiences at the meeting, the Task Force and the Advisory Committees dug ever deeper into the diagnostic problems that had been raised. We will return to some of these in the coming chapters.

The workshop discussions below are based on the edited "Summary Report" of all the events at the conference. The "Workshop Reports" section of this large report in turn rests on accounts from the recorders at each of the workshops. Thus there is very limited recapture of the actual give-and-take in any given workshop.

Before we turn to examining the discussions individually, it must be pointed out that in four of the six workshops the issues of the "disenfranchisement" of dynamic psychiatrists and the elimination of neurosis as a categorizing principle were again raised. The current DSM-II included a separate section entitled "NEUROSES." This large category of neuroses in DSM-II included the following: Anxiety Neurosis, Hysterical Neurosis, Phobic Neurosis, Obsessive Compulsive Neurosis, Depressive Neurosis, Neurasthenic Neurosis, Depersonalization Neurosis, Hypochondrical Neurosis, and Other Neurosis. The treatment of these nine conditions was the bread and butter of psychodynamic psychiatrists and psychoanalysts. Of these diagnoses, Depressive Neurosis (sometimes called Neurotic Depression) was used especially frequently.[16] However, the abandonment of this section of the classification was part of the radical philosophical revision of American psychiatry that Spitzer was proposing. Spitzer's varied attempts to achieve the transformation of psychiatry played out in negotiations between the Task Force and other constituencies during the three years after the Midstream meeting.

We will now deal sequentially with the workshops, starting with the one on Schizophrenia. Two basic questions were raised:

1. What should be the symptoms that qualify an individual for the diagnosis of schizophrenia, and how long must they last before they can be judged relevant? (The duration of illness is important because people who are not schizophrenic can present with short-lived psychotic symptoms. An example would be a brief psychotic state as part of Borderline Personality Disorder. These issues were also significant because schizophrenia and affective disorders share many symptoms. However, schizophrenia usually has a worse prognosis than that of mood disorders, and there is usually a greater stigma attached to a diagnosis of schizophrenia.)
2. What are the subtypes of schizophrenia? (Schizophrenia was often overdiagnosed in the United States in the 1960s and 1970s, so one of Spitzer's goals for DSM-III was to reduce schizophrenia diagnoses by cutting the number of subcategories, for example, "borderline" or "simple" schizophrenia.) After the Midstream Conference "confusional" schizophrenia was also removed from the draft classification.[17]

Next, at the Personality Disorders Workshop, the following issues were discussed:

1. How do we deal with the fact that personality disorders are "fuzzy at the edges?" Pathology shades into normal problems of everyday life. Related is the question of how one distinguishes personality "disorders," which are pathological, from everyday personality "traits." These questions logically lead to the next point.

2. Is it possible in diagnosing personality disorders to have a diagnostic axis focusing on distinctions along a continuum (spectrum) of severity of impairment extending into normality (such as with high blood pressure, for example)? Of course, the spectrum concept does not easily lend itself to diagnoses based on discrete subdivisions, which were being espoused for DSM-III. Even if there were a spectrum, would such an axis be used by busy practitioners? (How to employ the spectrum concept to construct Personality Disorders diagnoses has been an important issue for the makers of DSM-5.)

3. Is there such an entity as Borderline Personality Disorder (BPD)? This was a hotly debated issue because of disagreements over whether there should be even a conception of "borderline" anything. See Chapter 9 for an account of how Spitzer and the Task Force approached this subject. (Today, BPD has taken on the mantel of a clear-cut diagnosis, especially in the context of early abuse.)

4. How should the clash be resolved between researchers, who wanted only categories supported by research evidence, and clinicians, who wanted categories frequently seen in everyday practice? Clinicians, especially analysts and psychodynamically oriented professionals, argued that if personality diagnoses were eliminated (a consideration for a while in 1976), how could they get paid by insurance companies for treating their "neurotic" patients who suffered from personality disorders such as Compulsive Personality Disorder? Another aspect of the researcher–clinician clash was that Personality Disorders had been put on a separate axis (Axis II) in the "Progress Report" draft. (This arrangement was finalized in DSM-III. Spitzer argued that he put these disorders on a separate axis so they would not be overlooked if the patient presented with both a florid Axis I diagnosis, such as schizophrenia, but had an underlying personality disorder.)

A result of the Midstream Conference was that the name "labile" personality disorder was changed to "impulsive" personality disorder in the draft classification. But the "impulsive" category never appeared in DSM-III.

At the Childhood Disorders Workshop, there was unanimous agreement that a multiaxial diagnostic system would be very welcome, but there was consensus on little else. Sample concerns were as follows:

1. What diagnostic labels would enable family psychotherapists to be reimbursed by third-party payers?

2. What would be the acceptance of the new diagnosis of "Infantile Autism?" (Childhood and Adolescent Disorders were greatly expanded in DSM-III.)

3. Some participants asked that an adolescent "identity confusion" diagnosis be provided, but this diagnosis did not appear in DSM-III.

4. Some argued that there was also a need for a "Core Gender Identity" disorder. (Psychoanalysts had identified eighteen months to three years as the period when core gender identity was set. A category for Gender Identity Disorders (GID) appeared in DSM-III under Psychosexual Disorders. GID will be removed from

DSM-5 to be replaced by "Gender Dysphoria," which most regard as a positive step toward respect for transgendered individuals.)
After the Midstream Conference, the list of childhood and adolescent disorders grew further.

The discussion in the Workshop on Mood Disorders was lengthy. Moreover, members of the Childhood and Adolescent Disorders Workshop joined the session.

1. An immediate topic for discussion was on the name "Mood Disorders." Should it be "Affective Disorders"? There was much debate. Spitzer, who was present at the workshop, offered a compromise, which was accepted: use the name "Affective Disorders" but stress in the text "that a central clinical feature is a pervasive disturbance in emotion or mood."
2. Should the terms *unipolar* and *bipolar* be used in reference to episodic (recurring) Affective Disorders? *Unipolar* perturbed some therapists because to them the term carried an implication of biological etiology, so the term was dropped.
3. What term should be used to designate patients who do not have episodic mood disorders? There was no closure on this question because to some participants various terms carried etiological connotations. There was so much concern about this issue that the workshop returned to discuss it at the end of the session, but there was still no agreement. The resolution of this diagnostic matter was seen as "the major problem" confronting the Affective Disorders Advisory Committee. (Ultimately, DSM-III had a category of Major Affective Disorders, which was subdivided into Bipolar Disorder [mixed, manic, or depressed] and Major Depression [single episode or recurrent]).
4. Under what broad category should children and adolescents with depressive symptoms be classified: Childhood Disorders or Affective Disorders? (This issue reached a dramatic stage a decade ago with the controversial use by some psychiatrists of the diagnosis of Bipolar Disorder in young children.)
5. Similar to the disagreement over criteria for Personality Disorders, should the nomenclature for Affective Disorders be limited to those diagnoses for which there are "data and agreement," or "include other categories that clinicians feel comfortable using but for which there is less data and less consensus?" (We will see that Spitzer ultimately opted for the latter when he decided on the policy of inclusiveness for diagnoses that were important for clinicians in their daily practices.) This topic is dealt with further in Chapters 9 and 10. The commitment to inclusiveness was an important philosophical decision that Spitzer made, to the dismay of the Wash. U. psychiatrists. The decision has had an impact on the DSMs ever since.

The discussion at the Workshop on Sexual Disorders was also very lengthy. Much debate revolved around decisions regarding the best category in which to situate sexual disorders since they were often intertwined with other disorders.

1. There was an announcement that the diagnosis of "Gender Role Disorder", although prepared by the Sex Advisory Committee, would henceforth be listed under Childhood and Adolescent Disorders. But "Gender Identity Disorder" ultimately appeared under Psychosexual Disorders in DSM-III.
2. There was a report on Spitzer's announcement to remove the criterion of "subjective distress" as necessary to the definition of a mental disorder. This issue was discussed in Chapter 7.
3. It was stated that the Sex Advisory Committee had dropped the term "perversion" because it had acquired a pejorative connotation. A replacement name had not yet been decided upon. (Ultimately, the replacement name was " paraphilia.")
4. Various subcategories of sexual disorders in the "Progress Report" were criticized or otherwise debated. It was agreed that the text as presently conceived needed considerable revision.
5. The subject of Sexual Orientation Disorder (the diagnosis that had replaced homosexuality in DSM-II) was extensively discussed. (It is clear from the deliberation that the issue of homosexuality as pathology was still not completely resolved. A much-debated "Ego-dystonic Homosexuality" diagnosis eventually appeared in DSM-III. The fierce battle over this matter is presented in Chapter 10.)
6. "One discussant argued that [sexual] disorders which are characterized by the commission of criminal acts, should be dropped from the psychiatric nomenclature and left to the courts." It was felt that a psychiatric diagnosis should not be used in the defense of criminal acts. (Nevertheless, Pedophilia and Sexual Sadism [possibly applicable to rape] were left in DSM-III.)

Lastly, the discussion in the workshop on Organic Mental Disorders (OMD) took place over several hours. OMD was the only diagnostic category that had some definitely known etiologies.

1. It was urged that psychiatrists "avoid the use of prognostic terms, particularly those which imply irreversibility." Also, terms like *psychotic* or *nonpsychotic* should not be used.
2. The main concerns of the workshop were with clinical applications, not research.
3. Where possible, it was argued, etiology should be identified.
4. There was much discussion concerning the many types of drug reactions. (Tobacco Dependence was a new controversial category. This matter is discussed in Chapter 12.)
5. How was the term *dementia* to be used and defined? There was considerable debate about this, and the workshop kept returning to this question. "It was decided that dementia is impairment, while senile dementia is a disorder."
6. It was agreed that the multiaxial approach was "particularly valuable [in OMD] because often a biological change is influenced by social stress as well as...the appearance of concomitant physical disease."[18] (In DSM-III "concomitant physical

disease" appeared on Axis III, and "social stress" was dealt with on Axis IV. Axis III was not controversial, but Axis IV raised certain problems that are discussed in Chapter 12 in connection with the field trials.)

With these workshops, the first day of the Midstream Conference came to a close.

The Final General Session on the second day of the meeting was divided into a "Preliminary Discussion," where there were spontaneous remarks, followed by the comments of "Invited Speakers." The original plan was to have only invited speakers, but the obvious discontent of the analysts required giving them some time to speak. It was at this session that probably the psychoanalysts' most strongly worded public protest at the conference took place. Dane Prugh led off the session by expressing his "concern that the Task Force would decide on something that was not a consensus of this Conference or of the psychiatric profession in general." Prugh asserted that "he saw a tendency on the part of the Task Force to take the position that 'if you can't feel it or touch it, it doesn't exist.'" He specifically objected to the removal of the neurotic disorders and worried, like other analysts, if there would be problems with third-party payers if DSM-III remained as planned in the "Progress Report."

The Task Force responded to the challenge by the analysts. Donald Klein replied bluntly that the Task Force was trying to improve communication among psychiatrists and therefore wished to "replace terms which carry excess baggage." "Neurosis" has been removed, he declared, because it suggests an etiology, "a 'causation' common to the categories [that had been] subsumed under [that] term [e.g., depressive neurosis]."[19] The Task Force, he asserted, wanted to "reduce confusion." Jean Endicott seconded Klein's comments but in a more conciliatory fashion. The specific diagnoses that used to be placed under Neurosis would still appear, she pointed out, just assigned to other categories. It was only Neurosis as an organizing principle that had been dropped, she explained. (In DSM-III, Depressive Neurosis came to be listed under Affective Disorders as Dysthymic Disorder [or Depressive Neurosis].) There are other principles "which are more useful and less confusing," Endicott finished. Spitzer spoke up in support of her and Klein.

However, the analysts would not be stilled on the issue of neurosis. Paul Chodoff now urged the Task Force to reconsider their plan. "Neurosis" was "commonly accepted in the psychiatric community and does indicate an underlying organizing principle." Otto Kernberg (an expert about borderline personality disorder, b. 1928) added his voice. He believed that "most outpatients have some kind of neurosis" so that subcategories should be listed under that term. Neurosis was a "sound" organizing principle, and he asserted that it need not suggest etiology. At this point the opposing sides had had their say, and the session was returned to the Final General Session with the invited speakers.

The invitees included five psychiatrists and three psychologists. All were either research oriented or represented the APA or the American Psychological Association. The group included two Task Force members and two researchers from the NIMH. The analysts and those who did psychodynamically based psychotherapy were effectively sidelined. The remarks of the eight speakers were essentially complimentary. There was praise for the work done by the Task Force thus far, including the "organization and openness of the process." Worries about third-party payers, it was said, should not deter the development of DSM-III. One speaker averred that DSM-III was not all that revolutionary. It just clarified "the currently used phenomenological system," and therefore the Task Force should "go ahead full speed."

The invited speakers at this final session declared that the multiaxial system would not only make for better patient care all around, it would be especially useful in gathering information that would both predict the length of stay and the best possible treatment in inpatient facilities. DSM-III would enable a "computer supported clinical information system," and with the "greater objectivity" provided by the diagnostic criteria, diagnosis via computers could be improved. Now large-scale studies of patients could be conducted "in order to validate, test, and extend DSM-III concepts."

With regard to compatibility with ICD-9, a speaker declared that American progress was more important than international collaboration. (This belief was stated over and over again in the months to come.) Moreover, DSM-III would facilitate research on etiology and outcome of treatments and would ease the way for administrative and clinical decisions. Now what was needed, urged one of the invitees, were field trials for "de-bugging" of DSM-III and more meetings like the present one to get greater acceptance of the new manual.[20]

As the conference started to wind down, Spitzer spoke to ask for continued financial support from the APA. He stated that the conference had provided useful feedback and increased the number of people the Task Force could rely on for help. To soothe all the participants, he "noted that the clinicians are demanding that if a change is made that we be sure it is worth it [and] that the researchers" were emphasizing that there not be new categories if there is no external validity for them. He concluded by declaring that "he was pleased to see much good will at the meeting."[21] Thereupon a member of the Task Force, Morton Kramer, proposed a resolution—whether spontaneous or planned is difficult to tell—urging that things "get done." The resolution called for further work on DSM-III, the developing of the multiaxial diagnostic system, the testing of the classification before its finalization, training of potential users on how to use DSM-III, and "sufficient resources" to enable the Task Force to carry out these activities. The resolution was passed unanimously.

Following this, the analyst Paul Chodoff was allowed to speak once again before adjournment. He pointed out what was obvious to all, that the Task Force was heavily loaded with researchers and academics and had few clinicians or analysts. What was needed, Chodoff argued, was a classification system for the actual patients who come into psychiatrists' offices. While this might be more difficult to do than diagnosing inpatients, it was "critical," precisely because of third-party payers. (We have seen that this was a repeated major concern of many psychoanalysts and psychodynamically oriented therapists. They did not see how psychodynamic contact with patients lent itself to diagnosing according to precise criteria. Would the insurance companies pay on the basis of traditional psychodynamic formulations, they worried?) Then, with a brief comment from the audience, the meeting concluded.

Looking back at the St. Louis conference, it is notable that those speakers who were happy with the descriptive, nonpsychoanalytic approach being proposed for DSM-III were far more positive in their estimation of the general mood and accomplishments of the meeting than were the psychodynamically oriented individuals. These latter participants had voiced only complaints and fears and saw little good in the advocated changes for their patients or themselves.

A KEY EDUCATIONAL ARTICLE FOLLOWS
THE MIDSTREAM MEETING

Keeping with his goals of openness and the education of American psychiatrists about DSM-III, Spitzer had not only planned the Midstream Conference but also, together with a colleague, written an information-laden article that was published three months after the St. Louis meeting.[22] The article appeared in *Psychiatric Annals*, a journal devoted to continuing psychiatric education; each issue was dedicated to a particular topic of current psychiatric interest. In September 1976 it was "Classification in Psychiatric Disorders." John K. Wing, an English psychiatrist who shared many of Spitzer's concerns, was the guest editor of the issue. Wing wrote in his commentary that "DSM-III in midstream [is] a promising venture that has already won much support and may well be influential internationally when it comes to fruition."[23] This was introductory praise for Spitzer's paper.

Spitzer considered it vital to communicate to a much larger audience than he had had up to this point. He believed a paper in *Psychiatric Annals*, in an issue devoted to the subject of classification in psychiatry, would be a key communiqué. He thought it so valuable that he referred to it often and even had it reprinted within another report. (Perhaps this strategic article at last put some fire under the analysts to contact Spitzer officially about their concerns. Even though an alarmed representative of the American Psychoanalytic Association had spoken up at the Midstream Conference in June for the establishment of an analytic liaison committee to the Task Force, it was not until December(!) that the chair of such a committee telephoned Spitzer's office about setting up a meeting.[24])

Spitzer announced in the article that his plan was to have the new manual "ready for use" by January 1979 because the ICD-9 was scheduled to go into effect throughout the world by that date. With each revision of the DSM, chairs of the DSM Task Forces have had to be concerned about the compatibility of their manual with the mental disorders section of the current version of WHO's International Classification of Diseases (ICD). This has frequently been part of the impetus to revise the current version of the American DSM because the U.S. government has a treaty obligation with WHO to collect mortality and morbidity statistics using the ICD, which requires some compatibility of diagnoses.

Spitzer presented the latest draft version (revised as of August 1, 1976) of the entire proposed classification that now had the addition of the contentious diagnoses of "borderline personality disorder" as well as "identity disorder of adolescence and young adult life," called for at the Midstream meeting.[25] The classification had been developed adhering to certain principles, he reported. All categories were "data-oriented, relying heavily on observation rather than on deductions from theory" (a boot to psychoanalysis). While the ultimate aim was to group disorders on the basis of eti-ology, "when etiology is unproven, obscure, or highly controversial, the basis for the sub-classification should be anchored in shared phenomenologic and natural-history characteristics, as is done in the rest of medicine," Spitzer argued.

There were several innovative features when compared to DSM-II, Spitzer pointed out. Descriptions of the disorders would be much more extensive, and there would be "operational criteria" for most disorders that would have both inclusion and exclusion criteria.[26] A sample of operational criteria for a manic episode was provided.[27] DSM-III would also contain a glossary defining all key diagnostic terms such as *hallucination*. Although Spitzer did not explicitly say so, it is obvious that this would be another tool he hoped would increase reliability. Another new feature would be a multiaxial clas-sification; Spitzer showed proposals for specific axes that were under consideration by the Task Force.[28]

Spitzer aimed at putting the creation of a radically new manual in an ideological and philosophical context. He acknowledged that DSM-III had become the subject of "intense controversy," and he sought to answer three major criticisms. The first was that DSM-III was "antihumanistic" because operational criteria fail to do justice to the complexity of the human mind and condition. "On the contrary," he argued, "clarity is not intellectually incompatible with humanism. Furthermore, if the use of operational criteria improves the reliability and validity of the diagnostic categories, this will result in more effective and patient-oriented treatment."

The second criticism was that DSM-III abandoned the legacy of Freud because the neurotic disorders were supposedly missing from the classification. However, the neurotic disorders were really there, he asserted, just under different categories— the Affective, Anxiety, and Hysterical Disorders. (This August 1976 classification was still very preliminary, and by the end of the process "Hysterical" had been changed to "Somatoform" and "Dissociative.")[29] Spitzer explained: the neuroses had been elimi-nated as an organizational principle because the analysts declared that the neurotic process of unconscious conflict was universal. But how then, he asked, could uncon-scious conflict be used as the basis for delineating a disorder? The Task Force had not rejected "Freud's psychologic insights," he maintained, but "unfortunately, the term 'neurosis' seems to have such symbolic meaning attached to it that for some it is a shib-boleth that distracts from an informed discussion of the issues."

Lastly, Spitzer answered the criticism that DSM-III was too extreme, being really just for researchers, not for clinicians. That fear was already being addressed, said Spitzer soothingly. "The Task Force is currently developing elaborate mechanisms for field debug-ging of DSM-III in a wide variety of psychiatric settings, including community mental health centers, the offices of private practitioners, and private psychiatric hospitals."[30]

Spitzer closed on a thoughtful note. The Task Force, he reported, was often over-whelmed by the amount of interest in its work. How should one account for this ava-lanche of reaction, he asked. He believed that all of the prominent issues facing the profession—third-party payments, defining a mental disorder, the very definition of psychiatric identity after a decade of social action by psychiatrists—were impinging on the making of DSM-III. "Turbulence," he concluded, "was only to be expected."[31]

THE ELITE TORONTO SYMPOSIUM AND THE
"GUIDING PRINCIPLES" OF DSM-III

The final subject we have to investigate in this chapter is an important symposium on psychiatric diagnosis that was held at the University of Toronto just two months after the *Psychiatric Annals* article. It is valuable to examine this symposium for three reasons: (1) it provides a further philosophical and organizational update to the status of DSM-III as a result of the Midstream Conference; (2) Spitzer's paper at the symposium, on the principles guiding the development DSM-III, was considered important enough to be republished in its entirety in the first official draft of DSM-III in April 1977; and (3) the panel discussion following presentation of the formal papers at the symposium provides one of the most helpful insights into issues psychiatrists were concerned with both a generation ago and today.

This small symposium, held in November 1976, attracted eleven of the biggest names in psychiatry and specialists in classification. Spitzer was there to defend the current draft of DSM-III, seconded by two other members of the Task Force. The other eight participants were a very select group of U.S. and European figures, including some we have met before: the brilliant Roy R. Grinker, a psychiatric polymath and the founder of the *Archives of General Psychiatry*; John K. Wing, a luminary in devising structured interviews; and George Winokur of Washington University fame. Also at the meeting were Robert J. Stoller, famous in the sphere of sexual disorders, and Paul H. Wender, a prominent student of schizophrenia and attention deficit disorder. The papers and the spirited and wide-ranging panel discussion were quickly made public in book form.[32]

In his talk, "Guiding Principles of DSM-III," Spitzer reported on the Midstream Conference, explaining that it had been attended by almost one hundred individuals with expertise in various aspects of classification; several national mental health organizations had also sent representatives. As a result of the discussions, Spitzer announced, "additional diagnostic categories were added, some were deleted, and a decision was made to proceed with the development of multiaxial diagnosis." The Task Force had been expanded and "liaison committees [were] now being set up with a large number of professional organizations representing psychiatry, psychoanalysis, medicine, neurology, pediatrics, psychology and social work."[33]

Since the St. Louis meeting, five months earlier, Spitzer had become more thoughtful about the matter of producing a manual that would fit all needs, and he had made an important decision. It was still the goal of the Task Force, he announced, to develop a classification that would be useful to all in the profession—clinicians, researchers, and administrators. But now he was more forthright in recognizing that each group had "special needs which at times may conflict." Nevertheless, he asserted that the Task Force would produce a manual that would meet every group's needs. First he acknowledged that "in research settings, it is important to minimize false positives since the purpose is to study homogeneous subgroups." But

> in clinical settings it is important to minimize false negatives which would deprive patients of needed treatment. Therefore, unlike the RDC [Research Diagnostic

Criteria] and the Feighner criteria [which are documents for research] a diagnosis can be made in DSM-III when the clinician does not have sufficient information to be certain that the patient satisfies the full criteria [as long as] it appears clinically probable.[34]

Spitzer had decided that clinicians needed a manual that would contain the diagnoses important to them in their everyday work with patients. This is why he had distanced himself from the Wash. U. position, which was to include diagnoses only if they were valid and to label everything else "undiagnosed."

Yet, he maintained, DSM-III would still benefit research. He candidly admitted that

many of the newer as well as traditional categories in DSM-III have insufficient evidence of predictive validity in the sense of providing useful information for treatment assignment or outcome. [But] by providing operational definitions of the disorders [that] will permit family, treatment and outcome studies, as well as systematic inquiry into etiology, the ultimate predictive value of the DSM-III diagnoses can be determined with an accuracy heretofore impossible.[35]

Spitzer also reported in Toronto that the Task Force had still failed to come up with an acceptable definition of mental disorder. However, he pronounced, out of the Task Force's discussions on this topic an important principle had arisen. In DSM-III, a distinction would be made between what constituted mental disorders and what "are variants of human behavior outside the direct professional responsibility of the psychiatric profession." He gave three examples of such division: (1) personality "traits" would be excluded (as opposed to personality "disorders," which give persons distress or impairment in social functioning); (2) simple bereavement would not be diagnosable (DSM-5 will include bereavement as a depressive disorder in their new classification, a decision that has excited worldwide protest); (3) separate incidents of antisocial behavior would be considered human variants (as opposed to Antisocial Personality Disorder, which required not only "persistent antisocial behavior but also persistent impairment in social and occupational function.")[36] We should note that after DSM-III was published, there were many who remained unconvinced about the efforts of the Task Force to accept variance and complained of the medicalization of normal life traits or situations. In recent years there has been a spate of books on this subject, and the makers of DSM-5 have found themselves in a maelstrom of criticism over their decisions to expand the spectra of other diagnoses, in addition to that of depression.

Spitzer announced further progress on the new manual. Once the use of the multiaxial system for diagnosis had been settled upon, the Task Force would decide on five axes and what they would represent. The Toronto symposium may have been the first public proclamation of the final version. To recap: Axis I would include all mental disorders except for the personality disorders. These latter disorders plus specific developmental disorders in childhood would be found on Axis II. Axis III would list "non-mental medical disorders that are judged to be pertinent to the etiology or management of the [patient's] psychiatric disorder" that appeared on Axis I or II. Axis IV would require the clinician "to indicate the severity of one or more psychosocial stressors which [might] have contributed to the development or exacerbation of the current episode of mental disorder…on Axis I." On Axis V the clinician could record "the highest level of adaptive functioning exhibited by the patient during the past year."[37]

In addition, operational criteria had been further developed, Spitzer declared, and as an illustration he presented the sample criteria for an episode of depressive disorder. Along with the expectation that operational criteria would greatly improve reliability among practitioners, he argued that they would prove to be important for research. Operational definitions of disorders, he forecasted, would encourage treatment and outcome studies as well as inquiries into etiology. Therefore, he boldly declared, "The ultimate predictive validity of the DSM-III diagnoses can be determined with an accuracy heretofore impossible. This will result in the refinement of some categories, the elimination of others, and the probable addition of entirely new categories."[38]

It is important to point out here that historically a major impact of DSM-III has been that it has influenced psychiatrists to think about mental disorders as quite discrete categories. This was the fruition of the goals of Robins and Guze, which were to devise homogeneous groups of mental patients for study to improve the validity of diagnoses. But their victory was not without costs. First, many psychiatrists turned away from conceptualizing particular mental disorders as part of a larger spectrum of disorders. Related to this, discrete categorization turned their attention away from focusing on the fact that many separate diagnoses actually share significant features and, therefore, their interrelationship with each other needs to be better interpreted. So, for example, the persons working on DSM-5 have stressed the evidence that many diagnoses share anxiety as a common feature and have significantly reoriented their classification as a result. Here, perhaps the obvious must be stressed: constructing a classification is like being on a perilous roadway fraught with potholes and landmines. And it often is difficult or impossible to foretell the outcome of a particular decision. For example, the emergence of the controversial diagnosis of Bipolar Disorder in children was unforeseen.

In Toronto, the panel discussion following the presentation of papers at the symposium was a heated debate, sometimes even acrimonious, as the panelists, acknowledged leaders in their specialties, wrangled over thorny problems confronting psychiatrists. The issues they addressed reveal some of the problems faced by Spitzer and the Task Force, the solutions for which would have a pragmatic effect on the diagnosing decisions of tens of thousands of psychiatrists.

Now that the results of the U.S.-U.K. study were in, panelists grappled with the challenge of defining schizophrenia. In an impassioned dispute about what constitutes the disorder, Roy Grinker, an elder statesman in American psychiatry, objected to the "representation of the spectrum concept in schizophrenia studies.…You can't be borderline [in the sense of there being a continuum] schizophrenic."[39] Paul Wender, a rising star in schizophrenia and hyperactivity studies, retorted, "The fact that the word 'spectrum' makes Dr. Grinker uncomfortable is irrelevant to its usefulness."[40] The two men clashed also over theories of biological vs. psychological etiologies of schizophrenia, Wender expostulating, "We have not found one datum indicating psychological etiological components."[41] Grinker did not mince words: "Sometimes at a meeting like this I feel as if I'm in a never-never land....No psychological factors in the aetiology of the schizophrenias. Now can anybody believe that?"[42] Some of the proponents of a biological etiology talked about the mechanism of genetics in mental illness—George Winokur was strong in this regard—but their opponents argued that the science in the field was still too unconvincing.

The related problem of distinguishing schizophrenia from an affective disorder also aroused animated dispute. Kraepelin's division of the two psychoses was never an unambiguous divide, and Kraepelin himself in his later years had wondered if his broad separation had been correct. American psychiatrists tried to square the circle by coming up with the diagnosis of Schizoaffective in DSM-I and II, for patients who presented with decided schizophrenic symptoms but yet had a severe mood disorder. Psychiatrists declared it a "type" of schizophrenia. We will see how the DSM-III Task Force debated this thorny problem at length and could not decide whether the diagnosis should be listed under Schizophrenia or Affective Disorders. After two years of shifting the diagnosis from category to category, they finally ended up with a Schizoaffective Disorder under the amorphous Psychotic Disorders Not Elsewhere Classified and with no diagnostic criteria, the only diagnosis in the manual without criteria. (DSM-IV kept the diagnosis but pushed it back under Schizophrenia.)

In the panel discussion, the ongoing dispute over the use of the word *borderline* continued, especially as it was used in Borderline Schizophrenia and Borderline Personality Disorder. We will look more closely at this in Chapter 10. Was the word just a synonym for *mild* or did it stand in its own right as a classifiable disorder? Spitzer asserted that he was not about to keep a diagnosis of Borderline Schizophrenia in DSM-III since there was no such thing as a "mild" case of schizophrenia. However, he argued for keeping the diagnosis of Borderline Personality Disorder because the diagnosis was important to so many clinicians and because, after several attempts, he had not been able to find a better term to replace it with. Winokur, representing the Washington University concept of diagnosing only "valid" disorders, immediately shot back: "And I, Dr. Spitzer, am very unhappy about it."[43] But then the panelists displayed a rare general agreement that once a diagnosis was entrenched, it was difficult to extirpate.[44]

Still, animosity was emerging over what was seen to be the inflexible diagnostic stands of Robins, Guze, Winokur, and their followers. Grinker was moved to refer to them as "the Washington University establishment" and a member of the audience asked, "Have we succumbed to pressure from the St. Louis group?"[45] Significantly, within the next year or two, Spitzer and the Task Force were to find Wash. U. psychiatrists, especially Guze, annoyingly obdurate on issues of validity and exact criteria.

Finally, in response to a question about ICD-9 from another panelist, Spitzer said that at first the Task Force had been worried that their mandate to be "creative," to craft a manual that fit the needs of American psychiatrists, would clash with the U.S. treaty obligation that the DSMs would be compatibile with the ICDs. But that worry, Spitzer reassured his audience, had been erased by the ability of DSM-III to be compatible with ICD-9 through the coding numbers of diagnoses.[46] Spitzer had met the letter of the law, if not its substance.

Thus closed the first two years of the making of DSM-III. The next three would bring seemingly unending challenges to the basic principles that had been laid down. Yet what seemed certain at this point is that the Feighner criteria, with their Wash. U. scientific (even if not all their philosophical) implications, had triumphed. For better or ill, they were about to overtake Western psychiatry as powerfully as Emil Kraepelin's schema of dementia praecox and manic-depressive illness had three-quarters of a century earlier.

Spitzer's intensified efforts to shape the diagnoses of the new manual in line with his descriptive vision occupied the coming two and a half years, from November 1976 to May 1979. Chapters 9 through 13 portray how he and the Task Force proceeded through deliberations, negotiations, clashes, and battles to create DSM-III.

9

THE ERUPTION OF DISCORD
FOLLOWING THE MIDSTREAM
CONFERENCE

Protestations against the Task Force's various undertakings began to take place almost immediately after the Midstream meeting and were to continue until the very day DSM-III was scheduled for approval by the APA's Assembly of Delegates. Most problems arose between various psychiatric constituencies and fit into two categories. The first category included disagreements over specific diagnoses and the best way to conceive of them and to label them. The second category encompassed deep philosophical rifts over what constitutes the very nature of psychiatry and how the human mind works. Sometimes, however, challenges arose from outside psychiatry, often having to do with professional rivalries. While most of these various contretemps were occurring simultaneously, they will be presented here as separate events, the better to understand them.

This chapter deals with three early contentions: the battle between Spitzer and the Assembly of Delegates, the APA group that represented local clinicians who were grouped into District Branches; the imbroglio with the American Psychological Association over the definition of a mental disorder (in Chapter 7 we saw the fight over the definition among psychiatrists themselves); and the issue of what diagnoses properly belonged in DSM-III, here centering around the Personality Disorders.

THE ASSEMBLY OF DELEGATES' QUEST FOR INCREASED
IDEOLOGICAL AND POLITICAL CONTROL

One of the first clashes after the Midstream conference involved both in-house politics and strong theoretical differences. Within three weeks of returning to the Psychiatric Institute (PI), Spitzer was hit with a broadside from Howard E. Berk, Chair of the APA's Assembly of Delegates' Liaison Committee to the DSM-III Task Force; Berk had been invited to the St. Louis meeting. Perhaps Spitzer should have been aware that something like the eight-page outburst he received from Berk might be in the cards. Right before the conference Berk had sent him a five-page memo complaining that the psychiatric profession, broadly speaking, was being denied input into the formulation of DSM-III. In this first missive, Berk inveighed against a process that, he said, was ignoring the "base of experience and knowledge" held by American psychiatrists. He charged that the proposed nomenclature had been stripped of "traditional psychiatric terms that are incorporated widely in psychiatric literature."[1]

Berk's accusations were due to the confluence of two situations. The first was that Berk, a psychodynamically oriented psychiatrist, was disturbed by the March 1976 "Progress Report" with its draft of a classification that clearly omitted "neurosis" and "psychosis" as organizing principles. He took note that the Report stated that the Task Force was developing a classification system "only secondarily...related to the ninth edition of the ICD," a manual that did include traditional psychodynamic terminology. Moreover, the "Progress Report" asserted that "the basis for classification should be...shared phenomenological characteristics," an approach often derided by psychoanalysts as "shallow."[2]

The second circumstance leading to Berk's outspokenness was that in the mid-1970s, the Assembly of Delegates had embarked on a path to assert its power in APA decision making. The Assembly was tired of years of charges that it was just a group of "political hacks" from the District (local) Branches. An opportunity to change this situation presented itself in the following way: after the APA meeting in Anaheim in 1975, some members of the Pennsylvania Psychiatric Society came away upset by Spitzer's presentation on the work of the Task Force up to that point. It seemed to them that DSM-III was veering away from "general psychiatric thinking." The Pennsylvania Society prepared an action paper urging that the Assembly should have the power to approve DSM-III "much in the same manner as any other policy of the [APA]." As a result, at the meeting of the APA in Miami the following year (May 1976), the Assembly voted to establish a liaison committee to the DSM-III Task Force.[3] According to Roger Peele (b. 1930), who was a member of the Assembly and later of the Liaison Committee, he and Dr. Oscar Legault (1915–2000), a psychoanalyst, proposed that the Assembly be able to approve DSM-III before other components of the APA gave their authorization.[4] Thus there was a political aspect to the Assembly's actions—a quest for power— as well as an ideological one revolving around missing psychodynamic explanations. The two strands came neatly together.

Whatever Berk's fears were before the Midstream Conference, they were severely deepened as a result of what he heard at the meeting. And it did not help that although he was on the platform at the final Plenary Session and thus expected to speak, he was the only one on the dais who was not called on.[5] As a result, Berk and Hector Jaso, another member of the Assembly Liaison Committee, wrote to Spitzer, eighteen days after the Midstream meeting had ended. They sent a long statement that they said they hoped would be included in the proceedings of the final session so that all participants would know their views. Their position paper was a stinging objection to what the Task Force was engaged in, and they mailed the document not only to Spitzer but also to everyone who had attended the Midstream Conference.[6]

What follows is a condensation of Berk and Jaso's detailed and dramatic attack, but the substance and style of their criticisms are rendered faithfully. To no surprise, the two men protested the removal of "neurosis" as a "massive exclusion of long held concepts in psychiatry," one that replaced "the castles of Neurosis...with a diagnostic Levittown." They praised the sophistication of ICD-9 that "reflects the greater reality of the diversity that does exist in life and in psychiatry," and quoted extensively from an earlier edition of the ICD to commend its differentiation between a classification and a nomenclature. A classification seeks to categorize and generalize about a group of cases and not individual occurrences, they wrote. A nomenclature is more primary and basic, portrays specific cases, and "is more creative and intuitive." Therefore, a classification is derivative and secondary to a nomenclature. The DSM-III Task Force, Berk and Jaso accused, was writing a derivative classification and seeking to force American psychiatrists to use it to diagnose individual cases. A "serious breach of validity" had occurred because the Task Force, in order "to achieve an a priori simplicity which the existing nomenclature does not permit, [had] achieve[d] a closure of their classification by expunging and mutilating…bowdlerizing…the offending nomenclature."

Holding back nothing, Berk and Jaso imaginatively charged that "the elimination of the [psychiatric] past by the DSM-III Task Force…can be compared to the director of a national museum destroying his Rembrandts, Goyas, Utrillos, van Goghs, etc. because he believes his collection of Comic-Strip Type Warhol's (or what have you) has greater relevance." They went on: the fact that members of the Task Force, including Spitzer, had said they were astonished by the feelings provoked by DSM-III illustrated their isolation from the mass of American psychiatrists. Berk and Jaso concluded that DSM-III as presently constituted might be beneficial for "investigation in a university setting, but [with] its narrowness and lack of eclecticism [it could not] fulfill the criteria for a national diagnostic and statistical manual."[7]

Within eight days, Spitzer replied with a "Dear Colleague" letter that he sent to all the Midstream conferees, essentially a rebuttal, item by item, of Berk and Jaso's accusations. In contrast to their indignation, Spitzer's tone was temperate. He first thanked all the participants at the conference and declared his satisfaction that the meeting had accomplished all that had been hoped for. He inserted a touch of levity referring to the Berk/Jaso attacks: "Wow!" Had they all attended the same conference? He then compiled a list of eleven "observations," keeping the moderate language. We will touch on just a few of these points here.

Spitzer addressed some specific diagnostic areas and expressed his confusion at the charge that DSM-III had no "psychological factors." What about the separate axis for categorizing psychosocial stressors, he wrote? He defended the elimination of "neurosis" and "psychosis" as organizing principles, something that he said ICD-9 might probably undertake as well. He rebutted the charge that DSM-III was a "simplification" of the classification: ICD-9 had 180 diagnoses that were described in forty pages, while DSM-III had 202 specific conditions described in several hundred pages. Moreover, Spitzer argued, the Task Force was not isolated. It not only responded to input from the profession—hence the dropping of the requirement of "subjective distress" for diagnosis of a sexual disorder—but did everything in its power to keep the profession informed via meetings and publications. Spitzer concluded that he was on the record at the May 1976 APA Annual Meeting for welcoming involvement from the Assembly of Delegates.[8]

These prompt "observations" from Spitzer are a further example of the energy and level of specificity he always brought to his position as Chair of the Task Force. Throughout his tenure, he tenaciously, but usually politely and often quite agreeably, defended his basic positions and remained a determined and skillful swordsman determined to parry the thrusts that he thought would endanger his basic goals.

As well as the letter to the Midstream participants, Spitzer also sent to three relevant APA officials and the director of PI, Edward Sachar, a copy of Berk and Jaso's charges. On his cover memo he wrote that "Dr. Berk's statement that DSM-III may be okay for 'university researchers' but not for the profession indicates the level of attack and the potential danger that it represents. Your help will be appreciated."[9]

We have witnessed the beginning of a series of seemingly never-ending parries and thrusts on the part of the Assembly of Delegates and Spitzer that only finally concluded with the emotion-charged approval of DSM-III by the Assembly three years later. As the interchange of letters, memos, and then face-to-face meetings began and continued, Spitzer made a political calculation that problems with the Assembly were there to stay and that he must deal with them one by one as the need arose. So, for example, after a couple of weeks had passed following Spitzer's immediate response to Berk, Spitzer began to think of ways of "offsetting" the opposition of the psychodynamically oriented psychiatrists. As we will see often in other negotiations, he was willing to consider compromise solutions as long as essential positions remained intact. Maybe, he mused now in a memo to the Task Force, clinicians could be given the choice of whether they wanted to use the DSM-III classification or the ICD-9 classification, so if they wanted to use the diagnosis "neurotic depression" they could use the ICD-9 codes. Then he wondered further whether DSM-III should include the ICD-9 classification to make it easier for practitioners to use. He concluded that in future contact with the Assembly "this would be further evidence of our reasonableness. *Let me know what you think*,"[10] he urged the Task Force (emphasis in the original.)

Spitzer continued his reasonable tone in a pleasant letter to Berk after a month passed. Knowing that the Assembly's Liaison Committee was going to report on their activities to the full Assembly of Delegates in Washington, DC, at the end of October, he proposed a meeting between himself and the Liaison Committee. "I would very much appreciate the opportunity of listening to your Committee regarding some of its concerns. It is possible that some of these concerns are based on misunderstandings which I would be able to hopefully clarify," Spitzer suggested. The Task Force, he said, would pay any travel expenses incurred by the Committee.[11] A meeting did occur the next month attended by Berk, Jaso, and Harvey Bluestone, another member of the Liaison Committee. The viability of the diagnosis of "neurotic depression," a category in DSM-I and II frequently used by psychodynamically oriented psychiatrists, but not in DSM-III, was an important subject of discussion. Spitzer and the Task Force were dedicated to getting rid of "neurosis" in diagnostic categories. Conversation revolved around what would be the equivalent of neurotic depression in DSM-III, and some tentative solutions were debated. Spitzer continued to mull this over and a few days later wrote to the Committee with yet another proposal, expressing his pleasure at the "very helpful discussion" at their meeting; he looked forward to the Committee's reply.[12] Thus did Spitzer attempt to smooth over disagreement without changing any categories in DSM-III. When Spitzer was given a copy of the report that the Liaison Committee had prepared for the full Assembly, he happily reported to the Task Force and key APA officials that its tone was "considerably changed from the initial document produced by this committee."[13]

Spitzer was right that the tone and language of the Assembly's Liaison Committee's twelve-page report to the entire Assembly were much more moderate than Berk's irate letter and memo to him that Berk had circulated to all the Midstream conferees. Yet Spitzer was not conveying to the DSM-III Task Force the fact that the Liaison Committee remained unhappy about DSM-III and spoke of "intense and deeply principled...discontents" among APA members. In the new report, there was still antagonism toward the elimination of diagnoses that were considered key, and there were worries that third-party payments were in danger. The report related that Spitzer had said that psychiatrists could choose whether they wanted to use ICD-9 or DSM-III, but the Committee said it had "serious objection" to this proposal because the official nomenclature of the APA "must be acceptable to...the preponderance of the membership of the APA." The Liaison Committee's recommendation was that use of DSM-III be put off for two years until ICD-9 went into force. Then, during this time, the DSM-III should undergo field-testing and national critical evaluation to determine whether the new manual accurately represented the views of the profession and was an improvement over ICD-9. The Liaison Committee reported that Spitzer was agreeable to this plan.[14] However, in Spitzer's official reply to the report, he declared that in his "initial view," he favored the plan for field-testing and critical review of DSM-III but said nothing about putting off use of DSM-III.[15] Moreover, the Liaison Committee recommended that, until the assessments of DSM-III had been completed, the present DSM-II be used along with a coding sheet that would allow DSM-II to be codable with ICD-9.[16]

In spite of the Liaison Committee's report and recommendations, Spitzer returned from the gathering in Washington upbeat and happy, writing to the Task Force, officials of the APA, Gerald Klerman, and Eli Robins that "we have definitely turned the corner." Spitzer related that the materials he had provided for the Assembly to read were received "extremely positively," and many members had told him "how much of an improvement the DSM-III material was compared to DSM-II or to the ICD-9 description of Schizophrenia.... The tone of the questions was friendly, and the audience seemed quite satisfied with the answers," Spitzer reported.[17] But Spitzer did not mention the section of the Liaison Committee's report about the "intense and deeply principled...discontents" among APA members, nor did he mention the Committee's recommendation that use of DSM-III be put off for two years while it was determined if DSM-III represented the views of the profession as a whole.

The Archives are silent on Assembly Liaison Committee matters for the next several months. There are references to a report from Berk to the Assembly Speaker (Chair) and to a March 1, 1977 letter from Berk to Spitzer that seem to have aroused feelings, but they are missing from the Archives. The next significant matter on record was that the Liaison Committee wanted to meet with Spitzer before they wrote their next report, which was to be presented at a meeting of the full Assembly in Toronto in April 1977. Spitzer replied to this request uncharacteristically sharply, saying that he had answered all of the questions in Berk's March 1 letter, and further, "it is not clear to me why you wish to have a meeting with me. I do not know what additional information I can provide to you that you do not now possess."[18] There matters rested until the Toronto meeting and the Liaison Committee's report to the Assembly.

The long report bristled with disappointment and anger, returning to the accusatory tone of Berk and Jaso's riposte to DSM-III after the Midstream meeting. Spitzer had misled the Liaison Committee, they declared, because he had recently set a deadline of July 13, 1977—just three months away—for all changes in terminology and coding in DSM-III, even though he had assured them in October that nothing would be settled until after 1978. Now, the Liaison Committee protested, no significant changes to DSM-III would be possible, even though many members still found the new manual "unacceptable." The Committee thus recommended "that the Assembly declare its wish that the deadline of July 13, 1977 for changes be rescinded." Furthermore, they complained, a new version of ICD-9 existed, the ICD-9-CM tailored for American physicians, and the Task Force was currently placing the current DSM-III draft into the mental disorders section of ICD-9-CM. Thus, ICD-9-CM was set to become the official U.S. nomenclature, yet, the Report continued, the Assembly of Delegates was filled with "apprehension" about the DSM-III draft which is still "in contention." To make matters worse, the report objected, this unsatisfactory draft was about to be field-tested. Because of this, the Committee was recommending that the DSM-III draft, "until approved by the Assembly, be kept the internal business of the APA, and that it be withdrawn promptly from the [new] ICD-9-CM."

The Liaison Committee proceeded to make a list of the objections to the DSM-III draft. These centered on unhappiness with "unjustifiable" elimination of and changes to terminology and diagnoses. There was renewed worry about possible disputes with third-party payers as a result of these eliminations and changes. Thus, the Committee pointed out, "Hysteria" was about to become a "Factitious disorder with its implication of willful deceit, [which] sounds like a term designed by an insurance company and reeks with invitation for third party challenge....Neurotic depression is no longer neurotic, and it is no longer a depression. It is an Adjustment disorder with a depressed mood. This too, seems very vulnerable to third party challenge and is certain of professional objection." Equally important, the Liaison Committee declared, DSM-III was putting obstacles in the way of U.S. psychiatrists and those in the rest of the world comparing diagnoses, thus preventing scientific communication. A "possible resolution," the Committee argued, would be to replace the draft of DSM-III with the mental disorders section in ICD-9.[19]

If we stand back from the fray, we can observe that economic and not just ideological differences existed between psychoanalytically minded clinicians, as represented by the Liaison Committee of the APA's Assembly of Delegates, and phenomenologists, who comprised most of the DSM-III Task Force. The phenomenologists were usually academicians and were salaried as medical school and hospital employees. They were not particularly concerned with getting paid by insurance companies. The clinicians, with private practices, had economic worries in a changed financial atmosphere in which insurance companies rather than private funds increasingly paid for care. As it turned out, the psychiatrists who worried about insurance coverage did indeed have reason to be fearful. But reduced coverage did not come about because of the specific diagnostic changes that concerned clinicians so greatly, but was rather based on the insurance companies' general claim that mental disorders, because their treatments were harder to assess, should not have parity with physical ills.

The Task Force, operating from a phenomenological orientation, had an intense desire to place psychiatry on a "scientific" basis to meet wide-ranging criticisms by physicians generally, as well as from other phenomenological psychiatrists, sociologists, lawyers, libertarians, and social advocates. Thus, Spitzer and the carefully chosen Task Force wanted a "data-oriented" psychiatry with no unproven etiological "theories" or "speculations." DSM-III, they promised, would be atheoretical (of course, an impossibility for this or any other classification). The psychoanalysts and their numerous psychodynamically oriented adherents responded that "data oriented" did not actually mean that a great amount of data had been gathered but rather that there existed only hopes that a manual based on description would gather useful data. Furthermore, being able to "prove" something, the analysts contended, was not the only heuristic principle that held truth. It should be noted that the belief that a radically revised manual would give psychiatry the scientific respectability it so desperately wanted has yet to achieve fruition; witness the clashes among psychiatrists and other clinicians and the disgruntlements among laypeople over the production of DSM-5 (although it should be stated that economic issues are also involved.)

The 1977 confrontation in Toronto between the Assembly and the DSM-III Task Force was to be the Assembly's last hurrah, as the locus of opposition shifted from the District Branch delegates directly to the psychoanalysts themselves. The Assembly Liaison Committee, which was reconfigured as a larger body under the chairmanship of Hector Jaso, turned out to be less confrontational than it had been under Howard Berk. Or perhaps Spitzer, with his dogged persistence, was wearing down the Assembly.[20]

Notwithstanding, the principle that the Assembly had to be given a voice in making important decisions had been established. In the spring of 1979, when DSM-III was up for a "yea" or "nay" vote, it was to the Assembly that all eyes were turned, as its approval was considered the largest hurdle to be surmounted before the acceptance of the revised manual.

THE PSYCHOLOGISTS RISE UP: THE DEFINITION OF "MENTAL DISORDER"

The more we continue to delve into the making of DSM-III, the more apparent it becomes that Spitzer always had many balls in the air. With his prodigious indefatigability and the capacity to make rapid decisions when necessary, he was always able to do a great deal of skillful juggling of the challenges that confronted him. Take, for example, the period in September and October 1976 when he was resolutely negotiating with Berk's Assembly Liaison Committee because of his concerns over what their first report to the full Assembly of Delegates in Washington would say. Just a few days before he received a copy of their report, a letter from Charles A. Kiesler, the Executive

Officer of the American Psychological Association, landed on his desk. The psychologists, it transpired, also had concerns with the direction DSM-III was taking.

Kiesler's letter was a masterpiece of careful and exact prose without a single word touching on the economic issues that psychologists had raised at the Midstream Conference. Kiesler stated that the Board of Directors of the American Psychological Association had reviewed and discussed the March 1976 DSM-III Progress Report and had conferred with "several experts." The conclusion they had reached was that the work on DSM-III thus far was "not sufficiently reflective of the most advanced and current knowledge of Nosology or of the prevailing perspective of professionals and researchers in the mental health community." The Board, Kiesler continued, had voiced its belief that since the APA diagnostic manual has an impact on mental health services and scientific inquiry into mental disorders, there was a need for "the most elegant and scientifically based statement of the art possible." In order to achieve this, a diagnostic manual used by all mental health professionals should portray a "consensus on...the nature of the human problems with which [they] work." The Board of Directors did not want "partisan conflict" between the two associations. "In that spirit," Kiesler wrote, "the American Psychological Association wishes to offer its complete services to assist the American Psychiatric Association in the further development of the DSM III." The DSM-III required a "collaborative effort" of psychiatrists and psychologists, the letter concluded.[21]

Spitzer's answer two weeks later was an equal work of art, cordial and welcoming. Since it is quite brief, it appears here almost in full.

> Actually, your organization is one of many professional organizations that we have decided to contact to suggest the formation of a liaison committee which would critically evaluate DSM-III. A copy of that letter which you would have received in a few weeks is enclosed.
>
> We certainly believe that the American Psychological Association is in a unique position to help us in our work, and we look forward to receiving information regarding your liaison committee.[22]

After this brief minuet of correspondence, there was a silence of over three months. While Spitzer went on to other things, the psychologists considered their options and decided to form a liaison committee to the DSM-III Task Force, as Spitzer had encouraged. Then, in February 1977, their executive officer replied to Spitzer's letter with a list of the names and addresses of the members of the liaison committee and requested that future draft versions of DSM-III and the classification and glossary of ICD-9 be sent to them.[23] A strategic contrast in mode of reaction is obvious: decision-making by any committee at the top organizational level, here that of the American Psychological Association, often results in delayed action, which can be detrimental to the group's efficacy. However, Spitzer had been given relatively free rein by the APA Trustees and had handpicked his task force. Furthermore, he only infrequently reported to the APA Council, to which he answered, so he could usually react swiftly to events as they arose. This situation, combined with Spitzer's proclivity for proceeding rapidly and decisively, often gave him a distinct advantage when dealing with other groups. This will be seen again in Chapter 11, in some of his contacts with the psychoanalysts.

Spitzer complied with the request for the draft of DSM-III by sending the psychologists' Liaison Committee the first official draft of DSM-III of April 15, 1977, three weeks before its formal debut. He enclosed with it the paper he had presented to the APA in Miami in May 1976 "dealing with the problems of defining mental illness, which I am sure will be of interest to you," he remarked blandly.[24] He closed by asking for comments on the materials he had sent, but he knew already that what he was sending— proposing mental disorders as a subset of medical disorders—was inflammatory.[25]

What draws our interest here is that Spitzer quite consciously was waving a red flag in front of the American Psychological Association, yet his main fight was not with its members but with the antipsychiatry movement. To contest the antipsychiatrists' influence was the chief motivation for Spitzer's seeking a medical definition of a mental disorder, and to start with, he pursued that goal with the psychiatrists.

Recall that Spitzer had been unhappy with the reception of his proposed definition of a mental disorder at the 1976 annual APA meeting. Although after this meeting he felt laid low by the negative reaction to his definition, he soon picked himself up and threw himself into the battle once more. He hoped that the research-oriented American Psychopathological Association (APPA), dedicated to having annual meetings on a distinctive cutting-edge psychiatric topic each year, would give a friendlier ear to his proposed definition of a mental disorder as a medical disorder.[26]

Spitzer very deliberately regarded a victory at the APPA meeting as opening the road to a victory against the antipsychiatry movement. He was one of the editors of the book that contained his and Endicott's paper at the meeting, and in the preface he took the opportunity to remind his readers of the blows psychiatry had endured in the 1960s and early 1970s: "The very concept of psychiatric illness," he wrote, "has been under considerable attack in recent years. This attack has largely depended upon studies derived from the social sciences. Some have taken the stand that what are called mental illnesses are simply those particular groups of behaviors that certain societies have considered deviant and reprehensible." Spitzer believed that this rejection of the legitimacy of psychiatry was partly owed to the fact that "no generally agreed upon definition of mental illness has been propounded that is not open to the criticisms of cultural relativism."[27] Thus, Spitzer conceived of DSM-III as a weapon that could repel psychiatry's cultural attackers if it demonstrated that psychiatry was a medical field.

One way to medicalize psychiatry was to have an unambiguous definition of a mental disorder as a medical disorder. Since in Spitzer's eyes the new manual had a potential of historic proportions, it was worth a fight with the psychologists to achieve this medical definition of a mental disorder.

The 1976 APA paper that Spitzer had sent the psychologists' Liaison Committee, with its definition of a mental disorder, jolted them, and their initial impulse was to draft a legal statement, a disclaimer, which they wanted Spitzer to include in DSM-III:

Although DSM-III is conceptualized here within the medical model it should be noted that while psychiatry is a subspecialty of medicine it is also one of the mental health professions, which includes clinical psychology, psychiatric social work and psychiatric nursing. For this reason, issues regarding the role of members of these professions in dealing with a specific disorder or group of disorders are to be considered within the framework of applicable legal statutes and regulations, as a function of the training and competence of the members of these professions.[28]

But for the moment this statement was not sent. Decisions were put off until the psychologists held their annual meeting in June 1977, when the American Psychological Association Board of Directors met and their Liaison Committee gave their report. Out of the discussions arose the decision that the President of the American Psychological Association, Theodore H. Blau (1928–2003), go over Spitzer's head and write directly to the President of the American Psychiatric Association. A lengthy letter was finally completed and sent on August 8, 1977.

The letter was prompted by the bombshell that had exploded when Spitzer sent the psychologists' Liaison Committee his May 1976 APA paper in which mental disorders were defined as a subset of medical disorders. Blau now informed Jack Weinberg (1910–1982), the APA's President, that the Psychological Association's Board of Directors was "quite perturbed" to learn of the proposal to place Spitzer's recent definition of mental disorders in DSM-III. Gone was the elegant phraseology of the original letter of nearly a year ago from the Executive Officer. Now the psychologists were blunt: "DSM-III and the proposed definition are immiscible.... The first is a scientific document dealing with nosology, while the other is concerned with professional, social, economic, political and interdisciplinary issues." The Board "strongly object[ed]" to Spitzer's proposed definition of mental disorders and argued that of the seventeen major diagnostic classes, at least ten had no known organic etiology. The proposed definition of mental disorder was "arbitrary."

Blau agreed that there were several positive features of DSM-III, and he ticked them off: the multiaxial diagnostic system, the use of operational criteria, the systematic descriptions for all disorders, the field testing of the drafts, the glossary of terms, and the attempted compatibility with ICD-9. But there he stopped and returned to his initial complaint. He listed again ten diagnoses that had no known organic etiology and pointed out especially that there was no justification for a medical label for Psychosexual Disorders. Moreover, Blau continued, Emancipation Disorders of Adolescence and Identity Disorder are frequently observed disturbances among adolescents, and "it appears absurd to include them as a subset of medical disorders," especially since the treatment "invariably" involves psychological and environmental approaches. In addition, the letter included a detailed appendage of disorders "obviously acquired through learning experiences." Blau concluded that mental disorders might be health disorders, but they could not be equated with medical disorders. Therefore, he wrote, "I would appreciate hearing from you that this matter has been resolved satisfactorily." Copies of Blau's letter also went to the presidents of the National Association of Social Workers, the American Nurses Association, and the National Education Association, whom Blau knew would be at one with the psychologists on the issue.[29] (Intriguingly, Spitzer did not share with his Task Force this challenging letter and the related correspondence until three months had gone by.)

Meanwhile, two months elapsed while the psychiatrists at the top organizational level considered how best to respond to Blau. Ultimately, it was decided that Spitzer should draft a reply for Weinberg to sign.[30] But in the interim, Spitzer and Joan Zaro, Ph.D., of the Professional Affairs Division of the American Psychological Association, had been talking on the telephone, and after one conversation, Zaro wrote a formal letter to Spitzer. The letter was quite conciliatory in tone, Zaro hoping that she and Spitzer could keep their discussion at a "low key and [as] constructive as possible." Nevertheless, Zaro emphasized the high level of concern of the leadership of the Psychological Association and sent Spitzer a copy of the legal "disclaimer" that had been drafted five months previously for inclusion in DSM-III. Zaro hoped that she and Spitzer could find "some satisfactory resolution to the problem," but she repeated the psychologists' requirement that Spitzer's definition of a mental disorder be taken out of DSM-III and the disclaimer put in.[31]

Spitzer was not about to be mollified. He soon prepared a draft of a letter for Weinberg to sign but at the same time wrote a heated letter to Melvin Sabshin, the Medical Director of the APA, who had recommended Spitzer's appointment as head of the DSM-III Task Force. Spitzer knew that Sabshin was supporting him in the revision of DSM-III as an empirical manual. Spitzer exploded. "These guys have chutzpah!" He proposed that the whole APA membership be openly apprised of the correspondence with the psychologists, in an article in *Psychiatric News*. Actually, he went on, if the membership knew of the negotiations, it would show that "DSM-III helps psychiatry move closer to the rest of medicine." He mentioned his "good relationship" with Zaro, and out of the blue decided that she was "embarrassed" by Blau's letter. (Was this wishful thinking on his part?) Finally, he wrote in a postscript that he had just finished talking to a reporter who had called him about the psychologists' concerns. Spitzer advised Sabshin that since "our troubles with the American Psychological Association are now public … we will have to make a public response."[32] Spitzer was not backing down.

Weinberg's letter was finally sent on November 3, 1977, three months after Blau had first written to him. Spitzer had drafted a lengthy four-page, closely argued reply for Weinberg's signature, simultaneously reasonable sounding and explanatory, yet at the same time unyielding, a typical example of Spitzer's style in a difficult situation. The letter is too long to summarize in detail, but it contains certain clear and definite points:

1. The American Psychiatric Association and the American Psychological Association each needed to respect the other's autonomy. Therefore, it was "inappropriate" for the Psychological Association to tell the APA how to conceptualize the disorders for which it assumes professional responsibilities.
2. The statement that the DSM-III classification of mental disorders is a subset of medical disorders would "certainly" be in DSM-III. However, the 1976 paper,

"Proposed Definition of Medical and Psychiatric Disorders for DSM-III," that Spitzer had sent to the Psychological Association's Liaison Committee would not appear in DSM-III.

3. It was not new that psychiatrists regard mental disorders as a subset of medical disorders. This has always been the case, but now it was being stated "explicitly." Weinberg wrote: "We believe that it is essential that we clarify to anyone who may be in doubt, that we regard psychiatry as a specialty of medicine."

4. Blau's letter had referred to DSM-III as a "scientific document dealing with nosology." Weinberg pointed out that "nosology means the study of the classification of *diseases.*"

5. Spitzer had explicitly stated in his 1976 paper that a particular condition could be a subset of more than one classification system. This claim was repeated: "The listing of a condition as a mental disorder...says nothing about whether it can also be appropriately conceptualized as a psychological disorder."

6. Wanting to demonstrate that the psychologists were being primarily motivated by economic fears, not science, Spitzer had Weinberg report that the Psychological Association Liaison Committee had "candidly" told Spitzer that its concern with the DSM-III classification stemmed from the possibility that a statement about mental disorders being medical disorders might be used against psychologists "in reimbursement for treatment."

7. Lastly, the APA did not wish to infringe on the rights of other mental health professions and would consider a statement to that effect to be placed in DSM-III.

It was not until after Weinberg's letter had been dispatched to Blau that Spitzer finally notified others of the contretemps, in a memo entitled "Complaint of American Psychological Association." This memo of November 14, 1977 went to the Task Force, the Assembly of Delegates Liaison Committee, the Chair of the APA Council on Research and Development, and the Director of the New York State Psychiatric Institute where Spitzer worked. Spitzer enclosed Blau's letter with Weinberg's response, which, of course, Spitzer had prepared, and concluded: "Trouble, trouble, trouble."[33]

Three weeks later, Blau replied to Weinberg. The proposed statement on the rights of other mental health professions might "be helpful" in the form that the psychologists had already written. (Recall that the legal statement that the psychologists had composed had by now been sent to the APA.) But, Blau continued, "Candidly DSM-III, as we have seen it in its last draft [4/15/77], is more of a political position paper for the [APA] than a scientifically-based classification....It would be irresponsible to produce a diagnostic system without an empirical scientific data base after so much scientific input by our many colleagues on both professions over the past thirty years." The American Psychological Association, Blau proclaimed, would "embark on [its own] truly empirical venture in classification of behavioral disorders [that would be] an interdisciplinary venture."[34]

A record of what transpired over the next several months is not in the DSM-III Archives. We only know that Spitzer and Zaro kept in touch, and that Zaro sent Spitzer the tentative report of an American Psychological Association Task Force on

"Descriptive Behavioral Classification," the plan for the psychologists' own diagnostic manual in response to the development of DSM-III. The new research-based classification was to be released in December 1981 and, not surprisingly, Spitzer had expressed interest in the project. Wilber E. Morley, Chair of the psychologists' own Task Force, in a summary of the report stated: "We believe that we have been able to demonstrate the feasibility of developing a behaviorally oriented approach which avoids some of the pitfalls inherent in the DSMs."[35]

What occurred next is in some dispute. Theodore Millon, the psychologist on the Task Force who has written about his experiences as a member, has dismissed the possibility that there was ever any chance that mental disorders might be defined as a subset of medical disorders. He paints a picture of serious discordance between Spitzer's intent and that of the DSM-III Task Force: "At no time would the task force have jeopardized acceptance of the substantive advances they had wrought in the DSM-III by including a statement so obviously provocative to one of the major mental health professions. Perhaps two or three task force members might have seen the fight as worth pursuing, but... when the concept was put to the test of a vote in February 1978, it was soundly and wisely defeated."[36] There are two problems with Millon's account. First, there is nothing in the Archives to indicate that such a vote took place in February 1978. Second, contrary to Millon's dating, in the Archives are minutes of a May 7, 1978 meeting of the Task Force in Atlanta at which the Task Force decided not to include in DSM-III a definition of mental disorders as a subset of medical disorders.[37] In the Archives, there is nothing between December 6, 1977 (Blau's answer to Weinberg) and May 7, 1978 (meeting of the Task Force) relating to this issue except Zaro's innocuous letter of February 15, 1978 to Spitzer.

What happened after Blau's letter to Weinberg? Was there intense behind-the-scenes negotiating between the American Psychological Association and the APA? What made the Task Force decide that it was best to give up on a medical definition of a mental disorder, even though Spitzer and the APA's Board of Trustees' had hoped to use such a definition to combat the antipsychiatry movement and the low status of psychiatry? We do know that the Task Force, from the start, was nowhere near as keen on producing a definition of a mental disorder as was Spitzer. Even if Millon is correct in his analysis that the Task Force did not want to risk their other achievements by holding out for the medical definition, we must not forget that he was a clinical psychologist, not a physician, and like many other clinical psychologists, he would not have wanted a medical definition. Thus one wonders if something is missing from the story, since there is a five-month lacuna in the written record coming after a period of intensifying correspondence. Then, seemingly out of the blue, comes a capitulation on the part of the APA.[38]

Attempts to discover what happened in those five months have not met with much success. Jean Endicott, who worked together with Spitzer on developing a definition of mental disorders as a subset of medical disorders, has no recollection of Task Force involvement during this period. Millon also remembers nothing specific and surmises that the eventual decision was a "personal" rather than a committee decision. Janet Forman (later Williams), who by this time was closely connected to ongoing events, states that she was not involved. Spitzer himself does not recall any further negotia-tions—neither within the APA (which seems to leave Melvin Sabshin out) nor with the American Psychological Association.[39]

In any event, consonant with the Task Force's decision of May 7, on May 26, 1978, Spitzer wrote to the Liaison Committee of the American Psychological Association: "This is to inform you that at a recent meeting of the Task Force on Nomenclature and Statistics, it was decided not to include in DSM-III any reference to the classification being a subset of medical disorders. It was the consensus of the Task Force that to do otherwise would be non-productive." Spitzer added that he understood that the issue of the disclaimer regarding professional responsibility for diagnosis and treatment still hung in the air.[40] There may have been still more negotiation, or at least the psycholo-gists were weighing an exact response, because it was not until six weeks later that there came a reply. "We were delighted," exclaimed Maurice Lorr, Chair of the Psychological Liaison Committee, "to hear that you have decided not to include in DSM-III any ref-erence to the classification being a subset of medical disorders. This decision is most constructive, and will do much to gain wide-spread acceptance of the revised nomen-clature, and to further good relations among the various disciplines." The matter of a separate disclaimer had not yet been decided, Lorr concluded.[41]

Finally, four months later, in November 1978, came the denouement, anticlimactic after two and a half years of posturing. "The decision reached," Lorr reported, "is that now that the medical definition has been removed from the Manual, there really is no need for a disclaimer. We assume, with this decision, that there will be no further problems concerning the medical definition within DSM-III."[42] And indeed, as Spitzer observed in the Introduction to DSM-III in a paragraph on liaison with other profes-sional organizations: "[The liaison] committees received drafts of DSM-III and were invited to make comments and suggestions and to express their concerns. In most instances, differences in point of view between a liaison committee and the Task Force were resolved to the satisfaction of all concerned."[43]

Yet it should come as no surprise that despite Spitzer's numerous failed efforts to get a definition of a mental disorder accepted by a wide variety of professionals, such a definition (although not a medical one) appeared nonetheless in DSM-III, first with an introductory caveat: "There is no satisfactory definition that specifies precise bound-aries for the concept 'mental disorder.'...Nevertheless, it is useful to present concepts that have influenced the decision to include certain conditions in DSM-III as mental disorders." Then came the definition:

> In DSM-III each of the mental disorders is conceptualized as a clinically significant behavioral or psychological syndrome or pattern that occurs in an individual and that is typically associated with either a painful symptom (distress) or impairment in one or more areas of functioning (disability)....When the disturbance is *limited* to a conflict between an individual and society, this may represent social deviance, which may or may not be commendable, but is not by itself a mental disorder.[44]

Several explanatory statements, qualifiers, and specific examples followed this definition.

A few last observations are required here. Spitzer and the APA had hoped to use DSM-III to cement the reputation of psychiatry as a medical subspecialty. While mainly owing to the psychopharmacological revolution, use of brain imaging technology, and genetic studies psychiatry has advanced toward that goal, to this day psychiatry is still often challenged and even mocked because the etiologies of most psychiatric illnesses remain unknown. On what scientific grounds, critics question, is a new diagnosis for DSM-5 being proposed?

Moreover, it is pertinent to recall that the actual construction of DSM-III was arranged in such a way that usually the advisory committees carried out the initial investigations and debates, then it was up to Spitzer and the Task Force to adjudicate and make final decisions. These policy matters were facilitated by the fact that Spitzer sat on all but three advisory committees, and in this role the enormous energies he possessed allowed him to "multitask," moving back and forth from one diagnostic disputation or resolution to another. Moreover, the advisory committees also usually contained representatives from the Task Force. A glimpse of the decision-making process of the Task Force is provided in the Minutes of the May 7, 1978 meeting: "Although there seems to be no perfect way to resolve disputes, it was suggested that many of them could be settled by votes or during conference telephone calls."[45]

At this point, a chronological context of events might be helpful: The contretemps between Spitzer and the psychologists took place from October 1976 to November 1978. The first draft of DSM-III was published on April 15, 1977, and the second one on January 15, 1978. Field trials testing the drafts began in 1977 and continued into 1979, the greatest part of them being funded by a grant Spitzer obtained from the NIMH. The field trials are discussed in Chapter 12.

While Spitzer was busy fighting partisan battles, he and the Task Force also had to make specific diagnostic decisions. Certain diagnoses were controversial—Borderline Personality Disorder was one—disliked by research-oriented psychiatrists but nevertheless cherished by many clinicians.[46] This controversy was part of a larger one: what diagnoses belonged in DSM-III?

WHAT DIAGNOSES BELONG IN DSM-III? ARE PERSONALITY DISORDERS VALID DIAGNOSES?

From almost the start of work on DSM-III, Spitzer was preoccupied with the diagnostic category of Personality Disorders (PD). This was a mine-strewn grouping because the very conception of personality disorders was contentious, raising the issue of the differing diagnostic needs of clinicians and researchers. There was a whole group of psychiatrists interested primarily in gathering "data" who disdained the PD diagnosis because of its amorphous and shifting nature and the lack of "hard evidence" for it. But it was a category for which psychoanalysts saw great merit, and, most importantly, it was a clinically popular diagnosis of nonpsychotic disorders that could be indicative of severe psychopathology. The category Personality Disorders had spawned eleven subtypes in DSM-II, including the debatable Asthenic Personality and Inadequate Personality. Also in DSM-II were the Paranoid, Cyclothymic, Schizoid, Explosive, Obsessive-compulsive, Hysterical, Antisocial (meant to be less pejorative than psychopathic), Passive-aggressive, and Other and Unspecified types. Spitzer removed four: Cyclothymic, Explosive, Asthenic, and Inadequate, and added five new ones: Schizotypal, Narcissistic, Borderline, Avoidant, and Dependent. Hysterical was renamed Histrionic. Ultimately, for DSM-III, Spitzer and the Task Force devoted most of their time to dealing with one new personality disorder diagnosis, Borderline Personality Disorder (BPD) and a somewhat related one, Schizotypal, to replace borderline schizophrenia.

From the start, Spitzer freely solicited advice on what to do about the cluster of personality disorders, and he was quite open to even unsolicited communications. In the first year of leading the Task Force, he began to wonder if DSM-III should include a new subtype, Depressive Personality Disorder, and sought the advice of Aaron T. Beck (b. 1921), a recognized expert on depression who had also done key studies on diagnostic reliability. But Beck was negative toward all personality disorders and bluntly wrote: such a "construct is so artificial and removed from observables, that it is probably of little utility and, even worse, it is probably a misleading fiction." Although trained as a psychoanalyst, he deplored what he considered to be the unwarranted explosion of Personality Disorder subtypes.[47] Thus, for a while, things hung fire.

Then, almost a year later, Spitzer was contacted by an analyst, Donald Rinsley (1928–1979), from the Menninger Clinic in Topeka, who urged introducing the controversial Borderline Personality Disorder into DSM-III as "a discrete, diagnosable entity, with related prognosis and therapeutic indications."[48] To analysts and other psychiatrists who used this characterization, BPD referred to a severe mental disorder, difficult to treat, and distinguished by many of the following: intense and unstable interpersonal relationships, black-and-white thinking, strong, inappropriate mood shifts or anger, uncertainty about self-image, physical self-damage, chronic feelings of emptiness, and impulsivity leading to self-destructive behavior. Brief psychotic episodes were possible. The psychoanalyst Adolph Stern (1879–1958) had introduced the name into the literature in 1938 to describe a group of patients who had what was seen to be a mild form of schizophrenia, on the "borderline" between neurosis and psychosis, and were regarded as "extremely difficult to handle effectively."[49] Soon after, in the 1940s, another analyst, Robert P. Knight, began to discuss these patients with their "borderline states," and his work popularized the concept.[50]

Spitzer and his colleagues had been wrestling with the problem of whether there could be "borderline" anything (not just personality), and Spitzer appreciated hearing from someone who might provide a rationale for BPD. Could Rinsley, he asked, supply him with "any specific descriptive criteria that could be used to capture the concept of borderline personality organization?"[51] After this request, Spitzer went off to the Midstream Conference, and the matter went into abeyance.

Then, a month after Spitzer had returned to New York, he and Donald Klein of the Task Force, in their personae as members of the "Personality Subcommittee," made a key announcement that surprised Spitzer's correspondents. Spitzer and Klein had decided it would be "useful" to include Borderline Personality in DSM-III "with careful specification" that the diagnosis be used only if no other personality disorder could be diagnosed. (This decision illustrates what other Task Force members already realized, which is how closely Spitzer and Klein often worked together.) "Don and I," Spitzer wrote to the whole Task Force on July 19, 1976, "have started work on the operational criteria based on some suggestions made by Dr. Donald Rinsley." Spitzer also wrote to Rinsley letting him know of the decision.[52]

In keeping with his action favoring the BPD interest of the psychoanalytic camp, Spitzer also wrote the same day to the analyst Alex Kaplan (1913–1996) that he had been impressed by Kaplan's comments at the Midstream Conference on the definition of narcissistic personality, which was not in DSM-II. Would Kaplan please send him "an edited version" of the definition?[53] Kaplan's discussion may have attracted Spitzer's attention because his second training analyst at Columbia, Arnold Cooper, had developed influential ideas about narcissism that Spitzer admired at the time.

Returning to the diagnosis of BPD, Spitzer's decision to incorporate the diagnosis into the new manual far from ended the debate surrounding this contested diagnosis; controversy swirled about it for the next two and a half years, as Spitzer was committed to seeing the issue through. One of the first matters Spitzer had to address was whether *borderline* should be used as a noun or an adjective. Did it describe a full-fledged disorder or did it merely mean a level of severity? Another issue that Spitzer had to untangle was whether there were episodes of psychosis associated with BPD; the profession did not agree on this question. The Archives do not contain evidence that indicates as much concern with other PD diagnoses as there was with BPD and the new Schizotypal diagnosis.

Spitzer determinedly kept working on the BPD diagnosis, which so many clinicians desired, because even though he had decided he wanted it in DSM-III, he wished to make it a clearer, firmer entity. To this end, Spitzer sought to elucidate two conceptions of "borderline" as put forth by researchers who worked in this area. To start with, he proposed that the borderline diagnosis most closely conceived of as "borderline schizophrenia" in DSM-II be called "Schizotypal Personality Disorder" in DSM-III. Spitzer was attempting to rid the nomenclature of excess and unwarranted schizophrenia diagnoses since schizophrenia was so overdiagnosed in the United States, with such dubious varieties as latent, prepsychotic, pseudoneurotic, pseudopsychopathic, or borderline schizophrenia.[54] His grounds for removing this assortment of schizophrenia types were that while these referred to patients with supposedly "schizophrenic" symptoms, the individuals had no history of a psychotic episode.

Then Spitzer turned to another conception of "borderline," this one envisaged as borderline personality "organization." This notion was the creation of the psychiatrist and analyst Otto Kernberg. It was this concept that Spitzer wanted to make into BPD, but with a different, more descriptive and meaningful name than "borderline."[55] He wrote to the Task Force in December 1976, five months after he had made the decision to put BPD in DSM-III, "We are desperately in need of a suitable term to identify the Kernberg Borderline Personality Disorder since we seem to have found a suitable term [Schizotypal] to express the other form of borderline....Could you please consult your thesaurus and come up with a suggestion....Don Klein and Jean Endicott have discussed this with me and we have come up with the term Unstable Personality Disorder....Comments?"[56] Spitzer also informed the Task Force that he was sending out a questionnaire to 4,000 APA members "to help firm up our criteria for these two forms of borderline." This remarkable move to solve a thorny problem demonstrates Spitzer's openness to feedback and his desire to make DSM-III a manual that clinicians would find acceptable and usable. He was always aware that he was serving two constituencies, researchers and clinicians, and he sought to both help and satisfy the two groups, but not always equally.

The APA members' answers to the questionnaire on rating "borderline" individuals yielded data on 808 patients and 808 controls that Spitzer and Jean Endicott subjected to a variety of statistical measurements. On this basis, Spitzer concluded that it was possible to find diagnostic criteria to describe both BPD and Schizotypal PD and that there was a measureable difference between the two disorders.[57] However, the questionnaire did not solve Spitzer's dilemma of how to add BPD to the nomenclature but with a better name, and he still was not satisfied that he had nailed the best description and criteria for this new addition. He began correspondences with specialists in the field that went on for another two years. One controversy that was not resolved until a few months before the manual was up for approval was whether brief psychotic episodes were found in BPD.

In late January 1977, there was a flurry of letters regarding a suggestion from Millon, whose great forte was personality disorders. The letters highlight comprehensively the disagreements over what to do about a so-called "borderline personality." Although Spitzer had already proposed a name for the "borderline" group of schizophrenias (Schizotypal), Millon had suggested that this group of disorders be named "schizoid." As for another name for BPD, Millon proposed "cycloid." This last suggestion was unwelcome to most because they thought it was too easy to confuse "cycloid" with a bipolar illness or other affective disorders. Michael Sheehy, on the Task Force and Personality Disorders Advisory Committee, also thought that the name "cycloid" would be indistinguishable from Histrionic (formerly Hysterical) Personality Disorder, which had been in DSM-II and which Spitzer was retaining in DSM-III.[58]

Spitzer had written to Kernberg, soliciting his opinion. Kernberg was pleased to be consulted but argued against Millon's designation "schizoid" since "most patients with borderline personality organization are not predominantly schizoid or related to the schizophrenia spectrum."[59] Kernberg also opposed the name "Unstable Personality Disorder" that Spitzer, Klein, and Jean Endicott had come up with and urged that Spitzer use Kernberg's own term of Borderline Personality Organization. He argued for keeping the word *borderline* because most people were familiar with what is meant by a Borderline Personality and because DSM-III would be "weakened" if its classification and terminology "deviate[d] too far from…present clinical understanding and practice."[60]

But Kernberg's position was far from being accepted. The letter reflecting quite emphatically the views of many psychiatrists who believed BPD was not a justifiable entity came from Donald W. Goodwin (1932–1999), a member of the Task Force, who had trained at the anti-analytic, research-oriented program of Washington University.

> The borderline syndrome is a mess.…"Borderline" in the rest of medicine refers to early, mild or atypical cases of a presumed illness. We will *never* agree upon

diagnosis if the prototype for the condition is based on early, mild or atypical cases....We are including under the rubric "borderline" early, mild and atypical symptoms of a number of psychiatric conditions, including schizophrenia, affective disorders, obsessional neurosis, patients supersensitized to their own mental contents by an excess of psychotherapy....In short, in my opinion, the borderline syndrome stands for everything that is wrong with psychiatry [and] the category should be eliminated and that simply renaming it will not help matters....I know there are a substantial number of psychiatrists in the country who would agree with [my] points, and they all didn't train under Sam [Guze] and Eli [Robins].[61]

Nevertheless, Spitzer was committed to the borderline personality concept, but he kept delving for another name for it. In the fall of 1978, Spitzer dispatched for reactions and comments a proposal for a new version of the BPD category by Larry Rockland, a member of the American Psychoanalytic Association's Liaison Committee to the Task Force. Spitzer asked several questions: Was Rockland's new name for BPD "Identity Diffusion Disorder" acceptable? Could Rockland's emphasis on disturbances in interpersonal relations easily confuse BPD with Narcissistic Personality Disorder? Were Rockland's diagnostic criteria based more on individual clinical experience than on empirical study? Would Rockland's draft win "widespread support within the community of [BPD] investigators" since it primarily represented the views of one analyst, Otto Kernberg, "whereas the DSM-III version is more general and non-specific?"[62]

Rockland's proposal garnered almost no support. Neither the four (out of eight) members of the Personality Disorders Advisory Committee nor the three outside experts who responded to Spitzer's questions were happy with the recommended revision. Above all, they proclaimed, they didn't think Rockland's new name for BPD—Identity Diffusion Disorder—was any better. One respondent said the name could be mistaken for Erik Erikson's formulation of the adolescent identity crisis. Moreover, it was argued, the present DSM-III draft descriptions and diagnostic criteria were superior; Rockland's could easily be confused with other diagnoses. One expert pushed his own name, "Psychotic Character."[63] Rockland's proposal died a quiet death, one more incident, the psychoanalysts thought, that showed a basic antagonism to their contribution to psychiatric knowledge. (The tempestuous interaction between Spitzer and the analysts is presented in Chapters 11 and 13.)

In any event, Spitzer was beginning to accept the reality that the name of BPD was going to remain Borderline Personality Disorder, although he continued to get complaints about using the term *borderline* even from those who agreed with the concept of the diagnosis.[64] But his quest to solidify the hallmarks of BPD did not rest. Right after the Christmas holidays of 1978, Spitzer wrote to John G. Gunderson, one of the experts on BPD to whom Spitzer had sent Rockland's psychoanalytic version of BPD.[65] Gunderson had aroused a great deal of interest with an article that he and Margaret T. Singer, Ph.D. published in 1975, containing a review of the literature on borderline patients and a suggestion of six features that could be used to diagnose borderline patients in the initial interview.[66] Gunderson was (and still is) affiliated with McLean Hospital in Belmont, MA, and Harvard. Spitzer, still on a quest after three and one-half years to secure convincing diagnostic criteria, was not sure whether or not to include "brief psychotic experiences" in the text description of BPD, episodes that Gunderson said did exist in BPD. Thus, he asked, would Gunderson please "provide several specific descriptions of such experiences?" The level of detail Spitzer went on to ask for is striking: samples of six to ten such incidents, information on whether the experiences were "limited to therapy or transference distortions, whether delusions or hallucinations were involved, and how long such episodes lasted."[67] Gunderson replied within the week, pleased that Spitzer was considering revising the BPD text with such information, but distinctly unpleased at having to be the one to do the rewriting. Nevertheless, he plunged in via a three-page letter.

Gunderson described five types of typical psychotic experiences that occurred in the absence of drugs and outside of the therapy context: (1) feelings of worthlessness and hopelessness; (2) the feeling of being outside one's body or perceiving changes in size and shape of themselves and others; (3) visual and auditory distortions; (4) paranoid beliefs; and (5) beliefs by patients that their minds could be read or that they could read the minds of others. Gunderson also included three more unusual experiences that had occurred in intensive therapy situations. He then concluded: "Psychotic experiences are a central characteristic of borderline personalities.... You have heard all this from me before. I am pleased that you are giving it the attention it requires."[68]

Spitzer answered ten days later with some conclusions he had reached about how to describe BPD. He decided that what had been preventing him from including psychotic experiences as a feature of the disorder was that it wasn't clear exactly how a psychotic experience should be defined. He reflected: "I think that to most clinicians the term 'brief psychotic episode or experience' conveys something much more disruptive of daily functioning than the kinds of experiences you have reported. [But] thanks for your letter... it clarifies what we may be disagreeing about." Spitzer reported that he would probably end up "noting in the Associated Features section of both Borderline and Schizotypal Personality Disorders that these kinds of experiences are frequently seen."[69] It should be noted that Spitzer's final decision came just three and a half months before the manual had to be voted on. Many affairs relating to DSM-III were not resolved until the last moment.

It is a measure of how difficult it was to describe BPD precisely that we find the following remarks in the description of this diagnosis in DSM-III: "There is instability in a variety of areas.... No single feature is invariably present.... Frequently this disorder is accompanied by many features of other Personality Disorders.... In many cases more than one diagnosis is warranted.... Transient psychotic symptoms of insufficient severity or duration to warrant an additional diagnosis may occur."[70] Even before Spitzer had fixed on the precise language, aware of the controversial nature of his decision, he had taken the precaution of attempting to convince American psychiatrists of the validity of the new Borderline and Schizotypal Personality Disorders. By April 1978, the *Archives of General Psychiatry* had accepted his article, "Crossing the Border into Borderline Personality and Borderline Schizophrenia: The Development of Criteria."

Outside of BPD, Spitzer paid relatively little attention to other personality disorders. He had come to a decision by September 1977 to return Passive-Aggressive

Personality Disorder to the nomenclature after having initially decided to eliminate it, although it had been in DSM-II.[71] And when Donald Klein wrote to him commenting on the Personality Disorders section in the second draft of DSM-III, January 1978, Spitzer dutifully sent out all of Klein's questions and comments and asked for reactions from the Personality Disorders Advisory Committee. Klein had raised issues about whether one could make a double diagnosis of schizophrenia and a personality disorder. He also had comments and suggestions on an assortment of the personality disorders: Passive-Aggressive, Histrionic, Narcissistic, Anti-social, and Avoidant.[72] The Archives are silent on the responses to Spitzer from the Personality Disorders Advisory Committee or the Task Force. However, we do know that at one of the few meetings when the Task Force actually met together, in October 1978, on the agenda under "Controversies" there was a discussion of Antisocial Personality.[73] Further, Roger MacKinnon, on the Personality Disorders Advisory Committee, wrote three months before the final vote on DSM-III with suggestions for fine-tuning the diagnostic criteria and description of Histrionic Personality Disorder.[74] We lack Spitzer's reply. Finally, just a few days before the Assembly's vote, Spitzer wrote to Allen Frances (eventual editor of DSM-IV) and Arnold Cooper, both psychoanalysts, about "how to justify the inclusion of Narcissistic Personality Disorder" because Klein had again raised questions about its description.[75] These few pieces are all there are in the Archives on personality disorders outside of BPD.

In DSM-III the Personality Disorders were placed on Axis II of the multiaxial diagnostic system and were listed after the Axis I disorders, the latter making up the bulk of all psychiatric disorders. Spitzer listed eleven specific types of personality disorders (similar to the number in DSM-II), to the satisfaction of many clinicians and certainly the psychoanalytic community, but much to the discomfiture of the "hard" researchers. Spitzer had these two discordant constituencies to keep in mind as he made decisions about the structure of DSM-III. In this case, the clinicians' desire for a popular diagnosis received primacy.

Nevertheless, an unfortunate situation arose. The insurance companies were less inclined to pay for treatment for Axis II disorders, since they consisted of lifelong personality patterns that required long-term, highly intensive, and therefore expensive treatment. But since a patient with a chronic personality disorder often had an Axis I condition such as depression, an anxiety state, or an adjustment disorder, the treating clinician sometimes filed for payment under these diagnoses. The insurance companies would pay more for acute episodes and exacerbations associated with Axis I diagnoses. However, this circumstance enhanced the probability of "comorbid" diagnoses, when the patient met the criteria for more than one diagnostic category. "Comorbidity" came to bedevil psychiatric diagnosis, as it confused the identification of individual psychiatric disorders, undermining the very raison d'etre of a psychiatric classification. It became the goal of the makers of DSM-5 to create more realistic and valid diagnoses that would incorporate the several disparate features of a given psychiatric disorder.

In this chapter we have learned about Spitzer's battle with the assertive Assembly of Delegates' Liaison Committee after the Midstream meeting; the vicissitudes of his attempt to define mental disorders as a subset of medical disorders; and his tenacious campaign both to turn the Borderline Personality Disorder diagnosis into a usable category for clinicians and to frame it in terms of diagnostic criteria he believed were necessary. In the following chapter we will see that the clinical–research divide appears again in conjunction with Spitzer's decision to split the age-old hysteria diagnosis into two new ones, Somatoform Disorders and Dissociative Disorders. In addition, disagreements over conceptualizations of human sexuality await us.

10

CLINICIANS VS. RESEARCHERS AGAIN AND NEW ANTAGONISMS OVER SEXUALITY

As Spitzer and the Task Force crafted DSM-III, certain themes became obvious. In the previous chapter we saw three: first, a strong clash between phenomenological and psychodynamic conceptions of mental disorders, as Spitzer and the Assembly Liaison Committee struggled for dominance; second, the intensity of the desire to use DSM-III in the fight against the antipsychiatry movement, even if that meant doing battle with the American Psychological Association; and the third, with the inclusion of Borderline Personality Disorder in the nomenclature, Spitzer had made a resolute decision that the new manual had to be responsive to the needs of clinicians, even though he was aware of the claims of the researchers.

The first part of the present chapter takes the clinician vs. researcher theme further in connection with Spitzer's abandonment of the diagnosis Hysterical Neurosis and formulation of two separate diagnoses to take its place. Here we see that Spitzer and the Wash. U. psychiatrists, while happily united on the usefulness of diagnostic criteria for making a diagnosis, were vigorously divided over which diagnoses belonged in a diagnostic manual and how many criteria were sufficient to make a diagnosis. The second and third parts of the chapter deal with issues directly related to human sexuality.

THE HISTORIC "HYSTERIA" TRANSFORMED AND THE ONGOING CONFLICT BETWEEEN CLINICAL AND RESEARCH NEEDS

The tension between the needs of clinicians and those of researchers was always palpable. It continues today as the DSM-5 Task Force and Work Groups attempt to craft a revision pertinent to the full range of the competing goals of psychiatrists. In the making of DSM-III, we can see the clinical vs. research tautness in a new category that Spitzer created for DSM-III, Somatoform Disorders. It would partly take the place of Hysterical Neurosis, which Spitzer had decided to eliminate from DSM-III. In DSM-II, Hysterical Neurosis was subdivided into two types: conversion type and dissociative type. (We should remember that "hysteria" was the disorder that first led Freud to develop psychoanalysis and the theory of "unconscious conflict.")

In DSM-II, the classification that had favored a psychoanalytic approach, the "conversion" type of hysteria, referred to physical symptoms such as blindness, deafness, anesthesias, and paralyses, for which no evidence of physical pathology could be found. The name was based on the psychoanalytic understanding that a psychological problem had been "converted" to a physical problem. The "dissociative" type of hysteria meant that there were alterations in the person's state of consciousness, for example, amnesia, or changes in his or her identity, which would manifest themselves as multiple personality. Spitzer replaced "Hysterical Neurosis" with diagnoses under the two new categories of "Somatoform Disorders" and "Dissociative Disorders." There was also a third new diagnosis, "Psychological Disorders Affecting Physical Condition." This was entirely separate from Somatoform Disorders, but it will play a part in our story.

The various new designations must be identified here for the sake of clarity: In DSM-III, there ultimately were five diagnoses grouped under the new, general Somatoform Disorders. These were Somatization Disorder, Conversion Disorder, Psychogenic Pain Disorder, Hypochondriasis, and Atypical Somatoform Disorder. We will refer to three of these:

- **Somatization Disorder**—The essential features of this were described as "recurrent and multiple somatic complaints of several years' duration for which medical attention has been sought but which are apparently not due to any physical disorder."
- For **Hypochondriasis**—"The essential feature is a clinical picture in which the predominant disturbance is an unrealistic interpretation of physical signs or sensations as abnormal, leading to preoccupation with the fear or belief of having a serious disease."
- **Atypical Somatoform Disorder** "is a residual category [unable to be diagnosed more specifically] to be used when the predominant disturbance is the presentation of physical symptoms or complaints…apparently linked to psychological factors."[1]

Separate from Somatoform was **Psychological Factors Affecting Physical Condition**. Here a clinician could "note that psychological factors [e.g., an argument or information of the death of a loved one] contribute to the initiation or exacerbation of a physical condition [e.g., migraine headache or sacroiliac pain]….This category [could] be used to describe disorders that in the past have been referred to as either 'psychosomatic' or 'psychophysiological.'"[2]

Our main focus here will be on the Somatoform Disorders and Spitzer's parting company with the Wash. U. psychiatrists on the portrayal of aspects of this new category. Not only was there a clinical–research divide, but there were also clashes between phenomenological and psychodynamic conceptions of mental disorders.

The story begins with Spitzer's wide distribution of the first draft of DSM-III in April 1977, one copy going to the Wash. U. psychiatrist, Samuel Guze. Within a few days Guze wrote to Spitzer to congratulate him on his "major accomplishment." Guze, one of the major developers of the Feighner criteria, egotistically stated, "I think that we agree that the single most important accomplishment of DSM-III will be the shift to operational criteria. Everything else is of lesser importance." Although Guze was congratulatory, he still had "a couple of minor points to raise," one of which concerned Somatoform Disorders, where he found unwelcome evidence of Spitzer's seeming reliance on the psychoanalytic idea of unconscious conflict. Guze complained: "I do not know what is intended by [the phrases] 'positive evidence that the symptom is a direct expression of the psychological conflict' and 'determination that the symptoms are *not* under voluntary control.'"[3]

Spitzer referred to Guze's position in a further memo of July12, 1977, as confirmation that the two men had "a real disagreement" about Somatoform Disorders. In reply, Guze took this opportunity to challenge Spitzer on the idea that there was "positive evidence" that symptoms are linked to "psychological factors." Guze argued that "from my knowledge of the literature, and based on my personal experience this criterion [positive evidence of psychological factors] is almost impossible to apply objectively and consistently. In fact, I believe that this is why I rejected the idea of defining conversion symptoms in terms of any hypothesized mechanism." He concluded by saying he was "pessimistic," but that maybe, after all, Spitzer would "propose useful criteria concerning the link to psychological factors."[4]

Paula Clayton, on the Task Force and also on the faculty at Washington University, seconded Guze and wanted to make it totally clear that there was a gulf between Spitzer and the psychiatrists at Washington University. "It is a philosophical issue," she declared.

> When we see a patient with an unexplained medical symptom we accept it as an undiagnosed psychiatric illness.... [W]e always keep an open mind that this may turn out to be a nonpsychiatric or a diagnosable psychiatric illness.... We prefer to live with uncertainty than evoke unconscious or conscious mechanisms that give us false security. We would consider a symptom unexplained (not diagnosed medical illness) if the patient has a satisfactory negative medical work-up concerning the symptom, or has a symptom that cannot be explained with medical knowledge, e.g., tunnel vision...or bilateral paralysis with no cord injury or insult.[5]

The issues surrounding Somatoform Disorders at this point seem to have disappeared from Spitzer's concerns until eight months later, when an unsolicited letter landed on his desk and again focused his interest on this new classification. A psychiatrist at Temple University, David Soskis, had seen the second draft of DSM-III, issued on January 15, 1978, in which hypochondriasis had been relegated to the category of an "Atypical Somatoform Disorder." Soskis urged the creation of a separate category of "Hypochondriasis" as an independent part of the Somatoform Disorders and enclosed reports from his own research and a proposed entry for the condition.[6] We know that Spitzer read every letter that crossed his desk. The result is that within the week he got a memo off to the Factitious and Somatoform Disorders Committee plus Task Force members Donald Klein, Nancy Andreasen, Bish (Z. J.) Lipowski, Jean Endicott, and the epidemiologist Lee Robins, asking them to study Soskis' proposal to include hypochondriasis as a separate disorder in DSM-III. There had been a Hypochondriacal Neurosis in DSM-II. Spitzer argued that Soskis had done "a very good job of separating hypochondriasis from Somatization Disorder," the first category under Somatoform. (In the 1978 draft of DSM-III, as a subcategory under the Somatoform Disorders, Hypochondriasis referred to recurrent and multiple somatic complaints not apparently due to any physical disorder.) Soskis, Spitzer asserted, had "avoid[ed] our removing a well-defined clinical entity from the [already existing] nomenclature." He added, "It does mean one more mental disorder, but that seems to be our fate."[7]

The Archives contain only a single reply to Spitzer's memo, that from Steven Hyler, a member of the Factitious and Somatoform Disorders Advisory Committee. Hyler liked Soskis' draft on Hypochondriasis and discussed the traits differentiating it from Somatization Disorder. Hyler enjoyed using Yiddish terms, sometimes mockingly, and at this juncture he added to his assessment of a separate diagnosis for hypochondriasis: "My 'gut' reaction as to the differentiation of these two disorders is that the young female 'hysteric' will receive the diagnosis of Somatization Disorder while the more mature male or female kvetch or noodge will receive the diagnosis of Hypochondriasis."[8]

Months passed as Spitzer consulted with various Advisory Groups and Task Force members and engaged in further correspondence. Finally, Spitzer determined that the diagnosis of Hypochondriasis would enter DSM-III, accepted Soskis' rewriting of the entry and, in vintage Spitzerian style, invited Soskis to become a member of the Factitious and Somatoform Advisory Committee.[9] In addition, Spitzer determined that a new diagnosis of Dysmorphophobia or Body Image Disorder would find a home in the category of Atypical Somatoform Disorder.[10]

In the last few months before DSM-III came up for approval, until the moment before the vote, Spitzer was forced to give added attention to Somatoform Disorders because of critiques from a variety of Task Force members, Advisory Group members, and the Wash. U. psychiatrists that related to Hypochondriasis and Somatization Disorders. During these same months, as we shall see, he was swept up by a wide array of crises, yet his ability to tackle competing demands never failed him. It is also remarkable how many diagnostic issues were not settled until the very last moments before the Assembly of Delegates voted on approval of DSM-III. The following section deals precisely with last-minute issues.

Although the inclusion of Hypochondriasis in the nomenclature appeared settled, James Brophy, a member of the Psychosomatic Disorders Advisory Committee, abruptly—or perhaps he had learned of the change much belatedly—wrote an emphatic memo to Spitzer denouncing the added diagnosis. Seemingly allied with the Wash. U. position, he wrote that it was "another wastebasket term that has hampered good patient treatment. Because of the assumed legitimacy of such terms (because we put them in the nomenclature) clinicians use them when the cause of a problem is not found and they (terms such as hypochondriasis and psychosomatic) become unassailable diagnoses. I strongly feel we should not include this as a diagnosis [underlinings in the original]."[11] When Spitzer chose to retain the Hypochondriasis diagnosis, Brophy wrote again three months later, just as Spitzer was preparing to go to Chicago for the decisive APA meeting, now stating his "unalterable opposition to the inclusion of the category 'psychosomatic' reaction [because] it is a regression from the whole thrust of the psychophysiologic committee.[12] I think the term 'Hypochondriasis' carries the same dangers."[13] Spitzer retained the Hypochondriasis diagnosis anyway, but it turned out that Brophy had not been alone about getting rid of "psychosomatic" at the last moment. On May 3, nine days before the Assembly was scheduled to vote, Spitzer wrote, "For some reason you were not given the good news that we are going back to 'Psychological Factors Affecting Physical Condition.' Relax."[14]

However, Spitzer could not deal as easily with last-minute concerns about Somatization Disorder, mainly because the Wash. U. group wanted the original and much more numerous Feighner criteria to be the diagnostic criteria for this disorder.

(Spitzer preferred fewer criteria, an amount that was more clinician-friendly.) About this, Guze wrote irritably to Spitzer:

> I am really at a loss about how to reply [to your letter]. Under no circumstances would I consider a sensation of a lump in the throat, or fainting spells, as conversion symptoms [Spitzer changed "lump in the throat" to "difficulty swallowing" but kept "fainting spells" in DSM-III].[15]
>
> I do not want you or anyone else to think that I am in any way comfortable with the proposed criteria for Somatization Disorder. If asked, I would only say that they represent your best effort to meet conflicting needs [of clinician and researcher], but that they do not represent what I consider to be the best criteria to use.[16]

However, even before Guze wrote, Spitzer had already queried the Task Force about the number of diagnostic criteria to include for Somatization Disorder. The Archives hold only two responses, from George Saslow and Henry Pinsker, and they both supported Spitzer's choice of fewer criteria. Saslow stated forcefully: "DSM-iii [sic] was not intended to be a document for research workers. Our decision to be inclusive [for clinicians] rather than selective [for researchers] established that intention, I thought. For this reason, I urge that we stay with the present DMI-iii [sic] criteria."[17]

In the final few days before the Assembly vote, Spitzer decided the time had come to make known clearly and resolutely his position and reasoning on an acceptable number of criteria for Somatization Disorder. In a quite lengthy memo to sent the Task Force, Guze, and Lee Robins (the Wash. U. psychiatric epidemiologist), Spitzer reviewed the history of the Wash. U. group's unhappiness with the latest DSM-III criteria for Somatization Disorder, based on their argument that the equivalent in the Feighner criteria had a very good reliability score. He then recounted how the Task Force had tried to develop more comprehensive criteria, the better to "approximate the original Feighner criteria" but yet establish criteria that would remain "clinically acceptable." But Guze and Robins were not satisfied with the Task Force's modifications and still argued for the original, more numerous Feighner criteria to be placed in DSM-III. So Spitzer related how he had reworked the Somatization Disorder criteria yet again, still keeping in mind that clinicians should be able to remember the groupings of the symptoms "without having the criteria in front of them." Spitzer found the reliability score of these more recent criteria to be quite good and added, with obvious annoyance, "It is hard to know what else could be wrong with an individual who has at least 14 unexplained physical symptoms [as in the DSM-III draft]. If this is not some form of Somatization Disorder, then what is it?"

Ultimately, the diagnostic criteria for Somatization Disorder included "a history of physical symptoms of several years' duration beginning before the age of 30 [and] complaints of at least 14 symptoms for women and 12 for men, from [among] 37 symptoms." The thirty-seven symptoms were distributed among seven categories: belief in sickliness; conversion or pseudoneurological symptoms (e.g., difficulty swallowing, loss of voice, fainting), gastrointestinal symptoms; female reproductive symptoms; psychosexual symptoms; pain; and cardiopulmonary symptoms.[18]

Spitzer emphasized that the DSM-III criteria "are far more usable clinically than requiring that the original Feighner research criteria be used." He reiterated that "our concern is that by including the Feighner criteria, unmodified, they will not be used by clinicians" and that, therefore, the Task Force had to take "a broader view" than did the Wash. U. group. He concluded significantly: "We believe that the scientific merits of the revised criteria can be defended on their own grounds. However, we should like to add that given the current political situation with DSM-III [he meant the still ongoing battle with the psychoanalysts over the elimination of "neurosis" from the nomenclature], there is hardly any advantage in asking clinicians to make diagnoses based on 20 to 24 symptoms in nine out of ten categories."[19] Henry Pinsker, perennially protecting the interests of the clinician, resoundingly seconded Spitzer:

> The St. Louis people don't have to be any more content than the analysts. DSM-III is not the embodiment of science, nor is it the popular version of RDC [Research Diagnostic Criteria].... For clinical purposes, the softer standards for somatization order are fine; for research on the condition, one may want to use the more rigorous criteria.... The Feighner criteria are deficient for clinical purposes because they do not admit the early case.... Clinically, we must handle such problems. For research we must avoid them. As it is, asking people to make a diagnosis on the basis of fourteen points is possibly beyond the frontier of what is acceptable.[20]

Pinsker had summed up the philosophy of many on the Task Force. DSM-III was to be a manual of inclusiveness. Spitzer had no compunction adding diagnoses if they were of great use to clinicians, as long as they could be described by clear diagnostic criteria. Description—the phenomenological approach—was key to the making of DSM-III, which meant that etiology, including the views of the psychoanalysts, was held in abeyance for a future day, except in the unambiguous case of the organic brain disorders.

The episodes just related unambiguously illustrate Spitzer's forcefulness when he was set on a path he deemed essential to his conception of DSM-III. When thus determined, he was willing to take on formidable constituencies, whether they be his ostensible allies at Wash. U. or the psychoanalysts who still held powerful positions in American psychiatry. We will see his resolve and tenacity next, on an issue that startled many.

DIAGNOSING HOMOSEXUALS DISTRESSED BY THEIR ORIENTATION . . . AGAIN

At the same moment that Spitzer was urgently sending out a questionnaire to a sizable chunk of the APA membership on how to label and define Borderline Personality Disorder, and just when the controversy with the American Psychological Association over the definition of a mental disorder was heating up, intense disagreement burst out over the approach that should be taken to homosexuality in DSM-III. Spitzer, it became clear, was planning not only to retain in the manual's new edition a separate diagnosis referring to homosexuals who were troubled by their sexual orientation but also to coin a new name for this situation. He had the intention of replacing his own 1973 inspired "Sexual Orientation Disturbance" that had been in DSM-II. The "acrimonious dispute" (Spitzer's own words), although generating a voluminous correspondence, remained within the confines of the profession—the gay community did not get involved.[21]

The debate over the place of homosexuality in the new manual highlights the clinical (and perhaps also social) ambivalence psychiatrists continued to feel in the wake of the decision to remove the diagnosis of homosexuality from DSM-II. After the 1974 vote by APA members to depathologize homosexuality, the public may have thought that psychiatrists had settled the issue once and for all. But the bitter dispute over whether there should be any diagnosis in DSM-III referring to homosexuals troubled by their orientation shows that psychiatrists had come to no closure about the matter.

As we launch into an account of the controversy, it is useful to remember that most of the disputation revolved around three issues:

- Should there be a special diagnosis for homosexual individuals who were troubled by their orientation?
- If there should be a label, what should it be?
- Where under the broad heading of Psychosexual Disorders should the particular designation (if any) be listed?

As these questions were addressed, Spitzer faced a combination of disbelief, anger, and threats. There was at first predictable astonishment on the part of some. Why were homosexuals different from other depressed or anxious patients psychiatrists routinely encounter? Why should homosexuals' problems with sexual identity or enjoyment of sexual relations set them apart from heterosexual people with the same complaints? There was also strong opposition to the neologisms (e.g., homodysphilia) that Spitzer had coined to label homosexuals' problems. And finally, there were threats of resignation from the Psychosexual Disorders Advisory Committee to indicate general disapproval, as well as threats to take the matter to higher authorities within the APA.

Three psychiatrists in particular arrayed themselves against Spitzer's plan to include in DSM-III a diagnosis for homosexuals distressed over their sexual orientation. They were Judd Marmor (1910–2003), Professor of Psychiatry at the University of Southern California, a former President of the APA and a psychoanalyst who had argued for a decade against the idea of homosexuality as pathology;[22] Richard Pillard (b. 1933), Professor of Psychiatry at Boston University and one of the founders of the Gay Caucus within the APA; and Richard Green (b. 1936), Professor of Psychiatry at the State University of New York at Stony Brook and one of the members of the DSM-III Psychosexual Disorders Advisory Committee. There had been some low key grumblings from others in the summer of 1975 about a draft classification that declared "homosexual arousal" to be a sexual object choice disorder, since this raised fears that it might bring homosexuality back as a disorder in the nomenclature. However, the first real thunderbolts, in what was to become a determined attack against Spitzer's goals, were dramatically hurled by Green in an angry letter to Spitzer in December 1976.

Green's ire initially seemed pointedly personal. He wrote to Spitzer that as one of the original members of the Psychosexual Disorders Advisory Committee he believed he and his colleagues had been working fruitfully. Then the composition and activities of the committee had been drastically altered, he accused, when Spitzer had added colleagues from Columbia University. These individuals seemed to have taken over, he complained, and his own input had been correspondingly unsolicited or ignored. He had "formulated an extensive document on gender role disorders," and then heard nothing for a year. Now, suddenly, he had received a note wanting an immediate response on revisions to his document and also informing him that, without ever having consulted him, there was a new diagnostic term for homosexuals distressed about their homosexuality, "homodysphilia." Green exploded at the "neologism" and the way decisions were supposedly being made without involving him. He threatened to let the membership of the APA know that he was not responsible for those decisions, and he abruptly resigned from the Psychosexual Disorders Advisory Committee.[23] On this note, the war started.

Spitzer, although deeply immersed in sorting out the contentious BPD diagnosis, responded in two weeks with a densely packed three-page letter, initially as angry as Green's communication. He accepted Green's resignation, defended his choice of the additional members of the Advisory Committee, and accused Green of repeatedly not responding to memos that had been sent to him. Spitzer also explained in some detail how he had coined the new term "homodysphilia" in response to requests at presentations that he should come up with a term that was "more accurate and far more acceptable to the profession that the original term, 'Sexual Orientation Disorder.'" He further argued that Green did not seem to understand that all proposals and revisions, whether those of Green personally or the Advisory Committees, had to be "finally approved by the Task Force which had the ultimate responsibility for DSM-III." But then Spitzer, not one to burn bridges, expressed regret at Green's withdrawal from work on the Sexual Disorders Section of DSM-III and asked Green to let him know if he wanted to receive further drafts for his comments, even though he had resigned from the Advisory Committee. And, "one final detail": did Green want his name listed in DSM-III with his dates of membership in the Advisory Committee or did he prefer not to be listed at all?[24] It is obvious from later correspondence on this issue and others as well that Green continued to be a member of the Advisory Committee.

Aside from Spitzer's irate response to Green, the record is silent for almost three months. Then in March 1977—either hearing from Green or getting wind of the April 15, 1977 draft of DSM-III soon to be officially released—Pillard, a founder of the APA Gay Caucus, feared that a reversal of the 1973 APA decision that removed homosexuality as a diagnosis in DSM-II might be in the offing. He sent out letters to at least six psychiatrists who he thought might lend a sympathetic ear: Judd Marmor (Fig. 10.1), the analyst who had been President of the APA and a long-time critic of pathologizing homosexuality; Leon Eisenberg, who had served on the APA Board of Trustees; Marcel Saghir, a Wash. U. psychiatrist who had extensively studied male and female homosexuality; Harold Lief, an expert on human sexuality who was a member of the Psychosexual Disorders Advisory Committee; George Winokur, one of the leading neo-Kraepelinians; and Richard Green. All but Eisenberg and Lief were supportive, although Winokur, while sympathetic, was not prepared to get involved.[25] Marmor was especially encouraging and maintained a vigorous and eloquent presence throughout the whole controversy, taking on Spitzer and expressing vital clinical and philosophical ideas. In answering Pillard's letter, Marmor also sent copies of his letter to Spitzer and Green. (It should be noted that here, as well as in almost the entire correspondence of the debate, letters sent to one person were usually at the same time copied to all other interested parties.)

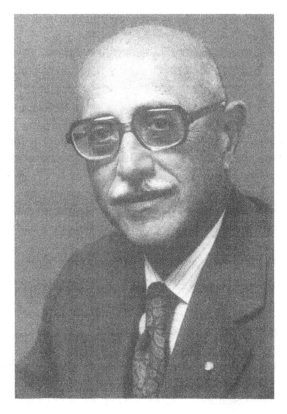

JUDD MARMOR, M.D.

FIG 10.1 Judd Marmor (1910–2003) was a pioneering voice for taking the diagnosis of homosexuality as pathology out of the DSM. He championed this position well before Spitzer worked to remove the diagnosis and to replace it with Sexual Orientation Disorder. Thus, Marmor tenaciously fought with Spitzer to prevent a new diagnosis in DSM-III for homosexuals who were troubled by their homosexuality. But Spitzer prevailed with the inclusion of "ego-dystonic homosexuality" in the revised classification.

Source: Reprinted with Permission from the *American Journal of Psychiatry* (Copyright © 1976) American Psychiatric Association.

Marmor found homodysphilia "unnecessary" and the concept behind it "archaic" and continued: "My own view is that a person's sexual orientation is irrelevant to the question of whether or not there is a mental disorder present." If a gay man or lesbian is distressed about his or her orientation, then the correct diagnosis should be the name of the underlying psychological disorder, for example, anxiety reaction or depressive reaction. Marmor concluded that if "Spitzer's group" insisted on keeping the concept of homodysphilia, he would be glad to join with Green, Pillard, and others to urge that the "equally meaningless" term "heterodysphilia be included as a balancing term" in DSM-III.[26] Spitzer now had a lot on his plate. At the precise time that he was being confronted with increasing opposition over his positioning of homosexuality in the new DSM, he was facing the start of organized hostilities from the American Psychoanalytic Association. (This new contretemps will be discussed in Chapter 11.)

Meanwhile, sometime in March 1977, the first official draft of DSM-III (April 15, 1977) began appearing[27] with the term "dyshomophilia" (which had been substituted for "homodysphilia") listed under the Paraphilias (new term for perversions.) Next to Dyshomophilia in parenthesis was Homosexuality. The gay community soon learned officially of Spitzer's proposal because Spitzer sent a copy of the section discussing Dyshomophilia to Franklin E. Kameny (1925–2011), founder of the Mattachine Society, a pioneering organization for gay and lesbian civil rights. As always, Spitzer was quite open about his positions, but there is no record that Kameny weighed in at this point. (We should bear in mind that the terms "homodysphilia" and "dyshomophilia" were being used simultaneously.)

Then in May, at the 1977 annual APA meeting in Toronto, Green spoke to Spitzer who, no doubt having heard criticism from others as well, informed him that he was planning to remove Dyshomophilia from its place among the paraphilias.[28] This step did not satisfy Green, who also had contact with certain other psychiatrists at the meeting, all of whom agreed, he reported, that "homosexuality can be subsumed under a variety of other places in DSM-III including depression, anxiety, adult situational reactions...or somewhere else." This argument was made repeatedly throughout the controversy, but Spitzer would not be swayed by it. Also in Toronto, Judd Marmor suggested that those who were opposed to Spitzer's plan appeal to the Committee on Research and Development, to which the DSM-III Task Force reported. Green, meanwhile, said he planned to poll each member of the three DSM committees involved with human sexuality to find out if they wanted any kind of diagnosis referring to homosexuality in the new manual. The swirl of opposition was building.

Spitzer also took the time to reflect on his experiences in Toronto in a letter to Pillard and present his own justification for having such a diagnosis, arguing for the possibility of pathology: "For many of us, the issue as to whether or not at some level homosexuality is in some cases pathological is still not resolved. To remove the category entirely from the classification would be a way of removing the legitimization of therapeutic efforts to study its etiology."[29] Was this the same Robert Spitzer who had led the way in taking the diagnosis of homosexuality out of the DSM? Nevertheless, he ended his letter graciously: "Let's keep talking." We see in this communication a microcosm of how Spitzer often dealt with thorny issues: he both talked about possible compromise and staked out a position that he was determined to defend. The upshot of the whole homosexual battle bears out both of these observations.

As soon as he received a copy of Spitzer's letter to Pillard, Marmor wrote back in a sharp rebuttal. He argued that homosexuality is not pathology in "some cases." He labeled Spitzer's position as "regressive" and declared that he had "reverted" to a position in which he considered homosexuality pathology, no doubt owing to "unconscious homophobia," so frequent in his generation. Such bias, Marmor declared, was "basically moral and judgmental rather than scientific." He closed, "I plead again with your committee" to remove homodysphilia from DSM-III.[30]

The controversy continued to build over the summer as Green began polling the Psychosexual Disorders and Gender Identity Disorders Advisory Committees. He also declared that if "homosexuality (or whatever it is called)" were not removed from DSM-III, he and like-minded colleagues would bring the matter to the Council on

Research and Development.[31] Eleven days later Spitzer wrote to the Psychosexual Disorders Advisory Committee to poll them whether they would accept Dyshomophilia in DSM-III, not under Paraphilias but under the heading "Other Psychosexual Disorders." Here was Spitzer's first compromise, but he did not retreat from his overall goal. He argued that "in our current state of ignorance this is a scientifically defensible position [since] specific treatment programs are designed for this condition." If the Psychosexual Disorders Advisory Committee did not support this view, Spitzer threatened to bring the matter to the Task Force.[32]

Predictably, Marmor replied to attack Spitzer for his "arbitrary and unwarranted" stand, since every group in the APA governance had voted that homosexuality "did not constitute psychopathology." Marmor was strongly joined in his protest by John Money (1921–2006), a psychologist renowned for his work in sexual identity, the biology of gender, and sex change. He had coined the term "gender role" to replace that of "sex role," believing sexual identity is primarily a learned phenomenon.[33] Money wanted to delete Dyshomophilia from DSM-III, objecting not only to the term but also to the concept. "It is improper to single out homophilia from among all the other philias as the only one deserving of the prefix dys-, the addition of which turns it into a disease." Moreover, "the net result of including the term, dyshomophilia, in DSM-III is simply to readmit homosexuality into psychiatric nosology through the back door." Moral indignation, Money wrote, should not be the criterion of psychiatric classification. He repeated what was probably the most frequent position of Spitzer's critics. "Any homosexual who seeks treatment can be classified in exactly the same way as the heterosexual is classified, namely, on the basis of anxiety, depression, various neurotic symptoms, failure of the sex organs to function adequately in a sexual partnership." If the rival camps on the inclusion of dyshomophilia reached an impasse, Money suggested a term already in the literature be used, "gender dysphoria." There would be three subtypes: heterosexual, bisexual, and homosexual.[34]

By the fall of 1977 the crisis had not been resolved, and Spitzer and Marmor were in an intense correspondence. Spitzer argued, politically, that Dyshomophilia was just another more accurate name for Sexual Orientation Disorder that had been approved by the APA Trustees in 1973. "It is quite clear," he asserted, "that a proposal to remove homosexuality without a diagnostic category specifically for homosexuals distressed by their homosexual impulses would not have been approved at that time. I am also convinced that it would not be approved at the current time."[35] Marmor responded within a week, but addressing clinical and etiological concerns. He was adamant in his position, based, he said, on his considerable experience in treating troubled homosexuals over the years. "In the vast majority of these instances it was clear that their anxiety, or distress…stemmed primarily from the fact that as homosexuals they felt severely disparaged and excluded by the mainstream of society." Almost always, their distress was not over their impulses themselves but on the consequences of expressing their impulses. Then Marmor lectured Spitzer: "The only reason we treat individuals who feel distressed by their homosexual impulses as a separate diagnostic category is because <u>we</u> have not yet <u>fully</u> accepted the idea that homosexual impulses per se do not necessarily constitute psychopathology."[36] (Underlinings are in the original.)

Thus at odds, Marmor and Spitzer traveled (Spitzer from New York, Marmor from California) to Washington, DC, on September 16, 1977, to heatedly debate the issue before the APA Council on Research and Development.[37] After a lengthy discussion with the Council, the Chair, Lester Grinspoon, "made it clear that under no circumstances would the Council wish to become involved in the resolution of this issue."[38] The APA hierarchy was done with the issues surrounding homosexuality and was not about to reopen these topics. The matter was thus kicked back to Spitzer who either had to convince the Advisory Committee on Psychosexual Disorders to side with him or else bring the matter before the Task Force for a binding decision. Spitzer turned to canvassing votes from the members of the Advisory Committee. The Archives provide us evidence of one such attempt in a September 23, 1977 letter from Spitzer to Robert J. Stoller (1925–1991), a psychoanalyst and internationally known theorist on sex-identity issues. Spitzer appealed to Stoller to cast a vote for his (Spitzer's) position, after Stoller had already abstained on the issue of including a separate category for Dyshomophilia.[39] Stoller answered in a thoughtful scholarly letter, exploring the issues at stake, but still not committing.[40]

Six months had passed since Pillard and Marmor had taken their clear stand against Spitzer (and nine months since Green's outburst). Opposition to Spitzer's position remained unabated, and he had been unable to achieve any consensus on either his position of there being a separate diagnosis for homosexuals upset by their orientation or a category with the name Dyshomophilia. Feelings continued to run high on both sides.

Spitzer, indomitable as always, sent out another poll on October 5 to the Advisory Committee on Psychosexual Disorders. Giving no ground on the advisability of having a separate diagnostic category for the disorder he was proposing, he offered the committee a choice of three names for the condition: Dyshomophilia (his term), Distress About Homosexual Impulses (Marmor's very reluctant term), and Homosexual Conflict Disorder (a new suggestion from a member of the Advisory Committee.) Spitzer's accompanying memo was laced with humor, in an attempt to defuse the tense situation.[41]

The poll proved a bust. The Advisory Committee again could not reach a consensus and Spitzer made the decision to bring the matter to the Task Force. On October 18, 1977, Spitzer sent out a ballot to the Task Force offering the members four choices toward resolution of the dispute: (1) Homosexual Conflict Disorder (HCD) will appear as a separate category; (2) HCD will appear as one of the examples noted in Other Psychosexual Disorders; (3) The Task Force should meet with the interested parties for further discussion; (4) Other_____.[42]

Now that the Task Force was involved, matters began heating up even further, if that were possible. The Task Force, which included a number of forceful individuals, were not content with Spitzer's options and began raising all sorts of objections to them and offering their own strong views. But, paradoxically, because of this situation, and the fact that the Task Force had been appealed to as a court of last resort, events finally began to move to a climax.

In a lengthy memo to Spitzer in early November, Donald Klein, always out-spoken and an influential Task Force member, made a strong case for there being certain circumstances in which conflicted homosexuality (psychopathology) occurs, thus siding with Spitzer. Klein also pointed out, "Once we have gotten the issue of whether to consider "dyshomophilia" an illness out of the way, there remains the question of what the label should be and where it should be within DSM-III." As to its placement, and upholding Spitzer' argument, he urged that the diagnosis be in a separate category in order to facilitate communication among psychiatrists. As to a label, he endorsed yet another of Spitzer's verbal creations, "ego-dystonic homosexuality."[43] Four days later, Spitzer received another boost from Jon K. Meyer, a sexual-disorders expert at Johns Hopkins on the Psychosexual Disorders Advisory Committee, seconding Klein on the need for a separate category for homosexuals distressed by their orientation.[44] And one week later, Robert Stoller came off the fence and endorsed a separate category for "Homosexual Conflict Disorder," an important victory for Spitzer.[45] Then, as Thanksgiving approached, Spitzer abruptly sent a terse memo to "Participants in Homosexual Conflict Disorder Category [sic]." He declared that "a new formulation of Homosexual Conflict Disorder is in the making. Therefore, Task Force members should not vote until they have had ample time to consider this new proposal."[46]

Still the Green–Spitzer imbroglio did not cease. The day after Spitzer's memo, Green angrily wrote to Spitzer that he believed the majority of participants did not share Spitzer's viewpoint, and if the issue was not resolved soon, he was prepared to go to the APA Assembly of Delegates.[47] Spitzer wrote back (with copies to everyone) that Green did not know how to count and enumerated the majority that he, Spitzer, had on the need for a specific category.[48]

Events overtook Green as Spitzer moved on December 20, 1977 to formulate a new draft for "ego-dystonic homosexuality," which was now listed under Other Psychosexual Disorders.[49] This was a clear shift away from the original placement of Dyshomophilia under the Paraphilias in the April 15, 1977 draft. The revised draft shifted the focus of the diagnosis from the alleged psychopathology of the homosexual person—the "dyshomophilia"—to his or her distress over the impairment of heterosexual functioning. Many saw this as an attempt on Spitzer's part to compromise. The draft beneath the subheading "Predisposing Factors" read as follows:

> Since homosexuality itself is not considered a mental disorder, the factors that predispose to homosexuality are not included in this section. The factors that predispose to Ego-dystonic Homosexuality are those negative societal attitudes towards homosexuality which have been internalized. In addition, features associated with heterosexuality, such as having children and socially sanctioned family life, may be viewed as desirable and incompatible with a homosexual arousal pattern.[50]

This discussion of "Predisposing Factors" is a shift from the 4/15/77 draft where homosexuality and hence "Dyshomophilia" were attributed to a dysfunctional family constellation between the child (the future homosexual individual) and his or her parents.[51]

With the new draft of December 20, Spitzer released a "Ballot on Ego-dystonic Homosexuality" to be completed by the members of the Task Force and the Advisory

Committee on Psychosexual Disorders. It allowed for three plans and general comments:

> Plan A: Inclusion of Ego-dystonic Homosexuality in DSM-III with the possibility of the respondent's suggesting minor revisions.
> Plan B: No separate category at all. Instead include conflicted homosexuality under "Psychosexual Disorders Not Elsewhere Classified."
> Plan C: Other (Specify)
> Comment also on the suggestion for a category called "Psychosexual Relationship Capacity Disorder."[52]

Richard Green continued to object: "I cannot accept the logic of ego-dystonic homosexuality."[53] Judd Marmor acquiesced, though noting, "I would have preferred no separate category at all."[54] Henry Pinsker, on the Task Force, was willing to come to terms with Spitzer's Plan A but argued that the decision to remove homosexuality from the list of mental disorders "has created problems in nosology which simply can't be overcome.... We have stood on our heads to maintain that homosexuality both is and is not a disorder. It doesn't work." But he took refuge in the belief that "our Diagnostic Manual is not a logical system [and] includes conditions which may or may not be diseases. [Hence] we can include ego dystonic homosexuality without feeling silly about such a contrived and inconsistent disease entity."[55]

The diagnostic criteria for Ego-dystonic Homosexuality in DSM-III were two:

> A. The individual complains that heterosexual arousal is persistently absent or weak and significantly interferes with initiating or maintaining wanted heterosexual relationships.
> B. There is a sustained pattern of homosexual arousal that the individual explicitly states has been unwanted and a persistent source of distress.[56]

Thus the great homosexuality fight of 1977 came to an end, not with a bang but with a whimper. Pillard and Green objected to the end but realized that any future debate was futile. With his revisions, Spitzer was ultimately able to win over Judd Marmor. The Task Force accepted Spitzer's final formulation and was glad to see the issue achieve closure.[57] Spitzer had prevailed in getting a separate diagnosis for homosexuals disturbed by their orientation but, in a compromise, had had to shift the broad categorization and conceptualization of the diagnosis in order to satisfy his critics. Such a conclusion to an "acrimonious dispute" was not atypical. Spitzer may have had to bend and twist, but he did not "give away the store."

TWO CODAS

The first ending to our story is that seven years after Ego-dystonic Homosexuality appeared in DSM-III, the controversial diagnosis was removed from DSM-III's revision, DSM-III-R, while Spitzer was chairing its Task Force.

The second is that in 2001 Spitzer conducted a study in which he interviewed 200 gay and lesbian individuals and concluded that it was possible to undo homosexuality through "reparative therapy," psychotherapy that could lead to heterosexuality. He published this study in the *Archives of Sexual Behavior* in 2003.[58] In 2012 he concluded that he had been wrong and that his study was flawed. He wrote a letter to the *Archives* retracting his study.[59] He was then featured in a dramatic video in which he apologized profusely to all gay individuals and their families whom he may have harmed by his publication.[60]

WOMEN'S CRITIQUE OF PSYCHOSEXUAL DISORDERS AND OTHER DIAGNOSES

The issue of changing psychiatry's attitudes toward homosexuals turns our attention to similar struggles of other groups that faced discrimination. Battles to expand the rights and opportunities for Americans being discriminated against were a visible part of life in the United States after the end of World War II, starting with civil rights for African Americans. This civil rights struggle inspired other minority and disadvantaged groups to campaign for the remedying of their unequal status. The 1960s saw the beginning of crusades by or on behalf of gay individuals, mental patients, Latinos, and women, as well as attempts to curb police powers. As Spitzer worked to construct DSM-III, he heard from women who focused especially on issues relating to Gender Identity Disorders (GID) and Psychosexual Disorders.

There was an uptick of involvement as various female psychiatrists and sociologists began to respond in May 1977 to the April 15, 1977 draft of DSM-III that Spitzer had widely distributed, avidly looking for feedback. Any controversy that emerged was fine with him, since contention itself did not usually disturb him. Thus, Spitzer always welcomed the reactions of interested individuals, even if he ended up rejecting the changes they suggested. Yet, at the same time, he was usually willing to consider various concerns and perhaps compromise on them, as long as positions he deemed essential remained intact. This two-fold strategy was very effective in achieving his desired results, although it sometimes angered his challengers or opponents, to whom, at first encouraged by his openness, it appeared that he would accept their proposals.

As far as women's interests were concerned, the largest group of documents in the Archives are letters to and from Ann Laycock Chappell, M.D., a member of the APA Committee on Women. Chappell had apparently been sent a copy of the DSM-III draft, and she, in turn, had duplicated sections about which she was troubled and sent them to various professional women for comment. It is obvious from the correspondence that she received many answers, but the material in the Archives contains only some of them. Nevertheless, it is still possible to report on the issues raised because they are remarkably similar from letter to letter. The Archives also contain an exchange of letters between Chappell and Spitzer that chronicle a winning exchange in the making of DSM-III.

Much attention in the opening letters was focused on the diagnosis of "Gender Identity or Role Disorder of Childhood" under the broader heading of "Psychosexual

Disorders." Chappell's responders expressed concern with the psychiatric labeling of children who like to partake of activities mainly enjoyed by the opposite sex, such as boys who like to play with dolls and girls who play a lot of sports. (We must remember that this was in 1977 when it was still not common for girls to be as active in a variety of sports as they are today.) Deviation from cultural stereotypes, it was argued by Chappell's colleagues, should not be pathologized, especially as relating to girls, who were pressured to eschew traditional "masculine" interests and pastimes. Elaine Hilberman M.D., also on the APA Committee on Women, suggested that "Essential Features" of the Gender Identity Disorder should contain a statement that "girls often wish they were boys becuase [sic] of the social realities that boys have more options and power regarding how they will live their lives." Pauline Bart, a sociologist (whose comments reflected the views of two psychologists as well), asserted that "females should be removed from this category because tomboyism is associated with healthy functioning in females and we would not want in any way to discourage such behavior." Carol Nadelson, M.D., a widely known expert on women's psychological issues (and eight years later President of the APA), declared that "the entire section [of Essential Features of GID] warrants rewriting and rethinking. The sex stereotyped material should be eliminated. It perpetuates stereotypes which produce anxiety in children and adults who view the specifically defined behaviors as normal or abnormal. There is abundant literature on this subject."[61]

There were other criticisms as well. The women welcomed the replacement of the prejudicial term "hysterical" (from the myth that hysteria is a specific disorder of women) by the term "histrionic" in Personality Disorders. However, Chappell's colleagues complained that the good had immediately been undone by adding "Hysterical Personality" in parenthesis right next to "Histrionic Personality Disorder." Then there were strong objections to the new discussion of "Sexual Sadism," listed under Paraphilias, with its broad definition of "sexual activity with non-consenting partners." The responders worried that many rapists would be placed in this category, thus falsely turning rape into a crime of passion and away from the realization that rape is an aggressive crime against women. A violent, criminal act, it was argued, should not be turned into a mental disorder. The description should not lead one to the conclusion that "all rapists are pathological," one of Chappell's correspondents concluded."[62] The issue of determining the boundary between psychopathology and crime is still being debated.

Finally, Nadelson took issue with the language in "Somatization Disorder (Briquet's Syndrome)." "Briquet's Syndrome," an alternate term for hysteria, was introduced by Paul Briquet (1796–1881) in 1859 and much preferred by the Wash. U. psychiatrists. Under "Age at Onset," the DSM-III draft referred to the association of Somatization Disorder with "menstrual difficulties." Under "Complications and Impairment" the text mentioned "women undergoing non-cancerous hysterectomy." Nadelson called hysterectomy for psychopathology "a unilateral situation and interpretation. Clearly there is collusion or support on the part of the physician which encourages such symptomatology."[63] What Nadelson appears to be saying is that it is the responsibility of a physician, when faced with a patient's physical problem for which there appears, after thorough investigation, to be no pathology, to interpret the patient's symptoms more accurately, rather than prescribing needless medication or surgery. If guidance or psychotherapy appears to be indicated, the physician should take that position rather than taking the sometimes easier way out—offering a possibly useless or dangerous physical remedy.

Chappell sent all the replies she had received to Spitzer, who appeared both bemused and taken aback by the large volume of material and chose to deal with the situation humorously. "I have decided to become famous by editing a book on the correspondence regarding Gender Disorders of Childhood. Since you are largely responsible for engineering this literature, would you like to be co-editor? On a more serious note, I am, to say the least, a little overwhelmed by all of the input from your female network. Can I expect to get from you a summary of what you think we should do with specific rewriting of the offending section?"[64] This being the early days of the feminist movement, Spitzer was obviously unfamiliar with the seriousness with which some women viewed the unequal status of women. But the women criticizing the DSM-III passages saw the unequal status reflected in the descriptions that appeared under Gender Identity or Role Disorder, Histrionic Personality Disorder, Sexual Sadism, and Somatization Disorder. The commentators regarded the language in these disorders as perpetuating falsities that handicapped women in much the same way that gay individuals regarded the pathologizing of homosexuality by psychiatrists, also categorized under Psychosexual Disorders.

We should also note that with the women's objection to the Gender Identity descriptions we see another favorite tactic of Spitzer when he faced complaints about material in DSM-III. He turned to the objector and asked her or him to provide specific changes and rewritten text for himself and the Task Force to consider, thus placing the burden on the critic, who many times withdrew.

But that did not happen this time. Chappell replied in a week with a three-page letter, which unfortunately is missing page 2 in the Archives. But on the first page there is a long discussion of the "Gender Identity Disorder of Childhood" repeating twice the "potential for harm" that was contained in the category as written. Moreover, Chappell declared:

> A major concern is that the category tries, but fails, to differentiate true identity confusion with failure to follow sex stereotyped roles....Such a failure is unforgivable and unacceptable. There is a real philosophic argument on how to impart gender identity without imparting sexual stereotypes [but] it does become imperative...that in these criteria we must remove all sex-stereotyped material.

Chappell, doing what Spitzer had asked, presented a solution:

> Either we must separate the discussion and criteria by sex or omit girls altogether from this category. I would strongly recommend the latter course in view of the paucity of research criteria and the potential for great harm. Girls should not be

included until research gives us criteria by which to delineate girls with pathological outcomes from normal, vigorous tomboys.

Helpfully, Chappell offered to "write a paragraph which..." And here the missing page
terminates her thought.

On page 3 Chappell informed Spitzer that she was sending him copies of all letters
that had been received and closed, by saying, "Please contact me or any of the respondents if we can be of further assistance in smoothing out these areas or correcting the
deficiency."[65]

There is a good chance that Spitzer was somewhat bewildered by the passion behind
these words. His first response to Chappell had been to joke about her concerns. After
all, this was a man who had reassured the APA Council on Research and Development
and the Reference Committee two years earlier that there were sufficient women
involved in the making of DSM-III, since there were already two women on the Task
Force and one on the Psychosexual Advisory Committee. The events described here
took place more than a generation ago, and it does not seem implausible to conclude
that Spitzer at that time might have been clueless and asked, along with Freud, "What
does a woman want?"

The Archives seem to bear out this supposition, in a handwritten and soothing
letter from Chappell to Spitzer expressing her regret over "the distress you describe in
your letter....I'm not personally angry with you. I am angry with some of the issues
raised by DSM-III....But the anger is not a personal one." The letter from Spitzer that
provoked such a response is missing, but it is clear that in this missing letter Spitzer was
expressing his upset at Chappell's stern lecture to him about the offending passages in
the DSM-III draft. For Chappell writes to Spitzer: "Many of my comments and phrases
were not in my own words—including...the captioned 'unacceptable and unforgiv-
able.' The thrust of most of the letters was not to exempt gender disorder entirely but
rather to do major reworking to exempt sex role stereotyped behavior....Additionally,
everyone was sufficiently concerned about potential damage to little girls." Chappell
closed, "Do take care."[66] Spitzer wrote back, "I feel better as a result of your July 13th
letter. I look forward to receiving your summary of specific suggestions for changes."
Signed, "Your faithful correspondent."[67]

The rest is almost denouement. Soon after his letter to Chappell, Spitzer made
serious efforts to carry out the women's proposals and objectives. He informed the
"Advisory Committee on Gender Identity" of Chappell's positions, enclosed the correspondence that Chappell had earlier forwarded to him, and asked the Committee
how the category could be "defined without reliance on stereotyped sex behavior,
which most of Dr. Chappell's respondents found objectionable."[68] Within two months,
Spitzer and Jon Meyer of the Psychosexual Disorders Committee rewrote the Gender
Identity Disorder of Childhood section and sent it out for comments from the people
who had originally written the section and from Chappell.[69]

If one compares the Gender Identity Disorder of Childhood section in the April 15,
1977 draft of DSM-III with the section in the revised draft of January 15, 1978, it is
readily apparent that almost the entire category had been reworked with an attempt to

meet the concerns of Chappell and the other critics. In the later draft, under "Essential Features" and "Diagnostic Criteria," the discussions of boys and girls were done separately. The new descriptions were written so as to stress the significant pathology of the disorder, and they explicitly declared, "There is not merely the rejection of stereotypical sex role behavior as, for example, in 'tomboyishness' in girls or 'sissyish' behavior in boys." The category "Sex Ratio" said only "No Information," which reflected the belief of the women responders that there was not sufficient research to make a statement about this section.[70]

After distribution of the revised draft, the Chair of the APA's Committee on Women requested a copy because of her Committee's interest in the revisions, and the chief of Women's Programs of the American Psychological Association wrote with the hope that there would be no sex bias in DSM-III. The Archives have no further correspondence from these women, so most likely they had no serious complaints.[71] The saga ends with a much-belated letter to Spitzer from Robert J. Stoller, who had taken part in the homosexuality controversy, replying to Spitzer's long-ago request for a rewrite on the gender identity disorders. Seemingly siding with the women critics, Stoller, a researcher on gender identity, averred: "I believe the issues are insoluble at present due to our lack of adequate information." "Identity" is a "vague" term, and "it is nothing more than a shorter way to say 'the mix of masculinity and femininity found within a person.' That always left the problem of the meaning of 'masculinity' and 'femininity.' These I have thought as being whatever an individual, a group, or a culture believed was masculinity or femininity."[72] One wonders if today, when there is clearer evidence of some genetic contribution to gender identity, Stoller would still take this position.

Eventually, in DSM-III, diagnostic criteria for Gender Identity Disorder of Childhood was divided into two sections, one for females and one for males. For females, the criteria included a "strongly and persistently stated desire to be a boy, or insistence that she is a boy (not merely a desire for any perceived cultural advantages from being a boy)." There also had to be "persistent repudiation of female anatomic structures [such as] she will not develop breasts [or] she has, or will grow, a penis." Finally, the onset had to take place before puberty. (Note that there is no reference to girls being tomboys.) For males the criteria included a "strongly and persistently stated desire to be a girl, or insistence that he is a girl." Second, there had to be "persistent repudiation of male anatomic structures" or "preoccupation with female stereotypical activities as manifested by a desire for either cross-dressing...or by a compelling desire to participate in the games and pastimes of girls." As with girls, the onset had to occur before puberty.[73]

In the 1960s a number of women became resolved to change many of the circumstances under which they worked, including their lower pay; lack of promotion to higher positions in government and industry; their ability to control the number of children they had; and the inequitable relationships many saw in their marriages. In short, these women wished to be regarded in the eyes of the world as equal with men. The APA in the 1970s had created a Committee on Women, and the women who served on this committee decided to make their voices heard in the revision of the

Diagnostic and Statistical Manual. On the whole, this was acceptable to Spitzer and the Task Force, and while all of the women's concerns may not have been addressed to the extent they wished, a great many were. Women's issues—in contrast to the other two matters we have just examined in this chapter—never became a battle during the making of DSM-III.[74]

Spitzer's relationship with women over the months of 1977–1978 was essentially a cordial one, unlike the one he was having simultaneously with representatives of the American Psychoanalytic Association. Psychoanalysts had dominated American psychiatry for almost three decades. But Spitzer, though trained as an analyst, was making it increasingly clear that he had fundamental differences with psychoanalysts over both their theories and their treatments. In this his Task Force stood behind him. They had made an early decision to steer psychiatry away from psychoanalysis, in favor of a Kraepelin-like descriptive system. The strength of their decision became apparent even at times when Spitzer moved toward a compromise position. The Task Force often remained obdurate and forced Spitzer's hand. The next chapter will chronicle the struggle over psychoanalytic dominance.

11

THE PSYCHOANALYTIC AWAKENING
TO DSM-III

Although not realized by the psychoanalytic establishment at first, Spitzer and the Task Force were determined to undo the psychoanalytic dominance of American psychiatry. They had decided at their very first meeting that the analytic influence had gone "too far," and they believed they could construct a "scientific manual" based on empirical findings. After the Midstream Conference there was skirmishing in this area with the challenges of the Assembly of Delegates' Liaison Committee to the Task Force, but Spitzer had been able to contain their demands.

As the Assembly of Delegates' Liaison Committee began to soften its grip, the American Psychoanalytic Association Liaison Committee commenced its own efforts to affect the construction of DSM-III.[1] The psychoanalysts started out with the expectation that through negotiating with Spitzer they would be able to influence at least some aspects of DSM-III. They also came to see, correctly, that even though DSM-III was not touted as a textbook, since it had only a small claim on etiology and none on treatment, the manual was going to become authoritative.

THE PSYCHOANALYSTS' ACTIONS FOLLOWING THE
MIDSTREAM MEETING

At the Midstream Conference of June 1976, some of the few analysts who attended recognized that it was necessary to become involved with the making of DSM-III. Clearly, DSM-III was not going to be a reprise of DSM-II (1968), as DSM-II had been a reprise of DSM-I (1952). Yet once the analysts had returned home, they did not immediately form a liaison committee, nor did they contact Spitzer. It was not until Christmas time, six months later, that Dr. Leo Madow (1915–2009) (Fig. 11.1), a prominent analyst and Chair of the Departments of Neurology and Psychiatry at the Medical College of Pennsylvania, called Spitzer's office to arrange a meeting. He asked specifically for a time three months hence, on a Saturday in March 1977. One cannot but wonder why the analysts were proceeding so slowly. The message that Spitzer's secretary left for Spitzer was ambiguous: Madow had said that a group of four to five people representing the American Psychoanalytic Association wanted "to find out about DSM-III, about what issues they have not yet decided." To whom did "they" refer—Spitzer or the analysts? In any event, Spitzer told his secretary that either March 19 or 26 would be suitable.[2]

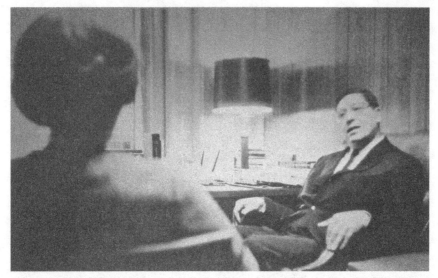

FIG. 11.1 Leo Madow, the, psychoanalyst who led the American Psychoanalytic Association's first subcommittee to the DSM-III Task Force. In trying to get the new manual to reflect various aspects of psychoanalytic thought, Madow faced Spitzer's driving empiricism and the uncompromising anti-psychoanalytic bias of the Task Force. This photo is a vivid contrast with the picture of Eli Robins in his lab (Fig. 3.4). Together they clearly demonstrate two different modes of psychiatric focus. *Source*: Drexel University College of Medicine Legacy Center

It is not clear whether the meeting took place at the end of March or the beginning of April, but it must not have gone too well because in a memo to the group thanking them for coming to meet with him, Spitzer wrote, "I apologize for some testiness on my part—a result of both battle fatigue and underlying personality structure." He then presented some thoughts about including psychodynamic material in DSM-III and asked for the Liaison Committee's responses. He promised that any material he received from them by April 29 could be considered for a May 1 meeting of the DSM-III Task Force.[3]

The analysts came away from the initial meeting quite perturbed by what they had heard. However, the DSM-III classifications, "bad as they were," were not what troubled them the most. Rather, it was the "superficial" nature of the text that accompanied the categories.[4] Madow submitted a report to the Executive Council of the American Psychoanalytic Association on April 28, the day before Spitzer had asked for analytic material to be delivered to him. Madow made clear to the Council that his committee did not consider the approach of the Task Force just "atheoretical" but actually anti-analytic, bringing "into question the central etiological assumptions of the psychoanalytic perspective."[5] The Task Force had included in the descriptive material only information that "could be proven statistically, which was...an antianalytic stance."[6]

Madow urged that the Executive Council hire an analyst to rewrite significant portions of DSM-III from a contemporary psychoanalytic perspective, which would highlight recent changes and advances in psychoanalytic theory. He maintained that this was the only avenue to effectively respond to Spitzer's repeated assertion that if a critic had complaints he should submit specific revised material. But some on the Council were dubious, and a discussion ensued. Surely "Spitzer could be reasoned with" if scientific arguments were made. Others were not so certain and thought that Spitzer was in a very powerful position. Otto Kernberg believed the situation was critical. He had been to the Midstream meeting, where he had felt a sense of "helplessness." Spitzer appeared to be flexible but had strongly negative feelings about psychoanalysis, he went on, and members of the Task Force and other advisers were even more hostile to the field. The analysts might want to dismiss it all as a "joke," but that would be dangerous. "The guns are pointed at us," Kernberg concluded. Yet, someone offered, perhaps the Assembly Liaison Committee could be counted on to stop Spitzer, and the way forward should be to support Howard Berk. In the end, the Council turned down Madow's suggestion that they deal with the situation by funding someone to prepare rewritten text to present to Spitzer. Instead, it was decided, they would ask for a larger involvement in the preparation of DSM-III and try to slow down the rate at which it was being developed.

Of course, they could not know it at the time, but the analysts were about to shut the barn door after the horse had escaped. They were just starting to get involved with DSM-III after the Task Force and the Advisory Committees had been working for over two years and had already made crucial decisions. Time would show that Spitzer and the Task Force could not be dealt with by "reasoning" with them and that neither greater analytic involvement nor attempts to slow down the process would work. It is unknowable if presenting substantial amounts of revised text—as Leo Madow had advised—would have had any effect at this particular juncture. Nevertheless, it might well have been more difficult for Spitzer and the Task Force to reject totally a large body of rewriting, especially if the suggested text had shown some regard for a descriptive approach and highlighted recent developments in psychoanalysis. We will see that later efforts offering short analytic revisions had little influence. In Spitzer, the analysts were facing a very determined adversary, and in the Task Force, a hostile one.

THE ANALYSTS PUT THEIR PLAN INTO ACTION

The day after the Executive Council of the Psychoanalytic Association made their decision, their President and President-elect sent a telegram to Louis Jolyon ("Jolly") West (1924–1999), Chair of the Council on Research and Development, the APA entity that Spitzer answered to. The two analysts asked that the APA "postpone taking any definitive actions on DSM-III until there has been more opportunity for study not only of its content but its methods and loci of evaluation" and that the psychiatry section of the ICD-9-CM be postponed for a year so that the Psychoanalytic Association could have more input into the classification.[7]

In response to these requests, the Council on Research and Development held "a lengthy discussion" but voted unanimously not to recommend to the APA Board of Trustees that the publication date of DSM-III be postponed. It was necessary, West explained, that the development of the new manual move swiftly in order to insert the terminology of DSM-III into ICD-9-CM, which was scheduled by WHO (not under control by the APA, West pointed out) to be published in 1978 and to become effective January 1, 1979. There would be many problems if DSM-III (now scheduled for approval in May 1979) and ICD-9-CM were in simultaneous use with "markedly different terminologies for psychiatric disorders." To temper his rejection of the analysts' request, West said he had sent their telegram to the American Association of Chairmen of Departments of Psychiatry, which then authorized the formation of a special ad hoc committee to review various concerns, including those of the analysts, regarding DSM-III. (Various former chairmen interviewed could not recall if this ad hoc committee had ever met. Nevertheless, as we shall see, it did get involved in an attempt to contribute to the Introduction to DSM-III.) West informed the analysts that his tenure as Chair of the Council was over and that in the future they should address any concerns to his successor, Lester Grinspoon (b. 1928).[8]

To counter the rebuff, the analysts scored what seemed to be a victory. Spitzer agreed to add two analysts, John Frosch, M.D., and his nephew, William A. (Bill) Frosch, M.D., to the Task Force. Explaining both of these choices later, Spitzer wrote, "Although committed to psychoanalysis, [John Frosch] had made clear his belief that psychiatry had suffered in the past from its failure to distinguish between etiological, dynamic and descriptive levels of analysis." As for Bill Frosch, Spitzer declared that he had [already] "demonstrated his capacity to work within the Task Force perspective by contributing to its work on substance abuse disorders.... He accepted the descriptive criteria-based approach to diagnosis."[9]

Spitzer also offered once more to review "specific suggestions for changes in the draft writeups [sic] for those categories that members of [Madow's Liaison Committee] felt were poorly written." The Committee promised the replacement sections by June 15, and on June 6, Spitzer wrote to Madow to ask if the substitute passages were forthcoming.[10] But again the Liaison Committee chose not to send material to Spitzer. "Unfortunately," Madow wrote to Spitzer on June 10, the Liaison Committee felt "somewhat discouraged" following the May 1977 Toronto meeting, where they had heard with dismay the preliminary results from the field trials and learned that DSM-III was to be incorporated into ICD-9-CM. Therefore, continued Madow, his committee "did not pursue actively the draft write-ups we had indicated we would submit to you by June 15. However, on rethinking," Madow wrote, "it is apparent to all of us that there continues to be value in our input; and I have encouraged...our President to look into this in order to participate as helpfully as possible in this work that you are undertaking."[11] What Madow had in mind, when his suggestions for major rewriting had already been turned down by the analysts' Executive Council, is puzzling.

While these events transpired, other psychoanalysts, quite separately, in the Washington, DC metropolitan area, were responding to sections of the April 15, 1977 draft. Roger Peele, the Acting Superintendent of St. Elizabeth's Hospital in Washington and a member of the APA Assembly Liaison Committee to the Task Force, had passed on to four analysts from the Washington Psychiatric Society sections of the draft for review. While Peele was not an analyst, he was sympathetic to psychodynamic thinking.[12] The analysts examined a great deal of the draft, though not all of it, they noted, and they gave Peele a prompt response, both to the general approach of the draft and to specific disorders.[13] They leveled a reproach, often to be repeated by analysts, that Spitzer and the Task Force had ignored "the large body of psychiatric knowledge about intrapsychic conflict and structure, accumulated over many years of clinical experience." They wrote that their major objection was to an underlying principle Spitzer had adopted: that it was justifiable to remove Neurosis as a separate category in DSM-III because intrapsychic conflict was to be found in many psychiatric disorders and that even well individuals had some measure of conflict. Therefore, Spitzer had concluded, Neurosis could not be used as an organizing principle. In addition to protesting against this reasoning, the analysts took issue with several specific descriptions of disorders in the draft and objected to the new terminology—often neologisms, they criticized—that replaced old language in common use. Why was "Somatoform" better than "Psychophysiologic" or "Psychosomatic," they asked? They ended by "strongly" opposing the inclusion of DSM-III in ICD-9-CM and urging the Washington Psychiatric Society, "in the strongest possible terms," to disapprove the further use of the new manual.[14]

Someone forwarded this report to Madow, who sent it on to Spitzer. In an answer to Madow, Spitzer summarily dismissed the report because it was an evaluation from four individual analysts, not from the analysts' official Liaison Committee. He also pointed out that while he disagreed with the Washington report, it did contain two specific references to weak spots in the draft, first in the language regarding Obsessive Compulsive Disorder and second in the conceptualization of the definition of psychosocial stressors in the multiaxial system. Spitzer said this was the kind of specific assessment he wanted. That is why he was "very disappointed" that he had not received critiques from Madow's Liaison Committee.[15]

We should note here that Spitzer seems to have been insisting that the only type of feedback he wanted was on individual points in the DSM draft.[16] He did not appear willing to change anything relating to basic philosophic differences that existed between him and the analysts. But this was exactly what the analysts wanted to critique and influence, and Spitzer's implacability was the source of their frustration and distress. Twice, it eventually turned out, Spitzer was amenable to a compromise with the analysts that involved modification of the multiaxial system, but determined members of the Task Force rejected any concession. Spitzer had chosen these people precisely for their devotion to a strict empiricism, and he now, ironically, reaped the fruits of his own planting.

THE ANALYSTS SUBMIT A "SPECIFIC" REVISION OF MATERIAL IN DSM-III

Throughout the summer of 1977 there was no reply from the analytic Liaison Committee. One wonders why they did not take Spitzer up on his offer with more alacrity. Was Madow still discouraged? A response from the Liaison Committee finally came in September in the form of specific recommendations, by Lawrence (commonly known as Larry) Rockland, M.D., for the inclusion of psychodynamic materials in the Anxiety Disorders section of DSM-III.[17] Spitzer was surprised that given "the importance with which it viewed this task, the Committee did not turn to an analyst of national prominence," but simply to a member of Madow's group. (Perhaps the Analytic Executive Council had been wrong to turn down Madow's proposal for a major revision by a specially chosen analyst. Would such a high-profile effort have carried significant weight, since Spitzer was a graduate analyst and had respect for some of the luminaries in the field?) On September 20, Spitzer forwarded Rockland's recommendations to the Task Force for their review and "judgment as to the value of including such material in DSM-III." He posed a series of four alternatives regarding inclusion for the Task Force to consider and asked for their replies within the next two weeks.[18]

These actions turned out to be the start of more than six months of complicated negotiating between Spitzer and the analysts. Both sides launched a variety of initiatives for possible psychodynamic contributions to DSM-III, none of which came to fruition.

The Task Force was willing to accept some of Rockland's descriptive changes but did not want to accept dynamic recommendations, for example, "that obsessive compulsive disorder represented a 'regression to anal conflict.'" These proposals were described as "simplistic and parochial" and only "anecdotal."[19] But the Task Force did not respond to Spitzer's requests for a timely decision from them. However, in answering Madow's inquiry of why he had not received a response after six weeks' time,[20] Spitzer did give him bad news from other sources. He reported to Madow that at his recent meeting with the Assembly of Delegates' Liaison Committee "there was a consensus that the inclusion of psychodynamic material in DSM-III...would be a mistake, as it would then require the inclusion of material from other schools of thought." Moreover, Spitzer continued, a member of the Liaison Committee of the Academy of Psychoanalysis had strongly objected to Rockland's material because he thought it would not be acceptable to members of the Academy.[21]

SPITZER REJECTS THE PROPOSED REVISON BUT OFFERS ALTERNATIVES

It was not until another full month later that Spitzer gave Madow the Task Force's verdict. In the third paragraph of his long and complex letter, Spitzer informed Madow that DSM-III "will not include detailed statements regarding proposed psychodynamic or other mechanisms to account for the disorders."[22] How so? The DSM-III classification, Spitzer wrote, was a descriptive classification because psychiatrists had reached no consensus on the etiologies and mechanisms of most mental disorders. At a later date, Spitzer wrote again to Madow, more specifically, that the Task Force had largely opposed the inclusion of psychodynamic material "on the grounds that the inclusion of such material was beyond the scope of DSM-III [because] to include such material we would have to also include other explanations of mechanisms to account for such disorders."[23] In addition, Spitzer declared that it was difficult to evaluate the psychodynamic data regarding "the mechanisms that account for psychopathology." This last judgment, of course, rejected the many psychoanalytic explanations of these mecha-nisms. Spitzer's argument had to have angered and exasperated Madow; the analysts had been thwarted again.

To cushion the blow, Spitzer offered some ameliorating promises. First, while the DSM-III text would not include detailed statements of psychodynamic or other mechanism to account for the disorders, there would be "acknowledgment of pro-posed hypotheses to account for the disorders." Spitzer gave the example of fetishism: "Some investigators have suggested that specific internal conflicts…predispose to the development of the disorder." But what Spitzer gave with one hand he took away with another: "Other investigators suggest that the phenomenon can be explained by condi-tioning or imprinting." To the analysts, it was an insult to put behavioral explanations on a par with psychoanalytic ones. In any event, no explanations about the etiology of fetishism ever appeared in DSM-III.

Spitzer also said that there would be a list of references in DSM-III, and "these refer-ences [could] include articles on some of the proposed mechanisms for understand-ing these disorders." Indeed, there were 121 references in DSM-III, and a respectable number of them contained psychodynamic thinking. However, the references were buried at the back of DSM-III in Appendix C, at the end of a comparative listing of DSM-II and DSM-III categories and diagnoses, hardly drawing a large number of read-ers. These references were not referred to anywhere in the table of contents, although readers who closely studied the DSM-II/DSM-III comparison could find numbers in the charts referring to the various references.

Next, Spitzer proposed that the instructions for coding Axis II Personality Disorders "could indicate that the clinician might wish to note prominent coping mechanisms [such as] projection and denial." In a separate letter to Rockland, Spitzer asked for his help in working on definitions for such coping mechanisms used by patients.[24] However, ultimately, there were no instructions in DSM-III for putting coping mecha-nisms on Axis II, although, as we soon shall see, it had first seemed possible that there might.

Finally, the "DSM-III would include in its Glossary of Technical terms, a list of coping mechanisms, their definitions and examples." While there was a glossary in DSM-III, no specific terms relating to coping mechanisms appeared there (e.g., projec-tion or denial). The argument could be made that the definitions of some of the terms listed included information that might be considered psychodynamic.

Undeterred by the tensions between the analysts' Liaison Committee and the Task Force, Spitzer maintained his cordiality. Controversy rarely caused him to burn his bridges. On the same day he wrote to Madow rejecting psychodynamic material, he wrote an ebullient letter to the President of the American Academy of Psychoanalysis, thanking him for his interest in having the Academy's members answer the question-naire on what to do about the contentious diagnosis of Borderline Personality Disorder. In his letter, Spitzer mentioned that the membership of the American Psychoanalytic Association was participating in the project.[25]

Even though Spitzer had written so negatively to Madow about the inclusion of psy-chodynamic material, a startling second thought occurred. Spitzer now wrote again to

Madow and told him that after speaking to the two analysts on the Task Force, Bill and Jack Frosch, he had found a way to overcome the Task Force's opposition. "Instead of mentioning specific conflicts involved in the various disorders [as Rockland had done], there could be a general statement indicating some investigators believed that various internal conflicts predispose to the development of the disorder."[26] Spitzer edited the Anxiety Disorders and Paraphilias sections according to this principle and sent the material to Madow.[27] Madow's Liaison Committee then met with Bill Frosch, who confirmed what Spitzer had said. The analysts were pleased and decided to revise other categories along the lines of Spitzer's editing of the Anxiety Disorders and Paraphilias. But when Spitzer met with the Task Force and showed them the editing he had done, they opposed his solution and convinced him, he later said, that he had erred.[28] Spitzer then telephoned Madow and gave him the news.[29] Madow later recounted how "quite defeated" he had felt. It seemed to him, he wrote to Spitzer, that Spitzer had wanted the analysts' participation, but now it appeared that they were "being blocked" in their efforts to contribute to the development of the new manual. "Is there any appeal mechanism?" he concluded.[30]

WOULD THE MULTIAXIAL SYSTEM PROVIDE SOME COMMON GROUND?

In response, Spitzer proposed a complex course of action involving further approval by the Task Force but, more concretely, reiterating his earlier idea of the clinician noting prominent coping mechanisms used by patients on Axis II.[31] He acted on this by calling a one-day meeting of the Glossary of Technical Terms Advisory Committee, since in the past they had discussed the inclusion of coping styles as an optional item in the multiaxial system. This meeting may have occurred in February or March 1978, soon after Spitzer had conveyed to Madow the the Task Force's rejection of Spitzer's compromise proposal (his editing of disorders to be in accord with the general notion that internal conflicts can predispose to the development of certain disorders.) To the Glossary Committee meeting he also invited four men: John Strauss, who had proposed his own multiaxial system and written on schizophrenia; Larry Rockland and Bill Frosch, the two analysts; and George E. Vaillant, also an analyst who had written on defense mechanisms, schizophrenia, and the reliability issue.

Vaillant (b. 1934) a highly recognized figure today, had known Spitzer for over a decade. Vaillant says they were both rebels but pragmatists, realizing that "American psychiatry was a mess and needed clarity in diagnosis," although they did not always agree.[32] Spitzer was aware that Vaillant was interested in coping styles and defense mechanisms, Vaillant having published his findings in this area since the early 1970s.[33] In 1977, Vaillant's book, *Adaptation to Life*, had appeared and established his reputation as an expert in coping styles and defenses in adult males. In the book, Vaillant postulated a four-level hierarchy of defense mechanisms, ranging from the pathological to the mature. Vaillant recalls a meeting with some New York analysts that Spitzer had organized "to plan for a possible axis VI (defenses and coping) for the new DSM-III." It is not clear whether Vaillant is referring to the 1978 meeting or an earlier analysts' meeting on this topic several months before. In any event, Vaillant reports that "after several hours, it was clear that we were unable to reach consensus on a list of the important defenses or to agree on their definition or their significance for psychopathology." It was a "Tower of Babel."[34] Nevertheless, the Glossary Committee recommended that there be a place for recording coping styles in the multiaxial diagnostic system.

Spitzer duly reported to the Task Force the recommendations of this committee and asked for the Task Force's "opinion and guidance."[35] He distributed ballots for the Task Force to vote on a proposal with three possible avenues whereby clinicians could include coping styles, and a last option for rejecting the idea totally.[36] He also sent a ballot to Madow's Liaison Committee.[37] The Task Force voted down all of the specific options for including coping styles, and at a meeting of the Task Force and the Assembly Liaison Committee together, the entire group agreed with the Task Force vote.[38] They allowed only the following statement to be put in the section of DSM-III that explains the use of the manual: "Axis II and description of personality features: Axis II can be used to indicate personality traits when no Personality Disorder exists. For example, compulsive traits [or] paranoid traits."[39]

However, at the same time, on March 28, 1978, Spitzer proposed yet another compromise, which was to add a separate axis for etiology. Spitzer appeared genuinely desirous of working out some way of satisfying the psychoanalysts that would not disturb his overriding goal of a descriptive manual. He sent a three-page memo to a wide range of people: the Task Force, George Vaillant, the Glossary Advisory Committee, the Assembly Liaison Committee, Madow's analytic Committee, the American Academy of Psychoanalysis' Liaison Committee, and the American Psychological Association (not clear to whom there specifically.)[40]

In his memo, Spitzer reported that Hector Jaso, the new Chair of the Assembly Liaison Committee, had "made a very interesting suggestion that I believe we should seriously consider…having an additional axis which would allow the clinician to express his concept of the relative importance of various etiological factors." The great advantage of such a proposal, Spitzer argued, was that it might "solve the problem that we have been struggling with of allowing psychodynamically oriented clinicians the option of expressing their views of the importance of intrapsychic factors." Spitzer envisaged that this axis could be used not only by analysts but also by other clinicians to articulate "major viewpoints." There would be no coding of the information to gather statistics, which was one of the traditional uses of classifications like the APA's DSMs or the WHO's ICDs. Spitzer believed that the various formulations would presumably "have some significant correlations with treatment recommendations." The axis would be good for teaching purposes to "structur[e] the supervision of clinical assessment."

However, Spitzer continued, since psychosocial stress would be one of the etiological factors used, the inclusion of a separate axis for psychosocial stressors would be redundant and, therefore, should be eliminated. Spitzer concluded:

One of the advantages of having this axis [on etiology] would be that it solves (?) [sic] the problem of coping styles and defense mechanisms. We could still allow the clinician the option of describing traits, or coping styles, in Axis I, II, and III, but defense mechanisms [would only be] appropriate for noting in the etiological formulation....Even when etiology is unknown, the clinician still is obligated to have some kind of formulation, and having such an axis would permit him to express it.

With this memo, Spitzer sent out a ballot that allowed four choices. The options were (A) Include a separate axis for etiological formulation; (B) Replace Axis IV, Psychosocial Stressors, with an axis for etiological formulation; (C) No axis for etiological formulation; (D) Other.

Bill Frosch later declared that the Task Force's discussion of this proposal, which he had supported, was "decidedly anti-psychoanalytic" and that "issues of content" were not talked about.[41] Spitzer appears to have asked all the many addressees of his memo to return the ballot to him, yet the Archives contain only thirteen replies and it is not possible to ascertain if any more were received. Within this limited response, the vote was nine nays, against a separate axis, and four yeas. There were also some very strong comments against the advisability of adding any more axes or changing the current configuration.[42] In any event, the axis for possible etiological formulations was defeated because at a joint meeting of the Task Force and Assembly Liaison Committee, on May 7, 1978, "the group upheld the Task Force vote not to include such an Axis."[43]

Nevertheless, Spitzer did not close the door on the issue entirely, which was not an unusual move for him. (Think, for example, of his persistence when it came to including in DSM-III a definition of mental disorder as a medical disorder.) On May 5, 1978, as part of a field trial questionnaire, he sent out to the participants a sheet entitled "Some Hot Issues for you to Think About."[44] "Here," he said, "are some hot issues that are now under consideration. If you have a strong opinion about any of them—let us know right away." There had been a suggestion, he wrote, that there be

> an axis that gives the clinician an opportunity to choose amongst a list of etiological factors and rank order the applicable categories in terms of their relative importance....The list of factors could include psychosocial stress, environmental reinforcement, intrapsychic conflict, constitutional factors, genetic factors, etc.
>
> Would such an axis be used? Would it be useful for planning treatment? Would it encourage useless speculation and detract from the largely descriptive approach taken in DSM-III?

Unfortunately, the Archives do not contain any of the raw data Spitzer received back on this communication, but we know the conclusion. The Task Force's voting down of an etiological axis stood. If the axis had been approved, it would have given the analysts and psychodynamically oriented psychiatrists a vehicle to list within the manual their etiological formulations. ("Formulation" was the word Spitzer preferred; he argued that the clinician was "speculating" since in most cases the etiology was unknown.)[45]

Thus, the analysts' and Spitzer's initiatives came to naught. In these instances, Spitzer had not been obdurate, but the Task Force had. Still, conflict continued. Soon, the May 1978 APA meeting generated another clash. From that date until the next APA meeting in 1979, where final decisions would be made, there was continual battle. A dramatic verbal duel even took place in front of the Assembly, immediately preceding the moment it was set to vote on the acceptance or rejection of DSM-III.

THE ANALYSTS BECOME AWARE OF THE
STRENGTH OF THE TASK FORCE

At the 1978 APA meeting, a panel on the relationship of DSM-III to psychodynamic thinking took place. Perhaps the planning of this forum was one of the responses of the analysts to their rebuff. In an undated document by Larry Rockland, which might have been composed for the APA panel, he argued for the place of psychodynamic thinking in DSM-III; it was entitled "Some thoughts on the subject: 'Should Psychodynamics be included in the DSM III?'" Judging from archival material, this is the only time an analyst effectively attempted to rebut Spitzer's assertion that because everyone has intrapsychic conflicts, these cannot be used as a basis for class formation (Neurosis) in DSM-III. Rockland argued persuasively that not all intrapsychic conflicts are of the same order of magnitude. Psychopathology is a function of the subject matter and severity of the conflicts in each individual. (The makers of DSM-5 themselves have sought a dimensional approach to the classification of personality disorders, that is, pathology exists along a spectrum.) Rockland was less persuasive when sought taking the familiar psychoanalytic position that psychoanalysis and psychodynamic theories had more to contribute than other schools and thus deserved a place in DSM-III.[46]

More direct psychoanalytic action following the 1978 APA panel took the form of a long, intense letter from Paul J. Fink, a member of the analysts' Liaison Committee and Chair of the Psychiatry Department at Jefferson Medical College in Philadelphia. He addressed his letter to Lester Grinspoon, a prominent Harvard researcher and Chair of the APA's Council on Research and Development. Leo Madow also wrote to Grinspoon at the same time.[47] The protests and grievances expressed by Fink and Madow were to be repeated by them and others throughout the months to come as Spitzer and members of the Task Force by and large clung to their positions and arguments.

In their letters, Fink and Madow recounted the failure of the analysts' attempts to gain input into the formulation of the DSM-III text, and much of their criticism centered on the Task Force. The Task Force was "skewed" and "prejudiced" toward a phenomenological and descriptive point of view and was "anti-psychodynamic." This "small group of people" was "arrogant" in their refusal "to incorporate some of the things which [psychiatrists] have learned over the past 70 years." The Task Force's way of arriving at a diagnosis was a "throwback." Just because phenomenology is "documentable" does not mean "that that is the only body of knowledge that is available to us." The analysts had hoped that the appointment of the analysts John Frosch and William Frosch to the Task Force would have had some effect, but the "overwhelming" majority of the committee had rendered these men "impotent."

The Task Force, of course, would not have used the same harsh language describing itself, but Fink and Madow were absolutely correct about its influence. Its members had been chosen for their empirical outlook, their predilection for "data," or as Jean Endicott had put it, their fondness for DOPS, or "data-oriented people." And we learned from Andreasen that on the very first day of the Task Force's meeting, they came together over their desire to undo the psychoanalytic dominance of American psychiatry. When Spitzer showed a willingness to compromise with the analysts, the Task Force had voted him down.

Fink was also critical of Spitzer, claiming that he channeled all correspondence through himself and did not call meetings of the Task Force frequently enough. Thus, Fink asserted, much of the final decisions were made by Spitzer, who often worked in tandem with Donald Klein, who was on the Task Force and was Spitzer's close colleague at the New York State Psychiatric Institute. Finally, Fink raised again the issue of third-party payers who might misuse the lists of very specific criteria. "These can be lifted out and used as a club with regard to payment at any time." Fink hoped Grinspoon and the Council on Research and Development would consider converting the diagnostic criteria into a more general paragraph format since he realized the Task Force would be loath to take such an approach. Moreover, he asked, could Grinspoon put the matter of how DSM-III was being made on the agenda of the APA Reference Committee? It was time for "groups within the APA to know what some of the negative aspects of DSM III might be," Fink asserted.

Grinspoon gave much thought to Fink's concerns and probably consulted others about Fink's letter, for he did not answer him for six weeks. Finally, he acknowledged that there had been some concern "that the proposed DSM-III does not reflect the importance of psychodynamic thinking in the practice of psychiatry in the United States." He declared, therefore, that he had reserved a full day for a discussion during the fall meetings of the Council on Research and Development. On that day, Spitzer, and any others he chose to bring from the Task Force, would "be available to those who wish to criticize and make suggestions about DSM III." Grinspoon invited Fink and those he might call upon to attend the session.[48]

SHOWDOWN IN WASHINGTON: THE MEETING WITH THE COUNCIL ON RESEARCH AND DEVELOPMENT

The Archives have preserved the minutes of Grinspoon's September 8, 1978 "Open Meeting on DSM-III"—all eighteen pages of them![49] The meeting was an all-day affair. The entire Council on Research and Development attended. Spitzer came with two persons he had chosen to bring, Edward J. Sachar (1933–1984), director of the New York State Psychiatric Institute and a renowned researcher who had trained as a psychoanalyst, and Janet Forman, his Text Editor and Project Coordinator of the Field Trials, whom Spitzer ultimately would marry. No one from the Task Force was present. Fink, by contrast, attended with a group of analysts and other supportive psychiatrists: Madow, William Offenkrantz, Anton Kris, Larry Rockland, William Frosch, Miltiades Zaphiropoulos, Chair of the American Academy of Psychoanalysis Liaison Committee to the Task Force, and Howard Berk from the Assembly Liaison Committee. In addition there was Jules H. Masserman (1905–1994), President of the APA, who was also an analyst. Frosch spoke from the point of view of both an analyst and a member of the Task Force.

Grinspoon opened the meeting by stating that there seemed to be three areas of concern to APA members in regard to DSM-III: (1) the lack of psychodynamic material; (2) "the implications of having rigid criteria to establish a diagnosis;" and (3) the "overinclusiveness" of DSM-III, particularly the diagnosis Tobacco Use Disorder. (This last complaint was due to much opposition to Spitzer's making this a disorder; many psychiatrists and their friends and family smoked and thought it ludicrous that what they viewed as a normal activity of everyday life should be deemed a psychiatric disorder. Spitzer obviously was well ahead of the crowd in this matter.)

Grinspoon asked Spitzer to start the proceedings by reporting on his NIMH Field Trials. Spitzer had come prepared, having three days earlier tallied up the answers he received from a June 28, 1978 questionnaire sent out to participants in the field trial he and Forman were conducting.[50] He talked at some length and cited statistics he had collected that indicated wide support of the proposed manual both by psychodynamic psychiatrists and by those not in this school. This approval, he reported, extended to innovations such as the diagnostic criteria and the abandonment of "traditional classifications of neurotic subtypes" such as neurotic depression. He added that "69% of psychodynamically oriented respondents felt that DSM-III represented a significant positive step in the development of scientific psychiatry." Moreover, he said, his statistics showed that DSM-III had much better reliability when compared to that of DSM-II. (It should be noted that the reliability of DSM-III was later challenged.)[51]

During the first part of the meeting, Grinspoon dutifully and determinedly went around the room asking for each person's comments, and initially calm prevailed, as little that was said drew provocative replies. When some acrimony began to surface, Grinspoon tried to rein it in and return to going around the room, so everyone at the meeting could have his say. All the arguments that had been leveled against DSM-III in the past three years were reiterated once again by the analysts present, Fink taking the lead. Yet Offenkrantz, Chair of the American Psychoanalytic Association's Peer Review Committee, said that his committee could work with any system of classification and diagnosis and astutely chided psychoanalytic clinics for not taking a greater role in the field trial: "Organized psychoanalysis [had] been asleep in regard to this issue." But Madow answered that organized psychoanalysis "felt that it was an exercise in futility to submit suggestions to the DSM-III Task Force." Spitzer repeated, as usual, that the Task Force wanted "specific suggestions" and pointed out several instances where the Task Force had made changes. For one, they had included personality traits, he declared, even though the research-oriented psychiatrists complained about such vague and subjective diagnostic material.

Speaking as an analyst, Frosch asserted that "the core membership of the Task Force had a frozen and predictable attitude." Spitzer conceded that the Task Force was not well balanced and that this was a result of his having been given "carte blanche." Still, he stated, he had asked for the participation of two eminent analysts in the beginning,

Theodore Shapiro and Arnold M. Cooper (1923–2011), and they both had declined. We should pause here to examine the significance of Spitzer's invitation to these two men. For one thing, it indicates that at the beginning Spitzer's mind was in flux as to the ultimate shape of DSM-III. Shapiro and Spitzer had been very good friends for a number of years. They had done their internships and residencies together, and their families were close.[52] Cooper had been Spitzer's training analyst during his analytic candidacy at Columbia, and at the time, Spitzer had greatly admired Cooper's skills and theoretical outlook. Although Spitzer was disenchanted with psychoanalysis for personal and professional reasons, the fact that he had asked these men to be on the Task Force shows that his mind was not closed to the psychoanalytic outlook. But he had chosen an anti-analytic Task Force, one often more rigid in their stance than he, and this had shaped Spitzer's thinking.

The other aspect of Spitzer's invitation to Shapiro and Cooper is that it is totally understandable that they declined. DSM-I and II had played absolutely no role in the analytic world, so who would have thought that DSM-III would be instrumental in the upending of that world? Aside from a few letters, no analyst or analytic institution paid any significant attention to what was going on in the construction of a new DSM for the first two years, and then, after the Midstream Conference, they took nine months to meet with Spitzer and discuss the situation. By that time the Task Force and the Advisory Committees had been meeting for two and a half years, and field trials had already been in place for two months. Any aspects of DSM-III that were inimical to psychodynamic thinking were as good as set in stone.

As the meeting wore on, it became a duel between Spitzer and the psychoanalysts. Grinspoon went around the room inviting people to speak. When their turn came, the analysts would say something critical, and Spitzer would defend his actions. Spitzer was a worthy opponent. When challenged, he invariably replied with a specific example or two in order to demonstrate that what the analysts accused him of was simply not true. The analysts became angrier and more hostile, digging up old reproaches but only infrequently countering Spitzer's arguments with evidence that was not just a laundry list of complaints. Spitzer was a master debater and did not mind controversy, and the analysts lacked a leader who was as skilled a tactician and strategist as he was. To Madow's worry that the Council on Research and Development would have to accept a "less than optimal" document because of time constraints regarding the publication schedule, Spitzer countered that three analytic clinics were participating in the field trials and giving him feedback.

When Grinspoon asked Madow to speak, the best he could do was to object that "psychodynamics was being placed on a par with 'god knows what.'" (By this he likely meant that Spitzer and the Task Force regarded psychodynamic ideas about etiology as equal to, say, behavioral ones. Madow was critical of the notion that if psychodynamic material was placed in DSM-III, room had to be made for other theoretical explanations that the analysts thought were certainly less important, if valuable at all.) Madow's comments were his entry point to criticizing the rejection of Larry Rockland's write-up of Anxiety Disorders. This rejection had deterred the analysts' Liaison Committee from making further contributions, Madow said. "In short, they were discouraged."

Spitzer pointed out that Rockland's descriptive material had been accepted. His psychodynamic material had been not accepted because "it gave an explanation reflecting a theory." Spitzer pointed to Rockland's ideas regarding panic attacks: that the object or situation the patient dreads is not in his or her conscious awareness, and this triggers the panic attack. Yes, said Spitzer, lots of clinicians believe this, but "there were a group of serious investigators who believed that the mechanism of panic attacks is biologic." Edward Sachar, a widely recognized psychoendocrinologist, added that panic attacks could be treated effectively with imipramine (Tofranil). And so it went, the atmosphere in the room heating up with each exchange.

When Spitzer became somewhat belligerent, declaring that "if various viewpoints regarding theories of behavior should be the charge of DSM-III, he would like instructions from the group assembled," Grinspoon tried to defuse the situation. He asked an analyst who had not yet spoken, Anton O. Kris, to give his comments. Kris was critical of DSM-III as it stood and accused it twice of being "shallow," as he and Spitzer sparred. Grinspoon again sought calm by continuing to solicit comments from people who had not yet spoken. This worked briefly, but the discussion had reached the simmering point where the participants began jockeying to voice and stress their individual concerns without regard for a formal process of a speaking order.

It is in this emotional atmosphere that Spitzer introduced an idea he had only recently formulated: "Project Flower," titled after Chairman Mao's "Let a Thousand Flowers Bloom."[53] Spitzer proposed that various organizations representing different schools of psychiatric thought—psychoanalysts, behaviorists, family therapists, psychopharmacologists, and the like—contribute to what might become a companion volume to DSM-III. Each group could provide a chapter explaining what additional information was needed to institute treatment once a DSM-III diagnosis was made. The idea fell flat among the analysts at the meeting who wanted to concentrate only on DSM-III, believing that DSM-III would become the profession's bible and no other publication could change that.

The minutes at this point become quite specific. Kris provocatively proposed that instead of Project Flower, "a separate introduction should be written by a group of people not involved in the DSM-III Task Force.... He was not at war," he maintained, but there needed to be "caveats" as to the "limitations of DSM-III in...arriving at a diagnosis." This prompted Spitzer to outrage: "The people who write DSM-III should write the introduction," he spat out. The minutes now quote Spitzer: "The argument that Doctor Kris was raising was not about content but really was an issue of trust. And, Doctor Spitzer thought it ad hominem. He found it surprising that there was no interest in Project Flower." Madow interrupted: "His group was concerned with DSM-III and...he did not feel that it was ad hominem to have a more objective introduction." Spitzer, of course, disagreed and stated "that to ask another group to write an introduction to DSM-III separately was offensive." At this boiling point Grinspoon interrupted and decided it was time to summarize the meeting.

In these final moments, Grinspoon tried both to soothe ruffled feelings and to emphasize the reality of what had occurred in the development of the new manual. He announced that the Council on Research and Development would consider the possibility of having a separate foreword by another group. Nevertheless, he addressed the participants: "We must accept that DSM-III is descriptive but...there is still considerable room for input of a descriptive nature." The analysts' Liaison Committee should "look at DSM-III and make suggestions regarding description." But Madow made a last challenge. Was the dropping of neurosis a "fait accompli?" Grinspoon replied that it "almost" was. Kris commented in resignation that while it had not been clear in the past what people were supposed to contribute to DSM-III, it "had become clear that the present document would be descriptive," and perhaps he and likeminded people could add something to the descriptive material. Grinspoon said he encouraged this, but there was no guarantee of its inclusion in DSM-III.

And so the meeting ended in a clear victory for Spitzer and the Task Force. In the chronology of the making of DSM-III this was eight months before DSM-III was to be presented for final approval. No doubt many in the APA hierarchy supported Grinspoon's actions. The Board of Trustees had decided that they wanted a revised DSM that would help American psychiatry regain its legitimacy and combat the antipsychiatry movement. The new Medical Director, Melvin Sabshin (1925–2011), had taken the post in 1974 with the explicit goals of ending "ideology" in American psychiatry, making psychiatry "scientific," and putting psychiatry squarely back in medicine.[54] Finally, following the day-long meeting of the Council on Research and Development, it held an executive session and decided to support the Task Force's inclusion of Tobacco Use Disorder (ultimately, Tobacco Dependence) in the new manual. Spitzer had triumphed across the board.

After the September 8 meeting, some went home to celebrate and others to lick their wounds and try again. The "losers" mounted two efforts to circumvent the Council's decision that DSM-III would be a descriptive manual and that if the analysts wanted to contribute to it, their material would have to deal with descriptive matters. One attempt to ameliorate the decision was a drive to have psychodynamic input to the Introduction to DSM-III. The other was a campaign to have a special appendix to DSM-III that would discuss how psychiatrists with a psychodynamic outlook could use DSM-III.

However, before describing the efforts to get a psychodynamic Introduction and then an Appendix into DSM-III, let us take in the finales of two ongoing dramas. First, by the end of 1978, John Frosch, the older of the two analysts on the Task Force, resigned his position, worn out by "the contentious stance of some of Spitzer's colleagues."[55] Second, Madow, too, decided he could do no more. He had failed in whatever efforts he had put forth and so delivered his final report as Chair of the Liaison Committee to the Executive Council of the Psychoanalytic Association in December 1978. The Council had twice rejected his requests for funds to underwrite the preparation of psychodynamically informed material. To his dismay, moreover, some psychoanalysts had collaborated in the drafting of descriptive material on the personality disorders, lured, in his view, by an ersatz "scientism." He urged the Analytic Association to reject Project Flower, since participation "in that effort could only provide a justification for the 'neo-Kraepelinian' approach of DSM-III."[56] The Executive Council, however, turned down Madow's advice on Project Flower and decided to endorse the writing of a chapter for the proposed volume. The war over DSM-III was drawing to a close on these two fronts, but not without some additional sallies on others. There were still five months to go.

WILL THE ANALYSTS CONTRIBUTE TO THE INTRODUCTION TO DSM-III?

After the Washington meeting, there was still an attempt to influence the final outcome by developing the Introduction to DSM-III. In the winter of 1977–1978, the American Association of Chairmen of Departments of Psychiatry (AACDP) had formed a Liaison Committee on DSM-III, but it had done very little, if anything at all. It may not even have met. But soon after the analysts had failed to influence the Council on Research and Development, it sprang into action in an attempt to affect the "values" of DSM-III. The AACDP was sympathetic to the analysts' cause. The upshot was a war of both sides trying to outflank each other.

The official initiative, the first shot, was a letter on October 16, 1978, from Robert Michels, M.D. (b. 1936), Chair of the Department of Psychiatry at the Cornell University Medical College to Peter C. Whybrow, M.D., Chair of the AACDP and the Psychiatry Chair at the Dartmouth Mental Health Center.[57] Michels, recognized broadly for his many activities, publications, and noteworthy achievements in psychiatry, psycho-analysis, and administration, argued that in the construction of a diagnostic scheme there needed to be an "executive body" whose role was "formulating the values and establishing the priorities that are to be served by the diagnostic system." Then there would be a "staff" to implement those values. "The group constructing the nomencla-ture…should see its role as implementing the profession's basic values, not determin-ing them." Michels proposed that to respond to "some of the troubling features of DSM-III" the role of the AACDP should be to weigh in on these, make suggestions for the future concerning DSM-IV, and, finally, make it "clear that we see [DSM-III] as a current statement, while we anticipate continued study of revision of our diagnostic system." A copy of Michels' letter went to many people, including Spitzer. The analysts were about to attempt an end run around the Task Force.

Spitzer, of course, was very angry over Michels' letter and wrote a fuming response, although in the Archives there is only the draft, so it is not possible to know if Spitzer ever sent an actual letter and to whom, Michels or Whybrow.[58] (In his response, Spitzer wrote sarcastically, "Perhaps Michels could head up the 'executive body.' I hope he would consider me for the 'staff' job.") Spitzer's real answer—his attempt to wrest the initiative—was to go immediately to New Orleans, where the psychiatry chairmen were to meet, so he could discuss the matter with them. Again, Spitzer had the energy and willingness to have a face-to-face confrontation. While there are no records in the Archives of this meeting, we do have a letter of thanks from Whybrow to Spitzer, which served only to anger him further. After initial cordialities of appreciation, Whybrow got to the point. Since no classification could ever be "perfect," "the notion of a detailed introduction is a very important one." Whybrow asked that the AACDP Liaison Committee be included in the writing of the Introduction. Whybrow offered

Spitzer the bait of a "formal endorsement" by the AACDP of DSM-III after such a joint introduction was developed.[59] After two weeks, Spitzer, ever the strategist, replied to Whybrow:

> We are both in agreement that the introduction to DSM-III is of great importance. In order to facilitate the contribution of AACDP to the writing of the introduction, may I suggest that your group...first meet without me and prepare a list of ideas or concepts that they believe should be included in the introduction....I will then respond by incorporating those suggestions into a draft which can then be reviewed by your group.
>
> Please let me know if this procedure is acceptable, and if so, when I can expect to hear from your committee.[60]

Not only was Spitzer not about to lose control of writing the Introduction, he tactically deflected the initiative to the AACDP Liaison Committee, which then had the burden of organizing a meeting and specifying their "ideas and concepts." Spitzer would wait to hear from them. To no great surprise, the Archives contain no record of suggestions about an introduction to Spitzer from the AACDP. Still, the AACDP, with its psychoanalytic links, tried one more time to challenge Spitzer and attempt its own end run. Under Michels' leadership they decided to write an introduction on their own, bypassing Spitzer, and to present this introduction directly to the APA, though to what APA group is not clear. Spitzer learned of this plan three months later when he telephoned to ask Michels where the suggestions from the AACDP Liaison Committee were.[61] Michels told Spitzer that the AACDP Liaison Committee was now communicating directly with the APA.

Spitzer was astonished and wrote an immediate letter of sharp complaint to the new President of the AACDP, Douglas L. Lenkoski, M.D., the Psychiatry Chair at Case Western Reserve, with a copy to Sabshin.[62] He demanded to know why, if the AACDP Liaison Committee had changed its function from serving as a liaison to the DSM-III Task Force, he had not been informed. He "seriously" questioned the appropriateness of this action of the AACDP. It was certainly "ironic," he went on, that the AACDP wanted to write the Introduction to all of DSM-III when it had not sought to provide any input to the making of the document over several years. How would the Assembly Liaison Committee to the Task Force, which had provided "input, guidance, and monitoring of the development of DSM-III...feel about your group taking it (sic) upon themselves the task of preparing an introduction to DSM-III?" Spitzer queried.[63] If indeed "Michels' committee" was preparing a separate introduction to DSM-III, Spitzer said he would communicate this to the Council on Research and Development and the Assembly Liaison Committee, "the APA committees that have the responsibility for monitoring the development of DSM-III." Spitzer asked for clarification. There is no further correspondence on this issue in the Archives. The AACDP's introduction to DSM-III died a quiet death as the analysts' and their psychodynamic sympathizers' focus shifted in the final months to the last subject of contention, the place of Neurosis in DSM-III. This is considered in Chapter 13.

WILL THERE BE A PSYCHODYNAMIC
APPENDIX IN DSM-III?

The analysts' second effort to override their rout by Grinspoon was their attempt to insert an appendix to DSM-III that would explain how psychodynamically oriented psychiatrists should use DSM-III. The APA's Reference Committee, consisting of important APA officers, discussed at its November 1978 meeting "the [analytic] opposition to the current draft of DSM-III and ways to overcome this opposition."[64] The Reference Committee suggested that "members of the Task Force who represent this orientation might prepare the draft of the appendix." Spitzer tried to counter this by arguing that it was the job of the Introduction to handle this issue and that a separate section for psychodynamically oriented psychiatrists "would stick out like a sore thumb and would have a devisive (sic) rather than a conciliatory effect." The tug of war here is obvious. The analytically oriented psychiatrists urgently desired to write something for DSM-III that would be written by them, that would represent their point of view. Spitzer, though, wanted to keep total control of the contents of the new manual securely in his hands.

Spitzer went to Sabshin for advice, and he suggested that Spitzer speak to the APA Board of Trustees at their next meeting and "convey to that group any reservations that the Task Force has about this [the Reference Committee's] directive." Spitzer was fortunate to have on his side a new Medical Director of the APA who was openly sympathetic to the type of revision DSM-III was undergoing and who was a quietly influential figure.[65]

To get further support for his position about the appendix, Spitzer asked the Task Force for a formal vote on the issue. He gave the Task Force three options, the first two dealing with approval of the idea of the appendix, and the last offering a rejection. Spitzer closed his memo to the Task Force by referring to Project Flower. If there was a positive response from the psychiatric profession, with each group writing its own chapter on treatment, "then clearly this idea for this appendix...would be obviated." The same day, November 16, 1978, Spitzer wrote to Alan A. Stone, President-elect of the APA, to ask for a meeting with the Trustees. He also alerted Stone to the possibility of the APA sponsoring a book on treatment that would render a psychodynamic appendix unnecessary.[66]

The Archives contain only one response to Spitzer's call for a vote on the appendix, that from Henry Pinsker, often fond of sending long missives explaining his thinking.[67] This time was no exception. Pinsker saw the issue as the old guard fighting desperately to hang on. "If my assumption that the fundamental issue is related to reform-conservative problems, nothing rational will work." He found the idea of an appendix both "stupid" and "absurd." To no surprise, the rest of the Task Force agreed. Spitzer had ringing support this time from an old nemesis, the Assembly Liaison Committee to DSM-III. But now the group had a new chair, Hector Jaso, who quickly wrote to Stone backing Spitzer's position that if one group got its theoretical ideas in DSM-III, every other group would expect to receive the same privilege.[68] Therefore, Jaso wrote, "At our recent meeting on November 18, 1978 [we] re-affirmed

[our] position of October 27, 1977 that no single theoretical orientation should be included in DSM-III. We are, therefore, respectfully requesting that the Board of Trustees and the Executive Committee of the APA rescind the directive [to develop a special appendix] to the Task Force on Nomenclature and Statistics." Jaso then gave his group's strong endorsement of "Project Flower." Moreover, in anticipation of the publication of DSM-III in January 1980, Jaso urged the Trustees to allocate funds to the DSM-III Task Force to devise educational materials to teach APA members how to use the revised manual.

In spite of this joint pressure, the Trustees shunted their advice aside and supported the action of the Reference Committee charging the Task Force to develop an appendix discussing the use of DSM-III by psychodynamically oriented psychiatrists. The Trustees directed the Task Force to report to the APA Council on Medical Education and Career Development as they prepared the appendix, not to the Council on Research and Development, which had been in charge up to that point. The Trustees also supported the concept of a separate volume on DSM-III and treatment planning (Project Flower) as well as the preparation of educational materials by the Task Force and authorized APA officials to seek outside funding for such educational matter on DSM-III.[69] William Offenkrantz, representing both the DSM-III Liaison Committees of the American Psychoanalytic Association and the American Academy of Psychoanalysis, immediately drafted an appendix and sent it to Sabshin.[70] Project Flower was also proceeding, and the same analytic Liaison Committees met with Spitzer to draft a chapter for "DSM-III Vol. 2: Treatment Planning," as Spitzer called it.[71]

Let us take stock. The time was three months before DSM-III was to go for an up-or-down vote by the Assembly of Delegates. On this attempt by the analysts to do an end run around Spitzer the score was 2 to 1 in favor of the analysts: the appendix was still in the works and the volume on treatment planning with a psychoanalytic chapter was taking shape. On Spitzer's side, he seemed to have scored with Project Flower, but he was still stuck with the appendix. Undeterred, he wrote again to Stone, with a copy to Sabshin, enclosing Offenkrantz's appendix and pressuring the President-elect who was to assume office in the same three months' time:

> Having this kind of an Appendix in DSM-III would not only be extremely embarrassing but extremely divisive....Its inclusion in DSM-III could only be viewed as an official endorsement by the APA of one school of thought. Can you imagine the reaction of our biologically oriented colleagues in the APA to the inclusion of such an Appendix in DSM-III? What do we do when the family or behavioral or group psychotherapy groups want their Appendix also?
>
> Who needs such trouble?

Spitzer was not giving up. On the same day, he wrote to Sabshin with copies to Stone, Grinspoon, Fink, Jaso, and Offenkrantz. As usual, Spitzer was hiding nothing. He wanted the analysts, Fink and Offenkrantz, to know exactly where he stood. Spitzer told Sabshin that he believed a misunderstanding had occurred. He argued that what actually happened at the December meeting of the Trustees, where Spitzer made a presentation about the Appendix, was that the Trustees decided "that the purposes for which the Appendix was designed could better be handled by a thorough discussion of the relevant issues of the Introduction to DSM-III, and that therefore a separate Appendix was not necessary." Spitzer told Sabshin that Stone agreed with Spitzer's memory of the events, also wanted the psychodynamic material in the Introduction, and believed the minutes of the meeting were wrong. Stone was going to write to Sabshin, Spitzer reported.

What should we think? We are gaining entree to the craziness of the days leading up to the big vote. The scrambling, the posturing, the pressures, the altercations, the surprises, the anxieties, the deal making—all were endless. So what was the outcome of the appendix vs. the introduction battle that Spitzer was waging? A whole month had gone by since Spitzer had last been in touch with Stone and Sabshin. Spitzer now wrote to Offenkrantz with copies to all parties involved.[72] Much seemed to have been resolved. Spitzer informed Offenkrantz that he was enclosing "an initial draft of a portion of the introduction to DSM-III that deals with how a psychodynamically-oriented clinical will need to obtain additional information towards the formulation of a treatment plan." Would Offenkrantz or his committee have any suggestions for improving the material? Spitzer disconcertingly added, this "in no way affects your committee's action regarding the possibility of a separate appendix or document in DSM-III for the use of psychodynamically-oriented clinicians." So had anything been resolved after all? Are we down the Rabbit Hole in Wonderland? Or had Spitzer gained an actual edge here?

LET A THOUSAND FLOWERS BLOOM

Simultaneously to these maneuverings, Spitzer was propelling forward Project Flower as a solution to the analysts' opposition to DSM-III. The idea first had arisen well before the Washington meeting with the Council on Research and Development. It had come from a psychiatric resident, Michael Mavroidis, who was spending a year as a fellow to learn how the APA works and was assigned to follow the activities of the Task Force. He wrote that he could not help but notice the "heated and divisive struggles" over DSM-III. This turmoil impelled him to come up with the idea that perhaps the organizations representing various psychiatric schools should all be allowed to publish appendices to the manual to take the pressure off the Task Force to incorporate their views in the text. Or maybe, he threw in, there could be a companion volume to DSM-III.[73]

The Task Force did not at all like the idea of appendices. But Spitzer was taken with the notion of a separate companion volume and conferred with Lester Grinspoon, Melvin Sabshin, and Lyman Wynne, M.D., Ph.D. (1923–2007), a pioneer in family therapy who had been added to the Task Force in 1976. These men supported Spitzer's idea of a book that would be called "DSM-III and Treatment Planning." Spitzer explained the new idea in a long memo to the Task Force and supplied them with a ballot to approve or disapprove the project.[74] Most of the Task Force approved, with greater or lesser enthusiasm, and so Spitzer launched his idea at the Washington meeting with the Council on Research and Development, where Leo Madow dismissed it as no substitute for analytic material in DSM-III itself. We will explore here the saga of the Psychoanalytic Association's initial relationship with Project Flower because the episode is emblematic of the analysts' dearth of appreciation for the realities of change occurring in the mental health field and their lack of awareness of the wider significance of their actions.

After the meeting with the Council on Research and Development, Mavroidis wrote directly to Madow to try to whip up his enthusiasm for Project Flower.[75] Mavroidis' central argument was that psychiatry was living in the "Age of Accountability." If the profession itself would not lay out exactly how it went about doing psychiatric and psychoanalytic assessments and precisely what was necessary in terms of time and cost to conduct successful therapy, the government and insurance companies would make those decisions and foist them on psychiatrists. Within a week Madow answered Mavroidis to explain to him why the project "falls short of dealing with our concerns about the DSM-III."[76] Madow's letter remains a key document in adding to our understanding of why the analysts ended up sustaining severe setbacks in the making of DSM-III. And we must not forget that this lack of success occurred in tandem with challenges already facing them: the efficacy of psychotropic medications, the therapeutic promises the analysts could not deliver on, competition from lower-charging psychologists and social workers, competing short psychotherapies, the analysts' failure to help the severely mentally ill, lack of parity in payment for psychiatric treatment, and managed care.

The first three of the four reasons for Madow's lack of interest in Project Flower were basically the same. Only material in the DSM-III would matter, he argued, because the descriptive material in DSM-III would come to function as a textbook. Allowing psychodynamic material to be "side-tracked" into Project Flower would defeat "a basic need in modifying the DSM-III itself." Psychodynamic material in Project Flower rather than in DSM-III would actually undo "accountability," making it more difficult "to establish the need for a psychodynamic or psychoanalytic approach to treatment." The last reason for Madow being against Project Flower was that "placing the concepts of psychoanalytic theory on a par with behavior modification, learning theory, etc....is a disservice to the contributions that psychodynamic theory have made to psychiatry."

This unwillingness to share space with allegedly inferior forms of clinical knowledge was part of the psychoanalytic mystique stretching back decades. But at this critical moment, the analysts' failure to assess their situation realistically, to take what there was to get, and to turn a losing position into a better, even if not an ideal, one was self-defeating. The analysts' Liaison Committee lacked that necessary strategist who could size up the situation, recognize what they were facing, and develop effective tactics. True, there was an unsympathetic, implacable Task Force on the subject of psychoanalytic explanation, so Spitzer would never entirely be a free agent. But, even so, he was a master strategist with inexhaustible energy.

The heart of Madow's argument was "DSM-III or bust," and bust it was to be. Yet it is understandable that to the analysts everything seemed unreal, and unfathomable.

They had been on top for decades, and they still occupied commanding positions in academic and organizational American psychiatry. How could this predicament with DSM-III have come about? Part of the answer, of course, is that they had not gotten involved with developing a revised manual from the start, never dreaming how much different DSM-III would be from DSM-II, which they had safely ignored. They waited nine months after the Midstream Conference to have their first meeting with Spitzer, even though the handwriting on the wall at that meeting was crystal clear. Or were their presumptions entirely understandable? We must acknowledge that it is never a simple matter to apprehend and interpret a crisis situation and the role of the players in it.

Although Madow had sent Spitzer a copy of his negative letter to Mavroidis, Spitzer remained undeterred and, after further consultation, sent out a letter on October 30, 1978, to the heads of six national organizations: the American Psychoanalytic Association, the American Academy of Psychoanalysis, the Society for Biological Psychiatry, the Association for the Advancement of Behavior Therapy, the American Family Therapy Association, and the American Association for Marriage and Family Therapists.[77]

Spitzer acknowledged that there had been criticism of DSM-III because treatment from a variety of perspectives requires information that was not necessarily contained in DSM-III diagnoses or the multiaxial system. One solution to this problem, he offered, could be the publication of a book that might be entitled "DSM-III and Treatment Planning." The purpose of the book would be "not to provide a forum for evaluating the relative merits of the DSM-III classification, but rather to provide each group with an opportunity to indicate what additional information is needed for a more comprehensive evaluation." Spitzer went on to say that he believed that "this book would [not only] go a long way towards resolving some of the divisiveness that has developed around the development of DSM-III, but would, more importantly, serve a critical educational purpose." Were the addressees interested in participating in the project? Copies of the letter were sent out to a wide array of psychiatrists, including Spitzer's former analyst, Arnold Cooper. Spitzer also sent a separate letter to the President of the American Psychological Association, inviting the psychologists' participation in the project "by insuring that one or two members from each of the committees of the participating national organizations are also members of the American Psychological Association."[78] He had learned a valuable lesson in the controversy over the definition of a mental disorder. Psychologists were a significant part of the mental health profession.

In various letters later on in the fall, Spitzer made it clear that if Project Flower got off the ground that would obviate the need for a separate appendix for psychodynamically oriented clinicians.[79] Hector Jaso, Chair of the Assembly Liaison Committee to DSM-III, also wrote a letter to Alan Stone, urging the Board of Trustees not to have an appendix in DSM-III for members with a psychodynamic orientation and "strongly" endorsing Project Flower.[80] Moreover, Spitzer sent a letter to the President of the American Academy of Child Psychiatry raising the possibility that a member of the Academy join each national organizational committee that would prepare a chapter for inclusion in Project Flower.[81] In December, the Trustees approved Project Flower but under the aegis of the Council on Medical Education rather than that of the Council on Research and Development. Were the Trustees sending a not so subtle message here? None other than Paul Fink, the analyst who had written the angry letter to Grinspoon denouncing the DSM-III Task Force and Spitzer, was Chair of Medical Education.[82]

By this time, in the early months of 1979, with the DSM-III vote looming ever closer, innumerable hotspots were demanding attention from Spitzer. Project Flower became one more. Once the formation of committees to write chapters for Project Flower got underway, problems began to arise. When Spitzer reminded the participants of his hope that a psychologist would sit on each of the committees, Alex Kaplan, President of the American Psychoanalytic Association, demurred.[83] "I feel," he wrote, "that this will complicate our task, adding a variety of other problems so that we cannot accept this suggestion." (He also made it clear that before his Association would agree to collaborate with the Academy of Psychoanalysis on the project, the Psychoanalytic Association alone would have to have the final word on the chapter. Spitzer accepted these terms.[84])

After notifying the psychologists that he was having difficulty with the analysts' allowing a member of the American Psychological Association to sit on their Project Flower committee,[85] Spitzer wrote to Kaplan, asking him to reconsider his position. He offered to put a statement in the book that would make it clear that the psychologists on the committees were there as consultants.[86] Meanwhile, Joan Zaro, Ph.D., of the Professional Affairs Division of the Psychological Association, indicated her organization's "disappointment" and "keen distress" over Kaplan's stance.[87] Every other organization preparing chapters was "cooperative and eager to have psychologists involved," she wrote. But Kaplan was unmovable. Writing directly to Zaro, he declared that the original letter from Spitzer about the analysts' involvement in the project had never mentioned the matter of a psychologist's inclusion.[88] He explained, as if that solved the problem, "the sub committee that was formed was taken from members of our Peer Review committee and at this time did not include any psychologists…I do not feel it will be useful to add another member [just] because of his specific professional background." On the same day, Kaplan wrote to Spitzer that he was "sorry" about so much feeling being expressed on this issue.[89] Nevertheless, he added, while the American Psychoanalytic Association had a number of "esteemed" psychologists involved in their organization, "there is no compulsion to include psychologists on all our committees." And there the matter ended. Spitzer wrote a long, peace-making letter to Zaro, citing his now revised views about the definition of a mental disorder as a medical disorder, welcoming the collaboration of all mental health professionals, and expressing his hopes for the endorsement of DSM-III by the American Psychological Association.[90]

The comments on this episode almost write themselves. Once again, the analysts had needlessly done their "thing," eliciting hostilities where none need exist. Furthermore, in a few years it was to become obvious that they were not realistically evaluating their position in the world of mental health care and were fighting a rear-guard action. In 1985, five years after the publication of DSM-III, the American

Psychological Association filed a class action suit against the American Psychoanalytic Association, along with other psychoanalytic organizations, as being in restraint of trade for their refusal to accept non-M.D.s for training. Three years later the psychologists won their suit; it was a scant decade after the incongruous imbroglio we have just witnessed.

But even as Spitzer was involved in negotiations with Zaro and Kaplan, he strove to bring Project Flower to fruition. He and Janet Forman spent a weekend working with the two analytic DSM-III committees on their chapter for the book on treatment planning. Remembering Spitzer's own account of his workdays—12, 14, even 16 hours— here is a good example. He notes in a prospectus of the volume that he and Janet Forman met with each one of the separate groups writing chapters in order to ensure the accurate focus of each chapter.[91] After the weekend, the Chair of the analytic group wrote to Sabshin of their progress and "pleasure at the mutually helpful collaboration" and, at Sabshin's request, sent him a preliminary five-page draft summarizing what the analytic chapter would look like.[92]

Project Flower was to have chapters on five major modalities of treatment: psychodynamically oriented psychotherapy, family therapy, group psychotherapy, behavior therapy, and somatic therapy. In the prospectus it was clearly stated that the goal of each chapter was to discuss "the kinds of information, above and beyond that required for a diagnosis, that would be necessary in order to evolve an adequate treatment plan."[93] All the groups were given very specific instructions: their goal was to show how to link the DSM-III diagnosis with planning for treatment in a particular modality. The chapters were not supposed to be turned into mini textbooks on the "how" of actual treatment.

Thus an elaborate plan had come about as a result of trying to win over the analysts to accept DSM-III just as it was, without special introductions or appendices written by them. But once DSM-III had been approved by the APA Assembly of Delegates, much of the impetus to develop the treatment planning volume was gone, so when problems with Project Flower began to arise, they were more likely to impede progress than if approval of DSM-III was still hanging fire. As time went on, it proved increasingly difficult to get all the chapters, written as they were by diverse committees, to be uniform in their approach.

THE WILTING OF THE THOUSAND FLOWERS

Matters began to fall apart when the Chair of the analysts' committee, William Offenkrantz, complained to the President of the American Psychoanalytic Association, Rebecca Solomon, M.D. Offenkrantz charged that Spitzer and the Task Force were "directing" the committee what to write and reported that Spitzer had said that the Task Force would critique the chapters submitted "to insure high quality."[94] Over the telephone, Spitzer assured Solomon that "your committee is free to decide on the content of the chapter," but he added, "provided that it is consistent with the objectives of the book." Still, Spitzer said he had not been issuing "directives," but was just trying to be "helpful."

The pace of problems picked up about the same time when Paul Fink, Chair of the Committee on Medical Education, to whom Spitzer was reporting in connection with Project Flower, decided that he could no longer work with Spitzer and his Task Force and wanted to appoint a new Task Force.[95] There is nothing in the Archives to indicate what the dissension was about, but Fink had been angry at Spitzer at least since Fink had written his accusatory letter to Grinspoon. Then at the Washington meeting, Fink had not been able to sway Grinspoon in his upholding of the decision that DSM-III would be a descriptive manual. This current clash between Spitzer and Fink was aired before a meeting of the Board of Trustees, and it was decided that Spitzer and the Task Force would still be in charge of Project Flower but now would report to the Council on Research and Development.

At this juncture, Spitzer appointed a subcommittee of the Task Force to review and critique drafts of Project Flower.[96] By then it was the end of May, and the project was starting to fall behind its original deadlines.[97] The analysts' subcommittee submitted the fifth draft of its chapter to Spitzer in September, a sign that it was having difficulty meeting the guidelines. Offenkrantz urged his committee to be careful to stick to the prescribed formula regarding treatment planning.[98] In the year from September 1979 to October 1980, Project Flower ran into increasing difficulties. (Recall that DSM-III was published in January 1980.) At this point, the project fades out of the main concern of this book, but below is a summation of subsequent events.

In July 1979, Donald G. Langsley (1925–2005), Chair of the highly placed Reference Committee and President-elect of the APA, had sent to all the members of his committee Spitzer's formal proposal for Project Flower. When Langsley had heard back from all his members, he sent them a long memo reporting their reactions.[99] While most felt that the concept of a book on treatment planning was a good one, they raised many objections about the actual volume thus far. They were concerned about the manner in which the book was being written and which organizations had been included and which were missing. Everyone agreed that the project was being developed in haste and lacked sufficient input from "many points of view and components of the APA." Langsley advised that the Council on Research and Development ask Spitzer and the Task Force to "reconsider the project" and "abandon any effort...to review a final draft in November."

Eventually, the Board of Trustees became directly involved and appointed a subcommittee to consider the drafts of each chapter and the various critiques that had been submitted.[100] Moreover, the Assembly of Delegates began to take notice of the project and wanted input. They were worried that a book on treatment planning would give "prescriptive commands for treatment and treatment plans [which] could cause all sorts of difficulties."[101]

In February 1980, the Board of Trustees' subcommittee submitted their report on Project Flower to the President of the APA, Alan A. Stone.[102] They reported that the various critiques they had read "ranged from mildly positive to strongly negative." The subcommittee was of the "unanimous opinion that the materials submitted to Dr. Spitzer and his committee are unacceptable for publication in their present form. Further [they did] not feel that additional editing of the present manuscripts [would] enhance their quality sufficiently to warrant publication." However, the subcommittee thought the idea a good one and suggested ways in which such a volume could be developed by the Council on Research and Development. Yet by May no new editor had been appointed.[103] Finally in October, there was a new editor, Jerry Lewis, M.D., but he reported directly to the Trustees, not to the Research and Development Council. Also in October the Assembly renewed its demands for input. Let's try to "keep this under the control of the Assembly," argued one member, "just like we carefully monitored DSM-III."[104] And there the paper trail in the Archives abruptly ends.

DSM-III and Treatment Planning never materialized as a companion volume to DSM-III, which was unfortunate for the psychoanalytic community. Madow and other analysts' strong belief that psychodynamic material, to be effective, had to be in DSM-III and nowhere else was erroneous. A companion volume, published by the APA in tandem with DSM-III, with a chapter on the relationship of a DSM-III criteria–based diagnosis to psychodynamic treatment planning, would have had a significant influence. It would have blunted the seeming "atheoretical" approach of DSM-III that contributed to the mistaken notion that all that was needed to make a diagnosis was a checklist of symptoms. This would have been particularly effective when it came to the education of psychiatric residents. Spitzer inserted an important caveat in the Introduction of DSM-III, but brief as it was, it was easy to ignore: "Making a DSM-III diagnosis represents an initial step in a comprehensive evaluation leading to the formulation of a treatment plan. Additional information about the individual being evaluated beyond that required to make a DSM-III diagnosis will invariably be necessary."[105] There followed four paragraphs giving examples of evaluations for psychodynamically oriented treatment, behavior therapy, family therapy, and somatic therapy. A chapter rather than a paragraph could have made a vital difference.

Project Flower appearing in the winter of 1980 would also have helped to hold the line against fifteen-minute "med checks," so beloved by managed care. In a related vein, *DSM-III and Treatment Planning*, by putting in cold print what kind of care was necessary for a particular DSM-III diagnosis, would have been an immediate weapon against the insurance companies' favoring limited treatments for a mental disorder. Project Flower was an opportunity lost.

Instead, two years later, the APA published a general volume entitled *Treatment Planning in Psychiatry*.[106] While the first chapter was written by Offenkrantz and his committee, the book lacked the immediacy and close tie to DSM-III and never had a substantial impact. Book reviews that would have linked DSM-III and treatment planning did not appear.

The war between Spitzer and the Task Force on the one side and the psychoanalysts on the other was ultimately not in the best interests of American psychiatry. It is true that in the early 1970s psychiatry was in a crisis situation for all the reasons we have discussed, and circumstances called out for a vigorous response. But the decision to revise the DSM in order to use it as a tool for "remedicalizing" psychiatry placed an exaggerated burden on its makers, pushing them to go to radical lengths in breaking with the past. There was nothing wrong with enhanced definition and description of disorders as a goal, but this did not have to mean the total extirpation of all psychoanalytic knowledge of how the mind sometimes functions. And while diagnosis has to be regarded as an essential part of psychiatry, Spitzer's resolve to make sharp divisions among most mental disorders and between mental disorder and normality pushed psychiatric conceptualization of mental disorder into clinically unsound extremes in certain diagnoses.

However, it was correct to seek to temper the psychoanalytic dominance of psychiatry, because this too had extended itself to an indefensible extreme, with unrealistic aims to make patients "weller than well" and the insupportable disregard of the severely mentally ill. Furthermore, when the analysts found themselves challenged by Spitzer, a more clear-sighted recognition of the ever-thinner ice on which they were skating would have led to a better outcome, certainly for a while. Of course, in the long term, the psychopharmacological revolution, competing effective short-term psychotherapies, and managed care would have taken their toll. But perhaps all this was beside the point for the psychoanalysts with at the time of the making of DSM-III. Almost no one surrenders power voluntarily.

12

THE FIELD TRIALS AND YET MORE
CONTROVERSIES

In this chapter, we will take a break from the high drama of the clashes between Spitzer and the psychoanalysts to focus on some important events that were occurring simultaneously. Then, after examining these circumstances, we will turn to the tense happenings of the final few weeks before DSM-III faced approval or rejection by the Assembly of Delegates during the 1979 annual meeting of the APA.

A variety of situations continued to challenge Spitzer. The first to be discussed here concerns the field-testing of the evolving manual in institutional and private settings, with close looks at the reactions of forensic psychiatrists and of psychoanalysts. The second pertains to one result of the field trials, namely the evidence that clinicians were having difficulties dealing with Axis IV of the multiaxial diagnostic system. This diagnostic variable involved the recognition and evaluation of any psychosocial stressors that were connected to the presenting psychiatric illness. Spitzer had high hopes for Axis IV, but he worried: would busy clinicians use it? We will conclude the chapter with brief surveys of some of the controversial diagnoses in DSM-III that have not yet been considered: Tobacco Dependence, Schizoaffective Disorder, Attention Deficit Disorder, and PTSD.

THE FIELD TRIALS

While Spitzer was occupied in 1977 with the various issues that have engaged our attention up to now, he enthusiastically began to conduct field trials, sending out material even before the official release of the first draft of April 15, 1977. Spitzer was determined to receive as much feedback as possible. As a result, he was able to present some tentative results at the 1977 APA meeting in Toronto that spring. This was bound to be impressive to his audience because a new DSM had never been publicly tested and there would be inherent interest in learning something of the results. These very early trials were preliminary to the more extensive testing that soon took place with a grant from the NIMH.[1] Spitzer was very proud of the trials, seeing them as the fulfillment of a long-standing conviction. When commenting on DSM-II soon after it appeared in 1968, he had declared then that DSM-III should be field tested before it was released.

Materials on the results of the field trials are not very extensive. From Spitzer and colleagues there are five published articles and a short appendix at the end of DSM-III. While the Archives contain many of the questionnaires and related memos and letters sent out during the NIMH trial, which followed the preliminary trial, there is only one document with raw data.[2] There is also one article by two forensic psychiatrists relating their experiences while participating in the preliminary field trials.[3] In addition, two sociologists have written a book that includes chapters on the trials. While it has some useful factual material, it is also a polemic against DSM-III.[4] Based on the statistics derived from the reliability sections of the questionnaires, the book is particularly an attack on Spitzer's assertion that DSM-III brought greater reliability to psychiatric diagnosis. The authors have some telling criticisms, but their bias leads them to some obvious distortions in their claims.

Spitzer made it very clear from the outset what his main goal was in conducting the trials. He told the NIMH that "the major purpose of the study is to identify and solve potential problems with the DSM-III draft."[5] Another important goal was to conduct reliability studies on psychiatric diagnoses made by the participants in the trials, which would include information on the five axes of the multiaxial diagnostic system. Spitzer was particularly interested in how the participants would deal with Axis IV, which asked for the ranking of the severity of psychosocial stressors that might have contributed to the disorder under question. More than any other axis, he was concerned with how readily this would be accepted by busy clinicians.

Spitzer also specified to the NIMH what the trials were not supposed to do: neither "insure that the types of facilities and patients be statistically representative in this country [nor] conduct a scientifically designed epidemiological study of the distribution of mental disorders in the population."[6] It is worth commenting here that Spitzer's disclaimer was problematic: if an investigator wants to establish that the sampling has good reliability then it is necessary to document a wide representation. Ultimately, the NIMH did come back to Spitzer toward the end of the trial to ask him for demographic information, and he had to return to the participants in the trial to ask them for some specific data.

Spitzer recruited participants for the trials by advertising in *Psychiatric News* and other journals, and he directly approached the Veterans Administration and the American Academy of Child Psychiatry to ensure he had representation from their patient populations. In addition, many letters went out to institutions and national organizations, including psychoanalytic institutes.[7] Any individual clinician who applied was accepted. There was no screening, thus some individuals without any "professional academic experience" were involved, although of course, these were very few.[8] Physicians received useful Continuing Medical Education (CME) credits for their participation. Spitzer started recruiting as early as the summer of 1976, after the Midstream meeting. The first welcoming letters with instructions, registration forms, and reporting forms for the NIMH trial went out on January 7, 1977. Psychodynamically oriented physicians were asked to identify themselves as such on the forms. All participants were given the most recent DSM-III classification of diagnoses and codes, dated January 4, 1977.[9] However, as of that time, the classification was not complete and Axes IV and V of the multiaxial diagnostic system were yet to be included in the reporting forms.

In his efficient manner, Spitzer established patterns of both making immediate changes to the original draft as soon as he received feedback he thought significant and sending out additional or revised instructions, diagnoses, or questionnaires as deemed necessary.[10] Admittedly, this process was not a scientific one, but getting the bugs out of the new manual was uppermost in his mind; any feedback was always welcomed and considered. Frequent directives sent to the participants were often made more palatable with good-natured humor, and Spitzer promised prompt responses to any concerns or questions. Whether deliberate or accidental, these various stratagems raised the enthusiasm of the participants and engendered better cooperation with Spitzer's ongoing requests of them.

Ultimately, after dropouts were excluded and late participants were added, the NIMH trials from 1977 to 1979 enlisted 467 clinicians in 123 facilities and 78 clinicians in private practice.[11] Spitzer published all their names in an appendix to DSM-III.[12] Adding in those who participated in the preliminary trials in 1977, clinicians saw a total of 12,667 patients.[13]

Phase 1 of the NIMH-sponsored field trials, with Janet Forman as Project Coordinator, began in September 1977 and included four separate studies:

1. Diagnostic Study: Each participant evaluated twenty patients using DSM-III diagnostic criteria. Results were recorded and problems noted.
2. Reliability Study: Private-practice clinicians were not involved in this study. Pairs of clinicians at any given facility independently diagnosed two of the twenty patients in the Diagnostic Study to determine the degree to which they agreed on the five multiaxial diagnoses.
3. Case Summary Study: The participants prepared case summaries of two of the cases in the Diagnostic Study. The summaries were then used to refine the diagnostic criteria and to evaluate controversial categories.
4. Debugging Study: Throughout the entire field trial, clinicians were asked to submit critiques of the DSM-III draft. In addition, after a few months—this turned out to be in June 1978—a questionnaire was sent to all participants asking specific questions about DSM-III and their experiences in the trial up to that point.

The clinicians were provided with various forms for recording their results.[14] In a number of episodic communications, Spitzer and Forman gently notified the participants as a group where they had fallen short and urged them on to better efforts.[15]

A WINDOW INTO RESULTS FROM THE FIELD TRIALS: THE SURVEY AFTER NINE MONTHS

On June 28, 1978, Spitzer and Forman distributed a questionnaire with thirty-six questions to all field trial participants; they tallied the answers on September 5. The survey covered a wide range of issues of special concern to Spitzer and was in essence a referendum on approval or disapproval of the current DSM-III draft. The questions were worded fairly. (The language is not reproduced verbatim here.) Large numbers of psychoanalysts did not participate in the trials, which somewhat skewed the results; we shall examine this situation in more detail presently. Below are five key questions and the results:

- **Question (Q):** What should be done about the problematic Axis IV, psychosocial stressors, of the multiaxial system? **Results (R):** The participants were given five choices, which scattered the vote. Still, 52% opted for keeping it and leaving it as it was. (Not surprisingly, the psychodynamically oriented participants gave Axis IV even more support—64%.)
- **Q:** Should the controversial diagnosis of Schizoaffective Disorder be listed in its own separate category, neither placed among the schizophrenia diagnoses nor among the affective disorders? **R:** 58% agreed while 26% were not sure. The psychodynamic clinicians' vote was not much different: 55% for the separate category and 24% not sure.
- **Q:** Should Neurotic Depression (Depressive neurosis) in DSM-II, a frequent psychoanalytic diagnosis, be replaced? Participants had a choice of two alternative depressive diagnoses or Adjustment Disorder with Depressed Mood. **R:** This was a hot topic. 56% said they approved of eliminating the neurotic diagnosis and chose an alternative, and 33% said they wanted to keep Neurotic Depression. But in the tally of psychodynamically oriented clinicians, 52% agreed with the new approach, and 42% wanted to retain Neurotic Depression. Here Spitzer had won by a small margin, but he had won.
- **Q:** Should the purely descriptive approach of DSM-III be retained or should psychodynamic formulations be added to the manual? **R:** Here Spitzer had a decisive victory. 75% supported the new descriptive approach (65% among the psychodynamically oriented participants) and 18% wanted to add psychodynamic formulations (28% among the psychodynamic clinicians.) 6% voted Other and were asked to explain what they meant.
- **Q:** Then Spitzer, leaving nothing out, addressed the delicate topic of third-party payers who, the analysts feared, might use the new diagnostic criteria to withhold payment on the analysts' diagnoses and approach. **R:** Only 3% (4% psychodynamic clinicians) voted to remove the criteria because their inclusion was "a real problem." 83% (78% psychodynamic) voted to retain the diagnostic criteria because they "represent one of DSM-III's major contributions."

The questionnaire ended with a twelve-question poll on the acceptance and rejection of the approach and usefulness of DSM-III. Without producing here all the raw data, it is quite accurate to conclude that the overwhelming number of respondents approved of the new manual in every category. With these results and statistics from other questions, Spitzer and Forman could confidently go to the September 1978 showdown with the analysts that was sponsored by the Council on Research and Development.

Before we proceed with further overall discussion of the field trials, however, two specific aspects need to be addressed. The first is the particular use of DSM-III by two forensic psychiatrists who participated in the preliminary trials. The second concerns the involvement of the psychoanalysts in the trials.

In Rochester, NY, two forensic psychiatrists, David Barry and Richard Ciccone, and a group of second- and third-year residents they supervised at a legal clinic evaluated for the field trial thirty cases of teenagers and adults with criminal charges pending. What the psychiatrists reported provides us with an immediate view of the early use of DSM-III that studying tallies of raw numbers from a questionnaire does not begin to approach. Of course, these were the experiences of only one group, and they were in the preliminary trial not the later NIMH one, so we cannot give undue weight to their testimony. Nevertheless, their frontline endeavors have the ring of authenticity and probably represent the experiences of some other participants in the field trials.

To start with, the group, inadvertently it seems, violated Spitzer's caution not to discuss diagnoses that were in the process of being formulated. Once a week the group held a conference meeting to consider specific cases, "focusing on the effect of differences in diagnosis between DSM-II and III on the offender's fate within the legal system."[16] Moving beyond this particular potential distortion of reported diagnoses, Barry and Ciccone made the significant observation that "some of the residents were assigning the diagnoses under DSM-III by looking for the category most closely approximating the patient's diagnosis in II, hoping to force a match." Barry and Ciccone concluded, "This will be an important source of bias among all of us experienced with DSM-II." What emerges from this particular awareness is the main reason why the residents tried to get a DSM-III diagnosis by looking at DSM-II: they wished to avoid the "icy plunge into the 350 pages of DSM-III." Confronted with almost triple the number of pages of DSM-III, compared with the 134 pages of DSM-II, an appreciable number of clinicians hoped they could fudge their way into a DSM-III diagnosis by avoiding actually reading DSM-III. Additionally, the psychiatrists pointed out, many residents failed to record Axes IV and V diagnoses, convinced that the axes gave them no more information than they had already collected in their diagnostic interviews and no added help in formulating a treatment plan. Axes IV and V, it was felt, were just there to aid researchers who wanted to investigate psychiatric subpopulations more easily. Barry and Ciccone predicted that the new axes would "wither away to become mere vestigial appendages of the new nomenclature."[17] Even Axis III, they asserted, would be used only infrequently, "and [was] likely to be viewed as a curiosity rather than a vital part of the diagnostic formulation." If these preliminary reports turned out to be true, DSM-III would face an uphill fight for acceptance.

However, there were positive aspects of DSM-III for forensic psychiatry. Barry and Ciccone welcomed the category of "V Codes," for diagnosing "conditions not attributable to a known mental disorder," such as marital problems or uncomplicated bereavement.[18] This had a welcome use in the courtroom. The "V Code" diagnoses "would allow [the users] to make note of the presenting problem without 'reaching' for psychiatric diagnoses or ignoring disturbing behavior by offering...a diagnosis of No Mental Disorder.... Thus, this category becomes an 'affirmative' diagnosis, rather than a wastebasket for incomplete diagnostic studies."[19] Moreover, psychiatrists who "scrupulously" diagnosed patients via DSM-III categories on Axes I and II would impress others in the courtroom by their "more objective" means of diagnosis. "Some of the hue and cry around the unreliability of our classificatory system may abate." Furthermore, the "still skeptical attorney" would be compelled to guide his or her questioning along the lines of the psychiatrist's diagnostic criteria. Thus, Barry and Ciccone concluded that once psychiatrists "steel" themselves and become familiar with this "tome," they would see that it has "far-reaching significance in their field," as well as for their connections with other related professions.[20] The implication here is clear: once forensic clinicians got used to DSM-III, which might take a year or two, they would see the advantages of the new diagnostic system.

What has just been described is valuable in gaining insight into the challenges Spitzer and the Task Force faced with the acceptance of DSM-III. Now let us turn to examine the results and significance of the NIMH questionnaire of June 1978 as related to the participation of the psychoanalysts in the trials. The statistics from the question-naire were affected by the fact that not many psychoanalysts, analytic training facilities, or psychodynamically oriented hospitals took part in the field trials. Appendix F of DSM-III contains the names of the participants in psychiatric facilities and those in private practice.[21] A total of 123 facilities participated; Spitzer had invited the analytic institutes to join the trial. While there may have been more analytic facilities taking part, we know for certain of the involvement of only three analytic institutes (Chicago, St. Louis, and Menninger) and three psychodynamically staffed hospitals (Institute of Living, McLean, and Sheppard and Enoch Pratt; also a fourth, although whether inpatient or outpatient is not clear, the Downstate Medical Center in Brooklyn). It was a tactical error on the part of the analysts not to have signed up for the trial in greater numbers. They might have been able to confront Spitzer and the Task Force on their home ground of using the aggregate, but now to the analysts' advantage. (Of course, it is understandable that psychoanalysts who worked with one individual for years did not appreciate the power of numbers; they did not routinely conduct studies of patient populations.) Leo Madow, Paul Fink, William Offenkrantz, and Alex Kaplan, analysts whose activities have been mentioned thus far in this book, were not on the list of par-ticipants in the trials. Nor were any of the other analysts who came with Madow to the eventful Washington meeting—Anton Kris, Larry Rockland, and William Frosch. The only place where we know that at least several analysts took part was Washington, DC, because we learn from Boyd Burris, President of the Baltimore-District of Columbia Society for Psychoanalysis, that analysts from his organization were in the field trials.[22] While ten facilities in New York City, which might have contained some analysts, par-ticipated in the trial, when checking the list of "Participants in Private Practice," we see that only three came from New York City, yet we know there were many analysts there.[23] It seems probable that Spitzer's statistics would have been different if a large quantity of analysts across the United States had taken part in the NIMH field trials.

THE NIMH FIELD TRIAL MOVES FORWARD

Let us return to the totality of the trials. More polls, small questionnaires, and requests for additional information, besides the ongoing reporting, continued to go out from

Spitzer and Forman over the rest of 1978 and into 1979: a call for ten more case summaries with requests for DSM-III diagnoses in order to check reliability further; a questionnaire to discover why certain registered clinicians had not started or completed the field trial; a questionnaire to learn more about the diagnosis of chronic mild depression; a request for fresh comments on controversial changes in yet another draft of DSM-III.[24]

The field trial advanced into Phase 2, as DSM-III slowly moved on the road to completion in 1979. Spitzer, the Advisory Committees, and the Task Force made decisions on one diagnosis after another as information was received from the field. Controversies were settled and problems solved. Only six weeks before DSM-III was to come up for approval before the Assembly of Delegates, Spitzer and Forman sent out a final questionnaire: Had participants ever changed a diagnosis after discovering their partner's diagnosis in a reliability study? Did the respondents approve of yet another change in the positioning of Schizoaffective Disorder? Had elimination of Neurosis as a diagnostic class been a mistake? What details should be included in Axis IV about psychosocial stressors? To satisfy a late request from the NIMH about the trials—we are now in late March 1979—would the respondents estimate the "social class distribution of patients evaluated" in the trial? And from what size population area had the patients come? Would the participants do a "personal favor" for Forman, who was working on her doctoral dissertation, and provide "some additional demographic data"?[25] Spitzer requested that the participants reply within a week because he had been asked to answer questions about DSM-III by an ad hoc committee of the Board of Trustees in April.

THE VEXING MATTER OF RELIABLE
PSYCHIATRIC DIAGNOSIS

Before closing our discussion of the ever-busy world of the field trials, we should investigate more closely the issue of whether DSM-III made diagnosing more reliable. Spitzer certainly thought so and wrote in DSM-III, "Perhaps the most important part of the study was the evaluation of diagnostic reliability by having pairs of clinicians make independent diagnostic judgments of several hundred patients. The results...generally indicate far greater reliability than had previously been obtained with DSM-II."[26]

However, it is no simple matter to write about the reliability portion of the NIMH field trial. For example, attempts to learn exactly how many clinicians and patients took part in the reliability studies run up against the complication that various official reports on this subject differ from one to the other. There is also some confusion about the number of reliability evaluations each clinician did. Throughout most of the original field trial documents and published accounts it is stated that each participant evaluated two patients. In Appendix F in DSM-III, Williams (Forman at the time of the trials) and Spitzer write that there were four assessments each. Yet in the same appendix, they declare that "approximately 300 clinicians evaluated a total of 670 adult patients."

Those perplexing numbers aside, it is probably more important to see just how reliable the diagnoses were in various axes of the multiaxial diagnostic system. Spitzer and Forman always kept in mind the accuracy of the reliability statistics and repeatedly queried participants about potential contamination of their diagnoses (with ready humor now and then to make the ongoing questioning more acceptable). Did you select a case because of an obvious "great" diagnosis? Was there a diagnosis already on some case material you read? Did you speak to your partner about your diagnosis after the patient interview? Did you change your diagnosis to be in accord with your partner's? Did you not send back a diagnosis because you and your partner disagreed?[27]

Spitzer and Forman expressed their reliability results in terms of a statistic called kappa. "Kappa is a measure of the extent of agreement between two clinicians diagnosing the same patients. The measure ranges from 0 to 1. [Kappa] factors out the proportion of agreement that could be expected by chance alone. Kappa is defined as the proportion of [agreement] actually obtained by clinicians, over and above chance agreement. 0 is only chance levels of agreement, 1 is perfect agreement."[28] Spitzer and Forman considered a kappa of .7 or above high and also counted as concordant the raters' agreement in the *class* of a diagnosis even if there was not agreement on the *exact* disorder. So, for example, if one rater made a diagnosis of paranoid schizophrenia and the other of catatonic schizophrenia, the fact that they both diagnosed schizophrenia was what mattered in measuring reliability.

There is no doubt that reliability was usually good when it came to diagnosing schizophrenia and major affective disorders on Axis I (Clinical Psychiatric Syndromes and Other Conditions). Kappa for schizophrenia when both clinicians interviewed the patient together was .82 and remained the same even when the two clinicians interviewed the patient separately (test-retest). Kappa for major affective disorders was .70 for a joint interview and .65 for separate interviews.[29] However, there were diagnoses for which agreement had been at best fair: schizoaffective (when clinicians were torn between a schizophrenia or affective disorder diagnosis), chronic minor affective disorder, and personality disorders in general (Axis II). The kappa for the latter was .61 for joint interviews and .54 for test-rests, which was somewhat improved over earlier studies but still only fair; for specific personality disorders kappa ranged from .26 to .75. Spitzer and colleagues admitted that "how to improve further [their] reliability is not at all clear."[30] They conjectured that the overall enhanced diagnostic reliability was owing to the "innovative" features in DSM-III: specifically (1) an improvement in the classification over DSM-II, (2) separation of Axis I and Axis II disorders, (3) the fuller and more uniform descriptions in DSM-III, and (4) the diagnostic criteria.

As mentioned earlier, two sociologists, Stuart A. Kirk and Herb Kutchins, have challenged Spitzer's reliability claims in many ways, arguing against the scientific credibility of DSM-III. Clearly, they were determined to blacken the notion that DSM-III brought greater reliability and that there existed validity in psychiatric diagnosis in general, questioning the "science" that supposedly underlay psychiatry. Their verdict is clear in the title of their book, *The Selling of DSM: The Rhetoric of Science in Psychiatry*. Yet their own rhetoric damages their credibility. They declare, for example, that "the majority of participants acknowledged that they made diagnoses without meeting all the criteria at least occasionally." Yet if one turns to the raw data of the June 28, 1978, Phase 1 Questionnaire (which are the only raw data that exist in the Archives), Kirk and Kutchins' statement is clearly untrue; the give-away lies in their distorting use of the words "majority...at least occasionally."[31] The actual numbers were that 63% "practically never" made diagnoses when the criteria were not met and 34% "occasionally." In another instance, the campaign the two authors mount against kappa is only weakly convincing.[32]

Nevertheless, Kirk and Kutchins make some telling points against the way in which the field trials were conducted. They point out that in certain cases the testers of DSM-III were also the makers; people on the Task Force and Advisory Committees took part in the field trials, hardly a satisfactory way to go about attaining reliability. In addition, they draw attention to the circumstance that most of the raw data collected were never published, which makes it harder to evaluate the soundness of Spitzer and Forman's conclusions. Kirk and Kutchins remind their readers that Spitzer accepted into the field trials everyone who had applied, without any screening of their background, training, or conflicts of interest.[33] Thus, the sociologists ask, despite the occurrences that compromised reliability, how could the big "selling" point of DSM-III be that at last it had brought reliability to the psychiatric profession? In response, we should note that in some areas psychiatric diagnosis has become more reliable. Probably a bigger problem with psychiatric diagnosis is that it lacks the certainty, the validity, that comes from biological tests.

THE "UNOFFICIAL" AXES IV AND V: WOULD THEY AFFECT TREATMENT AND PROGNOSIS?

Let us return once more to the field trials themselves. Spitzer and Forman singled out for special investigation with the participants the multiaxial system in general and, in particular, Axis IV and Axis V. These were not "official" diagnoses as Axes I through III were. (Axis III was for "conditions not attributable to a mental disorder that are a focus of attention or treatment.")[34] Axes IV and V were "available for use in special clinical and research settings" and were supplemental. They might be "useful for planning treatment and predicting outcome." But Spitzer realized that busy clinicians might pass them by, as happened with the forensic psychiatrists in Rochester. In any event, 81% of the clinicians participating in the NIMH field trial thought that the multiaxial system was "a useful addition to traditional diagnostic evaluation," although many made note that they had had "difficulty quantifying the severity of psychosocial stressors" on Axis IV.[35] Also, 68% approved of dividing disorders between Axis I and Axis II, and 74% found it useful to make note on Axis II of personality traits of individuals they had diagnosed on Axis I.

Let us briefly attend to Axis V first (the patient's "highest level of adaptive functioning [during the] past year"), since the history and use of Axis IV will require lengthier scrutiny. The kappa for Axis V was "quite good, " .80 when joint interviews were done and .69 when interviews were separate. Axis V was a measurement of disability and prognosis, and 63% of respondents found Axis V useful.

The reaction to Axis IV, which provided for recording "the overall severity of a stressor judged to have been a significant contributor to the development or exacerbation of the current disorder,"[36] was another matter. There the kappa for a joint interview was .62 and that for separate interviews was .58; that was judged to be "fair." Therefore, in their Phase 1 questionnaire, Spitzer and Forman offered several options of response about its utility. In the poll, 52% of the participants said to keep Axis IV as it is, 10% said eliminate it, and 30% opted for just describing the stressors but not calling for a discussion of whether they were clinically significant.[37] One group complained that the main problem with evaluating stressors was deciding how the hypothetically "normal" individual would respond to any given stressor. Another group objected to attributing any etiological significance of the stressors to the current disorder.[38] But since more than half of the clinicians said to keep Axis IV, Spitzer decided to retain it. He argued that there would have to be future studies to determine whether clinicians actually used Axis IV and its impact on patient care. Meanwhile, he believed the axis was worthwhile since "an individual's prognosis may be better when a disorder develops as a consequence of a severe stressor than when it develops after no stressor or a minimal stressor."[39]

THE SAGA OF "PSYCHOSOCIAL STRESSORS"

The new multiaxial system in DSM-III was a creation about which Spitzer and the Task Force were of one mind. By the winter of 1975 or early spring 1976, a proposed structure was in place. The Task Force and Spitzer had determined four out of the five axes that eventually appeared in DSM-III. Only what became Axis V (Level of Adaptive Functioning) was missing. The proposed Axis III was Intellectual Level, a category ultimately not part of the multiaxial system.

In this early model of the multiaxial system, what became Axis IV was at first Axis V. There is a treasure trove of documents in the Archives showing the scrupulous consideration given to implementing a multiaxial system and Spitzer's early preoccupation with "psychosocial stressors."[40] Spitzer was determined to get the axis dealing with the stressors into DSM-III and get it right.

We have notes from a remarkable meeting of what seems to be the Multiaxial Diagnosis Advisory Committee and guest consultants from the United Kingdom or perhaps a conference call including U.S. psychiatrists Dennis Cantwell, John S. Strauss, and David Shaffer and the well-known guest psychiatrists John E. Cooper, Michael Rutter, and John Wing.[41] It is clear that in early 1976 the axes were still fluid. As people discussed how the multiaxial system would work and what information should be on the various axes, Spitzer commented, "[Psychosocial stressors] must be included otherwise psychosocial areas will be overlooked."

At first, the participants debated various arrangements of axes and what these axes should cover. Much was proposed that did not end up in the multiaxial system. In this wide-ranging discussion Spitzer kept pushing to include psychosocial stressors in the diagnostic system. When the whole deliberation finally moved to psychosocial stressors, attention centered, with great specificity, on the many difficulties involved in creating such an axis.

At this point, spring of 1976, the Archives fall silent for several months. It seems likely that Spitzer, the Task Force, and the Advisory Committees shifted their focus to the upcoming Midstream meeting in June. There was a compelling need to get the lengthy and detailed progress report on DSM-III ready to send to all the conference's participants before the meeting. Some further resolution seems to have been made after the St. Louis meeting. By October 1976 the multiaxial system had been configured into its final form, although the details for the new Axis V were still not clear. In a memo on a variety of topics, Spitzer notified the Task Force:

> Further work on the multiaxial approach suggests the advisability of having the axis for intellectual level used to code usual level of social functioning when applied to adults. Some Task Force members had previously made such a suggestion, but the cogency of the arguments for including social functioning for adults previously seems to have escaped me.... The enclosed DSM-III classification sheet now includes the listing of the axis as currently conceived. Your response to this latest twist would be appreciated.[42]

Spitzer made the first public proclamation of the new multiaxial structure at the Toronto symposium on psychiatric diagnosis the next month (November 1976.) It appeared officially in the April 15, 1977 draft of DSM-III. The opening language describing Axis IV, Psychosocial Stressors, was very close to the definition that ultimately appeared in the published DSM-III.

But that did not mean Spitzer had decided on the final form of Axis IV. He was filled with doubt about the axis as it had appeared in the April 15, 1977 draft, being ever cognizant of the fact that busy clinicians might not want to take the time to make an Axis IV diagnosis. A steady correspondence and meetings on the subject began that went on for the next six months, through November 1977. At the end of August 1977, Spitzer explained his recent thinking in a letter to A. James Morgan, M.D., a member of the Multiaxial Diagnosis Committee from Philadelphia.[43] "It seems clear," he said, "reviewing the many comments... it will not be possible in the official multiaxial system to include ratings of severity.... The system will never work if it is complicated [and] no way of defining severity seems to be adequate." Spitzer did not desire "ratings of severity" because that would mean measuring and giving a label to the severity of the reaction of any individual patient to any given stressor. What he wanted was only the measurement of the "actual" severity of the stressor itself; in his examples, death of a spouse woud be "extreme," compared to pregnancy, which is categorized as a "moderate" stressor.[44] So he elaborated to Morgan:

> If we define [severity] as we defined it in the 4/15/77 DSM-III draft, then the very important clinical aspect of vulnerability [how the stressor affects the patient] is overlooked. On the other hand, if we include vulnerability, then it would appear as if we are measuring the patient's reaction, rather than the stressor itself. Therefore... the only viable system is to merely note the category [kind] of psychosocial stressor.

Or, as he had put it in the April 15, 1977 draft, "The patient's idiosyncratic vulnerability or reaction should not influence the rating."[45] Nevertheless, as we have observed, many clinicians in the field trial still found complying with Axis IV difficult; they had trouble keeping separate the rating of the stressor from the rating of the patient's reaction.

It seems logical to note on the basis of what we know about Spitzer—his disillusionment with psychoanalysis and his strong research interests—that his particular configuration of Axis IV leaned toward measuring the aggregate reaction—what was usual, the average, or the mean. His main focus was not on gauging the idiosyncratic response of the individual. As he put it in DSM-III, "This rating [the severity of the stressor] should be based on the clinician's assessment of the stress an "average" person in similar circumstances and with similar sociocultural values would experience from the particular psychosocial stressor(s)."[46] We should also point out, however, that there are hints that his psychoanalytic training remained alive: his reference to an individual being "vulnerable [as a result of] certain internal conflicts," and the remark about the clinician's judgment of an "etiologically significant" psychosocial stressor.[47] Like most human beings, Spitzer was a complicated person, never safe to pigeonhole.

A lot of the activity after the April 15, 1977 draft centered on the work of Frederic W. Ilfeld, Jr., a Harvard- and Stanford-trained psychiatrist. Ilfeld was a member of the Multiaxial Diagnosis Advisory Committee and was interested in the relationship between stress and psychological functioning. He was committed to educating others on the subject of patients being affected by psychosocial stressors. At the end of September 1977, he sent Spitzer a four-page letter arguing for the importance of Axis IV in response to criticisms from the Task Force that Spitzer had sent him.[48] The letter was accompanied by a seven-page draft modification of the Axis IV material that might be placed in the upcoming second draft[49] (which appeared on January 15, 1978). Ilfeld wrote at length on three major issues he had delineated: the purpose of having psychosocial stressors in DSM-III, the specific theoretical foundations of such a diagnosis, and how best to assess the severity of psychosocial stressors.

In Ilfeld's belief, Axis IV was needed because "stressors do contribute in large part to individual disorder and because their identification is of high utility in outlining treatment and assessing prognosis." The theoretical underpinnings of Axis IV were several, he explained. They came from the discipline of social psychology and particularly from the work of the German-American Gestalt psychologist Kurt Lewin (1890–1947). In psychiatry, Harry Stack Sullivan (1892–1949) had also been mindful of the effect of stressors. Moreover, community mental health efforts and research on psychosomatic disorders had shown the importance of being able to adapt to changes in one's situation. As to assessing the severity of stressors, "there is no final resolution" to the debate on whether to define severity as the effect on the "average" person or as the patient's idiosyncratic response to stress. Therefore, Ilfeld declared that the "middle path" in the April 15, 1977 draft was methodologically sound, that is, asking "the clinician to fuse his knowledge of potency of life stressors along with their particular impact upon a given patient." Ilfeld then rewrote parts of the April 15 draft, including a new coding system, and added an appendix that spelled out in astonishingly lengthy specificity the subtypes of possible psychosocial stressors.

Spitzer responded to Ilfeld's explanations and proposals with unbounded enthusiasm.[50] The material "is really terrific!" He was "quite sure that the reaction of the Task Force will be very positive.... [W]e will certainly include this revision in the next Draft." Ilfeld's revisions were sent to the Task Force, the Advisory Committee on Multiaxial Diagnosis, and the Advisory Committee on Childhood and Adolescence Disorders, and Spitzer asked for their reactions.[51] Moreover, Spitzer sent a copy to Bruce Dohrenwend, Ph.D., who worked in the areas of social psychiatry and epidemiology at the New York State Psychiatric Institute and had expertise in stress and psychopathology.[52] Spitzer asked him for "any suggestion that [he might] have in this terribly complicated area." None of the various committees' or individual's reactions to Ilfeld's draft can be found in the Archives. However, in spite of Spitzer's high praise to Ilfeld, it is clear from examining the DSM-III draft of January 15, 1978 and the published DSM-III that, while some of Ilfeld's proposals were kept, many were not. Additionally, the order of certain passages was changed, and Ilfeld's intricate coding system was sacked in favor of Spitzer's much simpler one. As Spitzer had written to Dohrenwend: "The system has to be simple if it is to be recommended for a routine clinical use."

Within a short time, it proved necessary to convene a special meeting "to come up with a clinically feasible application of the psychosocial stressor axis for use with children. Clearly [Spitzer wrote to a selected panel] the current proposal for the use of major categories of psychosocial stressors for adults does not make much sense for children."[53] After this, whatever concerns Spitzer had with Axis IV shifted to its use in the NIMH field trial and the feedback he received from the participants.

With the publication of the January 15, 1978 draft of DSM-III, the entry for Axis IV moved to its penultimate stage. Spitzer's desire for an axis on psychosocial stressors had been attained. The multiaxial system as a whole and the field trials to test it had been Spitzer's goals for many years and became his accomplishments in the new DSM.

In sum, it is true that full reliability had not been achieved. Psychiatry is an art as well as a science because of the limited knowledge about the etiology of many of its diagnoses. Because of these limitations, the Wash. U. psychiatrists had urged that there be only those diagnoses that had "validity" (at least in their eyes). But Spitzer was writing a manual for clinicians as well as for researchers and thus strove to make it inclusive of all diagnoses that the clinicians found useful, even if not totally valid. The field trials helped to fulfill a portion of Spitzer's goals, with their paramount emphasis being on debugging the entire diagnostic system that he and the Task Force had devised.

ADDITIONAL SUBJECTS OF NOTE

It is of course impossible, in a book like this, to consider all the aspects of the making of DSM-III. Here, however, is a quartet of topics that seem especially worthy of inclusion.

TOBACCO DEPENDENCE

Let us move from the field trials to one of the more controversial diagnoses that occupied Spitzer: the brand new Tobacco Dependence (its final designation). In the early

1970s, when approximately half the nation still smoked, despite the Surgeon General's warnings, this disorder subjected Spitzer to both outright ridicule from other psychiatrists and covert pressure by tobacco interests.

DSM-II had expressly eschewed any concern about tobacco dependence or addiction. Under the broad category Personality Disorders and Certain Other Non-Psychotic Mental Disorders, there was a general listing "Drug dependence." The opening sentence was unambiguous: "This category is for patients who are addicted to or dependent on drugs other than alcohol, tobacco, and ordinary caffeine-containing beverages."[54] Spitzer had decided very early on to confront the issue of the smoker distressed by his or her inability to stop cigarette smoking or had become visibly ill as a result of smoking but did not stop. (Sigmund Freud, who continued to smoke cigars after developing mouth cancer, smoking even as he underwent repeated disfiguring and disabling operations, would have qualified for Spitzer's new diagnosis.) Spitzer's proposal meant taking on the scorn of millions and the reproach of medicalizing "normal behavior.".

The Task Force had been meeting no more than a few months when Spitzer published in *Psychiatric News* his intent to have "drug withdrawal syndrome from tobacco" appear as a new diagnosis in DSM-III.[55] A week after this article was published, Spitzer received a letter from a psychiatrist in Montclair, NJ, who wrote, "At the risk of appearing querulous, I would like to suggest that [such] a diagnosis...appears punctilious and would hardly seem to warrant psychiatric evaluation."[56] But this or any jibes thrown Spitzer's way did not change his mind.

Nor did a letter six months later from Nakhleh P. Zarzar, director of the Division of Mental Health Services of the State of North Carolina.[57] This letter was actually the start of a careful and low-key, behind-the-scenes effort on the part of the tobacco industry to influence Spitzer, although there was no way he would have known that at the time. Some amorphous news about Spitzer's goal must have circulated because Zarzar wrote that he understood Spitzer was considering the addition of "compulsive smoking syndrome" to the manual. He somewhat bombastically warned: This would be "an unwise move," and might "unnecessarily complicate" state hospital reporting plus "possibly imply that state hospital physicians will have to treat all those with such a diagnosis." The Task Force should "not pass judgement on it lightly," he urged. Zarzar appended a letter from Richard Proctor, M.D., Chair of the Department of Psychiatry and Neurology (1960–1985) at Bowman Gray School of Medicine in Winston-Salem, NC, also raising objections to the new diagnosis. What Zarzar did not reveal was that Proctor was a paid tobacco industry consultant. Again, Spitzer brushed these protests aside. Two months later Sptizer announced in the March 1976 Progress Report that was used as the basis for the June 1976 Midstream Conference, that he had already formed the Advisory Committee on Alcohol and Drug Abuse. On the committee sat an expert on "tobacco use disorder," Jerome Jaffe, M.D., who was affiliated with New York State Psychiatric Institute.[58] Spitzer emphasized this appointment, specifically labeling Jaffe as his "special consultant" on this subject.

As we have seen, at the Midstream Conference the consciousness of many groups was raised about the reality of the omissions and additions planned for the new manual. The tobacco industry was no exception, although their leaders could not very well react openly. We know of their concerns and plans through tobacco industry documents unearthed in 2003 and made public in a 2005 article in the journal *Tobacco Control*.[59] An internal Phillip Morris (PM) memo describes PM's surveillance of Spitzer's and Jaffe's activities as early as October 1976 and adds the admonition: "Please treat this material in strictest confidence."[60] A week later Horace R. Kornegay, President of the Tobacco Institute (TI), the tobacco industry's Washington, DC–based lobbying and political arm, shared PM's concerns with the head lawyers of all the tobacco companies (Committee of Counsel) and some other high-level officials. Two weeks after this bulletin, Kornegay reported on a plan of action:

> I am please to advise that Dr. Richard Proctor, chairman of the department of psychiatry at Bowman Gray Medical School, has agreed to write a substantial number of his colleagues to object to this undertaking ["Compulsive Smoking Syndrome"]. This matter was called to Dr. Proctor's attention by Colin Stokes of RJR [RJ Reynolds Tobacco Company] and after talking with Mr. Stokes, Dr. Proctor is in full agreement that such a classification should not be included in the Diagnostic and Statistical Manual of the APA. Hopefully, the officers and directors of other companies are taking a similar interest to discourage this move by the APA.[61]

Within a week or two of this memo, Proctor began an always-polite correspondence with Spitzer. He wrote as a private citizen giving a home address instead of using Bowman Gray stationary. Proctor promised Spitzer, "I won't get into a 'debate' or prolonged correspondence with you about this matter of tobacco use" and then did just the opposite.[62] A blind copy of Proctor's letter went to "Mr. Colin Stokes, Chairman, R.J. Reynolds Industries, Inc." After an initial query, Proctor launched into circumspect assertions about the logical consistency of Spitzer's new diagnosis, which he put forward in two virtually identical letters a month apart. Proctor, trying not to tip his tobacco-connection hand, presented a very garbled, indirect argument, but it can be translated as follows: overeating (which he called a process) leads to obesity, a medical disorder in the ICD. Tobacco use (also a process) leads to carcinoma of the lung, also a medical disorder in ICD. If you can call tobacco use a psychiatric disorder, then, to be consistent, you should call overeating a psychiatric disorder, which you are not doing in DSM-III.[63]

Spitzer, ever the conscientious respondent, wrote back in a week—with a copy to Jerome Jaffe—defending his consistency: "Tobacco use is [only] considered a disorder when it directly causes some distress to the individual," not because it poses a risk for disease. He then added: "DSM-III does not include simple overeating leading to obesity as a mental disorder [because] our consultants…stated that there was no distinctive psychiatric syndrome associated with simple overeating that distinguished such individuals from individuals who do not overeat." Bulimia is in DSM-III only because "of its associated psychiatric symptoms." Nevertheless, Spitzer courteously thanked Proctor for writing "as it has helped sharpen our thinking in this very difficult area."[64]

Proctor continued in his attempt to help the tobacco industry by sending successive drafts of DSM-III to Frank G. Colby, manager of the RJR Scientific Information

Division. Moreover, he capitalized on the American Psychological Association's desire to prevent mental disorders in DSM-III from being defined as a subset of medical illnesses. In January 1978, in an article in *Psychology Today*, entitled "Who's Mentally Ill?," Proctor derided making tobacco use a psychiatric disorder by comparing tobacco use to drinking coffee and added, "I trust that, too, when the DSM-IV is compiled, missing a three-foot putt on the 18th hole will be classified as a psychiatric diagnosis. It would make about as much sense as the tobacco or caffeine classifications."[65] Proctor, trying to make a point, was artfully comparing apples and oranges. DSM-III has no diagnosis for drinking coffee. Under the broad category of Organic Mental Disorders, it makes a distinction between Substance-induced and Substance Use. Under "Substance-induced" is Tobacco withdrawal (292.00) and Caffeine intoxication (305.90), both states diagnosable by obvious physical signs and symptoms of impairment. Under Substance Use is Tobacco dependence (305.1)—the diagnosis the tobacco companies were fighting—but there is nothing about caffeine under Substance Use.

We hear no more about Proctor for over a year, until Spitzer writes to him and another psychiatrist, John Schwab, M.D., sending them the final draft of "Tobacco dependence" in DSM-III, eight days before the Assembly of Delegates was to vote on the acceptance of the new manual. The diagnostic criteria of the new disorder centered on the inability to stop tobacco use even though the individual had tried and on the individual's continued use of tobacco despite knowledge that it was contributing to a serious physical disorder. By now Spitzer was addressing his letter to Proctor at Bowman Gray School of Medicine, having learned about his psychiatric connection. We do not know the history of the Spitzer–Schwab relationship, but we do know that Schwab, in Louisville, KY, received funds from the Council for Tobacco Research in 1985.[66]

The last correspondence of note here is a lengthy letter from a New York City psychiatrist, Leonard Cammer, M.D., who wrote to Spitzer in reference to the rationale for Tobacco Use Disorder that Spitzer and Jaffe had presented. Cammer sent a copy to Proctor, so Cammer's letter has to be viewed as having a possible industry connection; it was sent to Spitzer at the same time that Proctor was writing to him. Cammer took a Szaszian approach:

> Long ago I came to agree with some civil libertarians. Every distress in life is not a sickness and the person should be free to make certain choices even if unhappily, such choices make him ill.
>
> To the extent that a behavior is part of social learning and serves a purpose in adaptation to the cultural milieu, such behavior is not usually considered a mental disorder....
>
> Psychiatry has been overextended, reaching into areas which might better be left to educators and some categories of psychologists, ecologists, sociologists and social workers.[67]

If one compares the diagnostic criteria of Tobacco Use Disorder (early draft) and that of Tobacco Dependence (final designation) from the years 1976 to 1980, the definition of Tobacco Dependence narrows over the serial drafts of DSM-III. It is impossible to prove that the tobacco industry was responsible for these changes, but we know for certain that the industry surreptitiously tried to influence Spitzer. Even after DSM-III was published in 1980, the industry continued its efforts to attack the inclusion of Tobacco Dependence as a psychiatric diagnosis in the APA manual.[68 69]

SCHIZOAFFECTIVE DISORDER

One of the more trying diagnoses to situate within the psychiatric classification is Schizoaffective Disorder. The problem is seen by the very name. How should a patient be diagnosed when he or she exhibits clear symptoms of both a psychotic disorder and a mood disorder? Which is the primary disorder? Under what broad category does the disorder belong? The diagnostic challenge lay within the heart of the Kraepelinian dichotomy between manic-depressive insanity and dementia praecox. Later in life Kraepelin himself began to question the surety of the distinct polarity, and the problem of the overlap of schizophrenia and major mood disorders has bedeviled psychiatrists ever since.

In 1933, seven years after Kraepelin died, Jacob Kasanin (1897–1946) addressed the challenging issue in the *American Journal of Psychiatry*.[70] It is possible that the enigma of "good prognosis schizophrenia"—why was some psychosis episodic and not as severe?—also affected Kasanin's thought. Later the authors of DSM-I and DSM-II decided to deal with the thorny diagnosis by classifying Schizoaffective Disorder as a type of schizophrenia, and the Task Force of DSM-III initially left it there, as can be seen in the April 15, 1977 draft of the manual. There were two subtypes, Schizoaffective Depressed and Schizoaffective Manic, each with its own operational criteria. However, the January 15, 1978 draft removed Schizoaffective Disorder from the schizophrenia heading and placed it in its own separate category with just one list of diagnostic criteria, but with an elaborate subtyping of nine forms. This subtyping is a clear indication of the struggle to delineate the disorder.

Spitzer and two colleagues published this classificatory decision in an article in *Schizophrenia Bulletin,* presenting it as the Task Force's final disposition of the matter.[71] They justified this resolution by indicating that much dissension had plagued their discussions:

> This is a compromise between two extremes: those who consider it a subtype of Schizophrenia and those who consider it a form of Affective Disorder....We believe that the evidence is not yet in to resolve this controversy, and our decision permits the group to be studied without premature closing as to its relationship to Schizophrenia and Affective Disorder, as well as the possibility that it represents a third independent diagnostic class.

But a stand-alone category was not to be its final resting place. No sooner had the January 15, 1978 draft appeared than William Carpenter, a psychiatrist on the Multiaxial Diagnosis Advisory Committee, suggested another way of looking at the situation, based on his conceptualization of the psychotic disorders.[72] Schizoaffective disorders did not belong alone, he argued, but rather with Schizophreniform Disorder, a type of schizophrenia sharing some of the same features as the schizoaffective diagnosis. (Schizophreniform resembled schizophrenia but was of shorter duration and perhaps acute and more resolvable.) Therefore, asserted Carpenter, Schizoaffective Disorder should be placed under Psychoses Not Elsewhere Classified, where Schizophreniform was found along with Brief Reactive Psychosis and Atypical Psychosis. The emphasis would thus be placed on the psychotic features of Schizoaffective Disorder. Carpenter's conceptualization centered around his criticism that the criteria of schizoaffective disorder in the January 15, 1978 draft were skewed toward drawing patients previously diagnosed with manic-depressive disorder into the schizoaffective class.[73] Spitzer circulated Carpenter's comments to select members of the Schizophrenic, Paranoid, and Affective Disorders Advisory Committee and to the Task Force, asking for their responses.[74]

The result was the creation of an increasingly heated debate over what shortly before had appeared to be a settled question. In a general account such as this of the disputed diagnostic issues it is impossible to cover all of the intense and detailed discussions that occurred over the next several months; a lengthy article or short monograph would be needed to fully examine the history of the schizoaffective concept and the extremely specific and sophisticated confrontation of the issues by the members of the DSM-III Advisory Committee and Task Force. What emerges most clearly in this debate is that the diagnosis and classification of Schizoaffective Disorder could only be considered in an effective manner by probing into a score of related theoretical, diagnostic, and clinical matters. What follows is a brief summary of topics that were considered and that provoked sometimes vehement argument:

- Could Schizoaffective Disorder (SD) be defined by the premorbid personality (the patient's state before the illness)?
- Could SD be diagnosed according to type of onset and duration of the disorder?
- Which psychotic symptoms are necessary for a SD diagnosis?
- Do SD and Schizophreniform Disorder belong together under the same general category of Psychosis Not Elsewhere Classified?
- How does one accurately differentiate between SD and Schizophreniform Disorder?
- Should SD be defined by a predominance of psychotic symptoms or affective symptoms?
- How does one distinguish between SD and an affective disorder with atypical psychotic features?
- Does SD belong among the affective disorders? (There was some very strong positive feeling about this and perhaps even a tentative decision to do so.)
- Since the NIMH-sponsored Research Diagnostic Criteria (RDC) have been used for the past four years with the current diagnostic criteria of SD, can the evidence from RDC studies be used to decide what to do about SD?
- How should mood-congruent and mood-incongruent psychotic features be used in the diagnosis and classification of SD?[75] [76]

It probably should be pointed out that for most psychoanalysts and many psycho-dynamically oriented psychiatrists in the 1970s these issues held little interest. The minute details of diagnosing, so necessary for research, did not hold the same deep significance for them as for the Task Force, and there were analysts who did not possess the knowledge to totally comprehend all the terms and concepts. These gaps in their knowledge did not perturb them since they did not conceptualize their patients' problems from the same viewpoint.

During the spring through fall of 1978, intense memos were sent out and meetings began to take place. Resolutions were achieved and then undone. At a Task Force meeting in October, there was "a rather heated discussion" followed by a straw vote that Schizoaffective Disorder should remain a separate category. The result being tentative, the decision was made to hand the issue over to a "special advisory committee" that was to offer suggestions for redefining Schizoaffective Disorder.[77] The special committee met at the end of October and had a six-hour discussion. They agreed that the category would not be abandoned, but they would explore alternative ways of defining Schizoaffective Disorder.

In his report back to the Task Force, Spitzer found it "not easy" to summarize the results of the committee's discussions.[78] Much of the debate revolved around making a differential diagnosis between Schizoaffective Disorder and a Major Affective Disorder, and various difficulties emerged. The committee discussed "whether to define Schizoaffective Disorder with precise boundaries, or whether to define it as an essentially residual [leftover] category." Ultimately they decided to do the latter because they were not able to agree on specific diagnostic criteria even though many were discussed. This meant that Schizoaffective Disorder would "no longer be considered a class of disorders, and its logical place [was] within the Psychoses Not Elsewhere Classified." Thus, William Carpenter's suggestion of six months earlier that had started the entire rethinking of Schizoaffective Disorder proved decisive. But since it was so hard to define Schizoaffective Disorder, the special advisory committee agreed that it was important to strengthen the criteria for Depressive Episode, Manic Episode, and Schizophrenia, and this was done.

Spitzer reported further on a debate over whether Schizoaffective Disorder should be subtyped, as had been done in the January 15, 1978 draft. Some proposals were made, but it proved impossible to define precisely some of the terms—for example, how chronic was chronic? Thus, "it appeared that subtyping...would actually impede the study of ways of subdividing this elusive condition.... There was no point in subdividing a category that was already acknowledged to be...undefinable." Spitzer concluded his report by declaring that the special advisory committee had been wise "in dealing with the category in a way that completely acknowledges our inability at this time to define the category more precisely."

Two weeks later, Spitzer added to his report still other changes that the committee suggested to Affective Disorder and Schizoaffective Disorder, and he asked the Task Force for responses.[79] But Spitzer did not wait long for other ideas and within four days prepared the entry for Schizoaffective Disorder for DSM-III. A category that had been described in numerous pages had been boiled down to three-quarters of a page, with no diagnostic criteria.[80] This was no small matter; early on Spitzer had taken the stance that a diagnosis would only be included in DSM-III if it was possible to develop precise diagnostic criteria for it. This requirement was at the heart of a descriptive manual. But for Schizoaffective Disorder Spitzer made an exception, so convinced was he that there were times when a clinician needed to have such a diagnosis available. Spitzer informed the Council on Research and Development about the decision and eventually received word that the Council was in agreement with the general approach that had been taken.[81]

Although the entry in DSM-III seemed to have been finalized, for Spitzer an issue settled did not really mean concluded. Four months later, at the end of March 1979, Spitzer sent a follow-up questionnaire to the participants in the NIMH field trial. He explained that in a revised draft that had gone out, the Task Force had "given up" on providing specific guidelines for Schizoaffective Disorder and had "relegated" it to the class Psychotic Disorders Not Elsewhere Classified. He asked if the participants agreed with this decision.[82] Even five days before the Assembly of Delegates' vote on DSM-III, Spitzer was still discussing the matter with Donald Klein and argued for leaving things stand. He concluded: "I think the basic issue is still whether we try to give specific criteria for Schizoaffective Disorder such as Ed [Sachar] suggests, or whether we fudge the situation and let the clinician, by and large, use the category" (the end of this sentence is missing from the Archives, but it is clear where Spitzer was heading).[83] This was made obvious when he explained to a letter writer after DSM-III had been approved: "Schizoaffective Disorder [can] be used whenever the clinician is unable to make a differential diagnosis between Schizophrenia and Affective Disorder."[84] Spitzer's attempt at a highly developed diagnosis, so typical of his approach in DSM-III, had come down to just such a bald statement.

In DSM-IV (1994) Schizoaffective Disorder is placed under Schizophrenia and Other Psychotic Disorders and contains diagnostic criteria. The diagnosis is typically used to describe a psychotic person with significant symptoms of depression and/or mania.

To look into the debate about Schizoaffective Disorder is to look into the heart and mind of conceptualization and diagnosis in psychiatry. The developers of DSM-5 have struggled anew to understand the relationship of various psychiatric disorders to each other, still without having laboratory tests to determine their etiology. Specifically, the Psychotic Disorders Work Group has proposed a new category of a very wide "Schizophrenia Spectrum and Other Psychotic Disorders," of which Schizoaffective Disorder is one part. Although this placement effectively keeps the disorder among the schizophrenias, the emphasis of this decision is on the concept of a spectrum. The work group is declaring that the attempt to sharply delineate certain psychiatric disorders may be falsely creating divisions where none or little exists.

PSYCHIATRY AND THE LAW

Psychiatric and legal matters are often intertwined, thus there is a distinct specialty of forensic psychiatry, to which we have already turned our attention. Not surprisingly, with the ongoing revision of DSM-II the American Academy of Psychiatry and the

Law (AAPL) formed a DSM-III Liaison Committee in 1976, and their Chair, Abraham L. Halpern, M.D., wrote to Spitzer that he was "convinced that our group will be able to be of considerable assistance in clarifying those aspects of DSM-III which relate to legal issues." He asked Spitzer to send to all members of his committee the next draft of DSM-III.[85] Spitzer duly complied and sent the draft of April 15, 1977. A few weeks later, Spitzer asked all the committees evaluating DSM-III to respond with their comments and critiques, and Halpern complied with a report that Spitzer found very helpful. He implemented most of the AAPL Committee's suggestions.

Halpern's committee was of the opinion that the legal profession had misused the first two DSMs, and they presented Spitzer with suggestions for dealing with this problem. They proposed that Spitzer put into the Introduction of DSM-III a "clarifying statement...that the terms used in DSM-III are for the purposes of diagnosis and treatment of mental disorder." They advised adding that a DSM-III diagnosis may be useful but not sufficient to be the deciding factor in legal issues concerning "criminal responsibility, competence to stand trial, capacity to make a will, competence to handle ones' affairs, etc."[86] Spitzer took their advice to heart, and we find in the Introduction to DSM-III this very clear caveat:

> The purpose of DSM-III is to provide clear descriptions of diagnostic categories in order to enable clinicians and investigators to diagnose, communicate about, study, and treat various mental disorders. The use of this manual for non-clinical purposes such as determination of legal responsibility, competency or insanity, or justification for third-party payment, must be critically examined in each instance within the appropriate institutional context.[87]

This warning has been modified and expanded to a longer statement on its own page in DSM-IV to stress that only trained clinicians can properly use the manual and that its diagnostic categories do not necessarily apply to legal situations. Gone is the statement about third-party payment, a tacit acknowledgement that it is understood that the manual is indeed used by insurance companies.[88]

Spitzer had discussed patients having an "irresistible impulse" in five disorders relating to impulse control: Pathological Gambling, Kleptomania, Pyromania, Intermittent Explosive Disorder, and Isolated Explosive Disorder.[89] The APPL Liaison Committee advised, however, that this wording had "a very special legal meaning and DSM-III would be likely...used in ways not intended by the Task Force" if left as is. They recommended that the term "irrestible impulse" be replaced wherever it occurred with the phrase "failure to resist an impulse." Spitzer, as usual, was very open to quite specific suggestions for refining the text and immediately made the changes, which appeared in the next draft of January 15, 1978.[90]

The APPL committee congratulated the Task Force on its achievement: "The spelling out of operational criteria and the multiaxial classification approach should at last make it possible to break away from the...practice in forensic psychiatry of viewing psychosis...as a prerequisite for the determination of significant psychiatric disability, incompetence, or 'insanity.'"

The forensic psychiatrists had indeed been of great assistance in clarifying certain problematic aspects of DSM-III to the betterment of the new manual. Spitzer's tactic of giving the drafts of the DSM-III a wide circulation reaped significant benefits in this instance.

ATTENTION DEFICIT DISORDER

Attention Deficit Disorder (ADD) was a new name for a childhood syndrome that had certainly been seen before. In the making of DSM-III, however, there was an attempt to clarify its conceptualization, hence its new title. ADD in DSM-III was a disorder characterized by developmentally inappropriate short attention, poor concentration, and impulsivity; hyperactivity was or was not present. The burgeoning of the diagnosis of this disorder as ADHD (Attention Deficit Hyperactivity Disorder), starting in DSM-III-R (1987), became a controversial subject in the 1990s, partly because of its frequent treatment by stimulants, most notably Ritalin (methylphenidate). The upsurge in the diagnosis of ADHD has continued to cause concern and speculation about its use, making the history of this entity of continuing note. Has an "epidemic" occurred, as some have maintained? But in the 1970s, ADD in childhood or adolescence was usually not a contentious subject, and the use of Ritalin was just beginning. The focus of argument then was whether DSM-III should contain a diagnosis of adult ADD (i.e., ADD Residual Type). We will see that strong feelings were aroused about this.

ADD received a significant upgrade in DSM-III. DSM-I (1952) contained no separate category for childhood and adolescent disorders. The nearest category for childhood diagnoses relating to ADD was under the broad title "Transient Situational Personality Disorders." There one could find Adjustment Reaction of Childhood with the category Neurotic Traits, one of which was "over-activity."[91] So it is no surprise that the committee that put together DSM-II (1968) added the broad rubric "Behavior Disorders of Childhood and Adolescence," although it appeared near the end of the classification. Under that they placed "Hyperkinetic Reaction of Childhood (or Adolescence)," with characterizations of overactivity, restlessness, distractibility, and short attention span.[92] In DSM-III there was not only the more elegant general heading, "Disorders Usually First Evident in Infancy, Childhood, or Adolescence," but also this category was placed at the very start of the "Text and Criteria" section of the manual.[93] ADD was the second of the nine childhood diagnoses found there with three subtypes: ADD with Hyperactivity, ADD without Hyperactivity, and ADD Residual Type (lasting beyond childhood). A battle occurred over whether this last phenomenon should be in DSM-III.

The drafts of April 15, 1977 and January 15, 1978 contained no mention of ADD Residual Type, but beginning in the spring of 1978 the addition of this diagnosis began to be fiercely debated because of suggestions by the psychiatrist, Paul H. Wender (b. 1934). Wender had been studying in the 1960s what was now being called ADD, and in 1971 had published the first monograph on the disorder, entitled *Minimal Brain Dysfunction in Children*. He had also published a book for parents of children with ADD,

The Hyperactive Child (1974). On April 6, 1978, Wender wrote to Spitzer outlining his ideas for an adult ADD diagnosis, a late date to be introducing new diagnoses given that field trials were well underway. Spitzer and others were taken aback by the suddenness of the plan, and Spitzer answered him, "What to do?" But he promised to send Wender's proposals "to other DSM-III mavens[94] who had a particular interest in this area."[95] Even though officially Spitzer was not on the Infancy, Childhood, and Adolescent Disorders Advisory Committee, he was now effectively involved. Spitzer voiced his misgivings to three members of the Committee (Wender, Rachel Gittelman, and Dennis Cantwell) as well as to Donald Klein and Michael Sheehy on the Task Force:

> I recall Paul saying that this category is appropriate to 15% of an adult out-patient psychiatric population....If that is the case, we are talking about a very common category whose inclusion requires major changes in our current conceptualization of mild psychiatric disorders. I don't think we should do this without some pretty compelling data.
>
> I certainly do not believe that we should include any category in DSM-III which cannot be tried out in the final stage of the Field Trial.[96]

Judith L. Rapoport, M.D., a child psychiatrist at the NIMH, quickly wrote back to Spitzer and and the others involved opposing the new entity, finding it "premature."[97] She stressed the difficulty in making an adult ADD diagnosis, arguing that prospective follow-up studies of children with ADD had not demonstrated much continued pathology, and a test screening adult patients for attention deficit would just as likely call forth schizophrenia and perhaps even Obsessive-Compulsive Disorder. Stimulant drugs had not been shown to be helpful. In general, Rapoport emphasized the problems of a differential diagnosis from other disorders and concluded with an antipsychoanalytic dig, but also a prescient caution: "ADD could replace oedipal anxiety as a new universal explanation; I urge restraint." Nevertheless, Spitzer developed an interest in the new adult diagnosis, abandoning his earlier caveats.

Unfortunately, the Archives do not contain the full correspondence on this subject, so any discussion here may be tentative.[98] But we do know that the debate between Wender and Rapoport continued throughout the spring and summer of 1978; a letter most likely from the child psychiatrist Dennis P. Cantwell to Spitzer (the second page is missing) refers to the ongoing issue of ADD Residual Type.[99] Wender himself had raised the possibility of this diagnosis being overused. However, Cantwell concluded, "I do think that these people do exist, and I think that they can be described every bit as reliably as some of the categories in DSM-III. I'm not bothered by the use of a term like attention deficit disorder because we can measure attention specifically."[100]

Wender and Cantwell together worked on developing and then revising operational criteria for ADD Residual Type, and four months after Cantwell's letter, they proposed their newly modified standards to Spitzer.[101] Adults with the residual diagnosis would have to have had both attention deficit and hyperactivity in childhood, which continued into adulthood. The criterion of impaired interpersonal relationships was removed. Wender offered further condensation if Spitzer required it.

Tinkering went on throughout the winter of 1978–1979 and in March 1979, two months before the Assembly vote on the new manual, there was a flurry of correspondence, now involving many of the members of the Childhood Advisory Committee (although Klein and Sheehy seem to have bowed out). Spitzer continued in a leadership role. On March 2, Gittelman and Joaquim Puig-Antich (1944–1989), also on the Advisory Committee, wrote to other members of the committee suggesting that Residual Type not have an age requirement, to provide greater flexibility in using the Residual diagnosis for adolescents and young adults.[102] It is clear that by now Spitzer was determined to have an adult ADD diagnosis in DSM-III. but Wender kept worrying about it, wondering how easily a childhood diagnosis could be applied to adults and whether adult psychiatrists would be willing to use a childhood diagnosis for the same disorder in an adult. Probably not, Wender thought. "Adult psychiatrists will have a strong predilection for not using the diagnosis of 'Attention Deficit Disorder' [since it carries] surplus semantic baggage from previous diagnostic phrases (such as 'Hyperkinetic Reaction of Childhood') which they would feel ipso facto could not exist in adult life."[103]

Spitzer and Wender continued writing back and forth,[104] Wender, adhering to his argument that even though the disorder in children is the same as that in adults, an adult psychiatrist wouldn't employ the ADD diagnosis unless it was listed among the adult personality disorders (Axis II). Spitzer remained adamant about retaining the ADD-Residual Type name. But still more kept the issue from being finally resolved. After almost a year, Rapoport and Wender were still at odds, just several weeks before the vote to approve the manual. Rapoport questioned whether ADD should even be in DSM-III; perhaps it needed to be postponed until DSM-IV so that the criteria, description, and differential diagnosis could be better worked out. Here, Wender, considering himself the "maven" on ADD, argued strongly that "there are more data and relevant supportive literature to support the notion of persistent and/or residual ADDs [than there are for] overanxious disorder, shyness disorder, introverter [sic] disorder, identity disorder....Whether or not ADDs is related to conduct disorders, as Judy observes, is problematic but not relevant to adult ADDs residual or otherwise."[105] Even after ADD Residual Type was removed from DSM-III-R and not included in DSM-IV, Wender continued to advocate for an "Adult Attention-Deficit Hyperactivity Disorder."[106]

Since the subject of diagnoses that appear and then disappear from the DSMs has gained critical attention over the years, this episode casts additional light on these events. The current development of DSM-5, with proposed diagnoses of an Autistic Spectrum Disorder and the new entity of Temper Dysregulation in children, has reawakened professional and public examination of this process of adding and removing diagnoses. In such situations, the APA Task Force on DSM-5 has often been challenged to justify its decision-making processes.

PTSD—POST-TRAUMATIC STRESS DISORDER

Before leaving this chapter, one additional diagnosis needs mention because our nation's attention is currently riveted on it: post-traumatic stress disorder (PTSD). PTSD found its way into DSM-III because of the casualties of the Vietnam War. It is another good example of the fact that strong social concerns and dedicated campaigns that enlist psychiatric support are occasionally reflected in the DSM.[107] One prominent circumstance in this category is the removal of the Homosexuality diagnosis from DSM-II. Sometimes, however, diagnoses are delayed or omitted because of organized support against them; for example, the inclusion of Premenstrual Dysphoric Disorder in DSM has received strong objections from some women's groups. (Its inclusion in the DSMs has been delayed, but it will appear in DSM-5.)

DSM-II did not contain a diagnosis that spoke to battle trauma. There had been one in DSM-I, Gross Stress Reaction, partly because psychiatrists were familiar with it from World War II and the Korean War. But as DSM-II was being constructed in the early days of the Vietnam War, it seemed that military psychiatrists were successfully treating "combat neurosis." Nevertheless, as the war wore on, and especially after news about the My Lai massacre came out in 1969, anecdotal evidence began to build that untreated war trauma was rife. Some psychiatrists began calling attention to it, notably Chaim F. Shatan, (1924–2001) Robert J. Lifton (b. 1926), and John A. Talbott. A social worker who worked at the Boston VA Hospital, Sarah A. Haley, also recognized numerous cases and published her experiences.[108]

When Spitzer was first approached about putting a relevant diagnosis in DSM-III, he rejected the request, citing lack of empirical data. But after some time, Shatan, Lifton, and Haley, plus other psychiatrists and war veterans who had combined their efforts and organized, were able to convince Spitzer to form an investigative subcommittee of the DSM-III Task Force. Spitzer asked Nancy Andreasen to chair the committee, and he and Lyman Wynne also sat on this group. Sufficient "hard" evidence was collected to convince Andreasen, a committed empiricist, of the validity of a diagnosis of combat-related stress, partly because she had had experience in treating burn victims and was highly aware of the traumas suffered by these individuals. In January 1978, Spitzer agreed to put the condition in DSM-III under the category Post-Traumatic Stress Disorder, which would cover other traumatic conditions as well as battle-related disorders. The first diagnostic criteria made the disorder widely applicable: "Existence of a recognizable stressor that would evoke significant symptoms of distress in almost everyone."[109] The concerted campaign for the inclusion of PTSD had succeeded despite the opposition of psychiatrists at Washington University who had argued that suffering veterans should be diagnosed under an existing diagnosis of depression, schizophrenia, or alcoholism.[110]

The path-breaking field trials and their various uses by Spitzer have been highlighted in this chapter, as well as certain controversial diagnoses. We have seen again how some issues were not finally resolved until the very last minute. As we are now approaching that crucial juncture, let us turn to examine pivotal events in the winter and spring of 1979.

Of the many stressful periods during the development of DSM-III, none could be compared to the emotional and intellectual pressures Spitzer faced during the final weeks leading up to the Assembly of Delegates vote scheduled for May 12, 1979. The psychoanalysts' efforts to make DSM-III contain a meaningful statement on psychodynamic theory and treatment were also now at a heightened pitch, as all parties faced the looming deadline.

13

THE FINAL WEEKS

As the new year of 1979 dawned, psychoanalysts and psychodynamically oriented psychiatrists began increasingly fervid endeavors to place in DSM-III a statement that reflected psychodynamic theory and treatment. While Spitzer was not totally opposed to the appearance of such material, he was adamant that he or those he appointed should be the ones to draft that statement and then negotiate its acceptance by the analysts. The analysts did not fully appreciate this resolute intent and continued to craft their own statements. In addition, many analysts and those in the psychodynamic camp began a grim and determined effort to derail acceptance of the entire manual.

The psychodynamic push coalesced around two specific goals. One was the endeavor to include in the classification itself an entire category of neurotic disorders. The other was to have a clear and full statement of psychodynamic thought, written by the analysts, either in a special appendix or as part of the Introduction. For a while it appeared that the APA Board of Trustees had mandated an appendix, but Spitzer, with the help of the Assembly Liaison Committee to the DSM-III Task Force, was able to get out from under such a decree. Melvin Sabshin, the APA Medical Director, probably also aided in this regard. As the final few weeks flashed by, efforts by the analysts intensified, leaving an expansive and explicit paper trail by which we can re-create their attempts to include in the descriptive manual a recognition that psychoanalysis had a special authority within American psychiatry. Thus Spitzer himself was faced with one demanding crisis after another. Simultaneously, he was going through the process of separating from his wife.

The initial protests against the new classification were directed against the Task Force's elimination of the eight categories of Neurosis that were in DSM-II. The President of the Baltimore–District of Columbia Society for Psychoanalysis, Boyd L. Burris (Fig. 13.1, Pictorial Essay), wrote to Spitzer objecting to exclusion of the term "neurosis." Burris asserted that it was understandable to have a descriptive manual for those disorders for which the etiology is uncertain but that this was not the case for the neuroses. He argued that "the contributions of psychoanalysis to the psychodynamic conceptualization of the neurotic disorders allows specific etiological considerations to be formulated" for these conditions.[1]

On the basis of a study of the DSM-III January 15, 1978 draft conducted by members of the Baltimore-DC Society who had participated in the field trials, Burris proposed to Spitzer a revision of several sections of the manual.[2] At almost the same time, the President of the Louisiana Psychiatric Association, F. A. Silva, also on the basis of a report of one of his Association's members, wrote to the President of the APA, Jules H. Masserman (1905–1994) predicting that the new manual would have "far-reaching" negative consequences for the treatment of mental disorders, the opinion of other medical specialties, and the payment of psychiatrists by third parties. DSM-III was such a "profound [issue] in its daily consequences," Silva hoped that each APA member would "be allowed to register by democratic ballot their personal response." He was not alone in calling for a vote by the membership of the APA. Holding the opinion that the new manual would yield only "more specific, codable diagnoses for research [Silva argued that] the actual practitioner of psychiatric medicine [had] little to gain and much to lose."[3]

Across the United States, many psychiatrists regarded the deletion of neurosis from DSM-III as unthinkable. They could not fathom how they would practice psychiatry without the bedrock diagnosis that meant an entire way of thinking. And beyond that, they feared that health insurance companies would deny them payment if they could not diagnose a patient using the particular diagnostic criteria in the new manual.

Another grass roots fear linked to insurance payment was that DSM-III was meant for computers and had an "anti-private practice and anti-psychotherapy bias" that would leave the psychotherapeutic "aspect of mental health work to the non-psychiatrists who are only too glad to pick up the slack, and to define their work as outside of the proper interest of psychiatry."[4] This same letter writer bemoaned that the "neurotic characters," meaning psychiatrists themselves and their patients who would "never qualify for a diagnosis in DSM-III," had been "left out" from the new manual, yet it was precisely these individuals who sought private psychotherapy.

A third lone voice, a professor of psychiatry at the University of Arizona College of Medicine, wrote directly to Spitzer and was careful to both state that he was not an analyst and praise DSM-III as a "heroic effort." Nevertheless, he went on, it was an error to eliminate neurosis because it could be defined "carefully," just as other diagnoses were in DSM-III, and he offered his very specific description. He concluded that "one of the merits of allowing the category to remain is that it allows for the fluid shift from one kind of neurotic disorder to another that we so frequently encounter in our practice."[5]

However, there were few individual endeavors to embark on any action. What the Archives mainly reveal are concerted, organized efforts. One was to halt DSM-III in its tracks when the Assembly of Delegates met to vote its acceptance or rejection. Another was to accept the manual's publication as long as it had a statement in which "dynamic psychiatrists...receive a significant explanation within DSM-III itself, and [a discussion of] how such psychiatrists can use the document."[6] The discussion in this chapter will veer between these two attempts by the analysts: one to stall any acceptance of a DSM-III that did not contain neurotic disorders within its classification, and the other to ensure that before the new manual could gain approval it had to include acceptable psychodynamic material. The correspondence in the weeks to come was frenetic; not all of it is in the Archives, although a lot can be learned from references in the extant documents to various events and people whose own communications are missing. Moreover, Spitzer and Ronald Bayer published an article in 1985, "Neurosis, Psychodynamics, and DSM-III," that quotes or refers to some documents not in the Archives.[7]

During all the negotiating and calls to action, Spitzer fought tenaciously to control what was or what was not to be in DSM-III. He wanted only himself or his appointees to write any psychodynamic additions to the manual. Proposals and counterproposals swirled about, the charged activity creating ever-increasing commitments and high tension. Throughout it all, let us remember that everyone involved was acutely aware of time passing, the date of May 12 fast approaching.

THE PSYCHOANALYTIC APPENDIX AND A MAJOR CATEGORY FOR THE NEUROSES

As discussed in an earlier chapter, the APA Board of Trustees had directed Spitzer to place an appendix in DSM-III that would explain how psychodynamically oriented psychiatrists could use DSM-III in their therapeutic work. In order to carry out this directive, Melvin Sabshin contacted William Offenkrantz (Fig. 13.2, Pictorial Essay), Chair of the analytic DSM-III subcommittee, and asked for a draft of such a statement. Working together with Spitzer, the subcommittee formulated a draft and sent it to Sabshin for his approval on February 19, 1979. The final revised copy was sent to Spitzer February 28. A few days later, to play it safe, Offenkrantz forwarded the statement to Lester Grinspoon, Chair of the Council on Research and Development, to whom Spitzer answered.

The analytic subcommittee's proposed appendix was a two-page, single-spaced document that discussed the data to be collected in an initial interview; the organization of the data based on "key" psychodynamic concepts; the theoretical constructs derived from the concepts; how the clinician could make a psychodynamic diagnostic formulation; and then how to assess all the information that had been gathered.[8] Two matters are noteworthy. The first is that at last the analysts were taking DSM-III seriously. Offenkrantz's subcommittee contained some major analytic luminaries. The second is that Spitzer, upon receiving the analysts' document, excised from it a sizable chunk devoted to the theoretical constructs of intrapsychic conflict; the consideration of when a conflict was considered neurotic; the goal of the neurotic symptom; and how "structural systems of mental life" emerged and became pathological. And then, as detailed in Chapter 11 in the section "Will There Be an Appendix for Psychodynamically Oriented Psychiatrists?," before even receiving Offenkrantz's appendix, Spitzer wrote to both Sabshin and Alan Stone, the APA President-elect. He claimed there had been an error, that the Trustees had actually mandated material in an introduction, not in an appendix. He was adamant that any statement should be in the Introduction to DSM-III.

Simultaneous with the efforts to add a psychodynamic appendix but completely separately John J. McGrath, the Area III member of the APA Board of Trustees, representing the states of New Jersey, Pennsylvania, Delaware, Maryland, and the District of Columbia, wrote to Boyd Burris (and most likely to presidents of Area III psychiatric societies) on March 13.[9] McGrath reported that the Area III Council had just unanimously approved a plan to counter the elimination of the neuroses as a diagnostic category in DSM-III when the Assembly would meet in May:

Once the motion calling for the vote on DSM-III has been made and seconded on the floor of the Assembly in Chicago, Area III will make a motion to amend (the main motion) specifically that "Area III opposes the elimination of the neuroses from DSM-III." As a subsidiary motion this will have to be voted upon before the main motion, and requires only a simple majority for passage.

Then, McGrath pointed out, the issue could be brought to a decisive vote. How to achieve this? He said there must be a stratagem to get out the necessary votes. Psychodynamically oriented leaders had at last realized that the situation they were in called for tactical thinking.

McGrath laid out a procedure. The delegates to the Assembly from each District Branch throughout the United States had to be instructed by the governing council of their local branches how to vote. So the time to act was now, he emphasized. All members concerned with the issue at stake needed to talk to their District Branch Councils or Assembly Representatives and express their views. "Coalition, and the exercise of our rights as APA members, are urgently needed; while the final vote is in May, the crucial processes are going on now at the District Branch level," McGrath exhorted.

A week later, Boyd Burris wrote to the presidents of all the analytic societies affiliated with the American Psychoanalytic Association, with copies to the President and President-elect of the Association, to William Offenkrantz, and to Oscar LeGault, the Area III deputy representative to the Assembly. Burris repeated the information McGrath had sent him and made a strong call for concerted action. A Neurotic Disorders category had to be in DSM-III, Burris asserted, essentially for three reasons. The first was "the need for continuity of the scientific research and thought which have gone into this category over the past several decades" (this would have made no impact on Spitzer); the second was the category was consonant with ICD-9 and thus with the international psychiatric community (only of secondary concern to Spitzer); and the third was the fact that "the large majority of American psychiatrists are psychodynamically oriented" (nevertheless, Spitzer's statistics from the field trial meant that he could argue that this group was accepting of DSM-III). Burris believed there was a "groundswell" for retaining Neurosis in DSM-III and urged fellow psychiatrists everywhere to "exercise [their] responsibilities as APA members."[10]

At the same time that the McGrath/Burris initiative was being made, three more challenges on the issue of the neuroses surfaced. First, Lyman Wynne, on the Task Force, suggested that "neurotic disorders could be defined descriptively by the presence of distressing symptoms [with] no need to incorporate psychoanalytically derived assumptions about etiology or psychodynamics."[11] The second person to take issue with Spitzer was the well-connected Roger Peele (b. 1930) (Fig. 13.3, Pictorial Essay); he was the representative to the Assembly from the Washington Psychiatric Society, a member of the Assembly Liaison Committee to the DSM-III Task Force, a member of one of the DSM-III Advisory Committees (Factitious and Somatoform Disorders), and Deputy Superintendent of St. Elizabeth's Hospital in Washington, DC. Peele wrote to Spitzer about "a groundswell of sentiment to preserve [the term] neurosis."[12] He offered his own classification that became known as the "Peele Proposal." Peele himself believed that "the term *neurotic* did not require an assumption of intrapsychic conflict." He supported the advances DSM-III had brought and thought that a *descriptively defined* (emphasis added) "neurosis" would avoid an unnecessary break with the past and would be consonant with ICD-9. Active in APA affairs, Peele sought to bring the membership together. Peele did not want to see a major clash in the Assembly, nor a struggle between the Assembly and the Board of Trustees. He also wanted to avoid a "divisive referendum of American psychiatrists" and thus "urged a pragmatic course on Spitzer." The third challenge was from psychiatrists in New York, who were sympathetic to DSM-III but nevertheless informed Spitzer they would vote for the position of Area III.[13]

With all this erosion of the backing for the elimination of neurosis in DSM-III, Spitzer became convinced that he could not ignore the situation. He later wrote, "The task…was to preserve the structure of DSM-III classification and its descriptive orientation while yielding some ground to those committed to the classification *neurosis*."[14]

PICTORIAL ESSAY

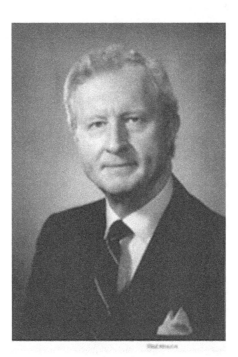

FIG. 13.1 Boyd L. Burris, 1980s. Burris, President of the Baltimore–District of Columbia Psychoanalytic Society, was a leader in the winter-spring 1979 fight to get "Neurosis" in the DSM-III classification. He correctly predicted an "upheaval" in American psychiatry if DSM-III was adopted. Courtesy Dr. Boyd L. Burris

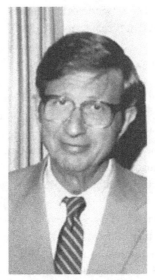

FIG. 13.2 William Offenkrantz, c. 1980. Offenkrantz was Chair of an American Psychoanalytic Association subcommittee to prepare a chapter on psychoanalytic evaluation of a new patient for "Project Flower," a volume to be entitled *DSM-III and Treatment Planning*. The subcommittee also sought in vain to get psychoanalytic material in either the Introduction or a special appendix in DSM-III. Courtesy Dr. William Offenkrantz

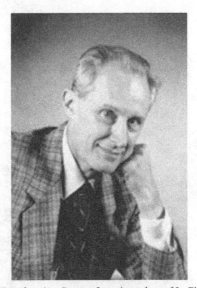

FIG. 13.3 Roger Peele, 1977, at that time Deputy Superintendent of St. Elizabeth's Hospital (NIMH) in Washington, DC. Peele, a leading member of the APA Assembly of Delegates Liaison Task Force to DSM-III, played a large role in the attempt to find a compromise solution to the problem of how to present Neurosis in the DSM-III classification. Right before the dramatic Assembly vote on whether or not to accept DSM-III, Peele argued the case for including Depressive Neurosis as a main diagnosis in the Affective Disorders. Courtesy Dr. Roger Peele.

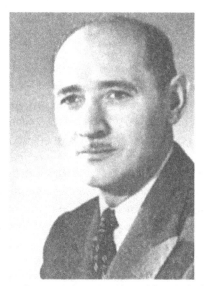

FIG. 13.4 Jules H. Masserman (1905–1994) was President of the APA in the final months before the approval of DSM-III and made clear his hostility both for Spitzer and the proposed new classification. By permission from Galter Health Sciences Library Special Collections, Northwestern University.

SPITZER'S "NEUROTIC PEACE TREATY"

While these protests to one of Spitzer's bedrock visions for DSM-III were mounting, plans had also been laid for Spitzer to meet with Hector Jaso's Assembly Liaison Committee and Offenkrantz's psychoanalytic committee at the Psychiatric Institute in New York on April 7 "to attempt to resolve what seemed to be an impasse" on the neurosis issue.[15] Spitzer tried to head off the upcoming meeting with two initiatives. The first was to send Offenkrantz a draft of a passage to be included in the Introduction that dealt with the information a psychodynamically oriented clinician needed to collect in order to formulate a treatment plan.[16] Spitzer gave Offenkrantz the jolting news that the passage had been prepared by Arnold Cooper and Allen Frances, the same two analysts who sat on Offenkrantz's committee that had prepared the psychodynamic appendix. But, Spitzer added to Offenkrantz, Cooper and Frances "made it clear that this help in no way affects your committee's action regarding the possibility off a separate appendix or document in DSM-III for the use of psychodynamically-oriented clinicians." Nevertheless, with the use of the words "possibility" and "or document," Spitzer was trying to dislodge the notion that the appendix would indeed appear.

Spitzer's second plan was to propose a "neurotic peace treaty," which, if all involved agreed to it, would obviate the need for the April 7 meeting. Copies of this plan also went out to Burris and Oscar LeGault (deputy Area III representative in the Assembly). Additionally, the treaty was the vehicle Spitzer had devised to deal with the array of challenges on the neurosis issue. The treaty was a complex three-part measure that would involve changes and additions to the classification (Axis

I and II), the Introduction, and the Glossary of Technical Terms. Spitzer proposed the following:

1. Immediately following the title of the classification the following statement would appear: "The neurotic disorders include the following: Anxiety Disorders of Childhood or Adolescence; some Affective Disorders; Anxiety, Somatoform, and Dissociative Disorders; and some Psychosexual Dysfunctions." (The exact placement of this key passage would later be fought over.)
2. There would be a long statement in the Introduction elaborating on five points: Freud's use of the term "psychoneurosis;" problems with the present-day definition of the term; a definition of the term "neurotic disorder" when used descriptively; a discussion of the "neurotic process"; and an explanation of why the neurotic disorders in DSM-III were not grouped together as in DSM-II.
3. In the Glossary of Technical Terms, Neurotic Disorder would be defined as stated in the Introduction. Under "Symptom Neurosis" (a frequently used psychoanalytic term) it would say "See Neurotic Disorder." Under "Character Neurosis" it would say "See Personality Disorder." Neurotic process would be defined at length.[17]

With this proposal, Spitzer asked, was there still a need for the meeting? He urged the potential attendees to let Jaso and Offenkrantz know their reactions. Spitzer closed by saying, "My own personal view is that this approach is not merely a compromise, but is, in fact, preferable to the previous approach taken by the Task Force toward this very difficult problem." We know that the "neurotic peace treaty" was circulated well beyond the immediate addressees and reaction came from several directions.[18] But the upshot was that the treaty did not at all satisfy the critics nor resolve the impasse, so the meeting was held as scheduled. It became one of the major confrontations between the two sides.

To complicate his negotiations further, Spitzer was now faced with rebellion from the Task Force. He had tried to convince them that his "neurotic peace treaty" was not capitulation or undoing vital progress, but not all were persuaded. Donald Klein, in particular was most vociferous. In a memo to the entire Task Force, Klein "accused Spitzer of usurping the authority of the task force" by not first consulting them before extending the "peace treaty" to his critics.[19] Klein charged that Spitzer was weakening in the face of those who wanted a psychoanalytic influence in DSM-III. Those arguing for a descriptive treatment of the neuroses in reality wanted "the term reinserted because they wish a covert affirmation of their psychogenic hypotheses. This is all too painfully "obvious," Klein went on. He accused Spitzer of engaging in a political maneuver that was "unworthy of scientists who are attempting to advance our field via classification and reliable definition."

Spitzer tried to persuade the Task Force by return memo that Klein had misread the situation and had not taken into consideration that they were only six weeks away from the final vote and the possibility of DSM-III going down to a serious defeat in the Assembly. The Task Force, Spitzer asserted, had to have an alternative to the Peele Proposal (descriptively defined Neurosis) or risk that the Assembly and Board of

Trustees would vote to have "neurotic disorders as a *diagnostic class* into DSM-III."[20] Ultimately, Spitzer was able to convince the Task Force that his "peace treaty" was the best response so as to not lose the basic orientation and organization of DSM-III they had developed and field tested over the past four and a half years.

SHOWDOWN AT THE PSYCHIATRIC INSTITUTE

Spitzer now had to prepare for the important April 7 meeting and sought the advice and support of other APA officials. He wrote to Grinspoon on April 2, "Because of the importance of the neurotic disorders controversy, I would like the [opinion] of the Council on Research and Development on the relative merits of various proposals for resolving this controversy in terms of preserving the *scientific* value of the classification."[21] He also told Grinspoon that he was inviting the director of the New York State Psychiatric Institute, Edward J. Sachar, to the meeting. Sachar, a highly respected biological psychiatrist, had previously spoken in favor of the Task Force's development of DSM-III.

Two days later, Spitzer traveled down to Washington to meet with Sabshin. They spoke about a number of issues, including the upcoming meeting at PI, although the formal focus of their deliberations was on the steps that needed to be taken as DSM-III wound its way through the approval process by the APA hierarchy. Because the material to be included in the Introduction remained a controversial issue, Spitzer agreed to mail each member of the Board of Trustees a draft copy of the proposed Introduction. Then, at an upcoming meeting of the Trustees, Grinspoon and he would formally present Spitzer's proposal. (The Trustees' meeting eventually took place on April 21–22, at which time more contention was stirred up because Spitzer presented his introduction while Offenkrantz presented a psychoanalytic appendix. We will return to the unforeseen results of that meeting.)[22]

Before the PI meeting Spitzer also approached Roger Peele, who advised him that "if you will simple [sic] follow Area III's advice, you'll stay out of trouble." Peele informed Spitzer in a follow-up letter that some "Washington private practitioners" had seen Spitzer's "neurotic peace treaty," but Peele had not heard their reactions. Then Peele gave Spitzer his own opinions about Spitzer's proposal and suggested some revisions.[23] Amidst these other initiatives, Burris weighed in with a letter full of dissatisfaction to Sabshin, with a copy going to Jules Masserman (Fig. 13.4, Pictorial Essay), the APA President.[24] While it may be difficult to keep track of all these events happening at once, perhaps more important here than following each thread is to appreciate the intensity of crisis felt on both sides, as well as the fierce determination and feverish activity that dominated the thoughts and actions of all the players. The stakes for each side were indeed high, and time was running out. No one was sure of the outcome.

The April 7 meeting at PI on the subject of the inclusion of neurosis as a diagnostic class went forward as planned, and a large contingent of guests attended, including Burris and some members of the Baltimore-DC Psychoanalytic Society.[25] Roger Peele, as a member of the Assembly Liaison Committee, came up from Washington as well, hoping to bring both sides together. Also in attendance were at least two members of the Task Force, Donald Klein and Jean Endicott, and perhaps others. Offenkrantz and some members of his psychoanalytic committee were there, including Arnold Cooper, Spitzer's former analyst. Unfortunately, there are no minutes or discussions of the meeting in the Archives.[26] However, six years later, Spitzer published some of his recollections (1985), which included 1982 interviews with many of the key players. Peele emerges as being most dedicated to a harmonious reconciliation, sensitive to the goal that American psychiatry not be plunged into divisive antagonism. This is borne out by his role over the next five weeks, right into the final debate in the Assembly. In 2010–2011, Peele supplied yet more memories that enhanced what was in Spitzer's article and in the Archives.

It was a long meeting, the room was crowded, and exchanges were often testy. Peele recalls that Klein was "fairly antagonistic," insisting that the content of DSM-III was a scientific issue and non-scientists in the Assembly (local District Branch representatives) should not be involved. Peele answered him, arguing that the Assembly had every right to be involved since it represented the people who would be using the manual, so it was not just a scientific issue. Sachar kept walking around, making comments as events proceeded.[27] Spitzer remembers that "much of the meeting was taken up with disputes over the placement of words, the use of modifiers, the capitalization of entries....Each adjustment, each attempt at fine tuning, carried with it symbolic importance to those engaged in a process that was at once political and scientific."[28]

A compromise eventually emerged. Illustrative of the close textual work of the long day, one of the key agreements was to move Spitzer's proposed statement in the DSM-III classification about what the neurotic disorders include from the head of the classification to a place in the middle, right before Affective Disorders. The psychodynamic contingent thought this placement would have greater significance. There also were proposals for new wording in the classification, wording that Spitzer and those members of the DSM-III Task Force who were present accepted. Spitzer said he would present the new language to the full Task Force and believed they would also accept it. Spitzer's bottom line, that Neurosis not be a separate category in the classification, held firm.

Thus, as Burris and Peele talked together on their return trip home, they felt that no agreement had been reached, since there had been no accord on the existence of a category of Neurotic Disorders in the classification. Peele especially objected to the classification's lack of the specific diagnosis Depressive Neurosis, perhaps the most common diagnosis used by practitioners in the Washington Psychiatric Society.[29] Burris wrote to Jaso after the PI meeting that he had had a busy weekend responding to telephone inquires about the outcome of the meeting. Burris reported that "the talk of referendum is still very much in the air. Many practitioners note that they will have no convenient way of coding...depressive neurosis...and anxiety neurosis....They wonder why the APA cannot have the same convenient nomenclature that is so readily available in ICD-9-CM. We shall see!"[30] To buttress his views, Burris sent Jaso copies of two letters from psychiatrists who supported retaining the neuroses in DSM-III. One letter is of particular interest because it confronted Spitzer on his home turf, something rarely done by his opponents—that is, on the validity of using the statistics generated by the field trials. First, though, the author declared:

> My viewpoint is that a vitally important issue such as DSM-III should not, under any circumstances, be decided by a plebiscite. It is a scientific issue. [But then, he argued] the proponents of DSM-III are saying that the field trials are "validating" DSM-III, when, in fact, they amount to no more than ratification of an artificial document. In effect, Dr. Spitzer and his committee are imposing their own implicit theories of psychopathology on psychiatry and the related mental health professions.[31]

This is the only documented expression of such views about the significance of the field trials. The writer's particular arguments do not seem to have found a larger audience.

THE ANALYSTS APPEAL DIRECTLY TO
THE BOARD OF TRUSTEES

Also unhappy with the results of the April 7 meeting, Offenkrantz's analytic committee decided to put direct pressure on the APA Board of Trustees. Two days after the PI meeting, Offenkrantz wrote a letter to each member of the Board of Trustees.[32] He reviewed the history of the Appendix that his committee had sent to Spitzer on February 28, in accordance with the Trustees' decision that such a statement appear in DSM-III. He then solicited the Trustees' support of that document at their next meeting on April 21. Offenkrantz reported that Spitzer, in a memo to all the groups preparing a chapter for Project Flower, had circulated the analysts' Appendix. It turned out that Spitzer had severely edited it, with only two paragraphs of the two-page, single-spaced narrative remaining. Offenkrantz was asking the Trustees to recommend the inclusion of the complete (underlining in the original) statement. He soberly and patiently explained how the analysts' document had summarized in a brief space dynamic psychiatry's fundamental premises and the resulting concepts, including their relevance to DSM-III diagnoses. Offenkrantz pointed out that the Appendix showed how the presence of the concept "intrapsychic conflict" could "be inferred in a clinical interview." He then launched into his formal appeal and final stand:

> Our statement provides an opportunity to demonstrate the linkage between basic premise, derived construct and converging data from multiple sources within the clinical interview. This is why we regard [the statement] as a seamless integration, whose coherence must be preserved for its educational and scientific value—thus, worthy of inclusion as it stands, or not at all.

To facilitate Spitzer's acceptance of their document, Offenkrantz's committee offered what it considered a meaningful compromise. Since their committee deemed the document so important, they offered "to forgo both authorship and attribution in

DSM-III." This move was not as trivial as it might appear. One of the battles between Spitzer and the analysts was over control of the authorship of what went into DSM-III. Spitzer wanted everything to come either from him, the Task Force, the Advisory Committees, or an appointed consultant. The analysts had attempted several times to wrest this control from Spitzer and had always been beaten back. Thus, their surrendering formal authorship represented a significant step.

Offenkrantz's letter was successful. The Board of Trustees agreed to put the issue on the agenda for their next meeting, a week and a half hence.[33]

In any event, the "neurotic peace treaty" was never ratified, so it did not matter that the Task Force agreed, with minor modifications, to what had been negotiated at the April 7 meeting.[34] Still, Spitzer optimistically sent off his revised Introduction and Classification to Grinspoon. Of course, the analysts had never been won over by those documents.

At this point, the Assembly's scheduled vote was less than a month away. On April 18, three days before the Trustees were to meet, Burris wrote an eloquent and gloomy letter to Masserman, who was finishing up his term as President of the APA. Burris had earlier written to Sabshin expressing his unhappiness with events concerning DSM-III and had sent a copy to Masserman. Masserman in turn had written back to Burris, noting his own dissatisfaction with many aspects of DSM-III as currently configured. Masserman was also an analyst and did not hide his dislike of Spitzer's modus operandi.[35] (Masserman was a significant figure in American psychiatry; he was president of four national psychiatric groups and one analytic one.)[36]

Burris' letter to Masserman is perhaps the most accurate, full, and expressive statement we have of the analysts' thoughts as the deadline of May 12 approached. Therefore, several segments will be quoted.

> It is heartening to note that you, too, are unhappy with many aspects of the current version of DSM-III. As you know, our Society is particularly concerned with the fact that DSM-III makes no provision for a section on specific Neurotic Diagnoses in its Classification. The April 7 changes on Neurotic Disorders, now being recommended by the Task Force...although in the right direction, falls [sic] far short of our Society's position, which is aimed at ensuring a suitable terminology for the use of psychiatrists in diagnosing the conditions that are encountered in their patients.
>
> Our Society has repeatedly offered the Task Force a reasonable and convenient outline for including Neurotic categories in DSM-III. We believe our suggestions are based on scientific fact and psychiatric usage and research going back several decades....Our outline is generally consonant with the thinking of the international psychiatric community and with the listing on Neurotic Disorders in ICD-9-CM.

At this point, Burris appealed to Masserman for his direct support and involvement: "We believe that our outline can be quickly integrated into the present Classification if

289 The Final Weeks

the Association [APA] decides that the Council and Task Force should include specific Neurotic Categories in DSM-III." If this did not happen, Burris asserted, American psychiatrists would rebel.

> We are increasingly convinced…as a result of our contacts with psychiatrists around the country…that the rank-and-file membership of the APA has significant dissatisfactions with the current version of DSM-III and in particular will attempt to satisfy its needs for specific Neurotic Diagnostic Categories through the orderly instruction of its elected APA officials. Should this general approach go fruitless, I believe that such news will move a majority of the same rank-and-file to exercise its democratic right to having available a Diagnostic Nomenclature of maximum usefulness.

In conclusion, Burris was dispirited, offering Masserman a dark prophecy: "Unfortunately for us all, DSM-III in its present version would seem to have all the earmarks for causing an upheaval in American psychiatry which will not soon be put down."[37][38]

Burris' prognostication would not have been at all disheartening as far as Spitzer and the Task Force were concerned. An upheaval in American psychiatry was exactly what they desired. Rather than the situation being unfortunate, to them it was liberating. In truth, American psychiatry was at a crossroad, and only time would tell what lay in store for it.

Burris did not keep his complaints, proposals, and predictions at all private. He sent copies of his letter to Spitzer, to Sabshin, and to to Alan Stone, incoming APA President, to Jaso and to Alex H. Kaplan, President of the American Psychoanalytic Association; and to his own Society Executive Committee. Burris' letter was not without effect, as he and others no doubt had hoped, especially when combined with Offenkrantz's appeal to the entire Board of Trustees.

THE TRUSTEES MEET

The Trustees met over two days, April 21 to 22, and their agenda item on DSM-III covered an entire page. In it, the history of the appendix vs. the introduction matter was reviewed, and it was noted that a "preponderance" of the Trustees had favored an introduction over an appendix for the material. "This was supported by action of the Council on Research and Development," it was observed. Spitzer, who had challenged the Trustees' decision that directed him to include a psychodynamic appendix, had won the battle of appendix vs. introduction. The question now was who—Spitzer or the analysts—would write any psychodynamic portion of the Introduction.

The history in the Trustees' agenda item went on to recount that the Task Force had been preparing the Introduction with assistance from the Assembly Liaison Committee. However, it stated that Offenkrantz had contacted the Trustees to ask "that a statement developed by [the analysts] be included in its totality in the introduction," not just part of the statement.

The Trustees planned that at their meeting Spitzer and Grinspoon would present Spitzer's Introduction. The agenda stated that the Board then had to make three
decisions:

1. approve in principle the concept of an introduction;
2. approve in principle the introduction prepared by the Task Force; and
3. approve the current process for the completion of the document."[39]

Finally, it was determined that at the coming May APA meeting in Chicago, the
Assembly Liaison Committee would present a report to the Trustees on the agreements
that had been made with the Task Force at the April 7 PI meeting.

The result of the Trustees meeting was to create a great crisis for Spitzer. Our source
of information about this session is a long memo from Spitzer to the Task Force. (This
is the only account of the meeting in the Archives.) He went to the Board meeting in
Washington on a Saturday, April 21, with confidence.[40] In Spitzer's mind the issue of
Neurosis had been resolved on April 7; the Board would be "overjoyed," he expected,
that there would be no bloody battles. But he found at the meeting "the entire cast of
characters," as he put it: Burris, Douglas Logue, an analyst, who at that time might
have been affiliated with Burris' Baltimore-DC Society, and Offenkrantz. Spitzer was
then shocked to learn of Offenkrantz's letter about the appendix to the Trustees. His
own Introduction, which Spitzer was convinced was "dynamite," had been sent to the
Trustees, but to his surprise, that was not what they were focused on.

Spitzer and Grinspoon made their presentations on the proposed Introduction to
the Board, but in Spitzer's opinion the Board ignored these and concentrated on the
material Offenkrantz had sent them. Alan Stone came to Spitzer's rescue and spoke
in favor of the section in Spitzer's Introduction that explained how DSM-III was to
be used by psychodynamically oriented clinicians. According to Spitzer's account,
Stone argued that Offenkrantz's material "was not pertinent" to that subject but was
"in the nature of 'this is what I believe.'" But the Board passed over Stone's comments,
Spitzer reported, and the discussion "deteriorated even further under the able leadership of our current President," Spitzer sarcastically wrote. Clearly, there was no love
lost between Masserman and Spitzer.

Masserman proposed that "there be an introduction to DSM-III," much to the
"perplexity" of all, Spitzer sneered. The motion passed, and had the "saving grace" of
declaring that the analysts' material would be in the Introduction and not in a separate
appendix. Now, with final certainty, the appendix was out.

What would come next? Spitzer imagined the scene, albeit with ridicule, showing
he was well aware of the antipathy he aroused in some:

> Consider yourself a Board of Trustees member, not familiar with DSM-III, not
> having read the introduction to DSM-III, and you are faced with the responsibil-
> ity for very quickly evaluating DSM-III. Bob Spitzer has the reputation of being
> able to sell used cars, with or without engines, and Bill Offenkrantz says that he
> has some material that ought to be included in the introduction to DSM-III. What

would you do? Clearly, you would want to have a committee appointed to review the situation and to determine what portion of Dr. Offenkrantz's material should be inserted into the introduction. (In addition, you might not have liked the tone of Bob Spitzer's voice or his charming manner.)[41]

What followed was much discussion among the Trustees of whether or not to have such a review committee, with arguments both for and against. Ultimately it was decided that no committee would be set up; instead, the Board members would study the Introduction and send their comments to the Task Force. It was also resolved that Spitzer should give a two-hour presentation on DSM-III to the Trustees on May 17 at the annual meeting (after the Assembly vote) so they could thoroughly review the manual in its final form. Spitzer breathed a sigh of relief—no committee!—and left Washington. Monday he went back again and learned that Sunday morning, after he left for New York, the Trustees had met again and returned to discussing DSM-III. They had held a straw vote as to whether or not DSM-III in its current form was preferable to DSM-II. To Spitzer's amazement, only one member of the Board, Alan Stone, had voted in favor of DSM-III. Based on this lopsided vote, an ad hoc committee was formed to review DSM-III and to report back to the Board on May 17, the same day Spitzer was to make his presentation.[42] The committee was to be chaired by Board member H. Keith H. Brodie (b. 1939), Chair of the Department of Psychiatry at Duke University, and had three other members.[43] Masserman was to be an ex officio member. Spitzer couldn't resist another jab at Masserman about "his great interest in nosology." The typical analyst in the 1970s, we must remember, looked down on the DSMs as merely compilations of statistics and believed diagnosis was not a vital issue.

Spitzer calmed down a bit, however, after speaking to Brodie. He came to the conclusion that all the ad hoc committee wanted to do was to review the litany of complaints that had been made about DSM-III, have Spitzer respond, and then become thoroughly familiar with DSM-III themselves so they could report back to the full Board and "justify a recommendation of approval." The ad hoc committee would meet May 4–5, and Spitzer was invited to come on May 5. He decided to send the committee the results of the NIMH Field Trial as well as favorable letters he had received. For the full Board meeting on the May 17 he invited people who would speak positively about the new manual, and he asked the Task Force to attend with him.

At this point, the volume of communications multiplied. There were attempts to influence the ad hoc committee, as well as increased activity from Burris' allies to firm up the plans for the Assembly's vote on May 12. The mood of the various letter-writers took on more urgency, with more than one or two letters being sent the same day (there is no record of the informal meetings and the phone calls that must have taken place). For us to make sense of the furor during this time, we will not follow the exact chronological order over the next pages. We will begin instead with the attempts to win over the ad hoc committee, thus diverting our attention for a moment from the analysts' plans to affect the May 12 vote of the Assembly.

THE AD HOC COMMITTEE

In focusing on the saga of the ad hoc committee, we learn more about Masserman's dislike of Spitzer. Masserman wrote a short letter to Brodie after the Trustees meeting, thanking him for his support. Masserman confessed that he had been leery at first of the straw vote of the Trustees on DSM-III, which Brodie had suggested:

> I anticipated that it might indicate the Board's practically unanimous dissatis-faction with DSM-III—something that Spitzer would inevitably learn about. Knowing him, he might start a self-righteous propaganda campaign to counter his "lack of appreciation" and thereby try to create more divisiveness in the APA, on various pleas ("his years of work...the large investment," etc.) to [sic] much of which already exists. However, I am sure your Ad Hoc Committee will also handle this aspect effectively.[44]

The next day Masserman sent a memo to the entire membership of the ad hoc com-mittee with his comments on past drafts of DSM-III and on the present one being evaluated.[45] This document is a combination of some reasonable suggestions and Masserman's sheer vexation and exasperation. One has to wonder if he was worn out by his year as president during such trying and taxing times. In a few more weeks and he could turn over the reins to Alan Stone.

In his memo, Masserman thanked the ad hoc committee "for undertaking this intellectually demanding and organizationally delicate, but highly important task." A tirade then followed. He criticized the current version of DSM-III (and Spitzer) in a variety of ways: on its very title; on the Introduction, including its authorship; and on the terminology and classification throughout. His criticisms and revisions were numerous; there is room for only some of them here. Masserman asserted that the title needed to be changed to accommodate "the clinically vulnerable connota-tion of 'disorder.'" Because of the term *disorder*, would third-party payers question "compensation of the therapy of a heavy smoker, a distraught housewife, or a wor-ried businessman?" (Did Masserman not know about the long and complex negotia-tions with the American Psychological Association that resulted in use of the term *disorder*?)

The authorship of the Introduction, Masserman continued, needed to indicate "the collaboration of other components of the APA and multidisciplinary consultants." (Who the latter were is not clear.) In the Introduction itself Masserman called for spe-cific revisions throughout, including a more accurate term than "multiaxial" ("a math-ematical rather than clinical term"). He challenged the reported results of the field trials and said their significance should "be limited to accommodating feedbacks of precon-ceptions rather than proof of validity (recall the Malleus Malificarum [sic])."[46] How could Spitzer claim, Masserman declared, that DSM-III did not deal with the etiologies of mental disorders when it included Axis IV on stressors and the whole category of Adjustment Disorders? Then another critique: Spitzer's Introduction concluded with

"Evaluation for Treatment Planning," four separate paragraphs on the formulation of treatment planning by clinicians considering psychodynamic, family, behavioral, or somatic treatments. At this point Masserman's cavil rang reasonable from a conceptual standpoint: "Here begins the artificial and misleading fractionation of 'treatment,' rather than making clear that modern comprehensive psychiatric therapy integrates biologic, psychodynamic, 'behavioral,' familial, social and cultural (including mystical) in various and often indistinguishable combination."

In a concluding section on "Terminology," Masserman became satirical. One senses a certain lapse into comic relief, both to vent and to soothe his ire. He derided the new category of tobacco abuse [sic] ("When is a Senate Committee wreathed in cigar smoke after a three martini lunch judged to have the additional Mental Disorder 305.1x [Tobacco Dependence]?") and queried if an antinuclear demonstrator has an "Anxiety Disorder." And "does Hugh Hefner have 302.82 [Voyeurism]? Conscientious priests 302.71? [Inhibited Sexual Desire]"? As for himself, Masserman declared that he had the particular Adjustment Disorder "309.28 [with mixed emotional features] over DSM-III."

Masserman's voice was joined by other negative letters to Brodie from Board members. Spitzer later talked of "their profound dissatisfaction with DSM-III;" they were either aligned with the pro-neurosis forces or concerned about "the politically divisive impact of adopting DSM-III without the concept of neurosis." He added, "It was clear that a compromise solution was a matter of some urgency."[47]

On the positive side, Judd Marmor, who had been President of the APA from 1975 to 1976 and who was on the Board of Trustees in 1979, wrote to Brodie to mount a strong defense of DSM-III and to praise Spitzer's accomplishments.[48] Even though Marmor had been vigorously opposed to Spitzer's desire to have a separate diagnosis for homosexuals troubled by their sexuality, he did not let that imbroglio keep him from declaring that DSM-III was an advance over DSM-II. He argued that "it is more precise in its descriptive approach to mental illness and I am convinced [that it] will ultimately lend itself to effective clinical usage."

Marmor was fond of evaluating events in psychological terms. Just as he had told Spitzer that he thought his position on homosexuality was due to an unconscious homophobia, he now wrote to Brodie that he believed the resistance to DSM-III was predominantly one of human beings' discomfort with change, "threatened by the new and the unfamiliar. After years of familiarity with DSM-II the shift creates anxiety in many people." Moreover, one could not evaluate DSM-III without reading "the explanatory material that goes along with the diagnostic terms used in DSM-III. I suspect," wrote Marmor, "that many of the Board members and many of the critics of DSM-III have not taken the time to study [that] material."

Marmor closed his letter with a persuasive statement that is worth quoting because it exudes a reasonableness and common sense that could not but help be appealing. Spitzer himself could not have done better. (It can be said that taking into consideration both Marmor's position during the homosexuality conflict and his arguments in this last minute crisis over the approval of DSM-III, one must conclude that he was an impressive leader in American psychiatry.)

"The Task Force," Marmor asserted,

> has worked hard and long and has employed many of the best minds in psy-
> chiatry in the course of its deliberations. It has consulted freely with psycho-
> analysts as well as with psychiatrists of other orientations. Its views have been
> presented to countless District Branch meetings...and discussed to a degree
> that is unprecedented....The APA has invested an enormous amount of time
> and money in it. To discard all of this and go back to DSM-II would not be only
> a regressive step but would make our Association a laughing stock in the eyes
> of the media.

The ad hoc committee, Marmor urged, should "examine all of the legitimate criticisms...and try to incorporate them constructively and creatively into the existing
document without destroying its essential unity."

The next communication came from Keith Brodie himself, addressed to the
three members of the ad hoc committee and Masserman (ex officio). Brodie confirmed their schedule to consider DSM-III and hear from Spitzer and alerted the
committee to all the additional materials they would receive in the mail. In addition to other preparations for the meeting, Brodie had contacted individually the
members of the Trustees, asking them to prepare a brief statement of their positions
on DSM-III.[49]

The plan was to convene in New York City May 4 and 5, a week before the Assembly
vote. On the May 4 they would spend the day deliberating among themselves. Brodie
hoped that Sabshin and Henry Work (1911–2007), the Deputy Medical Director of
the APA, would join them. The following morning they would meet with Spitzer
and then by themselves in the afternoon to finalize their recommendations for the
full Board of Trustees, gathering at the annual meeting in Chicago five days hence.
(Ultimately, the May 4–5 meetings were pushed up to May 7–8, or perhaps May 8–9,
making the entire procedure assume a more perilous air.) We cannot help but note
the increasing rounds of deliberations in various cities around the country as well
as the plethora of reading materials descending on all those involved on the ad hoc
committee and the larger Board of Trustees. We must also wonder how scrupulous
each psychiatrist was in reading the overwhelming amount of data raining down on
him or her. What would actually determine what positions they took? And what was
Spitzer thinking and feeling?

Spitzer turned to the APA Central Office to send to the ad hoc committee the most
up-to-date versions of several sections of DSM-III, which he supplemented the next
day with (1) the latest classification, "just in case;" (2) the Field Trial Questionnaire
Number 1, which contained statistics that Spitzer claimed showed a high acceptance of
DSM-III; (3) two articles on the field trials, soon to appear in the June issue of the
American Journal of Psychiatry, with reliability numbers Spitzer considered favorable;
and (4) the ICD-9 glossary, which Spitzer believed was not particularly friendly to the
psychodynamically oriented clinician. Spitzer also sent copies of this material to Stone,

Sabshin, and Donald Langsley, the Vice-president of the APA, who had given Spitzer some helpful advice.[50]

THE PEELE PLAN

While waiting for the verdict from the ad hoc committee, let us turn back to the plans of the analysts to affect the May 12 vote of the Assembly. Immediately after the Board decided to create the ad hoc committee, Roger Peele, a member of the Washington Psychiatric Society, sent a letter on the Society's letterhead to the entire legislative structure of the APA.[51] Copies also went to the ad hoc committee members, Spitzer, and Robert Campbell, the Speaker of the Assembly of Delegates. Recall that Peele was both a deputy representative to the Assembly from the Washington Society and a member of the Assembly Liaison Committee. He also was a member of the Factitious and Somatoform Disorders Advisory Committee for DSM-III. In 1979 he was still Acting Superintendent of St. Elizabeth's Hospital, a public mental institution then part of the NIMH.[52] He was not an analyst but played an increasingly significant role in challenging Spitzer in the weeks before the Assembly vote. Peele is still active in APA affairs, currently Secretary of the APA and on the Task Force for DSM-5. As a member of the Assembly, he has believed for a number of years that the Assembly should play a strong role in APA governance. Moreover, as head of St. Elizabeth's and supervising a residency program, he was one of the more scientifically involved members of the Assembly and hence gravitated toward its involvement with DSM-III.[53]

Peele's position on the issue of neurosis in the DSM-III classification was that there was no need to remove it since it was a term used all over the world in a descriptive sense and not in any psychoanalytic sense, including communist countries like China and Russia. The diagnosis of Depressive Neurosis in particular, he thought, should remain because of its widespread use.[54] Peele is also a political and fair-minded man. He "thought it an error, given the huge number of psychoanalytically-oriented psychiatrists in the APA at that time, to anger that many members more than necessary" over the diagnosis of depressive neurosis.[55] Thus, Peele warmed to Burris' initiative to keep neurosis in DSM-III.

There were no secrets about the organizing efforts to amend the motion to accept DSM-III in the Assembly, because the amendments to be proposed were designed, Peele carefully said, so as not to "violat[e] the basic structure of DSM-III that has already been carefully and thoughtfully developed." (He approved of DSM-III overall and had paid "a lot of attention" to the manual in draft form.)[56] Peele's letter was written to drum up widespread support for two amendments. If passed, the first, Proposal A, would give the clinician the option of employing the diagnostic entity Neurotic Disorder when he or she thought it would be useful to do so.

Proposal B was a bit more complex. Peele explained that it was formulated to deal with the current situation that clinicians, on an everyday basis, found the diagnosis Depressive Neurosis (coded 300.4 in DSM-II) useful, but it had not received a place in DSM-III.[57] In the particular draft of DSM-III that was extant in April 1979, Peele pointed out, there was a category "301.12 Chronic Depressive Disorder (Depressive Personality)" where many patients with "Depressive neurosis" would fit. Moreover, the code 301.12 was listed under the heading "Chronic Minor Affective Disorder." But, Peele argued:

> The terms and coding are undesirable. Patients and clinicians do not perceive of their problems as "minor" and the common connation in medicine that "Chronic" equates with "incurable" is also undesirable—and far from true with most of these patients. It also makes no economic sense to label entities either "Minor" or "Chronic." [Again the subject of third-party payment raised its head.][58]

Moreover, he went on, using the description "Depressive Personality" was not consistent with the usual clinical understanding of a personality disorder. Therefore, his Proposal B substituted "Pervasive Affective Disorders" for "Chronic Minor Affective Disorders" and brought back the DSM-II "300.40 Neurotic Depression" in place of the DSM-III "301.12 Chronic Depressive Disorder."

Peele argued that what he was suggesting was consonant with DSM-III's own aims of "acceptability to clinicians," "maintaining compatibility with ICD-9," and "avoiding the introduction of new terminology…except when clearly needed." Voting for his two amendments to the forthcoming motion in the Assembly to accept DSM-III would enable the manual to achieve its stated goals, he concluded. Peele's was a voice for mediation.

SPITZER'S REJOINDER TO PEELE'S PLAN

When Spitzer received Peele's letter, he thought about it, consulted several Task Force members, and decided to send out a "Dear Colleague" letter of his own to the same APA legislators whom Peele had addressed and to the entire Board of Trustees. He offered his own thoughts on the two amendments and on "our old friend Neurotic Depression,"[59] keenly aware that in a short twelve days the psychiatrists reading this letter would vote.

About Proposal A (optional use of Neurotic Disorder at will), Spitzer roguishly "wonder[ed] if it [was] not more political than clinically useful as compared with the statement now in the DSM-III classification section: Neurotic Disorders: These are included in Affective, Anxiety, Somatoform, Dissociative, and Psychosexual Disorders." Proposal A, he asserted, does not help the clinician know what portions of the DSM-III classification encompass the neurotic disorders, whereas the new manual does exactly that.

As for Proposal B, Spitzer readily agreed that the term "Chronic Minor Affective Disorders" needed to be replaced. As for the codes, he was fine with using the familiar 300.40 code instead of the new 301.12. And the term "Chronic Depressive Disorder" could definitely be avoided, he amiably responded. He did think Peele's suggested "Pervasive Affective Disorders" was "descriptively inaccurate," but Peele's point was well taken. Thus, he suggested, what about "Other Affective Disorders" as a more suitable heading for "Chronic Minor Affective Disorders"? Here Spitzer was displaying his typically positive reaction to suggestions for specific proposals that would improve or correct a problematic entry. He clung to his basic conceptualizations of DSM-III—he was not "giving away the store"—but he was very responsive to ideas for tweaking a particular piece of text.

However, Neurotic Depression was another matter entirely. Its elimination from DSM-III reflected a fundamental outlook Spitzer had about the new manual, and two-thirds of his letter was devoted to this ticklish subject. His arguing points were based on two items: the reports he had gathered from the field trials and his proposal for a whole new term for the familiar and thus desired DSM-II 300.40 code. To begin with, Spitzer said, he had received valuable information from the numerical breakdown of diagnoses when participants in the trials were asked to give both DSM-II and DSM-III diagnoses in evaluating a specific patient. Statistics had shown that "the DSM-II concept of Depressive Neurosis is not really equivalent to the DSM-III category of Chronic Depressive Disorder." What should be done about this disparity, he asked?

Spitzer proposed that the 300.40 category be called "Dysthymic Disorder (Neurotic Depression)."[60] This plan was a typically Spitzerian approach to a problem, imaginative and creative, but somewhat of a gamble, like "homodysphilia." First, he offered a compromise. This new formulation "would mean that the recommended term is Dysthymic Disorder, but the term Neurotic Depression [in parenthesis next to Dysthymia] may also be used and is an official term in the ICD-9-CM—the version of the ICD for American physicians—for this code number."

Spitzer then launched into his justification for this new terminology based on a name that already existed, he carefully pointed out, "dysthymia." This word could be found in both psychiatric and lay dictionaries. In psychiatry, it meant "depression of less intense degree than seen in manic depressive psychosis." In *Webster's Revised Unabridged Dictionary* it was defined as "afflicted with chronic melancholy, depressed in spirits." The source, he assiduously indicated, lay in Greek etymology from *dys*, meaning bad, and *thymos*, meaning spirit. "We know," Spitzer concluded, "that new terms seem strange at first. Initially, Somatization Disorder [SD] seemed a strange name for what had been called by many Hysteria, and by some Briquet's Syndrome. However, with use [SD] had become an accepted term, and its meaning is clear and descriptive." The same potential existed, he believed, for Dysthymic Disorder. Spitzer's prediction was an accurate one. Dysthymic Disorder not only made its way into DSM-III but also remained in DSM-IV. Many years later, Peele commented that the essence of the Task Force/psychoanalytic split had come down to one last issue: which term would be the main diagnosis and which would be in parenthesis, Dysthymia or Depressive Neurosis.[61]

THE AD HOC COMMITTEE MEETS WITH SPITZER

Meanwhile, Spitzer awaited his meeting with the Board of Trustees ad hoc committee. Would it turn out to be the nonthreatening session he had imagined when he first heard about the creation of the committee? The committee met on May 7 (pushed forward three days from the original date set)[62] and spent the day reviewing the various comments and questions the Board of Trustees had articulated about DSM-III. The committee also planned the exchange they would have with Spitzer about many aspects of the manual. Spitzer met with them the next morning, May 8, and was responsive to their concerns and gave acceptable explanations of why certain aspects of DSM-III had been fashioned in the manner they were.[63] In the afternoon, the committee discussed what would appear in their report to the full Board, and Brodie afterward wrote a long letter to Spitzer, detailing their conversation earlier in the day about the specific concerns of the Board.

On the whole, Brodie wrote, the committee was supportive of Spitzer and appreciative of the clarifications he had provided about many matters.[64] The range of issues that had drawn the interest of both the Trustees and the committee was broad, including all manner of perplexities, worries, and fears. The subjects covered included third-party payment; the wording of mental "disorder" vs. mental "disease;" attention deficit disorders in children; acute vs. chronic organic mental disorders; substance use disorders; the reversibility of dementia; schizophrenia; the neuroses; explanations about "borderline;" the V Codes (situations not deemed to be mental disorders); and rewriting of the Introduction to be more positive and less defensive. There were also highly specific requests for the tweaking of particular terminology. It is apparent from Brodie's letter that Spitzer had been conciliatory and responsive to all matters the ad hoc committee had raised. In addition, he was persuasive in arguing for his positions on topics about which the Board had doubts. Three times Brodie wrote "I believe you convinced our Committee that …."

A few of these subjects bear further attention. The committee voiced approval of the diagnostic criteria and the "good inter-rater reliability" they had produced. But, they also were "pleased" that Spitzer stressed that the criteria were not the final word, but "that clinical judgement is of paramount importance in making a diagnosis." This concept, Brodie wrote, would help with third-party payment "by a carrier intent on showing that a patient did not exactly conform to the criteria listed." Again, keeping remuneration in mind, the Board wished that "appropriate language be placed in the introduction to protect those treating Axis 2 [sic] disorders from arbitrary cutbacks in third party reimbursement." Economic fears had been a constant leitmotif of the clinicians who conceptualized treatment in psychodynamic terms since the Midstream meeting in 1976, three years earlier.

Protective of their reputation, the committee members hoped that the APA membership would "be acquainted [by Spitzer] with the reality that the…Ad Hoc Committee was not charged to rewrite DSM-III but only to show areas of concern expressed by Board members to you for further study by your task force." Moreover, being mindful that the issue of the neuroses was tearing apart the APA, the committee described itself as being "delighted with your inclusion of neurotic depression in parentheses following dysthymic disorders and would hope that you would consider placing in parentheses" the word *neuroses* next to other appropriate diagnoses. This would seem to be a reference to a compromise plan proposed by John Talbott,[65] a member of Brodie's committee, that Spitzer eventually did come to accept. "Phobic, anxiety, obsessive-compulsive, hysterical, and depersonalization neurosis were to appear in the new nomenclature as parenthetical terms following the appropriate DSM-III entries. An explanatory note would indicate that the *neuroses* were being included to facilitate identification with the terms used in DSM-II."[66]

In conclusion, Brodie urged Spitzer to review with the Task Force all the issues raised by the ad hoc committee so that "your presentation on May 17 [to the Board] could reflect your awareness of the Board's concern with regard to these issues and any changes which you might have been able to achieve in response to these concerns."

Spitzer immediately took Brodie's admonition one step further. No sooner had he received his letter than he wrote personal letters to each Board member who had expressed his or her disquiet on a specific matter. Spitzer explained to each how he had addressed their particular questions and the changes he had made in DSM-III to meet their objections.[67] Spitzer's alacrity in this matter speaks both to the pressures he felt at this time—72 hours before the Assembly's vote—and the level of precision and energy he brought to all matters.

In spite of the seeming cordiality and spirit of compromise, the reality was far from serene. Everyone was well aware of the challenges planned for the May 12 Assembly vote in Chicago. Could they be headed off by a last-minute deal? There were many who hoped so. But was there a way to solve the problem of the neuroses?

THE TALBOTT PLAN

On May 8, after meeting with the ad hoc committee, Spitzer sent a mailgram to Boyd Burris with copies to certain APA officials and APA members who were immediately involved in the crisis.[68] Spitzer laid out his proposals to resolve the impasse. Since Brodie, as Chair of the pivotal ad hoc committee, still played a leadership role, Burris and his allies replied directly to Brodie on May 10, stating that Spitzer's suggestions did not achieve most of their goals. It was now 48 hours before the Asembly's vote.

Burris did add, however, that a proposal by John Talbott, one of the members of the ad hoc committee, was "to be complimented for taking a bold step towards reaching a compromise."[69] (Talbott's suggestions later came to be viewed by many as a breakthrough in the negotiations.) The "Talbott Plan" (Fig. 13.5) of May 9 was very similar to what eventually appeared in DSM-III. Preceding the Affective, Anxiety, Somatoform, and Dissociative Disorders there was this statement: "In order to facilitate the identification of the neuroses included in DSM-II, the DSM-II terms are included in parentheses after the corresponding DSM-III categories." So, for example, under ANXIETY DISORDERS Talbott listed "Phobic disorder (Phobic neurosis)" or next to SOMATOFORM DISORDERS he proposed "(HYSTERICAL NEUROSES)."

But even with the Talbott Plan Burris declared, "We still have serious objections [because] the capitalized entry of NEUROTIC DISORDERS...has been deleted" from the classification.[70] For the analysts, the fight had come down to just this. Would there be a major category of Neurotic Disorders in the DSM-III classification? And if so, what exactly would be its form? Gone were the goals of a psychoanalytic appendix or a

Neurosis

Talbott Plan (as of May 9, 1979)

In order to facilitate the identification of the neuroses included in DSM-II, the DSM-II terms are included in parentheses after the corresponding DSM-III categories.

AFFECTIVE DISORDERS
Major affective disorders
Coding instructions as is.
    Major depressive disorder
296.2x   single episode
296.3x   recurrent
    Bipolar affective disorder
296.4x   manic
296.5x   depressed
296.6x   mixed

Other affective disorders
300.40   Dysthymic disorder (Depressive neurosis)
301.13   Cyclothymic disorder

Atypical affective disorders
296.82   Atypical depressive disorder
296.70   Atypical bipolar disorder

ANXIETY DISORDERS
    Phobic disorder (Phobic neurosis)
300.21   Agoraphobia with panic attacks
300.22   Agoraphobia without panic attacks
300.23   Social phobia
300.29   Simple phobia

    Anxiety states (Anxiety neurosis)
300.01   Panic disorder
300.02   Generalized anxiety disorder

300.30   Obsessive compulsive disorder (Obsessive compulsive neurosis)

    Post-traumatic stress disorder
308.30   acute
309.81   chronic or delayed
300.00   Atypical anxiety disorder (Atypical anxiety neurosis)

SOMATOFORM DISORDERS (HYSTERICAL NEUROSES)
300.81   Somatization disorder
300.11   Conversion disorder
307.80   Psychogenic pain disorder
300.70   Hypochondriasis
300.71   Atypical somatoform disorder

DISSOCIATIVE DISORDERS (HYSTERICAL NEUROSES)
300.12   Psychogenic amnesia
300.13   Psychogenic fugue
300.14   Multiple personality
300.60   Depersonalization disorder
300.15   Atypical dissociative disorder

FIG. 13.5 The Talbott Plan, May 9, 1979. Used with permission from the American Psychiatric Association Archives, DSM Collection.

section of the Introduction prepared by the analysts themselves. The possibilities of a sixth axis in the multiaxial diagnostic system for coping styles or etiology had long since died. Clearly DSM-III was to be a descriptive manual with diagnoses based on observable signs and symptoms. Perhaps there still was, however, one possibility of retaining, in a limited way, psychodynamic principles. Thus those with a commitment to these concepts put their entire focus on keeping their base rock diagnosis of Neurosis and all it symbolized about the role of unconscious forces in certain psychiatric disorders.

Burris and colleagues countered the Talbott Plan with what they called their "modification." They said they had found Talbott's proposal seriously lacking as it merely placed the neuroses in parentheses but without Neurotic Disorders as a major (i.e., capitalized) entry. They proposed instead a classification that included a major section entitled "NEUROTIC DISORDERS," but offered a compromise. Under NEUROTIC DISORDERS, all the subsections would be first labeled "Disorders," and "neurosis" would appear in parenthesis, for example, "generalized anxiety disorder (Anxiety neurosis)." The reasons Burris gave for his plan had been repeated tirelessly: "To allow practitioners to code their neurotic diagnoses, to prevent possible denial of insurance claims by third-party payers, and to satisfy the demands of those who believe that neurosis should be represented as a distinct and recognizable entity in psychiatry." Once again, Burris threatened a referendum. "We American psychiatrists are the ones who will have to live with DSM-III .... If we do not exhaust every means available to secure the most useful DSM-III, then we will have served poorly our colleagues and the traditions and institutions of which they are a part." Copies of Burris' letter to Brodie went to Masserman, Spitzer, Jaso, Peele, and the Speaker of the Assembly, Robert J. Campbell, who would chair the Assembly when it voted two days hence.

Burris' arguments and threats did not sway Spitzer, although they did heighten the pressure to seek an acceptable compromise. The Burris plan, to no great surprise, was not acceptable to Spitzer and the Task Force. Its effect would be to undo one of the basic conceptualizations of DSM-III they had been wedded to from the start: to discard those categories in DSM-II that were considered "speculative," founded on ideas of the etiological role of unconscious internal conflict in mental disorder. DSM-III, they all had decided, would be a descriptive, empirically based manual. And as Spitzer had shown over and over again, he was not going "to give away the store."

ARRIVAL IN CHICAGO: TWO DAYS TO GO

On the same day that Burris rejected the Talbott Plan and put forth the analytic "modification," the Assembly Liaison Committee to the DSM-III Task Force convened; by now all the major players had arrived in Chicago for the annual meeting. In being able to determine the future of DSM-III, the Assembly had achieved its goal to be a significant body—in this case even pivotal—in the APA hierarchy. The plan of the Assembly Liaison Committee was to attempt to broker a compromise between the analysts and

Spitzer. The Liaison Committee met over two sessions: Thursday, May 10, from 6:45 P.M. until 10 P.M., and Friday, May 11, from 9 A.M. until 11:20 A.M. Jaso and nine members of his Committee were present, including Roger Peele. There were five guests at the first session: Spitzer, Janet Forman (by now Williams), Henry Work (Deputy Medical Director of the APA), Robert Campbell (Speaker of the Assembly), and Melvin Lipsett (Recorder of the Assembly.)[71] On Friday the Assembly Liaison Committee met without guests. The Thursday and Friday meetings were preparatory to the decisive vote in the whole Assembly on Saturday.

First on the agenda Thursday night was a historical review of the "considerable activity" regarding DSM-III that had transpired since the Assembly Liaison Committee had last met, on April 7 at PI. That occasion was the all-day gathering to consider Spitzer's "neurotic peace treaty" and to find a way to bring the warring parties to settle their outstanding differences. At that time, the Assembly Committee had expressed its wish to include Neurotic Disorders as a major category in the classification (although without psychoanalytic etiological implications). This review of events of the last few weeks concluded with a report on the letter that Brodie, Chair of the Trustees Ad Hoc Committee, had just sent to Spitzer on May 9. At that point in the evening, a "lengthy discussion" commenced on various proposals to "modify" the Assembly Committee's position of April 7.

After two sessions, Thursday night and Friday morning, the Assembly Committee "agreed to the following modifications:" "To enlarge the category statement for Neurotic Disorders in the classification, and to change relevant category terms accordingly."

The first alteration was to tack on Talbott's introductory sentence—about facilitating correspondence between DSM-II and DSM-III categories—to Spitzer's April 7 statement that the neuroses were included in Affective, Anxiety, Somatoform, Dissociative, and Psychosexual Disorders. This formulation was edging toward the eventual compromise declaration that appeared in DSM-III. Then, according to Peele, Spitzer agreed to an additional sentence that eventually became the third sentence in the final version of the paragraph "NEUROTIC DISORDERS" in the DSM-III classification: "These DSM-II terms are included in ICD-9-CM and are therefore acceptable as alternatives to the recommended DSM-III terms that precede them."[72] (All three sentences were published together in the final Classification in bold type under the heading "Neurotic Disorders.")[73]

In this last May 10–11 meeting it was agreed that subcategories would appear with "disorder" first and "neurosis" in parentheses. An example of the compromise diagnostic proposal the Assembly Committee had agreed to was "Conversion disorder (Hysterical neurosis, conversion type)." However, the Assembly Liaison Committee would not accept Spitzer's suggestion of "Dysthymic disorder (Depressive neuroses)" under "other affective disorders" but instead, influenced by Peele, agreed only to the reverse: "300.40 Neurotic depression (Dysthymic disorder"). Every inch of ground had been fought over; each word and its ordering were deliberately placed to reflect every nuance of meaning, each agreement symbolic of deeper philosophic beliefs. What words were ultimately going to appear in parentheses (Fig. 13.6)?

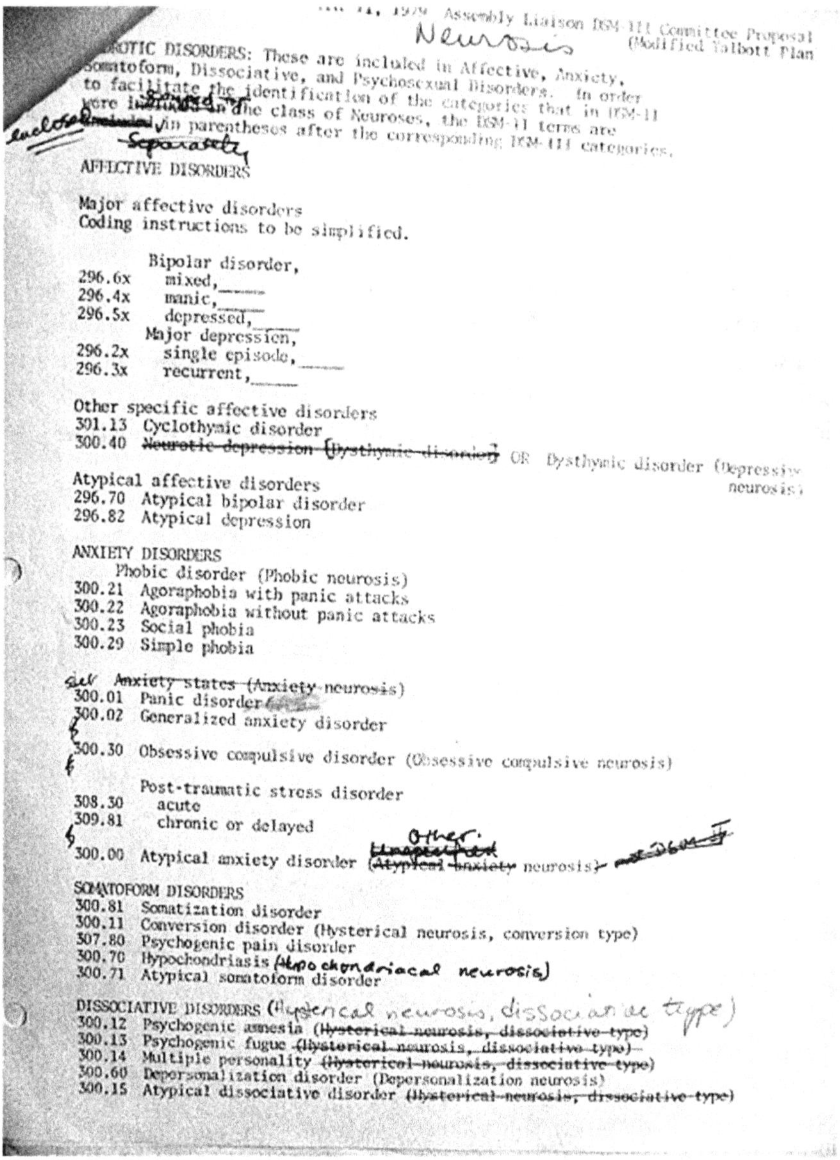

···· 14, 1979   Assembly Liaison DSM-III Committee Proposal
Neurosis   (Modified Talbott Plan)

~~ROTIC DISORDERS:~~ These are included in Affective, Anxiety,
~~Somatoform,~~ Dissociative, and Psychosexual Disorders. In order
to facilitate the identification of the categories that in DSM-II
~~were included in~~ the class of Neuroses, the DSM-II terms are
enclosed ~~reminded~~ in parentheses after the corresponding DSM-III categories.
~~Separately~~

AFFECTIVE DISORDERS

Major affective disorders
Coding instructions to be simplified.

Bipolar disorder,
296.6x   mixed,____
296.4x   manic,____
296.5x   depressed,____
Major depression,
296.2x   single episode,____
296.3x   recurrent,____

Other specific affective disorders
301.13   Cyclothymic disorder
300.40   ~~Neurotic depression (Dysthymic disorder)~~ OR Dysthymic disorder (Depressive
                                                                              neurosis)
Atypical affective disorders
296.70   Atypical bipolar disorder
296.82   Atypical depression

ANXIETY DISORDERS
Phobic disorder (Phobic neurosis)
300.21   Agoraphobia with panic attacks
300.22   Agoraphobia without panic attacks
300.23   Social phobia
300.29   Simple phobia

See ~~Anxiety states (Anxiety neurosis)~~
300.01   Panic disorder~~(...)~~
300.02   Generalized anxiety disorder

300.30   Obsessive compulsive disorder (Obsessive compulsive neurosis)

Post-traumatic stress disorder
308.30   acute
309.81   chronic or delayed

Other:
300.00   Atypical anxiety disorder ~~(Atypical anxiety neurosis)~~ ~~not DSM-II~~

SOMATOFORM DISORDERS
300.81   Somatization disorder
300.11   Conversion disorder (Hysterical neurosis, conversion type)
307.80   Psychogenic pain disorder
300.70   Hypochondriasis *(Hypochondriacal neurosis)*
300.71   Atypical somatoform disorder

DISSOCIATIVE DISORDERS *(Hysterical neurosis, dissociative type)*
300.12   Psychogenic amnesia ~~(Hysterical neurosis, dissociative type)~~
300.13   Psychogenic fugue ~~(Hysterical neurosis, dissociative type)~~
300.14   Multiple personality ~~(Hysterical neurosis, dissociative type)~~
300.60   Depersonalization disorder (Depersonalization neurosis)
300.15   Atypical dissociative disorder ~~(Hysterical neurosis, dissociative type)~~

FIG 13.6 A page from the minutes of the Assembly Liaison Committee for May 11, 1979. It shows
both the original committee decision of the classification of the neuroses (typed characters) as well
as the way things turned out, in the handwritten crossings-out and written changes. It still does
not, however, include the eventual third sentence (see Fig. 13.7) in the paragraph on top about the
"NEUROTIC DISORDERS." It is hard to know from whom this document comes, whether from
Spitzer or from someone on the Liaison Committee. Either could have recorded changes after the
full Assembly voted. The minutes give a good sense of the last-minute struggle that took place,
each side jockeying for the triumph of its terminology. Used with permission from the American
Psychiatric Association Archives, DSM Collection

At the Friday morning Assembly Liaison Committee meeting, 24 hours before the vote, representatives of the seven APA areas were present. Peele recalls that at this time five of these representatives supported having "Depressive Neurosis" as the primary designation and "Dysthymic" in parentheses. Peele was to give the speech supporting this arrangement at the full Assembly meeting, and he left the session thinking he was going to prevail when the vote on the matter took place the next morning.

However, Spitzer found "unacceptable" 300.40 Neurotic Depression (Dysthymic Disorder). Six years later he described his last-minute efforts: "Determined to have the assembly override its own committee's recommendations, he and his close collaborator on DSM-III, Janet Williams, met with the caucus of each area's representatives to the assembly. Using arguments well rehearsed during three years of debate, they sought to elicit support."[74] However, in these meetings Spitzer and Williams were unable to alter Peele's edge. "This degree of uncertainty," Spitzer recalled, "made it impossible to predict the outcome of the assembly's vote."[75]

The meeting of the Assembly Committee was adjourned at 11:20 in the morning of May 11. Now everyone awaited the gathering of the full Assembly, about 150 people, the next day. First on the agenda for the Assembly on May 12, Third Plenary Session, was "Item 5.G—Assembly Liaison DSM-III Committee Proposal (Modified Talbott Plan)."[76]

THE ASSEMBLY OF DELEGATES VOTES

The dry agenda item listed belied what was to be a session of high drama, a face-off between Roger Peele, as deputy representative from the heavily psychoanalytic Washington Psychiatric Society, and Spitzer. Peele and Spitzer had known each other for a few years, since 1975, when Spitzer came down to Washington to get Peele's assistance with writing up the diagnosis of "hysterical psychosis." While there, Spitzer decided that hysterical psychosis was no longer of prime importance, but two other diagnoses occurred to him: "brief reactive psychosis" and "factitious disorder." He asked Peele for a typewriter and, on the spot, "banged out" the essence of the new formulations. Peele could not help but be impressed at this initial meeting, regardless of any later perceptions about Spitzer's seeming enjoyment of conflict.[77]

Although not a psychoanalyst, Peele today still respects psychodynamic and analytic treatments where indicated, and thus at the Assembly meeting he argued for the primacy of "Depressive neurosis" as a bedrock analytic conceptualization. Other diagnoses of neuroses could be in parentheses, but not this one, he believed. Peele, as Chair of Psychiatry at St. Elizabeth's, kept the diagnosis of neurosis alive after 1980 when teaching the residents, so convinced was he of its usefulness.[78]

For the meeting of the Assembly, the Chicago Conrad Hilton had provided a ballroom with a two-tiered stage.[79] On the higher level sat the current Assembly officers, former Speakers of the Assembly, and some APA executive staff, including Sabshin. Campbell, the Assembly Speaker, stood behind a lectern at the front of this group. Right below, on a lower platform, sat the 14 Area and Deputy Area Representatives. On the floor was the body of the Assembly representing the District Branches and behind them the audience. A lectern with a microphone faced the audience. Up and down the aisles were microphones from which individual Assembly members could speak.

Campbell opened the meeting and then asked Spitzer to come to the front, to the lectern on the floor, to make some remarks and handle questions from the members. Spitzer also came prepared with handouts. After a while, Jaso made a motion that the Assembly approve DSM-III with one amendment: "Depressive Neurosis" was to be the main term and "Dysthymic Disorder" the secondary one. Following this, individuals came to the microphones on the aisles to speak. In this setting, Peele, sitting with other Assembly delegates, went to one of the aisle microphones and made a case for the vital significance to psychiatry of retaining Depressive Neurosis as a primary diagnosis. There was tension in the air, many people anticipating Peele's defense of Jaso's motion on the diagnosis of Depressive Neurosis.

Years later, when Peele was asked why he in particular was the main speaker for Jaso's amendment, he replied that as a member of the Assembly he believed the Assembly should play a role in the approval of important issues. He emphasized again that he "thought it an error, given the huge number of psychoanalytically-oriented psychiatrists in the APA at that time, to anger that many members more than necessary."[80]

In response to Peele, Spitzer argued that with "Depressive Neurosis" as the main designation, the consistency of the rest of the carefully planned manual was being violated. His message was that Peele's motion was undermining the whole direction of DSM-III.[81] He also suggested that opposition to the Task Force's recommendation "could be explained only in terms of emotional and political motivations." He pointed out that Depressive Neurosis could still be used in making the diagnosis, an argument which he believed weakened the Liaison Committee's position.[82]

Other members of the Assembly also spoke against the primacy of Depressive Neurosis. It is not clear who, if any besides Peele, spoke for it. Before the vote on the amendment, Peele came to the microphone again to answer Spitzer, but Campbell ruled him out of order, saying he had already had a chance to speak. The parliamentarian to whom Campbell had turned for a ruling on allowing Peele to speak again was Miltiades Zaphiropoulos, who was an analyst but also a past Assembly Speaker. Peele says Zaphiropoulos' ruling was a highly irregular move, seemingly in disregard of Robert's Rules of Order, but he decided not to take issue with it. He believed little would be gained, and even much lost, by challenging the popular past Speaker. While one would have thought an analyst would be in favor of Peele's amendment, Peele surmises that Zaphiropoulos may have made his ruling because "he very much wanted the Assembly to successfully process DSM-III." He also "generally liked to calm the waters," Peele avers.

Jaso's amendment was put to an oral vote, and it was resoundingly defeated. Spitzer's argument of preserving consistency on the issue of neurosis in DSM-III had been persuasive. There was also a strong feeling among many members that Spitzer's tremendous effort should be recognized.[83] Any other amendments proposed after Jaso's motion had failed were dealt with quickly. A general vote followed on DSM-III as a whole, and the decision to adopt it as the APA's new diagnostic manual was almost unanimous. Peele himself voted for it. Spitzer's eyes visibly watered, and the Assembly came to its feet with applause. For a vote, as opposed to the bestowal of an honor, to be followed by a standing ovation was almost unknown in the history of the body. Spitzer never lost the emotional feeling attached to that moment. Many years later, when he was interviewed for a *New Yorker* profile, he asked the interviewer to turn off the recording system as he wept in memory of that occurrence.[84] At the Assembly meeting, Peele went up to Spitzer to congratulate him. They spoke of the fact that Spitzer "had cleared the major hurdle" to the acceptance of DSM-III. Peele recalls that "there was warmth on both sides. It never got hostile between us."[85]

Peele believes that mixed in with the applause for Spitzer was recognition of the Assembly's achievement in having become a more significant body in the APA hierarchy. It had shown that it could effectively handle the approval of an important scientific document, Peele has argued. The Assembly had sought such a role since the early 1970s. By the mid-1970s, the Assembly had decided it wanted approval of the DSM-III to go through it, as a first step in the manual's achieving acceptance. Recall that by the time of the Midstream Conference in June 1976, the Assembly had already appointed a small liaison committee to the DSM-III Task Force, headed by the outspoken Howard Berk. (When Peele informed Spitzer that approval of DSM-III would have to go through the Assembly, Spitzer was none too happy about this situation.)[86] Later, the Assembly authorized a new larger liaison committee, headed by the less acerbic Hector Jaso of Rhode Island, on which Peele served. This newly organized committee was at times more cooperative with Spitzer, although not at the end on the issue of the placement of Depressive Neurosis. As a measure of the Assembly's ambitious reach, there was a referendum of all APA members in 1980, the year after the DSM-III vote, on a proposal to change the APA's governance structure so that the Assembly would become more dominant than the Board of Trustees. The proposal was defeated since a change in the APA's by-laws required a 67% vote, although 57–59% of the voters did approve the Assembly's plan.

While this bit of APA history is noteworthy and shows the multicausality of all significant events, the spotlight rightly shines on Spitzer. For five years, constructing DSM-III had occupied all his waking moments, and he and his carefully chosen Task Force had not as much revised the old manual as written a new one. Twelve- and sixteen-hour days were not unusual for Spitzer, and often they were spent meeting challenges and putting out fires. He was always juggling many balls. If there were confrontations, they did not slow him down. At all times, he kept in mind his essential goals and rarely departed from them. His marriage, however, foundered during these intense years.

Over crowded weeks and months, Spitzer had produced a 494-page descriptive manual based on highly specific diagnostic criteria and full definitions and discussions of each diagnostic category. Moreover, he had engineered the acceptance of an innovative multiaxial patient-evaluation system. He had enlisted the help of dozens of psychiatric specialists on Advisory Committees and inaugurated field trials in an effort to "de-bug" the new system. On difficult and challenging diagnoses, he had chased down experts so he could hammer out the final details. His prodigious labors were obvious to all. Recognizing these endeavors, of course, leaves out an assessment of the wisdom and long-term significance of his changes, creations, and omissions, which we have yet to address. But none could gainsay his adroitness and accomplishments.

After five long years—of committee meetings, discussions, telephone calls, polls, letter writing, questionnaires, arguments, presentations, and crises—Spitzer's vision had prevailed (Fig. 13.7).

SUBSTANCE USE DISORDERS

Code in fifth digit: 1 = continuous,
2 = episodic, 3 = in remission,
0 = unspecified.

305.0x Alcohol abuse,_____
303.9x Alcohol dependence
        (Alcoholism),_____
305.4x Barbiturate or similarly acting
        sedative or hypnotic abuse,
304.1x Barbiturate or similarly acting
        sedative or hypnotic
        dependence,_____
305.5x Opioid abuse,_____
304.0x Opioid dependence,_____
305.6x Cocaine abuse,_____
305.7x Amphetamine or similarly
        acting sympathomimetic abuse,_____
304.4x Amphetamine or similarly
        acting sympathomimetic
        dependence,_____
305.9x Phencyclidine (PCP) or similarly
        acting arylcyclohexylamine
        abuse, _____(328.4x)
305.3x Hallucinogen abuse,_____
305.2x Cannabis abuse,_____
304.3x Cannabis dependence,_____
305.1x Tobacco dependence,_____
305.9x Other, mixed or unspecified
        substance abuse,_____
304.6x Other specified substance
        dependence,_____
304.9x Unspecified substance
        dependence,_____
304.7x Dependence on combination of
        opioid and other non-alcoholic
        substance,_____
304.8x Dependence on combination of
        substances, excluding opioids
        and alcohol,_____

SCHIZOPHRENIC DISORDERS

Code in fifth digit: 1 = subchronic,
2 = chronic, 3 = subchronic with acute
exacerbation, 4 = chronic with acute exacerbation, 5 = in remission, 0 = unspecified.

        Schizophrenia,
295.1x disorganized,_____
295.2x catatonic,_____
295.3x paranoid,_____
295.9x undifferentiated,_____
295.6x residual,_____

PARANOID DISORDERS

297.10 Paranoia
297.30 Shared paranoid disorder
298.30 Acute paranoid disorder
297.90 Atypical paranoid disorder

PSYCHOTIC DISORDERS NOT ELSEWHERE CLASSIFIED

295.40 Schizophreniform disorder
298.80 Brief reactive psychosis
295.70 Schizoaffective disorder
298.90 Atypical psychosis

NEUROTIC DISORDERS: These are included in Affective, Anxiety, Somatoform, Dissociative, and Psychosexual Disorders. In order to facilitate the identification of the categories that in DSM-II were grouped together in the class of Neuroses, the DSM-II terms are included separately in parentheses after the corresponding categories. These DSM-II terms are included in ICD-9-CM and therefore are acceptable as alternatives to the recommended DSM-III terms that precede them.

AFFECTIVE DISORDERS

Major affective disorders

Code major depressive episode in fifth
digit: 6 = in remission, 4 = with psychotic
features (the unofficial non-ICD-9-CM fifth
digit 7 may be used instead to indicate that the
psychotic features are mood-incongruent),
3 = with melancholia, 2 = without melancholia,
0 = unspecified.

Code manic episode in fifth digit:
6 = in remission, 4 = with psychotic features
(the unofficial non-ICD-9-CM fifth digit
7 may be used instead to indicate that the
psychotic features are mood-incongruent),
2 = without psychotic features,
0 = unspecified.

        Bipolar disorder,
296.6x mixed,_____
296.4x manic,_____
296.5x depressed,_____

        Major depression,
296.2x single episode,_____
296.3x recurrent,_____

FIG. 13.7 A The place of "NEUROTIC DISORDERS" in DSM-III: the Neurotic Disorders are stated, but they are not a major category.

A. In bold face in the right hand column on p. 17 of DSM-III is the three-sentence compromise statement on the place of the "Neurotic Disorders" in the DSM-III Classification. Each sentence was painfully hammered out between Spitzer and the psychoanalysts. The entire paragraph was part of the so-called Talbott Plan, which emerged at the last minute before DSM-III was to be voted on by the APA Assembly of Delegates.

18   DSM-III Classification

Other specific affective disorders

301.13   Cyclothymic disorder
300.40   Dysthymic disorder
         (or Depressive neurosis)

Atypical affective disorders

296.70   Atypical bipolar disorder
296.82   Atypical depression

ANXIETY DISORDERS

Phobic disorders (or Phobic neuroses)
300.21   Agoraphobia with panic attacks
300.22   Agoraphobia without panic attacks
300.23   Social phobia
300.29   Simple phobia

Anxiety states (or Anxiety neuroses)
300.01   Panic disorder
300.02   Generalized anxiety disorder
300.30   Obsessive compulsive disorder
         (or Obsessive compulsive neurosis)

Post-traumatic stress disorder
308.30   acute
309.81   chronic or delayed
300.00   Atypical anxiety disorder

SOMATOFORM DISORDERS
300.81   Somatization disorder
300.11   Conversion disorder
         (or Hysterical neurosis, conversion type)
307.80   Psychogenic pain disorder
300.70   Hypochondriasis
         (or Hypochondriacal neurosis)
300.70   Atypical somatoform disorder
         (300.71)

DISSOCIATIVE DISORDERS (OR HYSTERICAL NEUROSES, DISSOCIATIVE TYPE)
300.12   Psychogenic amnesia
300.13   Psychogenic fugue
300.14   Multiple personality
300.60   Depersonalization disorder
         (or Depersonalization neurosis)
300.15   Atypical dissociative disorder

PSYCHOSEXUAL DISORDERS
Gender identity disorders

Indicate sexual history in the fifth digit of Transsexualism code: 1 = asexual, 2 = homosexual, 3 = heterosexual, 0 = unspecified.
302.5x   Transsexualism,_____
302.60   Gender identity disorder of childhood
302.85   Atypical gender identity disorder

Paraphilias

302.81   Fetishism
302.30   Transvestism
302.10   Zoophilia
302.20   Pedophilia
302.40   Exhibitionism
302.82   Voyeurism
302.83   Sexual masochism
302.84   Sexual sadism
302.90   Atypical paraphilia

Psychosexual dysfunctions

302.71   Inhibited sexual desire
302.72   Inhibited sexual excitement
302.73   Inhibited female orgasm
302.74   Inhibited male orgasm
302.75   Premature ejaculation
302.76   Functional dyspareunia
306.51   Functional vaginismus
302.70   Atypical psychosexual dysfunction

Other psychosexual disorders

302.00   Ego-dystonic homosexuality
302.89   Psychosexual disorder not elsewhere classified

FACTITIOUS DISORDERS

300.16   Factitious disorder with psychological symptoms
301.51   Chronic factitious disorder with physical symptoms
300.19   Atypical factitious disorder with physical symptoms

DISORDERS OF IMPULSE CONTROL NOT ELSEWHERE CLASSIFIED

312.31   Pathological gambling
312.32   Kleptomania
312.33   Pyromania
312.34   Intermittent explosive disorder
312.35   Isolated explosive disorder
312.39   Atypical impulse control disorder

FIG. 13.7 B   Note the words "neurosis" or "neuroses" in parentheses next to Spitzer's preferred labels on p. 18. A further compromise in June, after the Assembly's vote, led to the final addition of the word "or" within the parentheses, for example, "Anxiety Disorder (or Anxiety Neurosis.") After all the stormy negotiating, the parenthetical "neurotic" labels quietly disappeared from the next revision of the manual (DSM-III-R) seven years later (1987.) Reprinted with permission from the American Psychiatric Association (Copyright © 1980).

CONCLUSION

DSM-III was long awaited and was eagerly purchased when it appeared in 1980. It represented a radical revision of American psychiatry, the type of occurrence Thomas Kuhn (1922–1996) labeled a "paradigm shift." While initially Kuhn talked about such a shift to explain events in physics, for many years now Kuhn's notions of why this shift takes place have been applied to other scientific fields and have come to dominate the history of science as heuristic principles of change.[1] Kuhn downplayed the notion of science advancing by small accretions in knowledge. Rather, he spoke about an important new scientific development occurring because there was a "crisis" in a particular field of endeavor that traditional approaches could not successfully confront. Thus, events took a radical turn. In Kuhn's view, this was how science advanced.

KUHN'S PARADIGM SHIFT AND ITS APPLICATION TO AMERICAN PSYCHIATRY

There has been much discussion about the accuracy of Kuhn's formulation, and it is arguable that as far as psychiatry is concerned, a "hybrid" model of change is more accurate, for a number of reasons. A paradigm shift, in the original Kuhnian sense of "tradition-shattering" change in a "mature" science, is not totally applicable to modern psychiatry because of its observable cyclical nature. In the history of modern psychiatry, views of mental disorder have shifted back and forth, one era emphasizing the psyche, soul, or mind, and the next emphasizing the somatic, often the brain. There have also been shifts of looking at mental disorder as a spectrum from normal to abnormal, as opposed to viewing mental disorders as categories sharply delimited from each other and normality. (Of course, even as fundamental aspects repeat themselves, there also are clear distinctions from one psychiatric era to the next.)

Moreover, Kuhn's original idea of abrupt change has been modified to include a gradualist aspect. This is a return of the ancient "OTSOG" aphorism, progress "on the shoulders of giants," a principle of how change occurs slowly, brought again to twentieth-century attention by Robert Merton.[2] The sophisticated concept of incremental plus revolutionary change fits the creation of DSM-III. Change resulting because of a crisis is certainly an accurate template for psychiatry in the United States in the 1960s and 1970s. As we have seen, much was wrong, and dissatisfaction was great. Moreover, DSM-III can be seen as a radical *response* to the crisis in psychiatry. However, in terms of the manual's *development*, it would be incorrect to see it only residing in the years 1974–1979 when the Task Force was creating it. Actually, it was not de novo.

Therefore, contrary to the Kuhnian notion of science advancing only by a radical paradigm shift, DSM-III's new approach to diagnosis was many years in the making. The seeds were planted as early as 1927, when the Harvard physicist, Percy Bridgman, first enunciated the concept of gaining knowledge through "operational analysis." Scholars in various fields hailed Bridgman's vision as a way to make their work "scientific."[3] Mandel Cohen, a psychiatrist at Harvard, was likely influenced by Bridgman's ideas, as perhaps was Paul Dudley White, the Harvard cardiologist who collaborated with Cohen for a number of years.[4] Cohen transmitted his concept, of making psychiatry scientific through the use of "operational criteria," to one of his residents, Eli Robins. After his residency, Robins went to Washington University in St. Louis and there passed on Cohen's rubric to two co-workers, Samuel Guze and George Winokur. The three worked together tirelessly over the years to devise a way of making a psychiatric diagnosis through the use of "diagnostic criteria" (an alternative phrase to operational criteria). The Washington University psychiatrists then introduced the psychiatric world to their thinking via a galvanizing paper, known for its "Feighner criteria," in 1972. Through its wide dissemination, Feighner furthered the notion of using diagnostic criteria in clinical work, even though its original purpose was to spur on research. (Cohen lived until 2000 and thus had the satisfaction of seeing his ideas come to dominate psychiatry.)

Meanwhile, around 1971, Robins had met Robert Spitzer through an NIMH project, and he educated and excited him about the Washington University approach to psychiatry. Spitzer, who up to this time had been interested predominantly in biometrics and structured interviews, came away as from an epiphany. When the NIMH asked Spitzer and Robins to refine and expand the Feighner criteria, Spitzer enthusiastically responded to this new mandate. Together with Jean Endicott, a research psychologist, and Robins, Spitzer worked intensively to fulfill the NIMH's goals, and the three produced the Research Diagnostic Criteria (RDC). (Note the major role of the NIMH—an arm of the U.S. government—in the paradigm shift.) While Spitzer was developing the RDC, he was appointed by the American Psychiatric Association as the head of a task force to revise its *Diagnostic and Statistical Manual (DSM)*, and he brought to this project what he had imbibed from Robins, as well as his own plans and goals. Almost fifty years transpired between Bridgman's proposals and the first meeting of the DSM-III Task Force when it was swiftly decided to completely revise DSM-II and to use operational criteria (the term used in the first draft of DSM-III) as the means to arrive at a diagnosis.

KUHN'S EMPHASIS ON CRISIS AND ITS MANIFESTATION IN AMERICAN PSYCHIATRY

While the gestation of DSM-III was a gradual one, we should return to Kuhn because of his valuable idea that crisis in a scientific field presages radical change. By 1970 there assuredly was crisis in American psychiatry, though "crises" would be the better word, since the provocations and problems were ubiquitous. The early 1960s saw the start of an antipsychiatry movement that challenged the very legitimacy and competence of psychiatry. The validity of its diagnoses was disputed (Thomas Scheff); the authenticity and value of its therapy were scorned (Ervin Goffman); and it was argued that the practice of psychoanalysis and psychotherapy was not dealing with mental illness (Thomas Szasz). Psychiatry was also attacked by the deconstructionists of the period as having no inherent scientific legitimacy, being composed instead of social and cultural constructs that varied from era to era and place to place. Moreover, as the decade wore on, psychiatrists faced growing confrontation by lawyers and judges in commitment proceedings and were being overruled.

Psychoanalysis, the dominant form of American psychiatry, was losing its luster, even though analysts could point to many documented cases of success in improving patients' lives. Analysis had oversold its efficacy; drug remedies had been developed that appeared to give a faster result; competing effective psychotherapies had made their appearance, especially cognitive behavioral therapy (CBT); and there was obvious dissatisfaction with the failure of psychoanalysis to deal satisfactorily with severe mental illness. In addition, health insurance companies and government agencies began to demand the kind of accountability that many psychodynamically oriented psychiatrists were not providing. Coverage for long-term therapy decreased as insurance companies sought to maximize profits.

Phenomenologically oriented psychiatrists argued that because of psychoanalysis, psychiatry had moved far away from a testable empirical base. They contended that the analysts' distancing themselves from diagnosis and nosology had led to their de-emphasizing the traditional observation of signs and symptoms they regarded as necessary for the study of psychopathology. Further, they asserted that psychoanalytic theory had led to the mistaken belief in the near universality of mental disturbance (neurosis). They also maintained that the analysts tended to discount patients' self-reports of symptoms, so useful for diagnosis, in favor of the analysts' search for underlying meaning.[5]

Additionally, as many critics stressed, the reliability of psychiatric diagnosis was abysmal and hampered both biological and clinical research. In 1982, trying to account for the paradigm shift brought by DSM-III, the psychiatrist John S. Strauss (b. 1932) wrote about the "hunger" for reliability that marked psychiatric diagnosis in the 1950s and 1960s.[6] This lack of reliability was widely recognized both within the field and in medicine generally.

With regard to both the psychoanalytic predominance and the psychiatric involvement with social issues, many psychiatrists decried what to them seemed a drift away from psychiatry's medical roots. Both the reform-mindedness of the post–World War II era and the challenges to authority provoked by the Vietnam War affected numerous psychiatrists. Social psychiatry burgeoned, with its dedication to curing the mentally ill by eradicating socials ills such as poverty, slums, racism, and unemployment. But others asked: Were these laudable goals what the practice of psychiatry should be about? Melvin Sabshin, the new Medical Director of the APA, said his intention in taking this position was to wrench psychiatry free from the various "ideologies" that had captured it and make it an evidence-based, scientific, and empirical discipline based on the medical model.[7] To compound the various dissatisfactions, the deinstitutionalization of chronically ill psychiatric patients had overburdened limited outpatient treatment facilities, and many of those discharged were receiving no care at all. Homeless men and women were becoming a more frequent occurrence on city streets.

The lay public and organized medicine often showed low confidence in psychiatry. That judgment was only worsened by the publication in *Science* in 1973 of David Rosenhan's accusations that psychiatrists could not tell the difference between healthy and mentally ill individuals. In this atmosphere of confrontation, the APA Board of Trustees called a Special Policy Meeting to consider ways of reversing the general situation of criticism coming from many directions as well as the attempts by health insurance companies and government agencies to regulate psychiatric treatment. The Trustees made a number of decisions that they hoped would impact events in their favor, one of which was to call for the rapid publication of a new diagnostic manual that would link psychiatry more closely to medicine. In the meantime, only derision was evoked when later that same year the entire membership of the APA was polled on what many thought should have been a scientific issue, not a matter of votes: was homosexuality a mental disorder? Hence there was no doubt that psychiatry faced a deepening crisis, and under such a circumstance, radical change was surely a possible response.

THE INTERSECTION OF BROAD HISTORICAL FORCES AND LEADERS OF CHANGE

We come thus to the matter of how to envisage historically the making of DSM-III. Here, as in many important shifts and new directions throughout history, we have to ponder the role of broad forces of the time and that of the individuals who provided leadership, who were simultaneously the products of their age and the directors of change. (The role of the leader, often charismatic, is downplayed in the Kuhnian model.) The question of which was more important, the pressures of the time or the actors who led the way to transformation, is moot. What almost always occurred was a convergence of the personality, aspirations, ambitions, and aims of the individual with the stimulus of powerfully driven scientific, social, and economic circumstances.

We have outlined the circumstances: the slow but deliberate half-century march toward attempting to make a field scientific—from Bridgman and Cohen at Harvard to Robins, Guze, and Winokur at Washington University to Spitzer at Columbia. We have discussed the factors that produced a state of crisis in American psychiatry by 1970. Now we turn to the roles of individuals and the situations they faced in the creation of DSM-III. Before historically decisive events could occur, the union of many goals had to take place. Let us start with the word *dent*. Having been given the opportunity by their chairman to play a major part in the running of the psychiatry department at Washington University in the late 1950s, Robins, Guze, and Winokur dove in: "We wanted a broad research effort," Guze recalled, "and we wanted to put a tremendous emphasis on improving the diagnostic system in psychiatry....It was a very exciting and heady time. We thought, and it wasn't totally exaggerated, that maybe if we were lucky and lived long enough, we could really make a dent in American psychiatry."[8]

It was not by accident that Robins and Spitzer met. Martin M. Katz, chief of the Clinical Research Branch of the NIMH, knowing both men, decided they should meet. This was before the Feighner criteria paper was published. It certainly is possible to call Katz, with his great prescience of mind, the godfather who bestowed his blessings first on the RDC and then on DSM-III. The Wash. U. psychiatrists, left to themselves, even with the fame of the Feighner criteria, would not have affected American psychiatry in the way that Spitzer and the DSM-III made possible. Before DSM-III, sessions on diagnosis at an APA meeting were scheduled for the afternoon of the last day.[9] Spitzer, it may be remembered, related that when he was appointed as head of the Task Force for DSM-III, the Wash. U. psychiatrists were very pleased, knowing their ideas would find a welcome in the new manual.

ROBERT SPITZER AND THE CREATION OF THE PARADIGM SHIFT IN AMERICAN PSYCHIATRY

The two indisputable bookends of twentieth-century descriptive psychiatry are Emil Kraepelin and Robert Spitzer, both having actively propelled psychiatry toward empiricism, vigorous description, and the medical model. Certainly the vital importance of Sigmund Freud, especially in the middle of the century, should not be minimized, and many of his astute insights are for the ages. But the most influential psychiatrist in the last quarter of the century was Robert Spitzer. Let us now turn to his essential roles in the development of DSM-III.

Spitzer, given sole discretion, without any restrictions from the APA leadership, was free to appoint whomever he wished to the Task Force. He chose psychiatrists and psychologists whom he knew to be sympathetic to his goal for an empirically based manual. But interestingly, he at first approached two psychoanalysts with invitations, Arnold Cooper, his eminent former analyst, and Theodore Shapiro, a very close friend. Both turned him down. It was an important event in the making of DSM-III because it indicated that at the beginning, despite his ultimate appointments to the Task Force, Spitzer was flexible and to a certain degree open on the ultimate configuration of the manual.[10] The presence of psychoanalysts on the original Task Force is one of the great "might have beens" in the history of DSM-III and American psychiatry. Spitzer had been trained as an analyst and even practiced for a short while as one, and he never entirely rejected certain psychoanalytic concepts even though he was firm on the issue of the neuroses. He was willing to consider a sixth axis on coping styles or etiology in the multiaxial diagnostic system that the analysts would find congenial, but the Task Force, often openly antipsychoanalytic, turned these down. It was not the only time the Task Force determinedly forced Spitzer's hand when he was willing to compromise.[11] Donald Klein, anti-analytic and Spitzer's close colleague at the New York State Psychiatric Institute, whose opinion Spitzer respected greatly, was particularly vociferous at times.

Nevertheless, in spite of the crucial role of the Task Force in determining the direction of DSM-III, Spitzer clearly and decisively molded the manual from the moment of his appointment. DSM-III would have turned out very differently if another person had been chosen to head the Task Force. For example, the manual was hugely inclusive because Spitzer made the decision that this was the way to satisfy the needs of clinicians. Although Spitzer was enchanted by Robins' innovation of diagnostic criteria, he completely broke with him over the Wash. U. decision to have only a limited number of diagnoses on the grounds that many current diagnoses lacked validity. Spitzer opted for reliability over validity, a valuable undertaking, but with its own large risks. Spitzer knew he had two constituencies and tried to respond to both of them. For the researchers there were the diagnostic criteria, which were supposed to make it easier to find patients with the same disorder so that homogeneous groups could be formed for the study of mental disorders. For the clinicians there were the multiple diagnoses they used in everyday practice.

At all times, Spitzer brought an enormous will and energy to his new project. As we have seen, he immediately chose an empirically minded Task Force and began meeting with them, introducing swiftly the idea of having diagnostic criteria and a multiaxial system of diagnosing. He also informed them of his urgent desire for including a definition of mental disorder as a subset of medical disorders in the new DSM. (The Task Force was never enthusiastic about this last venture, a harbinger of events to come.) He appointed consultants in specific fields to write up new descriptions and diagnostic criteria for all diagnoses and vowed to publicize widely the steps being taken in the construction of DSM-III. To this last goal he was always faithful, with articles in *Psychiatric News*, panels at annual APA meetings, articles in psychiatric journals by him and members of the Task Force, wide circulation of the Progress Report in 1976 together with the catalytic Midstream meeting, and his own appearance on panels and symposia. He answered every letter he received, usually politely and enthusiastically, and even responded to phone calls. At all times he dealt with both conceptual and logistical issues with zeal and dexterity.

The subject of Spitzer's energy is worth a close examination. It is obvious in this book that Spitzer was a skilled politician. A basic aspect of this is the vast amounts of energy he could draw upon. He hardly had any match in the amount of time and sheer stamina he gave to revising the DSM. He came to live and breathe it 12, 14, 16 hours a day. Jean Endicott has pointed out that the revision was all he talked about with other people. He was also willing to rock his marriage in favor of tireless work on DSM-III. Eventually he and his wife divorced, and he married his text editor. He never obsessed over wording as he dashed off memo after memo, letter after letter, and complete definitions of diagnoses. Yet once done with the basic task, he was willing to get broad definitions and specific criteria just right, badgering experts and conducting field trials whose results, as they came in, he used to constantly modify aspects of the drafts of DSM-III. At one point he even polled a large number of APA members to get their views on the controversial Borderline Personality diagnosis. Until those last weeks in April and May of 1979, almost none of his adversaries matched the drive, dynamism, and passion he brought to constructing DSM-III, attributes that put these opponents at a distinct disadvantage. He could juggle a dozen balls simultaneously and be fresh and alert as he did so. In the last feverish weeks, he tended to crucial affairs and minutiae, as they cropped up, with equal vigor.

Spitzer's unrivaled energy was matched by his adroitness as an antagonist. Although quite cordial in most of the innumerable letters he penned, he burst forth when he felt incorrectly wronged or when he saw challenges to his authority as the leader of the Task Force. One of his traits, for better or worse, is that he never shrank from a fight. He actually enjoyed contention, readily admitting that he was a "troublemaker," and did nothing to avoid it. In recognition of this characteristic, Roger Peele, a deft and amicable man who has held and continues to hold many psychiatric leadership positions and had several contacts with Spitzer during the making of DSM-III, christened him the "happy warrior."[12] This aspect of Spitzer's personality was already obvious when he was an adolescent; he called himself "ruthless" when it came to opposing his teachers in high school.[13] Once set on a course of action, he always acted with determination and kept coming back again and again, if necessary, to achieve his goal. He rarely had to give way. Surrendering over the definition of a mental disorder as a medical disorder was one of the very few battles he lost.

SPITZER AND THE PSYCHOANALYSTS

In conjunction with any scrutiny of Spitzer as an adversary, there has to be an examination of his battles with the psychoanalysts. Such a discussion is independent of the question of whether Spitzer was incorrect in banishing all psychoanalytic influence from DSM-III. (To get ahead of our story, in some areas this exclusion led psychiatry astray.)

In the fall of 1974, Spitzer and the Task Force decided that since for most psychiatric disorders the etiology was unknown, they were going to write a descriptive manual that relied on observable signs and symptoms. In part this was the influence of the Wash. U. psychiatrists, who had spelled out in a much quoted 1970 paper what was necessary to establish an etiology and had observed that much of this information was currently unavailable.[14] Of course, the analysts had no way of knowing Spitzer and the Task Force's early decisions, first learning of them almost two years later with the circulation of the 1976 Progress Report and the Midstream meeting later that year. It is true that Spitzer had organized an informational panel at the 1975 APA meeting, but most analysts did not make a habit of attending the annual meeting, and even those who did were unlikely to attend a panel on the revision of the DSM, a small book they mostly ignored.

The analysts and psychodynamically oriented psychiatrists who attended the Midstream Conference were disturbed, some even appalled, by what they learned; for example, Howard Berk of the Assembly of Delegates Liaison Committee to the DSM-III Task Force was outraged. The Assembly Liaison Committee did meet with Spitzer four months after the Midstream Conference and were somewhat mollified by him, but they were not entirely happy. The analysts only slowly formed an ad hoc committee on DSM-III, and it was not until six months after the Midstream Conference that the Chair, Leo Madow, contacted Spitzer, asking for an appointment time, and then for three months hence. This plodding action makes it clear that the psychoanalysts did not think there were any problems that could not be easily negotiated, coming as they did from their position of dominance in American psychiatry. Madow, for example, was Chair of the Department of Psychiatry and Neurology at the Medical College of Pennsylvania, and many other analysts were also chairs of departments of psychiatry. Some occupied leadership positions in the APA. However, these individuals, as well as other analysts, had underestimated Spitzer's intentions and the skills he could employ to implement them. They also had no knowledge initially of the antipsychoanalytic bias of a number of members of the Task Force.

Spitzer was very clear in his own mind and expressed openly why he was eliminating neurosis as a classifying principle from DSM-III. Some form of neurosis was the standard diagnosis given by the analysts and used by most American psychiatrists as well. But Spitzer eschewed this. He argued that the concept rested on the existence of an unconscious conflict that is resolved by neurotic symptoms: "It's an interesting theory, but it's only a theory [and it's] untested." Psychiatry could only move forward as a scientific discipline, he asserted, if it relied on research using "a descriptive system that organized the classification on the basis of symptoms that are present."[15] He wrote in the Introduction to DSM-III that neurosis as a descriptive term still existed, subsumed under Affective, Anxiety, Somatoform, Dissociative, and Psychosexual Disorders. However, neurosis as an etiological concept, what he called the "neurotic process," had no place in a descriptive manual. He contended that there were several other theories about how neurotic disorders developed, stemming from the "social learning, cognitive, behavioral, and biological" schools of thought.[16]

There was nothing secretive about this position; Spitzer said repeatedly that he welcomed criticism in the form of very specific suggestions for changes or corrections. What he meant by this were ideas for rephrasing, clarifying the text, or removing particular objectionable terms, such as the proposals that the American Academy of Psychiatry and the Law and the APA Women's Committee provided him. In this way, he could ignore fundamental philosophical complaints, such as the psychoanalysts' desire to incorporate in the manual the subject of unconscious intrapsychic conflict and its concomitants. At various times the analysts attempted to include analytic thinking, whether in a particular diagnosis, in paragraphs in the Introduction, or in a psychoanalytic appendix. These he fought, and in later recollections he said he was amenable to compromise as long as it did not involve "giving away the store."

Why did Spitzer no longer find concepts about unconscious mental processes useful? After all, he had graduated from the Columbia University Psychoanalytic Clinic (today Center) and practiced as an analyst for a while. But psychoanalysis no longer claimed his loyalty. Over the years he tried various forms of therapy for himself— including Reichian, psychoanalytic, and behavioral—with ultimate disillusionment. And while he had graduated from Columbia, it was "just barely." After a short while as a graduate analyst, he came to the conclusion that he did not know "what the hell he was doing." He had had early success as a researcher when still a resident and while in psychoanalytic training continued his research interests in structured interviews and measuring change in psychotherapy. After his residency, he found his home in the Biometrics Unit at the Psychiatric Institute quite satisfying, with its stress on empirical verification.

Thus, half of the explanation of Spitzer's bouts with the analysts is clear. He was committed to empiricism. But why were the results of the battles so lopsided? In truth, Spitzer was a very skilled strategist and tactician, and the analysts had no equal. No one in the analytic camp devoted himself full-time to the analytic cause as Spitzer did to his project, and those who were at first involved in the analytic ad hoc committee lacked any coherent organization and a strategy. Again, it did not seem necessary because they believed themselves to be in an unassailable status. There also seemed to be no one to match Spitzer for sheer stamina and proactive thinking. Recall that he had scored a victory over the analysts at the September 1978 meeting in Washington with Lester Grinspoon and the Council on Research and Development. Soon thereafter he learned from a letter from Robert Michels that the Chairmen of the Departments of Psychiatry (to whose organization Madow also belonged) were going to attempt to use their clout to get at least some reversal of the analysts' loss. Finally, there were psychoanalytic efforts at organization and a considered plan. But upon finding out that the group was going to meet in New Orleans, Spitzer not only responded to Michels in writing, he also rushed to New Orleans to counter in person whatever the chairmen had in store, a move that surely they had not expected. Spitzer's zeal was unanticipated, as was his use of direct confrontation. This is only one instance where possible contention did not trouble him and where he was determined not to back down.

Moreover, Spitzer's nonpsychodynamic orientation toward DSM-III was not to be budged. The analysts took a very long while to realize this fact and so were unwilling to compromise on lesser issues, believing they could change the nature of the manual. In addition, the analysts not only felt at first they were in a position of dominance that would ensure them a successful outcome, they were also certain that their theoretical stance was the only correct one and that their kind of treatment was superior to all others. It could be argued that Spitzer should have been more up front with Madow's committee and made it perfectly clear what kind of suggestions he was interested in and what he did not want. But perhaps this was one confrontation Spitzer wished to avoid. Neither side acquitted itself well in this clash, with insensitive obstinacy the hallmark of both parties. And in Spitzer's camp there was the inflexible, non-negotiating Task Force.

Spitzer was left pulled between the analysts, for whom he seemed to wish some moderate compromise, and the Task Force, which at times was more recalcitrant than he would have preferred but whose basic orientation he shared. There is evidence in the Archives that Spitzer sought some compromise so he would be able to give the analysts an agreeable feature that would not violate the intrinsically descriptive nature of DSM-III. Thus, there is an element of tragedy in this story. Let us now recall certain illustrative events.

THE ONGOING CLASH

Several vignettes remind us of the thorny relationship between Spitzer and the analysts after their first formal meeting in late March or early April 1977. To begin with, when Spitzer released the April 15, 1977 draft of DSM-III, he asked all those who had received copies, including Madow's committee, to send him suggestions for changes by June 15. Aside from some brief textual recommendations for Intermittent Depressive Disorder, the analysts did not respond with material for substantive revisions.[17] Madow reported that the analysts had been discouraged by what they had heard at the annual APA meeting in May and therefore had not sent any "draft write-ups."[18]

But over the summer Madow's Liaison Committee acquired a new member, Larry Rockland, In the fall, Rockland submitted to Spitzer recommendations for the inclusion of psychodynamic material in the Anxiety Disorders section of DSM-III. Spitzer and the Task Force conferred for many weeks, and it was two months before Spitzer wrote to Rockland and Madow that there would be no extensive discussion of psychodynamic mechanisms under Anxiety Disorders. To cushion the rejection, Spitzer wrote that there were plans to include various coping mechanisms on Axis II.[19] Yet, such an aspect of Axis II never appeared, and the truculent Task Force also voted down a separate axis for coping styles. Spitzer also outlined to Madow certain measures that would be taken in lieu of including psychodynamic material in the new manual,[20] but the additions Spitzer promised never appeared. Some combination of his own predilections and pressure from the Task Force led to this outcome.

Still more vignettes illustrate the ongoing clash. At the Washington meeting of the Council on Research and Development, attended by Spitzer and the analysts, there was a brief discussion about "Project Flower" (*DSM-III and Treatment Planning*), for which Madow did not show much enthusiasm. Michael Mavroidis, the resident APA fellow, whose idea had stimulated Spitzer to propose Project Flower, wrote to Madow to urge him to throw his weight behind the companion volume, arguing that psychiatry had entered an "Age of Accountability."[21] The insurance companies and a variety of public officials wanted to know exactly what psychiatrists and psychoanalysts did in their evaluations and treatments, Mavroidis argued. Madow answered that Project Flower did not deal with the analysts' concerns about DSM-III. Psychodynamic psychiatry must have a home in the revised manual "to justify seeking dynamic therapy," he insisted.[22] But more than that, Madow asserted, other theories should not be accorded equal validity with psychoanalysis, which is what Project Flower was proposing. In essence, Madow had announced that psychoanalysis had the Truth, and compromise was not possible. He seemed to be willing to roll the dice on all or nothing, or perhaps he did not recognize that was what he was doing.

Project Flower foundered for more than one reason, but for psychoanalysis and psychodynamic psychiatry it was an especial loss. A companion book to DSM-III, appearing at the same time, would have showcased psychoanalysis, even if it had to share space with other treatment approaches. It would have been an effective teaching tool for residents and a helpful adjunct for negotiating with insurance companies. A treatment planning book was eventually published under new editors. The introduction briefly reminded readers that the descriptive philosophy of DSM-III was based on "signs and symptoms" and of the value of "reliable diagnostic criteria." However, there was no reference to DSM-III in the title. There was also no statement suggesting the use of the volume in residency training.[23]

Finally, there is the matter of the field trials. Spitzer invited all the psychoanalytic institutes to participate but got a very limited response. The analysts bring to mind the men who refused to look through Galileo's telescope because they were sure they knew the true heavens and did not want challenges and upsets.

SPITZER, NEUROSIS, AND CATEGORIES

Having emphasized the analytic part of the equation in the past few paragraphs, let us now turn to look at Spitzer. Many feel that his discarding almost every last bit of psychoanalysis in DSM-III was an error. Not all knowledge is testable empirically. The analysts were correct when they said they had amassed a great deal of usable knowledge and documented successes over the past seventy years. However, not all of their beliefs were of equal value. Therefore, part of the challenge of developing DSM-III should have been separating the wheat from the chaff and retaining what was valuable. The assurances Spitzer gave Madow in December 1977 about acknowledging proposed psychoanalytic hypotheses in certain disorders and including coping mechanisms in the glossary would have been even-handed recognition by the makers of DSM-III. Also, we have observed in Chapter 11 the possibilities of having an additional axis as a compromise with the analysts. Such an axis would not have detracted from the basic descriptive character of DSM-III.

Moreover, even though Neurosis was eliminated as a classificatory category so the manual could be descriptive, eradicating the notion of intrapsychic conflict as an *explanatory mechanism* for some psychopathology was short-sided. It is true that intrapsychic conflict exists in all individuals, but psychoanalysts point out there are many different varieties of intrapsychic conflict leading to different outcomes. Additionally, not all intrapsychic conflict is equal in the amount of suffering and disability that it causes.

Antipathy to virtually all of psychoanalysis did not serve the psychiatric profession well and perpetuated the profession's harmful pattern of extreme swings between material and non-material forms of knowledge. Furthermore, Spitzer's fascination with the Wash. U. stress on diagnostic criteria and on developing strictly homogeneous categories made him desert the dimensional way of thinking—the continuum from normality to psychopathology—that had been part of his psychoanalytic training.

It is this aspect of mental disorder that the developers of DSM-5 are trying so hard to recapture. For some diagnoses—Autism, for example—they are searching out the continuum along which various types of autistic disorders can be placed, thus blurring the sharp boundaries between them. While this can do away with some diagnoses, for example, Asperger's Syndrome, we may end up with a more realistic understanding of the nature of mental disorders and thus increased validity. (Of course, there might be a trade-off because stressing the dimensional aspect of mental disorder might make reliability harder to achieve, as subjective judgment is introduced—what one clinician means by "severe" may not accord with the evaluation of another.)[24] Problems with sharp categories have also been seen in DSM-IV, a categorical manual like DSM-III, where at times a single diagnosis may not suffice. Consequently, comorbidity (having two or more diagnoses) has skyrocketed, and certain diagnostic categories have expanded beyond usefulness and meaning.[25] Moreover, the number of patients given residual or atypical diagnoses, for example, Diagnosis X Not Otherwise Specified (NOS), has boomed. The makers of DSM-5 are proposing ways of dealing with comorbid diagnoses and residual diagnostic categories.

To sum up: Spitzer's extensive categorizing had mixed effects. Constructing a manual to meet the needs of researchers did help them to assemble homogeneous groups to study, and he did raise reliability for a large number of diagnoses, enhancing national and international cooperation. He also enabled vital advances in evidence-based psychopathology. But total empiricism was a perpetuation of cycles in psychiatry, which retards progress. Moreover, routing most psychiatric thinking into strictly categorical channels for almost a generation—another aspect of rejecting psychoanalysis—proved to be an unfortunate direction for conceptualizing all mental disorders.

DSM-III REDUX

When DSM-III first appeared in 1980 it rapidly sold out, and the APA had to print more copies. Since then, millions of copies of the various editions of the DSM have been sold worldwide, and their sale has been an unanticipated bonanza for the APA. Moreover, from the scientific point of view, the psychiatric portions of the International Classification of Diseases (ICD) and the DSMs have edged ever closer together. It is worth recounting who uses the DSM in the United States: psychiatrists, psychologists, social workers, patient advocacy groups, insurance companies, school administrators and teachers, guidance counselors, pastoral counselors, lawyers, judges, prisons, legislators, policy makers, government agencies, public and private grant giving bodies, and media organizations. If clinicians want to get paid by insurance companies, they submit DSM diagnoses.[26] If researchers are applying for grants, they phrase their proposals in DSM terms, although the NIMH is developing the Research Domain Criteria (RDoC) for research purposes.

Economic issues are involved in almost every single case where the DSM is used. Its use generates monetary benefits for the many professionals employing it, the local and national policy makers who interpret it, and the insurance and pharmaceutical companies who derive profit from it. Even the APA earns substantially from publishing the manual in many languages.

Revisions in the DSM make headlines in the general press, and patients and their families, wanting diagnostic changes, write urgently to the APA Task Force. Discussions of suggested alterations make for cocktail and dinner party conversations. In 2011, people were taken aback and late night comedians made sport when they learned that the DSM-5 Task Force was considering the elimination of Narcissistic Personality Disorder from the nosology. (For whatever reason, the Task Force did not remove it.) Furthermore, relying on knowledge of diagnostic criteria, individuals anxiously self-diagnose, and friends, husbands, and wives in arguments hurl diagnoses at each other. Clearly, beginning with DSM-III, the manual has exerted medical, societal, cultural, and economic influence in powerful ways.

Perhaps a book apiece could be written about the use of the DSMs by all these individuals and groups and the significance of this usage for masses of people all over the world because of the many translations. Just a few moments' thought on the ways in which the manual is put to use will readily bring to mind one or two of its impacts. To explore all of them is beyond the scope of this book, although some of them will be touched on as we sum up. Our discussion will focus most heavily on medical, philosophic, and economic aspects brought to the fore by DSM-III. Let us keep in mind that these subjects affect the lives of many millions of people here and abroad. Both positive and negative aspects of DSM-III will be highlighted.

THE POSITIVE ACHIEVEMENTS OF DSM-III

DSM-I (1952) and DSM-II (1968) were thin and spiral-bound, somewhere between thick pamphlets and dwarf-sized books. DSM-III was a large, thick, conventionally bound book of almost five hundred pages. This expansion was due to the inclusion of dozens of new diagnoses and extended descriptions of all the disorders plus their diagnostic criteria. No matter how one views the consequences and repercussions of the new manual, it must be acknowledged that it was a remarkable and painstaking effort to achieve reliability in diagnosis. Spitzer was a wordsmith, not only in coining new expressions but also in nuances of meaning and clarity. With regard to attaining reliability, he held that psychiatrists might disagree on what constituted depression but certainly not on "patient has no appetite." Specificity of criteria was one way to foster reliability.

To the extent that increased reliability in diagnosis was achieved, although not consistent across the board, it brought more uniformity of treatment and enhanced research. This was especially important in an era when psychopharmacology was offering some improved treatment. (Although improvement was not always the case. It has been demonstrated conclusively that the pharmaceutical industry has not infrequently developed new drugs that were not necessarily for the better.)

Beyond diagnostic criteria, DSM-III inaugurated the multiaxial diagnostic system, a royal road toward more sophisticated diagnosis—if it was used. It is true that some clinicians in the field trials found Axis IV challenging to work with, yet when it was employed, it led to better treatment. It meant the psychiatrist had to think about not only endogenous factors of the disorder but also what kind of exogenous stress the patient was under and whether this was worth investigating. Axis V also required some thought directed toward the level of adaptive functioning during the past year. Although Spitzer sagely indicated that these axes were useful for treatment planning and predicting outcome, he added that the axes were "available for use in special clinical and research settings," thereby indirectly discouraging their use.[27] Axis II was also valuable, put in to ensure that the clinician did not neglect underlying personality structures when dealing with the perhaps more compelling Axis I diagnosis. Unfortunately, some insurance companies began to place less value on Axis II disorders, wanting to reimburse the clinician predominantly for treatment of Axis I disorders. It is regrettable that good features of DSM-III were sometimes undermined for the sake of commercial gain. In DSM-5, the multiaxial diagnostic system will be discarded.

DSM-III contained some new diagnoses and eliminated some old ones. A number of these actions were beneficial to psychiatric progress. When the Task Force began meeting, American doctors were overusing the diagnosis of Schizophrenia, a fact that became only too apparent in the U.S.–U.K. studies comparing rates of diagnosis in the two countries.[28] One of Spitzer's stated goals was to reduce this overblown diagnosis, and he did so by eliminating certain questionable schizophrenia diagnoses. At the same time, the Task Force gave more weight to diagnoses of affective disorders, which could have signs and symptoms similar to schizophrenia, thus addressing the imbalance. Moreover, the addition of Borderline Personality Disorder (BPD), after much investigation, polling, and soul searching, was a plus for Spitzer. Despite the ire of the Wash. U. psychiatrists at this "unscientific" diagnosis, he realized that not including it would deprive clinicians of a key diagnosis. Time has borne out this valiant decision as increasingly more is learned about the childhood determinants, genetics, and treatment of BPD.

Additionally, in the 1970s, the Vietnam War and its suffering veterans vividly brought into focus the trauma of war, and Spitzer adroitly responded by putting a broadly defined Post-Traumatic Stress Disorder in DSM-III, another decision that has proved invaluable in our time. Finally, Tobacco Dependence was a pioneering diagnosis that initially brought much opprobrium and derision. Perhaps Spitzer was ideally suited to such an effort because confrontation almost never fazed him. We have also seen how the tobacco industry, worried about the loss of revenue, secretly attempted to sabotage inclusion of the diagnosis. A 2005 article in *Tobacco Control* raised the possibility that some of the industry's efforts might have succeeded in narrowing the extent and pervasiveness of the diagnosis.[29] If so, this is something Spitzer could not have known at the time.

Although DSM-III moved away from psychoanalysis excessively, at the same time the manual's empirical basis provided a comeuppance for psychoanalysts who fairly glibly assumed they knew more than they did. There are many examples. Without much justification, analysts wildly expanded the list of ailments they could treat. A theory of schizophrenia being caused by the "schizophrenogenic mother" is one example of rash overshooting.[30] Karl Menninger's declaration that psychoanalysis could make a person "weller than well" is another. Even though there was clear evidence that psychotropic medications could help alleviate psychic distress, some analysts, while medically trained, refused to prescribe drugs for patients, despite the possibility that they might bring relief. The theory was that relieving anxiety, for example, would harm the psychoanalytic process by taking away patients' suffering, thus reducing their motivation for therapy. Here bias got in the way of sound treatment.[31]

There are other positive achievements of DSM-III. Spitzer's idea of field testing any new manual, an idea he had as early as 1968 after working on DSM-II, strengthened DSM-III. For the first time for the APA manual, feedback from hundreds of clinicians meant that observable flaws in conceptualizations, clarity, and usefulness were remedied.

The Introduction to DSM-III was another good feature, a summing up of the essence of what Spitzer was trying to accomplish. He often has said that he was prouder of this than of anything he ever wrote. The concluding pages of the Introduction were especially useful but unfortunately mostly neglected. Spitzer made it very clear that using DSM-III to make a diagnosis was only the beginning of what needed to be done for a full evaluation of the patient and to plan treatment. He also noted that DSM-III was not the final word about the psychiatric endeavor, and he anticipated that many revisions and changes would be necessary to understand mental disorders.

Moreover, it was probably best in the long run that the focus of DSM-III turned psychiatrists away from the task of curing social ills as one of their foremost goals. Relieving social suffering was (and is) a laudable aim. However, this was not the best use of highly specialized psychiatric training. Certainly, within any practice, individual clinicians can dedicate themselves to alleviation of social injustice by the type of practice they devise and the fees they charge.

Another crucial issue is the "science" in DSM-III. Since 1980, there have been frequent criticisms that many of the diagnoses in the manual lack substantiation. Critics charge that there is no research, no literature to back up many of the decisions of the Task Force, that their pronouncements are the mere opinions of individuals musing around a table. This is a serious charge, and taken literally there is some truth to it. But the Archives tell a more realistic, nuanced story. They reveal that Spitzer, the members of the Task Force, the many Advisory Committees, and special consultants took their charge very seriously and worked diligently, sometimes in meetings that lasted many hours, to reach their conclusions. Spitzer took it upon himself to seek out the opinions of experts in the fields where Advisory Committees and Task Force members were having difficulties making decisions, One example is Spitzer's questioning John Gunderson about psychotic experiences in BPD. He pushed Gunderson on this matter so that he could clarify his own thinking about relevant diagnostic criteria.

Furthermore, some decisions had to be made where the literature and studies were weak, such as with Schizoaffective Disorder. The extensive debates over this elusive diagnosis—where did it fit in the classification, how should it be conceptualized, what criteria could be used to diagnose it—were at an especially high level, the diagnostic issues being deliberated at the heart of psychiatric discourse. This was not an easy matter to decide. First, in each draft separately and finally in the published DSM-III, Schizoaffective Disorder was located differently in the classification each time. It ended up as the only disorder in the new manual that did not have diagnostic criteria, a humbling position for Spitzer, who had vowed to put diagnoses in DSM-III only if they had clear criteria. But here clinicians in a bedeviling diagnostic situation, in the context of a highly categorized manual, needed a diagnosis. To eliminate the diagnosis made no sense, and the struggle to achieve an accurate conceptualization, with comparatively few scientific studies, should not be regarded as the product of superficial value judgments.

Moreover, Spitzer attempted to codify what constitutes a mental disorder. A definition of mental disorder is not necessary for the practice of good psychiatry, but it emphasizes an important concern for psychiatrists: What are normal and abnormal variants of human behavior? Where does normality end and psychopathology begin? This is both a psychological and philosophical question. Indeed, psychiatry will, for the foreseeable future, grapple with the question of what it means to be a functioning human being. This separates psychiatry from other medical specialties that need to focus on only particular aspects of human existence. Psychiatry ranks among the most difficult of all scientific fields because it attempts to study all at once what constitutes the entire functioning of human thought and behavior. That is precisely why there has been so much public attention to some of the disorders being investigated and labeled in DSM-5. What constitutes the essence of a human being? There is almost universal interest in this question, as the furor over whether to diagnose bereavement as a disorder in DSM-5 has clearly shown.

The answers to these questions involve biology and psychology, descriptive psychiatry and psychodynamic psychiatry, drug treatments and psychotherapy. True, there is always the allure of finding *the* magic bullet, whether in neuroscience, genetics, the human attachments that start at birth, or even spirituality and religion. But understanding human beings will never be reduced to a single overarching factor. The complexities of defining what is normal human behavior is also a philosophical question. Indeed, psychiatry in many respects is like physics, which is also philosophical: How did matter start? What was there before? Was there anything before it? How do we explain existence?

Finally, it should be noted that DSM-III created a feeling of optimism in many psychiatrists that American psychiatry was embarking on a path that could lead to forward-looking research and treatment. Many psychoanalysts and psychodynamically oriented psychiatrists had no such confidence. However, the applause that the Assembly gave Spitzer was a recognition of what had been created after a labor of five years and the hope—justified or not—that after two decades of attacks on psychiatry, a corner had been turned that would presage a better era.

DIFFICULTIES CREATED BY DSM-III

The positive achievements of DSM-III do not conceal the number of problems associated with it. Indeed, when recounting its admirable aspects, less favorable characteristics spring to mind. This is not surprising because rarely is a complex product flawless.

Perhaps the largest problem of DSM-III was its strict categorical approach, including its pivotal diagnostic criteria. This created several difficulties. False categories—separations that did not exist—were created, and sometimes patients were shoehorned into categories that did not really fit them. To avoid this, many psychiatrists found that they had no other recourse but to put their patients in those nebulous catch-all categories of Atypical, Residual, or Not Elsewhere Classified, essentially noninformative categories. From the perspective of the Wash. U. group, this lent support to their position that a significant number of patients were being given diagnoses of disorders that were not valid because the knowledge did not yet exist to categorize them and that "psychiatric illness unknown" was the more accurate diagnosis.

Moreover, sharp categorization meant not giving due emphasis to the fact that many discrete diagnoses actually shared significant features, thus their interrelationship with each other was too easily shunted aside. The co-chairs of the DSM-5 Task Force have specifically acknowledged these problems:

> The seminal article by Robins and Guze on diagnostic validity, which proposed a classification of psychiatric illnesses based...on external, empirical indicators, built a direct pathway to DSM-III....The resultant explicit criteria...did not come without [the] price [of their] reification....While diagnostic reliability has thrived, large-scale epidemiological studies have underscored the inefficiency of DSM's criteria in accurately differentiating diagnostic syndromes.[32]

The leading neuroscientist and former head of the NIMH, Steven E. Hyman, has emphasized the difficulties that have arisen from the reification of psychiatric diagnoses since 1980.[33]

A concrete example of an attempt to remedy such difficulties is that individuals working on DSM-5 place heavy weight on the evidence that many diagnoses share anxiety as a common feature, and they have reoriented their classification to reflect this important observation. (Interestingly enough, this brings these parts of DSM-5 full circle to the psychoanalytic stress on anxiety being central to mental disorders, even though DSM-5 specialists and the analysts probably disagree on etiology.) Moreover, concentrating on distinctive categories meant moving away from the notions of spectra and fluid concepts of psychopathology, another view held by psychoanalysts. Thus, DSM-III encouraged creating sharp dividing lines between illness and normality that do not exist.

Further, with reliability being an overriding goal of the DSM-III Task Force, arbitrary diagnostic criteria were fashioned, and validity was downplayed in favor of reliability. Yet validity is crucial to knowing what one is treating; ultimately, patient care is affected.

An additional drawback of DSM-III was placing so much emphasis on descriptive criteria, which easily devolved into "checklists"—if the patient is positive for two out of five criteria in category A and three out of six in category B, he or she qualifies for the disorder. The unintended yet foreseeable occurrence was that using a checklist of diagnostic criteria shifted the psychiatrist's focus away from getting to know a patient in a deeply meaningful way and from making a thorough-going evaluation of the complexities of that patient's circumstances. The multiaxial diagnostic system was supposed to prevent this from happening, but often it did not. Many psychiatrists either found Axis IV hard to use or skipped it entirely since it was not required for third-party reimbursement.

Nancy Andreasen, a pioneering expert on schizophrenia and former editor of the *American Journal of Psychiatry*, who was a sharp-edged empiricist on the DSM-III Task Force, has astutely recognized the troubling end results:

> Many of us are besieged by injunctions to interview and diagnose patients as quickly as possible, and sometimes even to eliminate our "old-fashioned" and "inefficient" narrative records that summarize present illness and past history, replacing them

with checklists of diagnostic criteria and symptom ratings. Many of us are being pressured to see ourselves as psychopharmacologists who prescribe medications to treat "brain diseases," at the expense of forgetting that the mind and person may need treatment with psychotherapy as well.[34]

The "pressure" undeniably comes from managed care, but succumbing to it has been aided and abetted by checklist psychiatry. This unholy alliance has enabled insurers to demand briefer sessions and briefer treatments for reimbursement, even when these shortened treatments were not in the best interests of particular patients.

There were additional unintended consequences of creating a plethora of new diagnoses and conceptualizing mental disorders in terms of specific diagnostic criteria. Both constructions proved a boon to the pharmaceutical companies, creating niches for the development of new medications, which were then relentlessly marketed to psychiatrists and the lay public alike, hence the vivid appellation "Big Pharma." Furthermore, Allen Frances, who directed the development of DSM-IV, has asserted that abuse of diagnostic criteria has created false epidemiological findings showing a greater amount of mental disorder in the population than actually exists. Large surveys of psychopathology in the populace, he declares, use poorly trained lay interviewers, hiring clinicians being too expensive. These interviewers do not know how to properly apply the diagnostic criteria.[35]

Finally, it was unfortunate that Project Flower did not materialize. It would have gone a good distance toward redressing the imbalance that existed in DSM-III. Capitalizing on Michael Mavroidis' idea, Project Flower was Spitzer's imaginative way to resolve the tension between him and the psychoanalysts. He had hopes that it would satisfy them sufficiently, especially after the Task Force had turned down a separate axis for coping mechanisms or etiology. His plan was that the book would bring to an end the analysts' insistence that there had to be psychodynamic material in DSM-III. While the Task Force did not greet Project Flower with great enthusiasm, it did not stand in the way of its realization.

However, the analysts were not positively disposed to the idea of a companion volume on treatment. They focused their fight on getting psychodynamic thinking into DSM-III proper, as they rightly realized the kind of impact that inclusion or exclusion of psychodynamic thought would have. They believed that they did not have to accept a compromise resolution of the issue, having little perception that they were already losing their leading and authoritative position in American psychiatry.

If Project Flower had come into being, it would have allowed the analysts to retain partial hegemony for a time before being irrevocably wounded by managed care, the pharmaceutical revolution, and the rise of measurably successful nonanalytic and briefer psychotherapies, for example, Cognitive Behavioral Therapy (CBT) and Dialectical Behavioral Therapy (DBT).[36]

PSYCHIATRIC MATTERS FOR CONTINUED ATTENTION

Many issues in contemporary psychiatry deserve attention. Following is a discussion of five that are relevant to the subject matter of this book.

Cyclical Nature of Psychiatry

One of the major difficulties with DSM-III lay in its total rejection of psychodynamic thinking. The Task Force was committed to dislodging psychoanalysis from its commanding place in American psychiatry. But prejudice interferes with sound judgment. In essence, the Task Force went to extremes in their pursuit of empiricism, preventing psychological thinking from having a home in DSM-III. This points to a crucial matter for psychiatry as a scientific discipline: the ongoing cyclical nature of psychiatry over the past two hundred years. This recycling has retarded progress by its big swings between emphasizing material (somatic-biological) and then non-material (psychical-psychological) approaches to conceptualizing and treating mental disorders. Each time a shift occurs, psychiatrists leading the new orientation deride and attack the current mode, a detrimental step for advancing forward.

This pattern is illustrated in the career of Mandel Cohen, who lived long enough to last through three cycles. Cohen first represented and was welcome in the biological/medical psychiatry that was dominant in the early part of his career in the 1930s and 1940s. Then psychoanalysis took center stage for almost three decades, and Cohen became persona non grata in the Harvard psychiatry department and was able to find a home only among the neurologists. However, starting in the 1980s, there was a swing back to the somatic emphasis. The descriptive approach became dominant once more, as signaled in DSM-III, and Cohen was welcomed back to the psychiatric fold. In 1999, the APA gave Cohen a Lifetime Achievement Award when Rodrigo Munoz, trained at Washington University, was President of the APA. Cohen had stood still while psychiatry had repeated its historical alternation between the material and the non-material.

The challenge in the revising of the DSM, the ICD, and major textbooks is to combine the best of each of these two avenues for looking at the human mind and the pathologies that afflict it. The optimal reappraisals today focus on bringing together the material and non-material, both of which are always applicable because of the very nature of the complex human being undergoing assessment. Ideally, both somatic and psychical conceptualization together have to dominate the search for etiologies and the understanding of pathological development. Psychodynamic and cognitive thinking fused with genetic and biological knowledge have the best chances of succeeding accurately. Emotions and feelings in human beings have been shown to make genes expressive, leading to overt psychopathology.

Pathologizing Normality

This matter is quite contentious. As we have seen, one of the main accusations of the antipsychiatrists was that psychiatry was guilty of pathologizing normal human variation. As Spitzer began adding numerous new diagnoses, he found himself open to this criticism, even by some psychiatrists. One point that must be noted, however, is that because of the advice of Paula Clayton on the DSM-III Task Force, an expert in affective disorders, Simple Bereavement was not included as a diagnosis. Instead it was placed in the V Code category: Conditions Not Attributable to a Mental Disorder that are a Focus of Attention or Treatment. As the revolution begun by DSM-III was assessed over the years, there were new objections. One charge was that nonpathological shyness had been turned into Social Anxiety and normal sadness had become a Depressive Disorder.[37] The authors of such criticisms also argued that creation of these diagnoses opened the way for pharmaceutical companies to develop medications that some of the newly identified patients might not really need. In subsequent years, it was discovered that the drug companies sometimes withheld information about efficacy and harmful side effects.

As we review the complexities of DSM-III, it seems logical to reflect on where American psychiatry is going in the area of diagnosis. Ironically, some of the same contentious issues that arose over DSM-III have returned in the making of DSM-5. For example, the new Task Force and some DSM-5 Work Groups have been criticized for the development of diagnoses that critics say would label many adults and children with psychopathology they do not have. The critics hold that these labeled individuals demonstrate no more than normal variants of human behavior. "Normality is being pathologized" has become again a frequent assertion. This argument holds that at a time when there is still a stigma to certain mental disorders and when diagnosed persons run the risk of being prescribed psychotropic medication with serious side effects, often by primary care doctors, pathologizing normality is no minor matter.

Allen Frances, the leader of the DSM-IV Task Force, often took this position, and he was not alone.[38] Frances was quite critical, for example, of the diagnosis of Psychosis Risk Syndrome in adolescents (which after field trials was relegated to a section for further study) and Temper Dysregulation Disorder in young children. DSM-5 introduced a bereavement diagnosis, with the possibility of bereavement becoming diagnosed as a major depressive disorder. This last decision raised so much controversy that the DSM-5 Task Force decided to append a caution to this diagnosis, to stress the importance of watchful waiting before making a diagnosis of depression. Frances' warnings found favor with many clinical psychologists and certain lay groups and leaders, in addition to a number of psychiatrists.[39] Division 32 of the American Psychological Association and the American Counselors Association have written Open Letters objecting to several DSM-5 diagnoses.

But the coming manual will have these and other contentious diagnoses, as well as a restructuring of diagnostic chapters, different from those in DSM-IV. The DSM-5 Task Force and a number of the Work Groups have argued that there is enough new scientific information since the last revision of the DSM in 1994 (text revision in 2000) to warrant significant updating. David Kupfer, head of the Task Force, has emphasized the neuroscientific and genetic advances in knowledge to justify revising psychiatric diagnoses.[40] The APA leadership and the makers of DSM-5 have also asserted that the includion of the new categories allows for early treatment of serious conditions, thus lessening or even preventing later affliction. Jeffrey Lieberman, APA former President, has rebutted criticisms of the revisions in a point-by-point "counter-argument."[41] Other APA officials and DSM-5 leaders have also refuted specific charges from time to time.[42]

Only time will tell how the revisions work out in practice. The law of unintended consequences will manifest itself in changes that were made—some not even originally controversial—as well as in areas that were simply left alone. Psychiatry is particularly vulnerable to problems associated with significant modification of its classification because of the complexities of understanding human existence.

Removing Diagnoses from the Nosology

The other side of pathologizing normality is whether conditions designated pathological should be taken out of the classification. An example comes from the DSM-IV category Sexual and Gender Disorders. (This was known as Psychosexual Disorders in DSM-III.) These decisions will always be controversial, just as was the ruling to remove homosexuality from DSM-II. In this instance, the question revolves around Gender Identity Disorder (GID) in Adolescents and Adults, that was Transsexualism in DSM-III. The debate here is whether or not some instances (some would argue for all) of GID are normal variants of human behavior. Transgender advocacy groups argue for the removal of GID, maintaining that being depathologized by the APA is a crucial milestone that will help to reduce the stigma and discrimination by society against transgender individuals, including the smaller, more specific group of transsexuals. However, those in favor of retaining the diagnosis of GID point to Criterion D of the diagnostic criteria for GID: "The disturbance causes clinically significant distress or impairment in social, occupational, or other important areas of functioning."[43] Criterion D must be fulfilled or the diagnosis of GID will not be made. Moreover, some advocacy groups argue that retaining GID will allow transgender individuals to receive needed medical care in state-run institutions.

With all these factors in mind, the DSM-5 Work Group on Sexual and Gender Identity Disorders has proposed replacing GID with "Gender Dysphoria," to reduce stigma. The name change will also place the stress not on the disorder but on the subjective feelings of the transgender individual in response to his or her particular situation. This calls to mind the battle that raged about Spitzer's firm desire to have a separate category for homosexuals who were distressed about their sexual orientation.[44] Spitzer was the victor and "Ego-Dystonic Homosexuality" appeared in DSM-III, but, significantly, disappeared from DSM-III-R and has been gone from the DSMs ever since (although it remains in ICD-10). The weight of the APA's decision on what constitutes normal variance in human sexuality and how it is labeled points to the wide social influence of the DSM. The APA's pronouncement is thus no minor matter.

Checklist Psychiatry

Another difficult diagnostic matter is that the DSMs risk collusion with third-party payers, meaning managed care of some variety, and Big Pharma. The pharmaceutical industry has an influence through its development and marketing of niche medications based on specific disorders and its advertising to clinicians and the lay public.

Can these connections be altered? It is unlikely that the insurance and pharmaceutical companies will change very much. Does that mean the onus is on the APA to mount a campaign urging that diagnosing and treating be based not only on diagnostic criteria but also on getting to know the patient better? Yet, is it realistic to hope that many psychiatrists will give up the lucrative practice of seeing patients for fifteen-minute med checks as long as insurers reward the clinicians for these brief visits? Will psychiatrists resist patient pressure consequent to pharmaceutical corporations telling the public: "Ask your doctor if _____ is right for you?" The vicious cycle, involving clinicians, insurers, and Big Pharma, is not an easy one to break apart. At least part of this cycle might be broken if psychiatrists took on the task of actively educating their patients to resist pharmaceutical marketing.

Suffering of Individuals with Mental Disorders

Our last matter also involves education. Critics of psychiatry of every stripe abound. In our story they have been the antipsychiatrists and the postmodernists of the 1960s and 1970s. Their charges then and now span the spectrum from being correct to being incorrect. But what is usually lacking from the critics is a realistic acknowledgement that the individuals under psychiatric care are suffering and that in most instances the clinicians treating them are trying to help to the best of their knowledge. This knowledge is usually used well, but even when it is incomplete or incorrect, the major aim in most cases remains: to help suffering. Thus there is a major task of tutelage awaiting psychiatrists—indeed, all mental health specialists—to teach about the suffering of their patients, which in mental disorders can include both emotional and physical agony. Of course, this has to be carried out in a way that does not downplay the progress that has been made in psychiatric treatments and certainly not in a way to stifle legitimate criticism.

THE IMPACT OF THE DSMS

The DSMs affect daily life in many ways.

It is commonplace to call the DSM the "Bible" of psychiatry. It is also not completely unthinkable to call it a Bible for the millions it affects, an actual holy book, whose verses guide professional authorities in many fields—the mental health clergy, if you will. Moreover, it is a book by whose injunctions, particular diagnoses, millions judge themselves and others. The gay population's insistence that homosexuality be removed from DSM-II is an illustration of the enormous authority and significance given to the APA's diagnostic system. The removal of the homosexuality diagnosis was considered the sine qua non of eradicating the opprobrium and discrimination from which homosexuals suffered, a foreshadowing of the potential effects of DSM-III and IV in other matters.

It is certainly true there are still stigmas attached to mental disorders. However, the DSM is steadily breaking down stigma by showing that previously disparaged conditions are actually illnesses. This more sophisticated view of mental disorders is being disseminated widely by making the DSM and its revision process available to a wide swath of people via the Internet. Although it often leads to unproductive self-diagnosing, this accessibility is educational and establishes the idea that the existence of some form of mental disorder is common and opens a path to the notion that perhaps it is treatable. And it is probable that as the years go by, even more treatments will be possible, although any optimism in our day is always qualified by uncertainty about economic conditions. Will treatment be affordable to masses of people in a world where there is poverty that is not easily remediable and where even developed countries are beset by economic woes?

Yet, for the foreseeable future, the revolution begun by DSM-III will continue, and its significance will remain. This can be seen in specific ways, and several illustrative examples should suffice since these instances easily affect the lives of scores of people. In the clinical area, patient advocacy groups representing mental disorders that are not in the DSM campaign for their putative disorders to be placed in the DSM so affected individuals can gain insurance coverage. Parents who want special services for their children in public schools agitate for a DSM diagnosis so that their special needs child will receive those services. Desiring that their patients receive insurance coverage so that they can be reimbursed for treatment, clinicians sometimes modify their diagnoses if another diagnosis brings greater benefits for their patients or clients. In the area of social welfare, community mental health providers make decisions about allocating housing and rehabilitation to needy individuals based on their DSM diagnoses. There are legal significances as well. In spite of clear DSM caveats, lawyers quarrel over whether their clients have or do not have DSM diagnoses in order to win their suits. In child custody hearings parents try to prove their former spouses have DSM diagnoses in order to deny them custody of their children. Other groups as well want the authoritative recognition a DSM diagnosis will confer. Fathers want Parental Alienation Syndrome (PAS) in the DSM so that their former wives who have child custody can lose custody for turning their children against their ex-husbands. But custodial women often insist these fathers are child molesters.

In any event, all societies have conceptions of normal and abnormal behavior, always in very basic ways that determine everyday life. In this regard, it is undeniable that the psychiatric revolution that began with the making of DSM-III has influenced the lives of ordinary people, the decisions of large corporations, and the shaping of governmental policies throughout North America and much of the Western world over the last thirty years. In some geographical areas, the impact of the manual actually extends beyond as well. DSM-III reverberates, sometimes unexpectedly, everywhere.

NOTES

All archival documents are from the American Psychiatric Association Melvin Sabshin Library and Archives (APA Archives), DSM Collection, and are used with permission. The documents in the endnotes are referred to as "Archives, DSM Coll." I accessed these documents at a time when they were not catalogued and were scattered in many boxes.

Chapter 1

1. Hannah S. Decker, "The Psychiatric Works of Emil Kraepelin: A Many-Faceted Story of Modern Medicine," *Journal of the History of the Neurosciences*, Vol. 13, No. 3, Sept. 2004, pp. 248–276. Kraepelin's greatest fame was his division of the severe psychoses into two categories, dementia praecox (later called schizophrenia, although the two are actually not identical) and manic-depressive insanity (bipo lar disorder). The term *schizophrenia* was coined by the Swiss psychiatrist Eugen Bleuler (1857–1939) as "the group of schizo-phrenias," indicating more than one. Moreover, Bleuler did not believe schizophrenia always ended in the severe deterioration that Kraepelin described. For further elaboration see Richard Noll, *American Madness: The Rise and Fall of Dementia Praecox*. Cambridge, MA: Harvard University Press, 2011.

2. Although it appears as if doctors returning soldiers to the front were not following the Hippocratic Oath, the battle-shocked troops were actually better off than comparable soldiers in World War I, who often returned home psychic wrecks, unable to live normal lives.

3. Meyer's wife, Mary Meyer, interviewed patients' families in what is considered the first psychiatric social work.

4. Gerald N. Grob, "The Forging of Mental Health Policy in America: World War II to New Frontier," *Journal of the History of Medicine and Allied Sciences*, Vol. 42, Oct. 1987, p. 413. I have found Grob's article about post–World War II psychiatry to be especially useful in writing the early part of this chapter.

5. For discussion urging the extension of analytic treatment, see works by the analyst Leo Stone, "The Widening Scope of Indications for Psychoanalysis," *Journal of the American Psychoanalytic Association*, Vol. 2, 1954, pp. 567–594, and *The Psychoanalytic Situation: An Examination of Its Development and Essential Nature*. New York: International Universities Press, 1961.

6. Karl Menninger, Martin Mayman, and Paul Pruyser, *The Vital Balance: The Life Process in Mental Health and Illness*. New York: Viking Press, 1964, p. 1.

7. Sigmund Freud, *The Psychopathology of Everyday Life*, trans. Alan Tyson. In *The Standard Edition of the Complete Psychological Works*, Vol. VI, ed. James Strachey. London: Hogarth Press, 1960.

8. To buttress his argument that reliance on diagnosis was unnecessary, Menninger quoted the philosopher Alfred North Whitehead: "Distrust the jaunty assurances with which

every age prides itself that it at last has hit upon the ultimate concepts in which all that happens can be formulated. The aim of science is to seek the simplest explanations of complex facts" (*The Vital Balance*, p. 34). (Yet, this argument could be turned against psychoanalytic reductionism.) Basically, "dynamic" psychotherapy does not depend on diagnosis for treatment decisions. But as we shall see, within the decade, the analyst or psychotherapist had to provide a diagnosis based on nosology in order to collect payment from an insurance company.

9. Such a heavy stress on mending the environment, of course, ignored the strong biological aspect of Freudian thought.

10. Alan A. Stone, "Psychiatry: Dead or Alive?," *Harvard Magazine*, Dec. 1976, p. 20.

11. Robert H. Felix, "Mental Public Health: A Blueprint," Lecture at St. Elizabeth's Hospital, Washington, DC, April 21, 1945, quoted by Grob, p. 417.

12. I taught history of psychiatry at the Tremont Crisis Center, which had been set up as one of the neighborhood centers envisioned in President Kennedy's Community Mental Health Centers Act of 1963.

13. Grob, p. 410.

14. Group for the Advancement of Psychiatry, *The Social Responsibility of Psychiatry: A Statement of Orientation*. Report 13. New York: GAP, 1950.

15. Less than fifteen percent of NIMH projects involved biological studies. See Grob, p. 425. One of the social scientists at work in the NIMH in the 1950s was the sociologist Erving Goffman, soon to become famous for his "antipsychiatry" book, *Asylums*, based on material he gathered during his stay at St. Elizabeth's Hospital. We will investigate Goffman's thought fully in this chapter.

16. Letter from Harry S. Truman to William C. Menninger, May 15, 1948, cited by Rebecca Jo Plant, "William Menninger and American Psychoanalysis, 1946–48," *History of Psychiatry*, Vol. 16, No. 2, 2005, p. 184.

17. William Menninger, "A Psychiatric Examination of the American Psychoanalytic Association," President's Address, May 1948, cited in Plant, p. 195. See discussion later in the chapter on the career of the psychoanalyst John Gedo.

18. Robin M. Murray, "A Reappraisal of American Psychiatry," *The Lancet*, February 3, 1979, p. 255.

19. Group for the Advancement of Psychiatry, *Medical Education*, Report 3. New York: GAP, 1948, pp. 2, 7, and 8; Group for the Advancement of Psychiatry, *Trends and Issues in Psychiatric Residency Programs*, Report 31. New York: GAP. 1955, p 1. For an additional synopsis see Mitchell Wilson, "DSM-III and the Transformation of American Psychiatry: A History," *American Journal of Psychiatry*, Vol. 150, No. 3, 1993, pp. 399–410.

20. Alan A. Stone, p. 17.

21. In the late 1950s in New York State, one-third of the annual budget was devoted to state hospitals. See Grob, pp. 427–428.

22. Grob, p. 412.

23. Albert Deutsch, *The Shame of the States*. New York: Harcourt, Brace and Company, 1948; Mary Jane Ward, *The Snake Pit*. New York: Random House, 1946; Albert Q. Maisel, "Bedlam 1946," *Life*, Vol. 20, May 6, 1948, pp. 102–118.

24. In a study published in 1970 a political scientist, Arnold Rogow, wrote, "Perhaps it is not too much to say that where the public once turned to the minister, or the captain of industry, or the scientist, it is now turning more and more to the psychiatrist." And the APA prepared a report in 1968 that was "an invitation to explore a career in mental health.... The psychoanalyst [will] find himself in tremendous demand." See Arnold Rogow, *The*

Psychiatrists. New York: Putnam, 1990, and the American Psychiatric Association, *Careers in Psychiatry*. New York: Macmillan, 1968, quoted in T. M. Luhrmann, *Of Two Minds: The Growing Disorder in American Psychiatry*. New York: Alfred A. Knopf, 2000, pp. 220–221. Yet, in 1964 the APA had issued a report finding that the training of psychiatric residents was inadequate regarding psychosis and the major psychiatric diseases, which psycho-analysis did not deal with.

25. Quoted in Grob, p. 444.
26. *The Atlantic Monthly: A Magazine of Literature, Science, Art and Politics*. Boston: The Atlantic Monthly Company, Vol. CCVIII, July–Sept. 1961, p. 62.
27. Roy R. Grinker, Sr., "The Sciences of Psychiatry: Fields, Fences and Riders," *American Journal of Psychiatry*, Vol. 122, No. 4, 1965, pp. 368–369, 371–372.
28. George N. Thompson, "The Society for Biological Psychiatry," *American Journal of Psychiatry*, Vol. 111, No. 5, Nov. 1954, pp. 389–391; Percival Bailey, "The Great Psychiatric Revolution," *American Journal of Psychiatry*, Vol. 113, No. 5, Nov. 1956, pp. 387–406.
29. I am indebted to Gerald Grob for these observations.
30. Benjamin Pasamanick, Frank R. Scarpitti, and Simon Dinitz, *Schizophrenics in the Community: An Experimental Study in the Prevention of Hospitalization*. New York: Appleton-Century-Crofts, 1967, see especially pp. 269–270.
31. Grob also noted this. I would add that social workers were also beginning to be competitors, and psychologists and social workers had the advantage of charging less.
32. Mitchell Wilson, "DSM-III and the Transformation of American Psychiatry: A History," *American Journal of Psychiatry*, Vol. 150, No. 3, March 1993, p. 402.
33. Alan A. Stone, "Psychiatry, Dead or Alive?" *Harvard Magazine*, Dec. 1976, p. 17.
34. There is a new book out on the antipsychiatry movement: Michael E. Staub, *Madness is Civilization: When the Diagnosis Was Social, 1948–1980*. Chicago: University of Chicago Press, 2011. Unfortunately, I learned of it too late to incorporate some of its information and ideas.
35. Nick Crossley, "R.D. Laing, and the British Anti-Psychiatry Movement: A Socio-Historical Analysis," *Social Science and Medicine*, Vol. 47, No. 7, 1998, p. 878.
36. Crossley, p. 878.
37. This seems, however, to be contradicted by Goffman's report that "I drank a few times on the grounds both with attendants and with patients." Erving Goffman, *Asylums: Essays on the Social Situation of Mental Patients and Other Inmates*. Chicago: Aldine Publishing, 1961, p. 267.
38. Goffman, p. x.
39. There is no unanimity on the extent to which Goffman had an influence on decisions to close state mental hospitals. For those who assert his significant effect, see Gary Alan Fine and Daniel D. Martin, "Humor in Goffman's *Asylums*," *Journal of Contemporary Ethnography*, April 1990, p. 90, and M. T. Berlim, M. P. A. Fleck, and E. Shorter, "Notes on Antipsychiatry," *European Archives of Psychiatry and Clinical Neuroscience*, Vol. 253, 2003, p. 65. On the other hand, Gerald Grob, with much expertise in this area, argues that the influence of Goffman's book on the closure of state hospitals must be examined within the larger context of the drug revolution and especially federal social welfare policies that devalued institutional care and were aimed at delivering psychiatric care through community-based mental health facilities. See Gerald N. Grob and Howard H. Goldman, *The Dilemma of Federal Mental Health Policy: Radical Reform or Incremental Change?* Rutgers, NJ: Rutgers University Press, 2006.
40. Fine and Martin, pp. 89–115.

41. Goffman, pp. 130, 132.
42. Goffman, p. 135.
43. Goffman, p. 140.
44. Goffman, p. 145.
45. Goffman's use of the word *mortifying* was later used by D. L. Rosenhan in what came to be a famous indictment of American psychiatry. We will discuss this at the end of this chapter.
46. Goffman, p. xiii. Goffman first used and defined the term *total institutions* in a 1957 paper, "On the Characteristics of Total Institutions," presented at the Walter Reed Institute's *Symposium on Preventive and Social Psychiatry*. The notion is not new, however. Bruno Bettelheim, in his 1943 discussion of the Nazi concentration camp, talked about the ways in which extreme situations could shape and mold the collective behavior of inmates. See his "Individual and Mass Behavior in Extreme Situations," *Journal of Abnormal and Social Psychology*, Vol. 38, 1943, pp. 417–452. The idea has been criticized for assuming that all institutions with patients, inmates, or prisoners are alike. I am indebted to Gerald Grob for these cogent observations.
47. Goffman, pp. 155–156.
48. Contrary to what some authors state, the antipsychiatrists quoted each other and in one case even met to discuss common interests. Goffman cited Szasz, and, as we shall see, Szasz had wide areas of agreement with Goffman. Furthermor, R. D. Laing, the Scottish antipsychiatrist, cited both the "labeling" theorist, Thomas Scheff (see later in the chapter), and Szasz and met personally with Goffman. Thus I am in strong disagreement with Berlim and colleagues who state that the "antipsychiatrists were such a disparate group of individuals with almost nothing in common with each other except that they were all, for different reasons, deeply critical of psychiatry and its professionals." M. T. Berlim, M. P. A. Fleck, and E. Shorter, " Notes on Antipsychiatry," *European Archives of Psychiatry and Clinical Neuroscience*, Vol. 253, 2003, pp. 61–67.
49. Goffman, p. 350.
50. Goffman, pp. 358–359.
51. In 1975 the Supreme Court held that no one could be involuntarily kept in a mental hospital if he or she was not receiving treatment.
52. Goffman here echoes the views of R. D. Laing.
53. T. S. Szasz, W. F. Knoff, and M. H. Hollender, "The Doctor-Patient Relationship and Its Historical Context," *American Journal of Psychiatry*, CXV, 1958, p. 526, cited by Goffman.
54. Goffman says that a "spontaneous remission may be a result of the patient's not having been sick in the first place" (p. 379). Here Goffman foreshadows the work of David Rosenhan, discussed later in this chapter.
55. Goffman, pp. 380–382.
56. In spite of there being some medication, when Goffman wrote in the late 1950s the country's mental hospitals still had a bulging population of over half a million, and the image of state hospital psychiatry was notoriously poor. It is true that in the 1950s and early 1960s the Food and Drug Administration (FDA) approved some effective psychotropic medications. In 1954 the FDA approved the antipsychotic drug chlorpromazine (Thorazine) and in 1960 and 1963 the "tranquilizers" chlordiazepoxide (Librium) and diazepam (Valium). As a result there were some discharges from state mental hospitals, but mass discharges did not start until 1965 with the passage of Medicare and Medicaid.

57. Thomas S. Szasz, *The Myth of Mental Illness: Foundations of a Theory of Personal Conduct*. Boston: Harper & Row, 1961.

58. Eric V. D. Luft, "Thomas Szasz, MD: Philosopher, Psychiatrist, Libertarian," *Upstate Medical University Alumni Journal*, Summer, 2001, http://www.szasz.com/alumnijournal.html.

59. Szasz, p. 3.

60. Szasz, p. 297.

61. Szasz, p. 5.

62. Szasz, p. 7.

63. Szasz, p. 14.

64. Szasz, p. 10.

65. Thomas Szasz, *The Second Sin*. New York: Doubleday, 1973.

66. Joel Paris, *The Fall of an Icon: Psychoanalysis and Academic Psychiatry*. Toronto: University of Toronto Press, 2005, p. 82.

67. Szasz, *Myth*, p. 11.

68. Luft, op. cit.

69. Szasz, *The Myth of Mental Illness*, p. 13.

70. Szasz, *The Myth of Mental Illness*, p. 4.

71. Szasz, *The Myth of Mental Illness*, pp. 13–14.

72. Szasz, *The Myth of Mental Illness*, p. 297.

73. Daniel Goleman, "Social Workers Vault into a Leading Role in Psychotherapy," *New York Times*, Science Section, April 30, 1985.

74. Thomas J. Scheff, *Being Mentally Ill: A Sociological Theory*. Chicago: Aldine Publishing, 1966, p. 7.

75. Scheff, pp. 7–9.

76. Scheff, p. 9.

77. Scheff, p. 23.

78. Scheff, p. 28.

79. Scheff, p. 32. Becker wrote that social groups create deviance. "Deviance is not a quality of the act the person commits, but rather a consequence of the application by others of rules and sanctions to an 'offender'." Howard S. Becker, *Outsiders*. New York: Free Press, p. 9.

80. Scheff, p. 81.

81. Goffman, pp. 155–156.

82. Scheff, pp. 81–82.

83. See, for example, the 1985 edition of Scheff's *Being Mentally Ill*.

84. Because of Laing's philosophy he objected to saying someone *has* schizophrenia, as though the person *had* a cold. He preferred talking about "the schizophrenic." See R. D. Laing, *The Divided Self: A Study in Sanity and Madness*. Chicago: Quadrangle Books, 1960, p. 35. In a later edition, Laing changed the subtitle to *An Existential Study in Sanity and Madness*.

85. Laing, *The Divided Self*, p. 24.

86. Laing, *The Divided Self*, p. 28.

87. Beginning in the mid-1950s until 1981, "the Foundations' Fund for Research in Psychiatry (FFRP) aided hundreds of researchers in fields related to mental health….Much of the research it sponsored during its early years was psychoanalytically oriented. In the 1960s it shifted to a more biological and social orientation. [In] its first decade …its research grants, fellowships, and support to departments of psychiatry helped to launch the modern era of psychiatric research." See M. Pines, "The Foundations' Fund for Research in Psychiatry and the growth of research in psychiatry," *American Journal of Psychiatry*, 1983, Vol. 140, pp. 1–10.

88. This interview can be found in Emil Kraepelin, *Lectures on Clinical Psychiatry*. Authorized translation from the second German edition. Revised and edited by Thomas Johnstone, third English edition. New York: William Wood & Company, 1913, Lecture III, "Dementia Praecox," pp. 21–29.

89. Laing, *The Divided Self*, pp. 29–31.

90. Laing, *The Divided Self*, p. 39.

91. R. D. Laing and Aaron Esterson, *Sanity, Madness, and the Family: Families of Schizophrenics*. Penguin Books: Harmondsworth, England; Baltimore, MD; Victoria, Australia, 1970 [1st ed. 1964].

92. Laing and Esterson, p. 18.

93. Laing and Esterson, p. 19. In the second edition of *Sanity, Madness, and the Family* (1970), Laing and Esterson took a more extreme position: "We do not accept 'schizophrenia' as being a biochemical, neurophysiological, psychological fact, and we regard it as a palpable error, in the present state of the evidence, to take it to be a fact. Nor do we assume its existence. Nor do we adopt it as a hypothesis. We propose no model of it." Laing and Esterson, p. 12.

94. Laing and Esterson, p. 27. A remarkable assessment, we must acknowledge.

95. R. D. Laing, *The Politics of Experience*. New York: Pantheon Books, 1967.

96 Back page blurb in the 1970 edition of *Sanity, Madness, and the Family*.

97. "In our 'normal' alienation from being, the person who has a perilous awareness of the nonbeing of what we take to be being (the pseudo-wants, pseudo-values, pseudo-realities of the endemic delusions of what are taken to be life and death and so on) gives us in our present epoch the acts of creation that we despise and crave." Laing, *The Politics of Experience*, p. 24.

98. Laing, *The Politics of Experience*, pp. xiv-xv.

99. Thomas Scheff, "Social Conditions for Rationality; How Urban and Rural Courts Deal with the Mentally Ill," *American Behavioral Scientist*, March, 1964, and "The Societal Reaction to Deviants: Ascriptive Elements in the Psychiatric Screening of Mental Patients in a Midwestern State," *Social Problems*, No. 4, Spring, 1964.

100. Laing, *The Politics of Experience*, p. 83.

101. Emil Kraepelin's *Lectures on Clinical Psychiatry*, 1906, quoted by Laing, *The Politics of Experience*, p. 73.

102. Erving Goffman, *Asylums*, quoted by Laing in *The Politics of Experience*, p. 75.

103. Laing, *The Politics of Experience*, p. 78.

104. Laing, *The Politics of Experience*, p. 83.

105. Laing, *The Politics of Experience*, p. 85. Laing and Rosenhan (see later in chapter) noted the unfortunate permanence of the label "schizophrenia."

106. Laing, *The Politics of Experience*, pp. 87, 89.

107. Laing, *The Politics of Experience*, p. 101.

108. Laing, *The Politics of Experience*, p. 12. Language like this had a special resonance at the height of the Cold War.

109. Laing, *The Politics of Experience*, p. 90.

110. See, for example, the writings of the psychoanalyst Theodore Lidz (1910–2001).

111. Here I will rely on a 1974 article that examines their journal evenhandedly: John A. Talbott, "Radical Psychiatry: An Examination Of The Issues," *American Journal of Psychiatry*, Vol. 131, No. 2, Feb. 1974, pp. 121–128. Talbott is a former President of the American Psychiatric Association.

112. From the *Radical Therapist*, quoted in Talbott, p. 122. Note the agreement with Szasz. The *Radical Therapist* was a very short-lived publication of two volumes spanning the years 1970–1972. All articles cited by Talbott are from the *Radical Therapist*, Vols. 1 and 2, 1970–1972.

113. Talbott, p. 122.

114. Talbott, p. 123.

115. To wit: "Paranoia is a state of heightened awareness....Depression is the result of intolerable alienation and deprivation..... Drug abuse is taught to children by their alcoholic, nicotinic, aspirinic, caffeinic elders....Schizophrenia is an experience saner than normality—in this mad world." *Radical Therapist,* quoted by Talbott, p. 124.

116. Quoted in Gerald N. Grob, "The Attack of Psychiatric Legitimacy in the 1960s: Rhetoric and Reality," *Journal of the History of the Behavioral Sciences*, Vol. 47, No. 4, Fall 2011, p. 408. I am relying heavily on Grob in this section for discussion of events in the legal profession.

117. Bruce J. Ennis, *Prisoners of Psychiatry: Mental Patients, Psychiatrists and the Law*. New York: Harcourt Brace Jovanovich, 1972, pp. vii–viii. Quoted by Grob, 2011.

118. Alan A. Stone, p. 19.

119. The "New Left" was the name associated with liberal, sometimes radical political movements that took place during the 1960s, often among college and university students. The term derives from an open letter of 1960 by the Columbia University sociologist C. Wright Mills entitled "Letter to the New Left." Mills wanted to move away from traditional "Old Left" emphasis on labor issues in order to focus on fighting alienation, anomie, and authoritarianism. The term "The Establishment" to identify prevailing authority structures stems from this time. Members of the "anti-Establishment" movement hoped to bring about a new kind of social revolution. Opposition to the Vietnam War and support of the Chinese Cultural Revolution marked the New Left. It both influenced and drew inspiration from various black civil rights and black power movements.

120. Alan A. Stone, p. 21.

121. E. Fuller Torrey, *The Death of Psychiatry*, Radnor, PA: Chilton, 1974. He went even further, arguing that "the psychiatrist has become expendable, he is left standing between people who have problems in living and those who have brain disease, holding an empty bag." A general practitioner or an internist, Fuller Torrey asserted, could take care of the relatively few patients with genuine brain disease, dispensing pills.

122. Center for Mental Health Services, *Mental Health, United States, 1996,* and *Mental Health, United States, 1998,* Washington, DC: Department of Health and Human Services, publications quoted in Allan V. Horwitz, *Creating Mental Illness*. Chicago and London: University of Chicago Press, 2002, p. 62.

123. American Psychiatric Association, *Training the Psychiatrist to Meet Changing Needs.* (Report of the Conference on Graduate Psychiatric Education held in December 1962.) Washington, DC: American Psychiatric Association, 1964. Gerald Grob called my attention to this publication in his article "The Attack of Psychiatric Legitimacy in the 1960s," 2011.

124. Judd Marmor, *Psychiatrists and Their Patients: A National Study of Private Office Practice*. Washington, DC: Joint Information Service of the APA and the NIMH, 1975. We will meet Marmor again, as he plays an important role in our story.

125. H. Keith H. Brodie and Melvin Sabshin, "An Overview of Trends in Psychiatric Research: 1963–1972," *American Journal of Psychiatry*, Vol. 130, No. 12, Dec. 1973, p. 1309.

126. Kate Mulligan, "Carter Commission Legacy Still Reaping Benefit," *Psychiatric News*, Vol. 38, No. 5, March 7, 2003, p. 14.

127. *Report to the President from the President's Commission on Mental Health*, Vol. 1: Number 040–000–00390–8. Washington, DC: U.S. Government Printing Office, 1978, quoted in Wilson, p. 403.

128. "Blue Cross VP Says MH Prospects Cloudy," *Psychiatric News*, Aug. 6, 1975, quoted in *Report to the President*, 1978.

129. "Javits says MH hurt by role confusion," *Psychiatric News*, Dec. 16, 1977, p. 1, quoted in *Report to the President*, 1978.

130. "Burden of MH coverage questioned at conference," *Psychiatric News*, Sept. 2, 1977, p. 18, quoted in *Report to the President*, 1978.

131. D. L. Rosenhan, "On Being Sane in Insane Places," *Science*, Vol. 179, Jan. 19, 1973, pp. 250–258.

132. Rosenhan later developed an interest in applying psychological methods to trial processes.

133. Rosenhan, p. 250.

134. Rosenhan, p. 251.

135. Rosenhan, p. 251.

136. Rosenhan, p. 252.

137. Rosenhan, p. 252.

138. Rosenhan, p. 253.

139. Rosenhan, p. 253.

140. J. Cooper, R. Rendell, B. Burland, L. Sharpe, J. Copeland, and R. Simon, *Psychiatric Diagnosis in New York and London*. London: Oxford University Press, 1972. The study is colloquially referred to as the U.S./U.K. Diagnostic Project.

141. Rosenhan, p. 255.

142. Rosenhan's usage of the word *depersonalization* is not the usual psychiatric usage. The psychiatric definition is "an alteration in the perception or experience of the self so that the feeling of one's own reality is temporarily lost. This is manifested in a sense of self-estrangement or unreality, which may include the feeling that one's extremities have changed in size, or a sense of seeming to perceive oneself from a distance." See American Psychiatric Association, *Diagnostic and Statistical Manual of Mental Disorders* (3rd ed.), 1980, p. 358.

143. The human potential movement of the 1960s originated with the concept of cultivating potential that its advocates believed to lie untapped in most people. Through the development of "human potential," human beings allegedly could experience an enhanced quality of life filled with happiness, creativity, and fulfillment. Moreover, the effect of individuals cultivating their potential was envisioned as leading to social change for the better.

144. The discussion of this epochal event draws mainly from two sources: Ronald Bayer, *Homosexuality and American Psychiatry: The Politics of Diagnosis*. New York: Basic Books, 1981, the most comprehensive and considered account, and Alix Spiegel, "The Story of How the American Psychiatric Association Decided in 1973 that Homosexuality Was No Longer a Mental Illness," *This American Life*, Chicago Public Radio, Jan. 18, 2002, http://www.this americanlife.org/Radio_Episode.aspx?episode=204.

145. Bayer, p. 102.

146. David J. Rissmiller and Joshua H. Rissmiller, "Evolution of the Anti-Psychiatry Movement into Mental Health Consumerism," *Psychiatric Services*, Vol. 57, No. 6, June 2006, p. 864.

The Rissmillers do not identify which opponents of psychiatry joined forces with the gay activists. They could have been former patients, Scientologists, or college students. There are a variety of possibilities.

147. Bayer, p. 103.
148. Bayer, p. 125.
149. Spiegel, 2002. Spiegel also reveals that there was a group of "concerned" psychiatrists in the APA who were eager to change the leadership and bring liberal reforms and were therefore sympathetic to the homosexual cause. Not surprisingly, her grandfather was among them.
150. Bayer, p. 126.
151. Bayer, pp. 132, 134.
152. Bayer, p. 136.

Chapter 2

1. George Mora, "The Historiography of Psychiatry and Its Development: A Re-evaluation," *Journal of the History of the Behavioral Sciences*, Vol. 1, 1965, p. 47.
2. Ilza Veith, *Hysteria: The History of a Disease*. Chicago: University of Chicago Press, 1965, p. 185.
3. Ernst von Feuchtersleben [1845], *The Principles of Medical Psychology: Being the Outlines of a Course of Lectures*, trans. H. E. Lloyd, rev. & ed. B. G. Babington. London: Sydenham Society, 1847, pp. 3–4, 8, 13, 75.
4. Hannah S. Decker, *Freud in Germany: Revolution and Reaction in Science, 1893–1907*. New York: International Universities Press, 1977.
5. Theodor Puschmann [1889], *A History of Medical Education from the Most Remote to the Most Recent Times*, trans. & ed. E. H. Hare. London: Lewis, 1891; New York: Hafner, 1966, pp. 441–442.
6. Siegfried Bernfeld, "Freud's Earliest Theories and the School of Helmholtz," *Psychoanalytic Quarterly*, Vol. 13, 1944, pp. 341–362; Paul F. Cranefield, "Freud and the School of Helmholtz," *Gesnerus*, Vol. 23, 1966, pp. 35–39.
7. Ernest Jones, *The Life and Work of Sigmund Freud*, Vol. 1. New York: Basic Books, 1953, pp. 40–41.
8. Jones, p. 42.
9. Fielding H. Garrison, *An Introduction to the History of Medicine*, 4th ed. Philadelphia & London, Saunders, 1929, p. 535.
10. Puschmann, pp. 441–444.
11. Wilhelm Griesinger [1845], *Mental Pathology and Therapeutics*. A Facsimilie of the English Edition of 1867. Introduction E. H. Ackerknecht. New York: Hafner, 1965.
12. Griesinger, pp. 9–10
13. With their unsubstantiated theories, the brain psychiatrists were being no less speculative than the practitioners of *Naturphilosophie* whom they had overturned.
14. Gregory Zilboorg, *A History of Medical Psychology*. New York: Norton, 1941, p. 441; Erwin H. Ackerknecht [1959], *A Short History of Psychiatry*, trans. S. Wolff. New York & London: Hafner, 1968, p. 66.
15. Zilboorg, p. 450.
16. Emil Kraepelin [1913], *Dementia Praecox and Paraphrenia*, trans. R. Mary Barclay. Edinburgh: E & S Livingstone, 1919; reprinted, Bristol: Thoemmes Press, 2002, pp. 3–4.

17. Bleuler's book was not translated into English until 1950. See Eugen Bleuler, *Dementia Praecox or the Group of Schizophrenias*, trans. Joseph Zankin. Foreword by Nolan D. C. Lewis. New York: International Universities Press, 1950. For many years, psychiatrists summarized Bleuler's contribution to the understanding of the disorder by saying he gave precedence to four symptoms (4 A's): Loosening of associations, disturbances of affectivity, ambivalence, and autism. However, recently it has been argued that this is a distortion of Bleuler's position. See Kieran McNally, "Eugen Bleuler's Four A's," *History of Psychology*, Vol. 12, No. 2, May 2009, pp. 43–59.

18. Karl Jaspers (1883–1969), the famous existential psychiatrist and philosopher, disagreed. Commenting on the psychiatric lectures, conferences, and journals at the end of the nineteenth century, he recalled that "frequently, the same things were bring discussed in different terms, in most cases in a very obscure manner. Several schools each had its own terminology.…There seemed to be no such thing as a common scientific psychiatry uniting all those engaged in psychiatric research." Quoted in P. A. Schilpp (ed.), *The Philosophy of Karl Jaspers*. New York: Tudor, 1957, p. 17.

19. In his "Self-Assessment" (*Persönliches*) written in his sixties, he noted: "The finer nuances of verbal expression have always been of great importance to me, and over the years, I have taken increasing pains to exploit the tools of language to the full." Kraepelin quoted in Eric J. Engstrom, W. Burgmair, and Matthias M. Weber, Emil Kraepelin's "Self Assessment:" Clinical Autobiography in Historical Context (Classic Text No. 49). *History of Psychiatry*, Vol. 13, 2002, p. 101.

20. Kraepelin, *Dementia Praecox and Paraphrenia*, pp. 5–73.

21. While descriptions of symptoms in DSM-III are full, they do not echo the diversity and evocative detail of Kraepelin's.

22. Kraepelin, *Dementia Praecox and Paraphrenia*, pp. 122–123.

23. Kraepelin, *Dementia Praecox and Paraphrenia*, pp. 26–28. Quoting from a letter Kraepelin illustrates not only the beliefs of persecution but also the incoherence of thought and loosened associations of dementia praecox: "I am in terrible anxiety. There is the greatest danger that my life is coming to an end with fear, because the whole institution is arranged like clock-work, which is managed, not by reason, but by crazy heads in the cells, which are regulated like toothed wheels, and not only are the cells so arranged that one must move to and fro in haranguations [sic] as on a telegraphic cobweb of nerves, also in the passages each square yard is a division that demands a hanging-man to appear from anywhere whether it is for a view or a brutal person." Kraepelin, p. 29.

24. Emil Kraepelin, *Manic-Depressive Insanity and Paranoia*, trans. R. Mary Barclay (from the 8th German ed. of the *Text-Book of Psychiatry*), ed. George M. Robertson. Edinburgh: E & S Livingstone, 1921; Bristol, England: Thoemmes Press, 2002, p. 36.

25. Kraepelin, *Manic-Depressive Insanity and Paranoia*, pp. 24–25, 77–78. For stuporous states see pp. 37 and 79–80, and for "melancholia gravis," involving hallucinations and ideas of guilt and sinfulness, see pp. 80–82.

26. Kraepelin, *Manic-Depressive Insanity and Paranoia*, pp. 27, 32, 55, 55–59.

27. Emil Kraepelin, *Memoirs*, ed. H. Hippius, G. Peters, and D. Ploog, trans. C. Wooding-Deane. Berlin: Springer Verlag, 1987, p. 61.

28. Quoted by Eric J. Engstrom in "Kraepelin, Social Section," in German E. Berrios and Roy Porter (eds.), *A History of Clinical Psychiatry: The Origin and History of Psychiatric Disorders*. London and New Brunswick, NJ: Athlone Press, 1995, p. 294.

29. Robert A. Woodruff, Jr., Donald W. Goodwin, and Samuel B. Guze, *Psychiatric Diagnosis*. New York: Oxford University Press, 1974, p. ix.

30. Engstrom, p. 294.

31. Engstrom, p. 294. It is of some interest that the Institute was opened in the middle of World War I.

32. Kraepelin, *Dementia Praecox and Paraphrenia*, p. 250.

33. Emil Kraepelin, *Clinical Psychiatry*. Abstracted and Adapted from the 7th edition of *Psychiatrie* (1904) by A. R. Diefendorf. New York and London: Macmillan, 1907; reprinted Bristol: Thoemmes Press, 2002, p. 127.

34. Kraepelin, *Clinical Psychiatry*, pp. 21–22; Kraepelin, *Dementia Praecox and Paraphrenia*, p. 244.

35. Kraepelin, *Clinical Psychiatry*, pp. 458–459.

36. Kraepelin, *Manic-Depressive Insanity and Paranoia*, pp. 258, 264.

37. Emil Kraepelin, *Lectures on Clinical Psychiatry*. Translated from the second German edition by Thomas Johnstone. New York: William Wood and Company, 1913, p. 345.

38. Emil Kraepelin, "The Manifestations of Insanity" (Classic text No. 12), trans. D. Beer in *History of Psychiatry*, Vol. 3, 1992 [1920], p. 29; Emil Kraepelin, "Patterns of Mental Disorder," trans. H. Marshall, in S. R. Hirsch and M. Shepherd (eds.), *Themes and Variations in European Psychiatry*. Bristol: John Wright & Sons, 1920, p. 528.

    Eugen Bleuler (1857–1939), the famous Director of the Bürghölzli Clinic in Zurich, gave dementia praecox the name "schizophrenia" in 1911, and Kraepelin seems to have picked it up here, though in his textbook and clinical lectures he always said "dementia praecox."

39. Paul Hoff, "Emil Kraepelin and Forensic Psychiatry," *International Journal of Law and Psychiatry*, Vol. 21, 1998, p. 350.

40. Kraepelin's book "does not enter upon a critical review of contradictory views of other writers; thus he would do his work and his readers a great favor if he should give his material the benefit of monographic publication. In the meantime the conscientious critic must refrain from comparisons unless he have as many or more records of patients collected with the principles in view which Kraepelin has brought forth for the first time." Adolph Meyer, "Review of Kraepelin, E. *Psychiatrie: Ein Lehrbuch fur Studierende und Aertze*, Funfte Auflage," *American Journal of Insanity*, Vol. 53, 1896, pp. 299–300; Adolph Meyer, "In Memoriam: Emil Kraepelin," *American Journal of Psychiatry*, Vol. 151 (6 Supplement), 1927, p. 142.

41. Kraepelin, *Memoirs*, p. 159.

42. Kraepelin, *Memoirs*, pp. 123–124. Conducting follow-ups is one area in which the neo-Kraepelinians could have an advantage over Kraepelin because they developed a structured interview format and, as time went on, they could rely on computers for onerous computations and statistical analyses.

43. As it turns out, these prognoses are somewhat oversimplified. Some schizophrenics, not most, recover and have good lives. And although severe affective (manic and/or depressive) episodes remit and there is a recovery, in some people the intervals between episodes shorten and the frequency and severity worsen. It may not be the same as a schizophrenic deterioration, but it can lead to the diminution or ending of life.

44. Eric J. Engstrom, *Clinical Psychiatry in Imperial Germany: A History of Psychiatric Practice*. Ithaca: Cornell University Press, 2003, p. 144.

45. Engstrom, p. 144.

46. Matthias Weber and Eric J. Engstrom, "Kraepelin's Diagnostic Cards: The Confluence of Empirical Research and Preconceived Categories," *History of Psychiatry*, Vol. 8, 1997, pp. 375–385.

47. Unfortunately, during the Nazi period (which began seven years after Kraepelin died), some of the science at the Institute was used to support Nazi racial ideas.

48. We know, of course, that Kraepelin could be sorely tempted to consider etiology based on personal and social factors. He wondered at length if "life's hard blows" were the cause of paranoia later in life. However, after much debate whether paranoia was due to life's exigencies (personal and social) or degeneracy (hereditary in origin), he opted for degeneracy.

49. Some examples would include Eugen Bleuler (1857–1939), Theodor Ziehen (1852–1950), and Oskar Vogt (1870–1959).

50. Schilpp, 1957, p. 16.

51. Emil Kraepelin [1917], *One Hundred Years of Psychiatry*, trans. W. Baskin. New York: Citadel Press, 1962, pp. 117, 150.

52. Which was itself a reaction to brutal imprisonments and the almost universal stigma of madness and social rejection of the mentally ill.

53. Josef Breuer and Sigmund Freud [1895], *Studies on Hysteria*, in *The Standard Edition of the Complete Psychological Works of Sigmund Freud*, Vol. II., ed. and trans. James Strachey, Anna Freud, Alix Strachey, and Anna Tyson. London: Hogarth Press, 1955, p. 305.

Chapter 3

1. Robert A. Woodruff, Donald W. Goodwin, Samuel B. Guze, *Psychiatric Diagnosis*. New York: Oxford University Press, 1974, pp. ix–x. The author (Goodwin) continued: these terms "are sometimes invoked by physicians to explain the unexplained. They usually mean 'I don't know,' and we try to avoid them." This included psychoanalytic etiologies such as "unconscious conflict."

2. W. Mayer-Gross, Eliot Slater, Martin Roth, *Clinical Psychiatry*. London: Cassell and Company, 1954.

3. E. T. O. Slater, "Obituary: W. Mayer-Gross, M.D., F.R.C.P.," *British Medical Journal*, Vol. 1 (5225), Feb. 25, 1961, p. 596.

4. Does Mayer-Gross make this analogy because he would argue that in both instances the physician is doing it because he or she has no effective treatment?

5. Samuel B. Guze, "The Need for Toughmindedness in Psychiatric Thinking," *Southern Medical Journal*, Vol. 63, June 1970, pp. 662–671.

6. Guze, p. 670.

7. Lee Robnis carried out "longitudinal studies of psychopathology, beginning with a land-mark study of sociopathy. [She devised] sophisticated survey instruments that were to become world-wide standards [and conducted] epidemiologic studies that would serve the field of genetics as well." Richard W. Hudgens, "The Turning of American Psychiatry," *Missouri Medicine*, Vol. 90, No. 6, 1993, p. 288.

8. David Healy, *The Psychopharmacologists III: Interviews*. London: Arnold; New York: Oxford University Press, 2000, p. 399.

9. Telephone interview with Nancy Andreasen, M.D., February 17, 2012.

10. Paula J. Clayton, "Training at the Washington University School of Medicine in Psychiatry in the late 1950's, from the Perspective of an Affective Disorder Researcher," *Journal of Affective Disorders*, Vol. 92, 2006, pp. 13–17. Paula Clayton went on to become the first female chair of a department of psychiatry.

11. John P. Feighner, "The Advent of the Feighner Criteria. This Week's Citation Classic," *Current Contents*, No. 43, Oct. 23, 1989, p. 14. Lithium is used to treat mania.

12. Kenneth S. Kendler, Rodrigo A. Munoz, and George Murphy, "The Development of the Feighner Criteria: A Historical Perspective," *American Journal of Psychiatry*, Vol. 167, No. 2, Feb. 2010, pp. 134–142.

13. Kendler et al., p. 136.

14. John P. Feighner, Eli Robins, Samuel B. Guze, Robert A. Woodruff, Jr., George Winokur, and Rodrigo Munoz, "Diagnostic Criteria for Use in Psychiatric Research," *Archives of General Psychiatry*, Vol. 26, Jan. 1972, pp. 57–63.

15. Feighner, "The Advent of the Feighner Criteria," p. 14.

16. Roger K. Blashfield, "Feighner et al., Invisible Colleges, and the Matthew Effect," *Schizophrenia Bulletin*, Vol. 8, No. 1, 1982, pp. 1–2.

17. Eli Robins and Samuel B. Guze, "Establishment of Diagnostic Validity in Psychiatric Illness: Its Application to Schizophrenia," *American Journal of Psychiatry*, Vol. 126, No. 7, Jan. 1970, pp. 983–987.

18. Robins and Guze, pp. 983–987.

19. Robins and Guze, p. 983. Three years before publication of this paper, Robins published an early attempt to establish operational criteria in a personality disorder. See Eli Robins, "Antisocial and Dyssocial Personality Disorders," in Alfred M. Freedman and Harold I.Kaplan (eds.), *Comprehensive Textbook of Psychiatry*. Baltimore: Williams & Wilkins, 1967, pp. 951–958. For the idea that Kraepelin himself was primarily a diagnostic clinician rather than a classifier (nosologist) see Eric J. Engstrom and Matthias M. Weber, "The Directions of Psychiatric Research: Introduction," *History of Psychiatry*, Vol. 16, 2005, pp. 345–364.

20. Feighner et al., "Diagnostic Criteria for Use in Psychiatric Research," p. 57.

21. American Psychiatric Association, Committee on Nomenclature and Statistics, *Diagnostic and Statistical Manual of Mental Disorders* (2nd ed.; DSM-II), 1968.

22. Feighner et al., "Diagnostic Criteria for Use in Psychiatric Research," p. 57.

23. Donald W. Goodwin, Samuel B. Guze, and Eli Robins, "Follow-Up Studies in Obsessional Neurosis," *Archives of General Psychiatry*, Vol. 20, Feb. 1969, pp. 182–187. See also Samuel B. Guze, "The Role of Follow-up Studies: Their Contribution to Diagnostic Classification as Applied to Hysteria," *Seminars in Psychiatry*, Vol. 2, No. 4, Nov. 1970, pp. 392–402.

24. Eli Robins and Samuel B. Guze, "Classification of Affective Disorders: The Primary-Secondary, the Endogenous-Reactive, and the Neurotic-Psychotic Concepts," *Recent Advances in the Psychobiology of the Depressive Illnesses: Proceedings of a Workshop*, 1972, pp. 283–293.

25. Feighner et al., "Diagnostic Criteria for Use in Psychiatric Research," p. 57.

26. The quotation from Scott appeared in both Donald W. Goodwin, Preface, in Robert Woodruff, Donald W. Goodwin, and Samuel B. Guze, *Psychiatric Diagnosis*. New York and Oxford: Oxford University Press, 1974, p. x, and Goodwin et al., "Follow-Up Studies in Obsessional Neurosis," p. 182.

27. Woodruff et al., *Psychiatric Diagnosis*.

28. Woodruff et al., *Psychiatric Diagnosis*, p. ix.

29. Nevertheless, as we shall see, personality diagnoses found their way into the DSM-III on Axis II in the multiaxial system introduced in DSM-III.

30. Healy, Vol. III, p. 407.

31. Feighner et al., "Diagnostic Criteria for Use in Psychiatric Research," p. 59. The illnesses covered by Feighner, et al. were depression, mania, secondary affective disorder, schizophrenia, anxiety neurosis, obsessive compulsive neurosis, phobic neurosis, hysteria, antisocial personality disorder, alcoholism, drug dependence (excluding alcoholism), mental

retardation, organic brain syndrome, homosexuality, transsexualism, anorexia nervosa, and undiagnosed psychiatric illness, pp. 58–62.

32. Healy, Vol. III, p. 408.

33. Feighner et al., "Diagnostic Criteria for Use in Psychiatric Research," p. 62; Feighner, "The Advent of the Feighner Criteria," pp. 1173–1174. On his own, Feighner later discussed a six-stage diagnostic model that included treatment outcome studies.

  A clear summary of the beliefs of the Wash. U. psychiatrists is provided in a short article written by Robins for internists and family doctors: Eli Robins, "New Concepts in the Diagnosis of Psychiatric Disorders," *Annual Review of Medicine*, Vol. 28, 1977, pp. 67–73.

34. Kendler et al., pp. 136–138.

35. Gerald L. Klerman, "The Evolution of a Scientific Nosology," in John C. Shershow (ed.) *Schizophrenia: Science and Practice*, Cambridge, MA: Harvard University Press, 1978, pp. 104 ff.

36. E-mail from Robert Hirschfeld, M.D., November 25, 2008.

37. See Gerald L. Klerman, Myrna M. Weissman, Bruce J. Rounsaville, and Eve S. Chevron, *Interpersonal Psychotherapy of Depression*. New York: Basic Books, 1984; also Myrna M. Weissman, "A Brief History of Interpersonal Psychotherapy," *Psychiatric Annals*, Vol. 36, No. 8, Aug. 2006, pp. 553–557.

38. Gerald L. Klerman, *Hastings Center Report*, Vol. 2, No. 4, Sept. 1972, pp. 1–3.

39. David Healy, *The Psychopharmacologists, II: Interviews*. London: Chapman and Hall, 1998, interview with Myrna Weissman, Klerman's co-worker and later wife, pp. 521–542; Hannah S. Decker, personal interview with Robert M. A. Hirschfeld, M.D. (b. 1943), March 2008. Hirschfeld was Klerman's protégé and co-worker and is now Chair of the Department of Psychiatry at the University of Texas Medical Branch in Galveston.

40. George Winokur, Paula J. Clayton, Theodore Reich, *Manic Depressive Illness*. Saint Louis: C.V. Mosby, 1969.

41. Winokur et al., *Manic Depressive Illness*, pp. 145–146

42. Healy, Vol. III, p. 405. Robert Spitzer at the time refused the label altogether. See "Letters to the Editor," *Schizophrenia Bulletin*, Vol. 8, No. 4, 1982, p. 592.

43. Klerman, "The Evolution of a Scientific Nosology," pp. 104–105. In the discussion that followed the presentation of his paper Klerman added: "Very few of the investigations I have mentioned are personally interested in, or willing to entertain, on principle, a developmental or psychogenic causation to the major psychoses.... The neo-Kraepelinians ... are just vitriolic about [developmental causation]." Klerman, p. 118.

44. Eugene Garfield, "A Tribute to Eli and Lee Robins—Citation Superstars. A Citationist Perspective on Biological Psychiatry," *Current Comments*, No. 46, Nov. 13, 1989, p. 321.

45. Kendler et al., p. 135.

46. Guze incorrectly said that Robins' analysis was with Hanns Sachs. See Healy, Vol. III, p. 398, interview with Guze. Both Hudgens (p. 288) and a psychiatrist at McGill University in Montreal, Joel Paris, state that Robins had a year's analysis with Helene Deutsch. See Joel Paris, *The Fall of an Icon: Psychoanalysis and Academic Psychiatry*. Toronto: University of Toronto Press, 2005, p. 76.

47. Paris, p. 76. Hudgens (p. 288) says Robins told him "the [analytic] process was useless."

48. Cohen was right about a physical diagnosis but probably was wrong about the actual diagnosis. See Mandel Cohen's remarks at the memorial service for Robins, February 4, 1995, "In Memoriam and Memorial Service," *Annals of Clinical Psychiatry*, Vol. 7, No. 1, March 1995, p. 3.

Joel Paris, a Canadian psychiatrist, tells a different version of what seems to be the same basic story: As a medical student, Robins had developed a paralysis and was hospitalized. A psychoanalyst-consultant said Robins was suffering from hysteria. But a psychiatrist working in the neurology department, Mandel Cohen, did not agree. Paris deduces that Robins was actually showing the first symptoms of MS. Paris gives no source for the story, but it may have come from either Richard Hudgens, a former Wash. U. psychiatrist, or Robert Cloninger, a former chair of the psychiatric department at Washington University. Guze, in his interview with David Healy, said that in retrospect he thought the episode was the beginning of Robins' MS.

49. Cohen, p. 3. Paula Clayton, who trained under Robins at Washington University, thinks it possible that Cohen's stand against a psychological explanation of Robins' paralysis may also have turned Robins away from analytic training. Hannah S. Decker, personal interview with Paula Clayton, January 29, 2007.

50. W. B. Kannel, T. R. Dawber, and M. E. Cohen, "The Electrocardiogram in Neurocirculatory Asthenia (Anxiety Neurosis or Neurasthenia): A Study of 203 Neurocirculatory Asthenia Patients and 757 Healthy Controls in the Framingham Study," *Annals of Internal Medicine*, Vol. 49, 1959, pp. 1351–1360. Another data-driven study was W. L. Cassidy, N. B. Flanagan, M. Spellman, and M. E. Cohen, "Clinical Observations in Manic-Depressive Disease: Quantitative Study of One Hundred Manic-Depressive Patients and Fifty Medically Sick Controls," *JAMA: Journal of the American Medical Association*, Vol. 164, 1957, pp. 1535–1546.

51. Cohen had graduated from Yale in 1927 and then finished Johns Hopkins Medical School in 1931.

52. Charles L. Rich, "Editorial: Swan Song," *Annals of Clinical Psychiatry*, Vol. 15, Nos. 3/4, September/December 2003, p. 143. Other information in this section of Chapter 3 also comes from Rich, pp. 143–144.

53. Winifred (Dia) Hamlen Black, granddaughter, "In Memoriam—Mandel E. Cohen," *Annals of Clinical Psychiatry*, Vol. 15, Nos. 3/4, September/December 2003, p.158.

54. Maurice Victor, M.D., neurologist, in Black, p. 151.

55. Black, p. 151.

56. Sheehan quoted in Healy, Vol. III, p. 498.

57. Healy, Vol. III, p. 499.

58. Hannah S. Decker, "Operational Criteria," unpublished paper. It has long been thought that Cohen got his ideas from his work with Paul Dudley White (1886–1973), the famous cardiologist. But this does not seem as probable as Cohen imbibing Bridgman's thought directly. It is possible that White was influenced by Bridgman at the same time. White and Bridgman were contemporaries, both men being in their forties when Bridgman's notions began to achieve popularity.

59. P. W. Bridgman, *The Logic of Modern Physics*. New York: Macmillan, 1932.

60. Bridgman, pp. 4–6.

61. David Healy, "Mandel Cohen and the Origins of the Diagnostic and Statistical Manual of Mental Disorders, Third Edition: DSM-III," *History of Psychiatry*, Vol. 13, 2007, pp. 210–215.

62. Telephone conversation with Anne Cohen, M.D., Mandel Cohen's daughter, also a psychiatrist, March 11, 2012.

63. Healy, Vol. III, pp. 500–501.

64. James J. Purtell, Eli Robins, and Mandel E. Cohen, "Observations on Clinical Aspects of Hysteria: A Quantitative Study of 50 Hysteria Patients and 156 Control

Subjects," *JAMA: Journal of the American Medical Association,* Vol. 146, July 7, 1951, pp. 902–909.

65. Purtell et al., p. 902.

66. Purtell et al., p. 909. The paper was reported in *Time,* although the magazine focused on just one aspect of the paper, that the authors had found that hysteria was a different illness in men than in women. "It's Different in Men," *Time,* Monday, June 9, 1952.

67. Eli Robins, *The Final Months: A Study of the Lives of 134 Persons Who Committed Suicide.* New York, Oxford: Oxford University Press, 1981.

68. Paris, p. 76; Hudgens, p. 287.

69. Healy, Vol. III, p. 402.

70. Rich, "Editorial: Swan Song," p. 143.

71. Richard W. Hudgens in C. Robert Cloninger (ed.) "In Memoriam—Samuel Barry Guze (October 18, 1923-July 19, 2000)," *Annals of Clinical Psychiatry,* Vol. 13, No. 1, March 2001, p. 4.

72. Samuel B. Guze, "In Memoriam and Memorial Service Eli Robins February 22, 1921-December 21, 1994," *Annals of Clinical Psychiatry,* Vol. 7, No. 1, March 1995, p. 7.

73. Samuel B. Guze, Oral History Project of the Washington University School of Medicine, 1994, Interview 4. http://beckerexhibits.wustl.edu/oral/transcripts/guze1994.html

74. Personal interview with Robert Spitzer, June 2, 2006.

75. Hudgens, p. 290.

76. Eli Robins' work on antisocial personality disorder drew from Lee Nelken Robins' work on the epidemiology of sociopathic personality. See Lee N. Robins, *Deviant Children Grown Up: A Sociological and Psychiatric Study of Sociopathic Personality.* Baltimore: Williams & Wilkins, 1966.

77. Eli Robins, "Antisocial and Dyssocial Personality Disorders," pp. 951–958; Marcel T. Saghir and Eli Robins, "Homosexuality: I. Sexual Behavior of the Female Homosexual," *Archives of General Psychiatry,* Vol. 20, Feb. 1969, pp. 192–201; Saghir and Robins, "Homosexuality: II. Sexual Behavior of the Male Homosexual," *Archives of General Psychiatry,* Vol. 21, Aug. 1969, pp. 220, 227; Eli Robins, 1981.

78. R. L. Spitzer, J. Endicott, E. Robins, J. Kuriansky, and B. Gurland, "Preliminary Report of the Reliability of Research Diagnostic Criteria Applied to Psychiatric Case Records," In A. Sudilovsky, S. Gershon, and B. Beer (eds.), *Predictability in Psychopharmacology: Preclinical and Clinical Correlations.* New York: Raven Press, 1975, pp. 1–47.

79. Garfield, "A Tribute to Eli and Lee Robins," 1989, pp. 321–329.

80. Personal interview with Robert L. Spitzer, M.D., June 2, 2006. For the history of the study, its description, and its goals see Martin M. Katz and Gerald L. Klerman [co-chairs of the NIMH-Clinical Research Branch Collaborative Program on the Psychobiology of Depression] "Introduction: Overview of the Clinical Studies Program," *American Journal of Psychiatry,* Vol. 136, No. 1, Jan. 1979, pp. 49–51. The program started in 1969.

81. Healy, Vol. III, p. 404.

82. Kendler et al., p. 139.

83. Interview with Paula J. Clayton, M.D., January 29, 2007.

84. Guze, 1994. In addition to this Washington University School of Medicine Oral History Project, see C. Robert Cloninger, ed., "In Memoriam—Samuel Barry Guze (October 18, 1923–July 19, 2000)," *Annals of Clinical Psychiatry,* Vol. 13, No. 1, 2001, pp. 1–10.

85. Healy, Vol. III, p. 396, and Hudgens, p. 288.

86. Healy, Vol. III, p. 396.

87. Kendler et al., p. 135.

88. Healy, Vol. III, p. 396.

89. Healy, Vol. III, p. 400.

90. Healy, Vol. III, pp. 399–400. It is possible that the Wash. U. psychiatrists coached their residents in this way because Mandel Cohen also had prepared the neurology residents at Harvard how to pass the psychiatry part of their boards at a time of psychoanalytic dominance. Robins may have carried the custom to Washington University. Telephone conversation with Anne Cohen, M.D., March 11, 2012.

91. Guze, 1994.

92. Hudgens, p. 287.

93. Hudgens, p. 289.

94. Healy, Vol. III, p. 400.

95. Joel Paris attributes this anecdote to Robert C. Cloninger, former Chair of the Department of Psychiatry at Washington. University. See Paris p. 78.

96. Guze, 1994. Yet they still had a long way to go. Guze recalled that before Robins became chair, "a senior person at the NIMH came to tell [Gildea] what a bad impression his department was getting because of the way Winokur, Robins and Guze were turning things."

97. Quantification and assessment of the severity of a patient's illness was formally made a part of DSM-III in Axis V of the multiaxial system.

98. Gerald L. Klerman, "Historical Perspectives on Contemporary Schools of Psychopathology," In Theodore Millon and Gerald L. Klerman (eds.), *Contemporary Directions in Psychopathology: Toward the DSM-IV*. New York and London: Guilford Press, 1986, p. 14.

99. Guze, 1994. Medical students interested in psychiatry were told by psychoanalysts to beware of Washington University.

100. Personal interview, January 26, 2007. Klein also came to the conclusion that his second analyst was a "dishonest fool." Personal e-mail from Klein, February 6, 2007.Without much more detailed information it is impossible to know who might have had a dogmatic and rigid analyst or who might have fled from psychoanalysis because of an unworked-through negative transference or some other transferential situation.

101. Allen Frances, Chair of the Task Force for DSM-IV and former chair of the psychiatry department at Duke University; Shervert H. Frazier, Director of the NIMH, 1984–1986, and former psychiatrist in chief, McLean Hospital; Daniel X. Freedman, Editor of the *Archives of General Psychiatry*, 1970–1990; John Gunderson, expert in both biological and psychodynamic aspects of borderline personality disorders; Thomas H. McGlashan, Director, Yale Psychiatric Institute; and Herbert Pardes, Director of the NIMH, 1977–1984, and President and CEO of the New York Presbyterian Hospital and New York Presbyterian Healthcare System. See Paris, pp. 121, 123–124, 128–131.

102. Paul Harris, "Obituary: Dr. Samuel B. Guze," *Psychiatric Bulletin*, Vol. 25, 2001, pp. 77–78.

103. Guze, 1994.

104. Michael J. Perley and Samuel B. Guze, "Hysteria—The Stability and Usefulness of Clinical Criteria: A Quantitative Study Based on a Follow-up Period of Six to Eight Years in 39 Patients," *New England Journal of Medicine*, Vol. 266, No. 9, March 1, 1962, pp. 421–426; O. Arkonac and S. B. Guze, " A Family Study of Hysteria," *New England Journal of Medicine*, Vol. 268, 1963, pp. 239–242; P. D. Gatfield and S. B. Guze, "The

Prognosis and Differential Diagnosis of Conversion Reactions: A Follow-up Study," *Diseases of the Nervous System*, Vol. 23, 1963, pp. 623–631; Samuel B. Guze and Michael J. Perley, "Observations on the Natural History of Hysteria," *American Journal of Psychiatry*, Vol. 119, 1963, pp. 960–965; Samuel B. Guze, "The Diagnosis of Hysteria: What Are We Trying to Do?" *American Journal of Psychiatry*, Vol. 124, 1967, pp. 491–498. Note that two of this series of papers were published in *New England Journal of Medicine*, the highly respected and widely read journal of general medicine.

105. Eugene H. Rubin, Charles F. Zorumski, and Samuel B. Guze, "Somatoform Disorders," in Theodore Millon and Gerald L. Klerman (eds.), *Contemporary Directions in Psychopathology: Toward the DSM-IV*. New York and London: Guilford Press, 1986.

106. Wilson M. Compton and Samuel B. Guze, "The Neo-Kraepelinian Revolution in Psychiatric Diagnosis," *European Archives of Psychiatry and Clinical Neuroscience*, Vol. 245, No. 4–5, 1995, pp. 196–201. Compton had gone to medical school and served his residency at Washington University. He was on the faculty of the psychiatry department at Washington University before moving to the National Institute on Drug Abuse at the National Institutes of Health (NIH) in Bethesda.

107. The main things Spitzer remembers about Guze is that he always looked "kind of stern" and was "always talking about [the] medical model." Personal interview with Robert Spitzer, June 2, 2006.

108. Samuel B. Guze, *Why Psychiatry Is a Part of Medicine*. New York: Oxford University Press, 1992, pp. 84–113.

109. Guze, pp. 80–83. Guze had been thinking of this for many years. See Samuel B. Guze and George E. Murphy. "An Empirical Approach to Psychotherapy: The Agnostic Position," *American Journal of Psychiatry*, Vol. 120, 1963, pp. 53–57.

110. Obviously, he no longer felt offended by Klerman's "neo-Kraepelinian" label.

111. Compton and Guze, 1995, p. 196.

112. Paula J. Clayton, "George Winokur: A Personal Memoir," *Journal of Affective Disorders*, Vol. 50, 1998, p. 77. See also Ming T. Tsuang, "Images in Psychiatry, George Winokur, M.D. 1925–1996," *American Journal of Psychiatry*, Vol. 156, March 1999, pp. 465–466. Tsuang says Winokur was born in Philadelphia.

113. Samuel B. Guze, "Obituary for George Winokur, MD, 1925–1996," *Archives of General Psychiatry*, Vol. 54, June 1997, pp. 574–575.

114. Guze, pp. 574–575.

115. Hudgens, 1993, p. 289.

116. George Winokur and Ming T. Tsuang, *The Natural History of Mania, Depression, and Schizophrenia*. Washington DC: American Psychiatric Press, 1996.

117. Tsuang, pp. 465–466.

118. Samuel B. Guze, "Validating Criteria for Psychiatric Diagnosis: The Washington University Approach," in Hagop S. Akiskal, et al. (eds.) *Psychiatric Diagnosis: Exploration of Biological Predictors*. Richmond, Australia: Spectrum Publications, 1978, pp. 47–59. Guze's chapter is an unusually helpful synthesis of the philosophy and work of the Department of Psychiatry at Washington University, emphasizing the necessity of the medical model in psychiatry, the vital role of diagnosis, and the lack of studies on the role of the "psychosocial" etiology of psychiatric illness.

119. Clayton is currently Medical Director of the American Foundation for Suicide Prevention.

120. George Winokur and Paula J. Clayton, "Family History Studies I: Two Types of Affective Disorders Separated According to Genetic and Clinical Factors," in J. Wortis (ed.), *Recent Advances in Biological Psychiatry*. New York: Plenum Press, 1967.

121. Winokur et al., *Manic Depressive Illness*, 1969.

122. George Winokur and F. N. Pitts, Jr., "Affective Disorder: I. Is Reactive Depression an Entity?" *Journal of Nervous and Mental Disease*, Vol. 138, 1964, pp. 541–547; Robert Woodruff, F. N. Pitts, Jr., and George Winokur, "Affective Disorder: II. A Comparison of Patients with Endogenous Depressions with and without Family History of Affective Disorder," *Journal of Nervous and Mental Disease*, Vol. 139, 1964, pp. 49–52; George Winokur and F. N. Pitts, Jr., "Affective Disorder: V. The Diagnostic Validity of Depressive Reactions," *Psychiatric Quarterly*, Vol. 39, 1965, pp. 727–728; George Winokur and F. N. Pitts, Jr., "Affective Disorder: VI. A Family History Study of Prevalence, Sex Differences, and Possible Genetic Factors," *Journal of Psychiatric Research*, Vol. 3, 1965, pp. 113–123.

123. George Winokur and E. Holemon, "Chronic Anxiety Neurosis: Clinical and Sexual Aspects," *Acta Psychiatrica Scandinavia*, Vol. 39, 1963, pp. 384–412; M. A. Stewart, F. Drake, and G. Winokur, "Depression Among Medically Ill Patients," *Diseases of the Nervous System*, Vol. 26, 1965, pp. 479–484.

124. George Winokur and Paula J. Clayton, "Family History Studies: II. Sex Differences in Primary Affective Illness," *British Journal of Psychiatry*, Vol. 113, 1967, pp. 973–979.

125. George Winokur, "Genetic Findings and Methodological Considerations in Manic Depressive Disease," *British Journal of Psychiatry*, Vol. 117, 1970, pp. 267–274; George Winokur and Theodore Reich, "Two Genetic Factors in Manic Depressive Disease," *Comprehensive Psychiatry*, Vol. 11, 1970, pp. 93–99.

126. George Winokur, "The Types of Affective Disorders," *Journal of Nervous and Mental Disease*, Vol. 156, 1973, pp. 83–96.

127. G. Winokur, R. Cadoret, J. Dorzab, et al., "Depressive Disease, a Genetic Study," *Archives of General Psychiatry*, Vol. 24, 1971, pp. 135–144; R. Cadoret, G. Winokur, J. Dorzab, et al., "Depressive Disease: Life Events and Onset of Illness," *Archives of General Psychiatry*, Vol. 26, 1972, pp. 133–136; G. Winokur and J. Morrison, "The Iowa 500: Followup of 225 Depressives," *British Journal of Psychiatry*, Vol. 123, 1973, pp. 543–548; George Winokur, "Division of Depressive Illness into Depresive Spectrum Disease and Pure Depressive Disease," *International Pharmakopsychiatrie*, Vol. 9, 1974, pp. 5–13; George Winokur, "Genetic and Clinical Factors Associated with Course in Depression," *Pharmakopsychiatrie Neuro-Psychopharmakologie*, Vol. 7, 1974, pp. 122–126; G. Winokur, R. Cadoret, et al., "Depressive Spectrum Disease vs Pure Depressive Disease: Some Further Data," *British Journal of* Psychiatry, Vol. 127, 1975, pp. 75–77; V. Tanna, G. Winokur, R. Elston, et al., "A Linkage Study of Depression Spectrum Disease: The Use of the Sib-Pair Method," *Neuropsychobiology*, Vol. 2, 1976, pp. 52–62.

128. George Winokur, "Unipolar Depression: Is It Divisible Into Autonomous Subtypes?" *Archives of General Psychiatry*, Vol. 36, No. 1, 1979, pp. 47–52.

129. George Winokur, Mark Zimmerman, and Remi Cadoret, "'Cause the Bible Tells Me So,'" *Archives of General Psychiatry*, Vol. 45, July 1988, pp. 683–684.

130. This is an example of the cyclical nature of psychiatry where once denigrated ideas return to favor. Here the judgment of the clinician, not just data-based evidence, plays a role in diagnosis.

131. Winokur, Zimmerman, and Cadoret, p. 684.

132. Winokur, Zimmerman, and Cadoret, p. 684. In response to Winokur's paper, even Spitzer back-pedaled from earlier positions, as will become obvious later in this work: "Diagnostic criteria can be interpreted very differently by different clinicians. DSM-III did not solve the problem of diagnostic reliability—it only improved it somewhat." E-mail from Robert L. Spitzer to Hannah S. Decker, December 3, 2006.

Chapter 4

1. Martin M. Katz and Gerald L. Klerman, "Introduction: Overview of the Clinical Studies Program," *American Journal of Psychiatry*, Special Section: The Psychobiology of Depression—NIMH-Clinical Research Branch Collaborative Program, Vol. 136, No. 1, January 1979, p. 49.
2. Katz and Klerman, p. 49.
3. Katz and Klerman, p. 50.
4. Interview with Robert L. Spitzer, June 2, 2006.
5. Robert L. Spitzer and Jean Endicott, "DIAGNO, a Computer Program for Psychiatric Diagnosis Utilizing the Differential Diagnostic Procedure," *Archives of General Psychiatry*, Vol. 18, 1968, pp. 746–756.
6. Jean Endicott, Robert L. Spitzer, J. L. Fleiss, and J. Cohen, "The Global Assessment Scale: A Procedure for Measuring Overall Severity of Psychiatric Disturbance," *Archives of General Psychiatry*, Vol. 33, 1976, pp. 766–771; Jean Endicott and Robert L. Spitzer, "A Diagnostic Interview: The Schedule for Affective Disorders and Schizophrenia," *Archives of General Psychiatry*, Vol. 35, 1978, pp. 837–844.

   In later years Spitzer, in conjunction with other authors, would create a Structured Clinical Interview for most DSM-IV Disorders diagnoses (SCID-I) and SCID-II for DSM-IV Personality Disorders diagnoses.
7. The collaborative study on the psychobiology of depression is still in existence, and Endicott remains a part of it.
8. Thomas S. Kuhn, *The Structure of Scientific Revolutions*. Monograph in the *International Encyclopedia of Unified Science*. 1962. This can be hard to locate, so the usual source is the second edition published by the University of Chicago Press in 1970.
9. David Riesman, *The Lonely Crowd: A Study of the Changing American Character*. New Haven: Yale University Press, 1950.
10. This information is in Riesman, *Faces in the Crowd: Individual Studies in Character and Politics*, in collaboration with Nathan Glazer. Abridged edition. New Haven: Yale University Press, 1965.
11. Jack Drescher, "An Interview with Robert L. Spitzer," *Journal of Gay and Lesbian Psychotherapy*, Vol. 7, No. 3, 2003, p. 104.
12. A name Spitzer today finds an anomaly since his father, as we shall see, was far from a worshipper of royalty. My own investigations into the matter are inconclusive. The only seeming explanation, yet unlikely, is that Spitzer was named after King Leopold II of Hungary (reigned 1790–1792), who granted a petition from the Jews there for equal treatment.
13. Telephone interview with Robert Spitzer, June 11, 2009.
14. Interview with Robert Spitzer, June 3, 2006.
15. Telephone interview with Louise Albert, July 7, 2009.
16. The New York Society for Ethical Culture was founded in 1876. Its chief supporters were Jews for whom traditional religion was not satisfying but who still wanted to join together to

353 Notes to pages 85–89

acknowledge and promote the importance of a secular moral life. It was an institution that had progressive and reformist agendas and was a strong supporter of social causes. An aim of the society, as set forth in its original charter, was to teach that morality is the highest ideal "above all human needs and interests." Ethical Culture societies continue to exist today.

17. Interview with Robert Spitzer, June 3, 2006.
18. Robert Spitzer, M.D., "DSM and Psychiatric Institute: A (Very) Personal History," Grand Rounds, New York State Psychiatric Institute (PI), January 6, 2006 (Transcript). Interestingly, Albert also remembers her brother getting this present, except she identifies this gift as a "chemistry set." One wonders why this incident stands out in her mind.
19. Telephone interview with Louise Albert, July 7, 2009.
20. Interview with Robert L. Spitzer, June 3, 2006.
21. Spitzer's declaration is in Riesman's *Faces in the Crowd*, p. 392.
    Without his parents' knowledge, Spitzer was being analyzed by a Reichian therapist who had him read Wilhelm Reich's *The Sexual Revolution* (1945), which preached the importance of sexual expression. (See Wilhelm Reich, *The Sexual Revolution*. 4th English Edition. Translated from the German by Theodore P. Wolfe. London: Peter Nevill, Vision Press, 1951.) The therapist also turned Spitzer against Soviet dogma.
22. Interview with Robert Spitzer, June 11, 2009.
23. Grand rounds, PI, January 6, 2006, and telephone interview with Louise Albert, July 7, 2009.
24. Riesman, *Faces in the Crowd*, p. 395.
25. Interview with Louise Albert, July 7, 2009.
26. Interview with Louise Albert, July 7, 2009.
27. Grand rounds, PI, January 6, 2006.
28. Telephone interview with Louise Albert, July 7, 2009.
29. Riesman, *Faces in the Crowd*, p. 351.
30. Riesman interview, *Faces in the Crowd*, p. 386.
31. Riesman, *Faces in the Crowd*, pp. 386–387. One may wonder whether this is only a rebellious act or also a display of emotional distancing, a trait that showed itself early in Spitzer's life and continued into adulthood. This is discussed in the following pages in more than one context.
32. Riesman, *Faces in the Crowd*, p. 387.
33. Riesman, *Faces in the Crowd*, p. 387.
34. Riesman, *Faces in the Crowd*, p. 387.
35. Riesman, *Faces in the Crowd*, p. 387.
36. NPR News, "All Things Considered," Profile: Effort by Robert Spitzer in 1974 to revise and update the *Diagnostic and Statistical Manual* for the American Psychiatric Association, and its impact on the understanding of human emotions. Reported by Alix Spiegel, August 18, 2003.
37. Interviews with Robert L. Spitzer, June 3, 2006, and June 11, 2009.
38. Riesman, *Faces in the Crowd*, p. 388.
39. Riesman, *Faces in the Crowd*, p. 353.
40. Riesman, *Faces in the Crowd*, p. 344.
41. Interview with Robert Spitzer, June 3, 2006. Wilhelm Reich, *The Function of the Orgasm*. New York: Farrar Straus & Giroux, 1973 [originally published in 1940.]
42. It is noteworthy that Spitzer told Alix Spiegel for a *New Yorker* article, the year before, that he had found Kronomeyer's approach "both soothing and invigorating....It greatly reduced [his] anxieties about his troubled family life....The sessions helped

him …'become alive.'" "Annals of Medicine. The Dictionary of Disorder: How One Man Revolutionized Psychiatry." *The New Yorker*, January 3, 2005.

43. Robert L. Spitzer, "Wilhelm Reich and Orgone Therapy: The Story of Robert L. Spitzer's Paper, 'An Examination of Wilhelm Reich's Demonstrations of Orgone Energy,'" *The Scientific Review of Mental Health Practice*, Vol. 4, No. 1, Spring-Summer, 2005; Grand Rounds, PI, January 6, 2006.

44. Telephone interview with Louise Albert, July 7, 2009.

45. Riesman, *Faces in the Crowd*, pp. 370–371.

46. Riesman, *Faces in the Crowd*, pp. 371–372.

47. Riesman, *Faces in the Crowd*, p. 369.

48. Riesman, *Faces in the Crowd*, p. 394.

49. Riesman, *Faces in the Crowd*, pp. 369 and 372.

50. Riesman, *Faces in the Crowd*, pp. 357, 376, 377.

51. Riesman, *Faces in the Crowd*, pp. 355 and 357.

52. Riesman, *Faces in the Crowd*, p. 357.

53. Riesman, *Faces in the Crowd*, p. 378.

54. Riesman, *Faces in the Crowd*, pp. 355, 358, 389.

55. Riesman, *Faces in the Crowd*, pp. 355 and 383.

56. Riesman, *Faces in the Crowd*, p. 378.

57. Riesman, *Faces in the Crowd*, pp. 395–396.

58. Telephone interview with Louise Albert, July 9, 2009.

59. Interview with Robert Spitzer, June 3, 2006.

60. In a *New Yorker* article of 2005, Alix Spiegel wrote that "the teen-age Spitzer had persuaded another Reichian doctor to give him free access to an orgone accumulator, and he spent many hours sitting hopefully on the booth's tiny stool.…" Alix Spiegel, "Annals of Medicine," 2005. But in an interview with him the very next year, Spitzer told me that he had sat in the booth only "a bit."

61. Wilhelm Reich, *The Discovery of the Orgone*. Vol II, *The Cancer Biopathy*. New York: Orgone Institute Press, 1948.

62. Spitzer's paper was entitled "An Examination of Wilhelm Reich's Demonstrations of Orgone Energy." The paper was published in 2005. See note 43.

63. Yale Kramer, Richard Rabkin, and Robert L. Spitzer, "Whirling as a Clinical Test in Childhood Schizophrenia," *Journal of Pediatrics*, Vol. 52, 1958, pp. 295–303.

   The other two medical-school papers were Robert L. Spitzer, Yale Kramer, and Richard Rabkin, "The Neck Righting Reflex in Children," *Journal of Pediatrics*, Vol. 52, 1958, pp. 149–151; Robert L. Spitzer, Richard Rabkin, and Yale Kramer, "The Relationship Between 'Mixed Dominance' and Reading Disabilities," *Journal of Pediatrics*, Vol. 54, 1959, pp. 76–80.

64. Robert L. Spitzer, "A Clinical Trial of Monosodium Glutamate (L-Glutavite) on Hospitalized Elderly Male Psychotic Patients," *American Journal of Psychiatry*, Vol. 115, April 1959, pp. 936–938.

65. Drescher, "An Interview with Robert L. Spitzer," p. 99.

66. Today, psychoanalysts no longer believe any analyst can remain a totally anonymous object. The analyst's very being and surroundings alone trumpet all manner of information about him- or herself. Analysis is regarded as a process whereby both the analysand and the analyst work together, each influencing the other in a myriad of

ways, all in the service of the analyst helping the patient to understand him- or herself better, moving toward the resolution of problems. Analysts call this joint effort "intersubjectivity."

67. Telephone interview, June 11, 2009.

68. Interview with Robert Spitzer, June 3, 2006.

69. Interview with Robert Spitzer, June 2, 2006.

70. Interview with Robert Spitzer, June 3, 2006. Bergler's book, *The Basic Neurosis, Oral Regression and Psychic Masochism* (New York: Grune and Stratton, 1949) spelled out his theory that our psyche is infused with unconscious masochism based on an unconscious willingness to continue to experience our negative emotions from childhood. See http://www.questforself.com/psychology_secret.html for a handy exegesis of Bergler's ideas.

71. Telephone interview, June 11, 2009.

72. Spiegel, "Annals of Medicine," January 3, 2005.

73. Interview with Spitzer, June 2, 2006.

74. Grand rounds, PI, January 6, 2006.

75. Interview with Robert Spitzer, June 2, 2006.

76. Robert L. Spitzer, "Images in Psychiatry," *American Journal of Psychiatry,* Vol. 158, July 2001, p. 1019.

77. Interview with Robert Spitzer, June 3, 2006.

78. Drescher, "Interview with Robert L. Spitzer," p. 99.

79. R. L. Spitzer, J. L. Fleiss, E. L. Burdock, and A. S. Hardesty, "The Mental Status Schedule: Rationale, Reliability and Validity." *Comprehensive Psychiatry,* Vol. 5, 1964, pp. 384–395; Robert L. Spitzer, "Mental Status Schedule: Potential Use as a Criterion Measure of Change in Psychotherapy Research," *American Journal of Psychotherapy,* Vol. 20, 1966, pp. 156–167; Robert L. Spitzer and Jean Endicott, " Assessment of Outcome by Independent Clinical Evaluators," in I. E. Waskow and M. B. Parloff (eds.), *Psychotherapy Change Measures: Report of the Clinical Research Branch Outcome Measures Project.* Rockville, MD: National Institutes of Mental Health, 1975, pp. 222–232.

80. Robert L. Spitzer and Jean Endicott, "DIAGNO: A Computer Program for Psychiatric Diagnosis Utilizing the Differential Diagnostic Procedure," *Archives of General Psychiatry,* Vol. 18, 1968, pp. 746–756; Robert L. Spitzer and Jean Endicott, "DIAGNO II: Further Developments in a Computer Program for Psychiatric Diagnosis," *American Journal of Psychiatry,* Vol. 125, January Supplement, 1969, pp. 12–21; Robert L. Spitzer and Jean Endicott, "Automation of Psychiatric Case Records: Boon or Bane?" *International Journal of Psychiatry,* Vol. 9, 1970, pp. 604–621; Robert L. Spitzer and Jean Endicott, "Automation of Psychiatric Case Records: Will It Help the Clinician?" *Diseases of the Nervous System,* GWAN Supplement, Vol. 31, 1970, pp. 45–46; Robert L. Spitzer and Jean Endicott, "An Integrated Group of Forms for Automated Psychiatric Case Records," *Archives of General Psychiatry,* Vol. 24, 1971, pp. 540–547; Robert L. Spitzer and Jean Endicott, "Computer Diagnosis in Automated Record-Keeping Systems: A Study of Clinical Acceptability," in J. Crawford, D. Morgan, and D. Gianturco (eds.), *Progress in Mental Health Information Systems: Computer Applications.* Cambridge: Ballinger, 1974, pp. 73–105; Robert L. Spitzer and Jean Endicott, "Can the Computer Assist Clinicians in Psychiatric Diagnosis?" *American Journal of Psychiatry,* Vol. 131, 1974, pp. 523–530.

81. Grand rounds, PI, January 6, 2006.

82. American Psychiatric Association, *DSM-II. Diagnostic and Statistical Manual of Mental Disorders.* Second Printing, Washington, DC, 1968. The guide to using the new

nomenclature was first published in the *American Journal of Psychiatry*, Vol. 124, No. 12, June 1968, pp. 1619–1629.

83. Karl Menninger, Martin Mayman, and Paul Pruyser, *The Vital Balance: The Life Process in Mental Health and Illness*. New York: Viking Press, 1964, pp. 9, 33.

84. Drescher, "Interview with Robert L. Spitzer," p. 102.

85. Grand rounds, PI, January 6, 2006.

86. Interview with Robert Spitzer, June 2, 2006.

87. "Biography of Dr. Theodore Millon." http://www.millon.net/content/tm_bio.htm.
    See also "A Blessed and Charmed Personal Odyssey," *Journal of Personality Assessment*, Vol. 79, No. 2, pp. 171–194, and S. Strack and W. Kinder (eds.), *Pioneers of Personality Science*. New York: Springer, 2006. It is impossible to tell how "central" Millon's role was, though Melvin Sabshin's autobiography (2008) discusses Millon's involvement. See *Changing American Psychiatry: A Personal Perspective*. Washington, DC: American Psychiatric Publishing.

88. Theodore Millon and Gerald Klerman (eds.), *Contemporary Directions in Psychopathology: Toward the DSM-IV*. New York, Guilford Press, 1986, p. 37.

89. Millon and Klerman, p. 38.

90. Donald Klein, quoted in Spiegel, "Annals of Medicine," 2005.

91. Interview with Robert Spitzer, June 2, 2006.

92. Interview with Robert Spitzer, June 2, 2006.

93. Grand rounds, PI, January 6, 2006.

94. Eli Robins and Samuel B. Guze, "Establishment of Diagnostic Validity in Psychiatric Illness: Its Application to Schizophrenia," *American Journal of Psychiatry*, Vol. 126, No. 7, January 1970, pp. 983–987; John P. Feighner, Eli Robins, Samuel B. Guze, Robert A. Woodruff, Jr., George Winokur, and Rodrigo Munoz, " Diagnostic Criteria for Use in Psychiatric Research," *Archives of General Psychiatry*, Vol. 26, January 1972, pp. 57–63. See Chapter 3 for further discussion.

95. Grand rounds, PI, January 6, 2006.

96. Telephone interview with Henry Pinsker, August 1, 2009.

97. Spiegel, NPR Profile, August 18, 2003.

98. Spiegel, "Annals of Medicine," January 3, 2005.

99. Spiegel, "Annals of Medicine," January 3, 2005

100. Interview with Robert Spitzer, June 3, 2006.

101. Grand rounds, PI, January 6, 2006.

102. Robert L. Spitzer, Principal Investigator, NIMH Contract #278–77–0022 (DB), DSM-III Field Trials, $93,286.00, September 19, 1977 to March 18, 1980.

103. Interview with Janet Williams, June 3, 2006.

104. Grand rounds, PI, January 6, 2006.

105. Robert L. Spitzer and Jean Endicott, "Computer Applications in Psychiatry," In Silvano Arieti (ed.), *American Handbook of Psychiatry*, Vol. VI, 2nd ed. New York: Basic Books, 1975, pp. 811–839; Robert L. Spitzer and Jean Endicott, "Psychiatric Rating Scales," in A. Freedman, H. Kaplan, and B. Sadock (eds.), *Comprehensive Textbook of Psychiatry*, Vol. II, 2nd ed. Baltimore: Williams & Wilkins, 1975, pp. 2015–2031; Jean Endicott, Robert L. Spitzer, J. L. Fleiss, and J. Cohen, "The Global Assessment Scale: A Procedure of Measuring Overall Severity of Psychiatric Disturbance," *Archives of General Psychiatry*, Vol. 33, 1976, pp. 766–771.

106. Robert L. Spitzer and P. T. Wilson, "Nosology and the Official Psychiatric Nomenclature," In A. Freedman, H. Kaplan, and B. Sadock (eds.), *Comprehensive Textbook of Psychiatry*, Vol. I, 2nd ed. Baltimore: Williams and Wilkins, 1975, pp. 826–845; Robert L. Spitzer, Jean Endicott, and Eli Robins, "Research Diagnostic Criteria," *Psychopharmacology Bulletin*, Vol. 11, 1975, pp. 22–25.

107. Robert L. Spitzer and Donald F. Klein (eds.), *Evaluation of Psychological Therapies: Psychotherapies, Behavior Therapies, Drug Therapies, and Their Interactions*. Baltimore: Johns Hopkins University Press, 1976; Jean Endicott, Robert L. Spitzer, J. L. Fleiss, and J. Cohen, "The Global Assessment Scale: A Procedure for Measuring Overall Severity of Psychiatric Disturbance," *Archives of General Psychiatry*, Vol. 33, 1976, pp. 766–771.

108. Robert L. Spitzer, "Letter to the Editor," *Schizophrenia Bulletin*, Vol. 8, No. 4, 1982, p. 592.

109. There is, of course, no diagnosis of Hallucinations. It is a symptom appearing in more than one diagnosis.

110. *Journal of Abnormal Psychology*, Vol. 84, 1975.

111. Interview with Robert L. Spitzer, June 2, 2006.

112. Robert L. Spitzer, "On Pseudoscience in Science, Logic in Remission and Psychiatric Diagnosis: A Critique of Rosenhan's 'On being Sane In Insane Places,'" *Journal of Abnormal Psychology*, Vol. 84, pp. 442–452. A further version appeared the following year: Robert L. Spitzer, "More on Pseudoscience in Science and the Case for Psychiatric Diagnosis: A Critique of D. L. Rosenhan's 'On being Sane in Insane Places,'" *Archives of General Psychiatry*, Vol. 33, April, 1976, pp. 459–470.

Chapter 5

1. Nancy C. Andreasen, "DSM and the Death of Phenomenology in America: An Example of Unintended Consequences," *Schizophrenia Bulletin Online*, 2006, p. 110. http://schizophreniabulletin.oxfordjournals.org/cgi/content/full/sb1054.

2. There is an amusing anecdote regarding the possibility of a single case being significant, which comes from V. S. Ramachandran, both a neurologist and psychologist, who directs the Center for Brain and Cognition at the University of California, San Diego: "Imagine I were to present a pig to a skeptical scientist, insisting it could speak English, then waved my hand, and the pig spoke English. Would it really make sense for the skeptic to argue, 'But that is just one pig, Ramachandran. Show me another, and I might believe you!'" Quoted in Norman Doidge, *The Brain that Changes Itself: Stories of Personal Triumph from the Frontiers of Brain Science*. New York: Viking Penguin, 2007, pp. 177–178.

3. Published in *JAMA: Journal of the American Medical Association*, Vol. 146, No. 10, July 7, 1951, pp. 902–909.

4. *JAMA*, Vol. 146, No. 10, 1951, p. 909.

5. Telephone interview with Nancy C. Andreasen, February 17, 2012.

6. Nancy C. Andreasen, *The Broken Brain: The Biological Revolution in Psychiatry*. New York: Harper & Row, 1984, p. 155.

7. Andreasen, p. 155.

8. Telephone interview with Andreasen, February 17, 2012.

9. Andreasen, "DSM and the Death of Phenomenology in America," p. 110.

10. Andreasen, "DSM and the Death of Phenomenology in America," p. 109.

11. Theodore Millon, "On the Past and Future of DSM-III: Personal Recollections and Projections," In Theodore Millon and Gerald L. Klerman (eds.), *Contemporary Directions in Psychopathology: Toward the DSM-IV*. New York and London: Guilford Press, 1986, p. 43.

12. Robert Spitzer and Michael Sheehy, "DSM-III: A Classification System in Development," *Psychiatric Annals*, Vol. 6, No. 9, Sept. 1976, p. 102. The theme of the entire issue of the journal was "Classification of Psychiatric Disorders."

13. Telephone interview with Henry Pinsker, August 31, 2009.

14. E-mail message from Nancy Andreasen, January 26, 2012.

15. E-mail message from Nancy Andreasen, January 26, 2012.

16. Telephone interview with Andreasen, February 17, 2012.

17. "Classification of Psychiatric Disorders," *Psychiatric Annals*, 1976, p. 39.

18. Theodore Millon, *Disorders of Personality, DSM-III: Axis II*. New York: John Wiley & Sons, 1981, p. viii.

19. Interview with Jean Endicott, January 26, 2007.

20. Interview with Jean Endicott, January 26, 2007.

21. Interview with Donald Klein, January 26, 2007.

22. Telephone interview with Allen Frances, June 28, 2010.

23. Robert L. Spitzer and Donald F. Klein (eds.), *Evaluation of Psychological Therapies: Psychotherapies, Behavior Therapies, Drug Therapies and Their Interactions*. Baltimore: Johns Hopkins University Press, 1976; Robert L. Spitzer and Donald F. Klein (eds.), *Critical Issues in Psychiatric Diagnosis*. New York: Raven Press, 1978.

24. Telephone interview with Henry Pinsker, August 31, 2009.

25. Donald F. Klein, "A Proposed Definition of Mental Illness," in Robert L. Spitzer and Donald Klein (eds.), *Critical Issues in Psychiatric Diagnosis*. New York: Raven Press, 1978, pp. 41–71.

26. Theodore Millon, "The DSM-III: An Insider's Perspective," *American Psychologist*, Vol. 38, No. 7, July 1983, and "On the Past and Future of DSM-III: Personal Recollections and Projections," *Contemporary Directions in Psychopathlogy: Toward DSM-IV*. 1986, passim.

27. Millon, *Disorders of Personality*, 1981, p. viii; Theodore Millon and Roger O. Davis, *Disorders of Personality: DSM-IV and Beyond* (2nd ed.). Oxford: John Wiley & Sons, 1996, p. xiii.

28. David Healy, *The Psychopharmacologists: Interviews*, Vol. I. London: Chapman & Hall, 1996, p. 343.

29. Interview with Donald F. Klein, January 26, 2007.

30. E-mail correspondence with Donald F. Klein, February 6, 2007. And a "complete idiot," he told David Healy, p. 347

31. Healy, Vol. I, p. 344. Freud also did not think psychoanalysis was suitable to treat schizophrenia. It was the analysts in the 1940s and 1950s who widened the scope of suitability, leaving themselves open to criticism. This expansion of treatment is discussed in Chapter 1.

32. Interview with Donald Klein, January 26, 2007.

33. Nancy C. Andreasen, *The Broken Brain: The Biological Revolution in Psychiatry*. New York: Harper & Row, 1984; Nancy C. Andreasen, *The Brave New Brain: Conquering Mental Illness in the Era of the Genome*. New York: Oxford University Press, 2001; Nancy C. Andreasen, *The Creating Brain: The Neuroscience of Genius*. New York: Dana Press, 2005.

34. The National Medal of Science is America's highest award for scientific achievement. Andreasen was recognized for her "integrative study of mind, brain, and behavior, by joining behavioral science with the techniques of neuroscience and neuroimaging in order

to understand mental processes such as memory, creativity, and mental illnesses such as schizophrenia." Wikipedia article on Nancy Coover Andreasen, http//en.wikipedia.org/ wiki/Nancy_Coover_Andreasen.

35. DSM-III, pp. 236–238.

36. Some information comes from Dr. Paula Clayton, who replaced Woodruff on the Task Force. She and Woodruff knew each other as medical students and psychiatric residents at Washington University. They were also fairly close because they lived near each other and drove to work together, their children played with each other, and the families socialized. Telephone interview with Paula Clayton, October 5, 2009.

37. Telephone interview with Paula Clayton, October 5, 2009.

38. Telephone interview with Nancy Andreasen, M.D., February 17, 2012.

39. Telephone interview with Paula Clayton, October 5, 2009.

40. We know Woodruff was still alive in March 1976 because he is listed as one of the Task Force members in the "Progress Report on the Preparation of DSM-III," p. 3.

41. Telephone interview with Dr. Henry Pinsker, August 31, 2009.

42. Personality disorders in DSM-III are Dependent, Histrionic, Narcissistic, Antisocial, Compulsive, Passive-Aggressive, Schizoid, Avoidant, Borderline, Paranoid, and Schizotypic. The list has been considerably narrowed in DSM-5, a move that has been the subject of much controversy.

43. Theodore Millon, "Personalized Assessment: Clinical Personality Instruments," http:// www.millon.net/content/instrumentation.htm. Millon says other people were misusing his ideas on personality so he was "driven" to do test construction himself.

44. Telephone interview with Henry Pinsker, August 31, 2009.

45. Telephone interview with Allen Frances, June 28, 2010. See also "Biography of Dr. Theodore Millon," under "Chicago Years (1969_1977)," http://www.millon.net/con-tent/tm_bio.htm.

46. Theodore Millon, "The DSM-III: An Insider's Perspective," *American Psychologist*, Vol. 38, No. 7, July 1983, p. 807.

47. Millon, "On the Past and Future of DSM-III," p. 60.

48. Theodore Millon, *Toward a New Personology: An Evolutionary Model.* New York: Wiley-Interscience, 1990.

49. Millon, "The DSM-III: An Insider's Perspective," p. 804.

50. Millon, " The DSM-III: An Insider's Perspective," p. 805.

51. Millon, *Disorders of Personality*, p. viii.

52. Telephone interview with Allen Frances, June 28, 2010.

53. Telephone interview with Henry Pinsker, August 31, 2009.

54. E-mail from Henry Pinsker, February 22, 2008.

55. Telephone interview with Henry Pinsker, August 31, 2009. See also "The Irrelevancy of Psychiatric Diagnosis or Psychiatric Diagnosis in the General Hospital," Unpublished paper presented at the Annual Meeting of the APA, May 1967, pp. 5 and 7.

56. Telephone interview with Henry Pinsker, August 31, 2009.

57. Henry Pinsker and Robert L. Spitzer, "Classification of Mental Disorders: DSM-III," in B. Wolman (ed.), *International Encyclopedia of Neurology, Psychiatry, Psychoanalysis, and Psychology*. New York: Van Nostrand, Reinhold, 1977.

58. Henry Pinsker, *A Primer of Supportive Psychotherapy*. Hillsdale, NJ: Analytic Press, 1997; Arnold Winston, Richard N. Rosenthal, and Henry Pinsker, *Introduction to Supportive Psychotherapy*. Washington, DC: American Psychiatric Publishing, 2004.

59. Millon, *Disorders of Personality*, p. viii.

60. Roland Atkinson, "Interview with George Saslow, M.D.," December 12, 2003. *Oregon Health Sciences University History Program, Oral History Project*, p. 4. Transcript on deposit in the library under call number W19 038 no. 90 2003.

61. "George Saslow, Ph.D., M.D., Academic Contributions," Oregon Health and Science University, 2004, http://www.ohsu.edu/psychiatry/faculty/saslow.htm. Also see transcript of interview with Roland Atkinson.

62. Jonas H. Ellenberg, "A Conversation with Morton Kramer," *Statistical Science*, Vol. 12, No. 2, May 1997, p. 103.

63. Morton Kramer, "Statistical Reporting," Section IV, pp. 52-72, and "Statistical Classifications of Mental Disorder," Section V, pp. 73-86. In American Psychiatric Association, *Diagnostic and Statistical Manual of Mental Disorders* (1st ed., *DSM-I*), Washington, DC, 1952; "Introduction: The Historical Background of ICD-8," "Statistical Tabulations," Section 4, pp. 53-63, and "Comparative Listing of Titles and Codes," Section 5, pp. 64-82. In American Psychiatric Association, *Diagnostic and Statistical Manual of Mental Disorders* (2nd ed., *DSM-II*). Washington, DC, 1968.

64. Telephone interview with Henry Pinsker, August 31, 2009.

65. Morton Kramer, "Some Problems for International Research suggested by Observations of Differences in First Admission Rates to Mental Hospitals of England and Wales and the United States," *Geriatrics*, Vol. 16, 1961, pp. 151-160.

66. Morton Kramer, "Cross-National Study of Diagnosis of Mental Disorders: Origin of the Problem," *American Journal of Psychiatry*, Vol. 25, Supplement, 1969, pp. 1-11.

67. Ellenberg, p. 106.

68. E-mail from Nancy C. Andreasen, January 26, 2012.

69. See Joshua B. Grossman, "Images in Psychiatry: Dennis Patrick Campbell, M.D., 1939-1997," *American Journal of Psychiatry*, Vol. 158, No. 4, April 2001, p. 546; James McCracken, "In Memoriam, Dennis P. Cantwell," Neuropsychiatric Institute UCLA, http://www.universityofcalifornia.edu/senate/inmemoriam/DennisP.Cantwell.htm; Peter E. Tanguay, "Dennis P. Cantwell, M.D. (1939-1997), Obituary," *Journal of the American Academy of Child and Adolescent Psychiatry*, Oct. 1, 1997.

70. Andreasen, "DSM and the Death of Phenomenology in America," p. 111.

Chapter 6

1. The issue of reliability is dealt with in some detail by Spitzer, Jean Endicott, and Eli Robins in "Clinical Criteria for Psychiatric Diagnosis and DSM-III," *American Journal of Psychiatry*, Vol. 132, 1975, pp. 1187-1192. They advocate achieving reliability through the use of diagnostic criteria.

2. For a full discussion see Robert L. Spitzer and Paul T. Wilson, "Nosology and the Official Psychiatric Nomenclature," in A. Freedman, H. Kaplan, and B. Sadock (eds.), *Comprehensive Textbook of Psychiatry* (2nd ed.). Baltimore: Williams & Wilkins, 1975, pp. 826-845.

3. Gerald Grob, "Origins of DSM-I: A Study in Appearance and Reality," *American Journal of Psychiatry*, Vol. 148, No. 4, April 1991, pp. 421-431.

4. Bénédict Augustin Morel, *Traité des Dégénérescences Physiques, Intellectuelles et Morales de l'Espèce Humaine*. Paris: J.B. Baillière, 1857.

5. This introductory section draws from the work of the historian of psychiatry German Berrios, in German E. Berrios and Roy Porter (eds.), *A History of Clinical Psychiatry: The*

Origin and History of Psychiatric Disorders. London and New Brunswick: Athalone Press, 1995. See the section on Mood Disorders in Chapter 15.

6. Emil Kraepelin, "The Manifestations of Insanity," Classic Text No. 12, transl. D. Beer, published in *History of Psychiatry*, Vol. 3, 1992 [1920], pp. 509–529. This article also appears as "Patterns of Mental Disorder," transl. H. Marshal. In S.R. Hirsch and M. Shepherd, *Themes and Variations in European Psychiatry*. Bristol: John Wright & Sons, pp. 7–30.

7. Today, the Massachusetts Mental Health Center.

8. Carl R. Doering and Alice F. Raymond, "Reliability of Observation in Psychiatric and Related Characteristics," *American Journal of Orthopsychiatry*, Vol. 4, 1934, pp. 249–257.

9. Doering and Raymond, p. 256.

10. Eliot Slater, "The Inheritance of Manic-Depressive Insanity," *Proceedings of the Royal Society of Medicine*, Vol. 29, Section of Psychiatry, February 11, 1936, pp. 981–990. Slater studied under Ernst Rudin (1874–1952), Kraepelin's choice of the genetics expert for his Psychiatric Institute in Munich. Slater was esteemed for his work in genetics—and by some for his advocacy of eugenics—and went on to co-author Mayer-Gross' psychiatry textbook so welcomed by the Wash. U. psychiatrists. Rudin, Slater's mentor, had a career as a geneticist and a proponent of eugenics and, later, "racial hygiene" under the Nazis. He had to flee for his life after World War II from the relatives of so-called genetically defective mental patients for whose murder his theories had provided "scientific" support.

11. Jules H. Masserman and Hugh T. Carmichael, "Diagnosis and Prognosis in Psychiatry: With a Follow-Up Study of the Results of Short-Term General Hospital Therapy of Psychiatric Cases," *Journal of Mental Science*, Vol. LXXXIV, No. 333, November, 1938, pp. 938–939.

12. Philip Ash, "The Reliability of Psychiatric Diagnosis," *Journal of Abnormal and Social Psychology*, Vol. 44, 1949, p. 275.

13. K. M. Colby, *An Introduction to Psychoanalytic Research*. New York: Basic Books, 1960.

14. B. Pasamanick, S. Dinitz, and M. Lefton, *American Journal of Psychiatry*, Vol. 116, 1959 (p. 127), quoted by Aaron T. Beck, "Reliability of Psychiatric Diagnoses: 1. A Critique of Systematic Studies," *American Journal of Psychiatry*, Vol. 119, 1962, pp. 210–216. See also W. A. Hunt, C. L. Wittson, and E. B. Hunt, "A Theoretical and Practical Analysis of the Diagnostic Process," in P. Hoch and J. Zubin (eds.), *Current Problems in Psychiatric Diagnosis*. New York: Grune & Stratton, 1953; G. A. Foulds, "The Reliability of Psychiatric, and the Validity of Psychological, Diagnosis," *Journal of Mental Science*, Vol. 7, Sept. 1956, pp. 1305–1312; V. Norris, *Mental Illness in London*, Maudsley Monographs, No. 6. London: Chapman and Hall, 1959; Seymour S. Kety, "The Academic Lecture: The Heuristic Aspects of Psychiatry," *American Journal of Psychiatry*, Vol. 118, 1961, pp. 385–397.

15. B. Mehlman, "Reliability of Psychiatric Diagnosis," *Journal of Abnormal and Social Psychology*, Vol. 47, 1952, pp. 577–578; R. L. Jenkins, *Journal of Clinical Psychology*, Vol. 9, 1953, p. 149; H. O. Schmidt and C. P. Fonda, "The Reliability of Psychiatric Prognosis," *Journal of Abnormal and Social Psychology*, Vol. 52, 1956, pp. 262–267; D. Bindra, "Experimental Psychology and the Problem of Behavior Disorders," *Canadian Journal of Psychology*, Vol. 13, 1959, pp. 135–150; P. Meehl, "Some Ruminations on the Validation of Clinical Procedures," *Canadian Journal of Psychology*, Vol. 13, 1959, pp. 102–128; Maurice Lorr, "Classification of the Behavior Disorders," *Annual Review of Psychology*, Vol. 12, 1961, pp. 195–216.

16. Aaron T. Beck, "Reliability of Psychiatric Diagnoses: 1. A Critique of Systematic Studies," *American Journal of Psychiatry*, Vol. 119, 1962, pp. 210–216.

17. A. T. Beck, C. H. Ward, M. Mendelson, J. E. Mock, and J. K. Erbaugh, "Reliability of Psychiatric Diagnoses: 2. A Study of Consistency of Clinical Judgments and Ratings," *American Journal of Psychiatry*, Vol. 119, 1962, pp. 351–357.

18. Interview with Paula Clayton, January 29, 2007. Dr. Clayton is a well-recognized expert in the fields of bipolar illnesses, bereavement, and suicide.

19. A. T. Beck, C. H. Ward, M. Mendelson, J. Mock, and J. Erbaugh, "An Inventory For Measuring Depression," *Archives of General Psychiatry*, Vol. 4, June 1961, pp. 561–571.

20. Martin M. Katz, Jonathan O. Cole, and Walter E. Barton (eds.), *The Role and Methodology of Classification in Psychiatry and Psychopathology*. Proceedings of a Conference held in Washington, DC, November 1965, under the Auspices of the American Psychiatric Association and the Psychopharmacology Research Branch of the National Institute of Mental Health. Public Health Service Publication No. 1584. Washington, DC: U.S. Government Printing Office, 1967.

21. Robert L. Spitzer, Jacob Cohen, Joseph L. Fleiss, and Jean Endicott, "Quantification of Agreement in Psychiatric Diagnosis: A New Approach," *Archives of General Psychiatry*, Vol. 17, July 1967, pp. 83–87.

22. The Swiss psychiatrist Eugen Bleuler (1857–1939) had published a book, *Dementia Praecox or the Group of Schizophrenias*, with this formula in 1911, but it was not translated into English until 1950. At that point, American psychiatrists began to use the four A's like a mantra. For a recent appraisal of Bleuler's four A's, see Kieran McNally, "Eugen Bleuler's Four A's," *History of Psychology*, Vol. 12, No. 2, May 2009, pp. 43–59.

23. See "Supplement. Cross-National Study of the Mental Disorders," *American Journal of Psychiatry*, Vol. 125, No. 10, April 1969. Also, J. E. Cooper, R. E. Kendell, B. J. Gurland, L. Sharpe, J. R. M. Copeland, and R. Simon, *Psychiatric Diagnosis in New York and London*. Maudsley Monograph Series, No. 20. London: Oxford University Press, 1972.

24. Gabriel Langfeldt, "Diagnosis and Prognosis of Schizophrenia," *Proceedings of the Royal Society of Medicine*, Vol. 53, Section of Psychiatry. June 14, 1960, p. 1051. (Looking at Langfeldt's four criteria, yet another diagnosis, as opposed to schizophrenia, would be a severe dissociative disorder.)

25. This approach today would be called a meta-analysis.

26. George E. Vaillant, "The Prediction of Recovery in Schizophrenia," *Journal of Nervous and Mental Disease*, Vol. 135, No. 1, July 1962, pp. 617–627.

27. In 1970 Robins and Guze published their key article on how to achieve validity of diagnosis using schizophrenia as a clinical example. Their criteria were clinical description, laboratory studies, delimitation from other disorders, follow-up study, and family studies. Robins and Guze declared that by using follow-up and family studies, cases with a poor prognosis could be validly separated from those with a good prognosis. They rightly concluded that schizophrenia with a good prognosis is not mild schizophrenia but a different illness. The 1970 study is where Robins and Guze pronounced that "classification is diagnosis."To review the Feighner diagnostic criteria for schizophrenia, see Chapter 3.

28. George E. Vaillant, "Prospective Prediction of Recovery in Schizophrenia," *Archives of General Psychiatry*, Vol. 11, November 1964, pp. 515, 517. In a 1966 study, Joseph H. Stephens and colleagues replicated Vaillant's work and conclusions. See Joseph H. Stephens, Christian Astrup, and John C. Mangrum, "Prognostic Factors in Recovered

and Deteriorated Schizophrenics," *American Journal of Psychiatry*, Vol. 122, April 1966, pp. 1116–1120.

29. John S. Strauss, William T. Carpenter, Jr., and John J. Bartko, "The Diagnosis and Understanding of Schizophrenia, Part III," *Schizophrenia Bulletin*, Issue No. 11, Winter, 1974, pp. 61–80.

   Moreover, that same year, Judith P. Kuriansky and colleagues postulated an actual change among the patient population at PI over two decades—the first decade from 1932 to 1941 and the second from 1947 to 1956—to account for the broadening of the concept of schizophrenia in the second decade. The conclusion of the study was that the patients in the first decade were more "hard-core" and in the second more "ambiguous." Judith B. Kuriansky, W. Edwards Deming, and Barry J. Gurland, "On Trends in the Diagnosis of Schizophrenia," *American Journal of Psychiatry*, Vol. 131, No. 4, April 1974, pp. 402–408.

30. Robert L. Spitzer, Joseph L. Fleiss, Eugene I. Burdock, and Anne S. Hardesty, "The Mental Status Schedule: Rationale, Reliability, and Validity," *Comprehensive Psychiatry*, Vol. 5, No. 6, December 1964, p. 384. When Spitzer wrote this paper he was unaware of the work on structured interviews being done by J. K. Wing in England. Wing was to become well-known for his structured "Present State Examination." See J. K. Wing, "A Standard Form of Psychiatric Present State Examinations (PSE) and a Method of Standardizing the Classification of Symptoms," in E. H. Hare and J. K. Wing (eds.), *Psychiatric Epidemiology*. London: Oxford University Press, 1970.

31. Like the Beck Depression Inventory, the Mental Status Schedule can be used to assess severity. See Kuriansky et al., "On Trends in the Diagnosis of Schizophrenia."

32. At this time, significantly, Spitzer was still in psychoanalytic training and was himself being analyzed, presumably using material from his unconscious.

33. Jean Endicott and Robert L. Spitzer, "A Diagnostic Interview: The Schedule for Affective Disorders and Schizophrenia," *Archives of General Psychiatry*, Vol. 35, No. 7, July 1978, pp. 837–844.

34. R. L. Spitzer, J. B. W. Williams, M. Gibbon, and M. B. First, "The Structured Clinical Interview for DSM-III-R (SCID) I: History, Rationale and Description," *Archives of General Psychiatry*, Vol. 49, 1992, pp. 624–629; J. B. W. Williams, M. Gibbon, M. B. First, M. Davies, J. Borus, M. J. Howes, J. Kane, H. G. Pope, B. Rounsaville, and H. Wittchen, "The Structured Clinical Interview for DSM-III-R (SCID) II: Multi-Site Test-Retest Reliability," *Archives of General Psychiatry*, Vol. 49, 1992, pp. 630–636; M. B. First, R. L. Spitzer, M. Gibbon, J. B. W. Williams, "The Structured Clinical Interview for DSM-III-R Personality Disorders (SCID II), Part I: Description," *Journal of Personality Disorders*, Vol. 9, No. 2, 1995, pp. 83–91; M. B. First, R. L. Spitzer, M. Gibbon, J. B. W. Williams, M. Davies, J. Borus, M. J. Howes, J. Kane, H. G. Pope, and B. Rounsaville, "The Structured Clinical Interview for DSM-III-R Personality Disorders (SCID II): Part II. Multi-Site Test-Retest Reliability Study," *Journal of Personality Disorders*, Vol. 9, No. 2, 1995, pp. 92–104.

35. Robert L. Spitzer, Janet B. W. Williams, Kurt Kroenke, Mark Linzer, Frank Verloin deGruy III, Steven R. Hahn, and David Brody, "Utility of a New Procedure for Diagnosing Mental Disorders in Primary Care: The PRIME-MD 1000 Study," *JAMA*, Vol. 272, No. 22, December 14, 1994, pp. 1749–1756; R. L. Spitzer, K. Kroenke, M. Linzer, S. R. Hahn, J. B. W. Williams, F. V. deGruy, D. Brody, and M. Davies, "Health Related Quality of Life

in Primary Care Patients with Mental Disorders: Results of the PRIME-MD 1000 Study," *JAMA*, Vol. 274, 1995, pp. 1511–1517.

36. R. L. Spitzer, M. Gibbon, J. B. W. Williams, and J. Endicott, "The Global Assessment of Functioning (GAF) Scale," In L. I. Sederer and B. Dickey (eds.), *Outcomes Assessment in Clinical Practice*. Baltimore: William & Wilkins, 1996.

37. R. L. Spitzer, J. Cohen, J. L. Fleiss, and J. Endicott, "Quantification of Agreement in Psychiatric Diagnosis: A New Approach," *Archives of General Psychiatry*, Vol. 17, 1967, pp. 83–87; R. L. Spitzer and J. Cohen, "Common Errors in Quantitative Psychiatric Research," *International Journal of Psychiatry*, Vol. 6, 1968, pp. 109–118; R. L. Spitzer and J. Endicott, "Automation of Psychiatric Case Records: Boon or Bane?" *International Journal of Psychiatry*, Vol. 9, 1970, pp. 604–621.

38. Robert L. Spitzer and Jean Endicott, "DIAGNO: A Computer Program for Psychiatric Diagnosis Utilizing the Differential Diagnostic Picture," *Archives of General Psychiatry*, Vol. 18, 1968, pp. 746–756; Robert L. Spitzer and Jean Endicott, "DIAGNO II: Further Developments in a Computer Program for Psychiatric Diagnosis," *American Journal of Psychiatry*, Vol. 125, 1969, January Supplement, pp. 12–21. See also R. L. Spitzer and L. M. Gilford, "UPDATE: A Computer Program for Converting Diagnoses to the New Nomenclature, of the American Psychiatric Association," *American Journal of Psychiatry*, Vol. 125, 1968, pp. 395–396.

   For the researcher in this subject, there are many additional articles on quantification in psychiatry and automated case records.

39. Robert L. Spitzer, Jean Endicott, Jacob Cohen, and Joseph L. Fleiss, "Constraints on the Validity of Computer Diagnosis," *Archives of General Psychiatry*, Vol. 31, August 1974, p. 203. Yet four years later Spitzer reported that the impact of computer programs "has been nil because the computer algorithms are not easily translatable into clinically useful rules." Robert L. Spitzer, Jean Endicott, Eli Robins, "Research Diagnostic Criteria: Rationale and Reliability," *Archives of General Psychiatry*, Vol. 35, June 1978, p. 782.

40. Robert L. Spitzer and Joseph L. Fleiss, "Re-analysis of the Reliability of Psychiatric Diagnosis," *British Journal of Psychiatry*, Vol. 125, 1974, pp. 341–347. Spitzer defined validity as "the utility of the system for its various purposes.... The purposes of the classification system [for psychiatry] are communication about clinical features, aetiology, course of illness and treatment." (p. 341)

41. Recall that the 15-year old Spitzer ("Henry Friend") characterized his behavior in class by saying "I squawk—yes I do, as any. The teachers are afraid of me—I'm sometimes too ruthless." See David Riesman, *Faces in the Crowd*, 1965, p. 369.

Chapter 7

1. "Summary Report of the Special Policy Meeting of the Board of Trustees, Atlanta, Ga., February 1–3, 1973" *American Journal of Psychiatry*, Vol. 130, No. 6, June 1973, pp. 732–738.

2. Presumably, the thinking was that there would be a revsion of DSM-II commensurate with its original size, categories, and features.

3. See *Dorland's Medical Dictionary for Health Consumers*. Philadelphia: Saunders, 2007, and *The American Heritage Medical Dictionary*. New York: Houghton Mifflin, 2007.Eventually a separate APA Task Force was created to deal with the matter of the Problem-Oriented Medical Record, with one of its members appointed as a liaison to the DSM-III Task Force.

4. Memo from Walter Barton, M.D., Medical Director of the APA, March 20, 1973. Quoted in Stuart A. Kirk and Herb Kutchins, *The Selling of DSM: The Rhetoric of Science in Psychiatry*. New York: Aldine De Gruyter, 1992, p. 80.

5. Robert L. Spitzer and Paul T. Wilson, "DSM-II Revisited: A Reply," *International Journal of Psychiatry*, Vol. 7, 1969, pp. 421–426.

6. Spitzer and Wilson, p. 425.

7. There was one area, however, where Spitzer pulled back somewhat while he was head of the Task Force: the importance of the congruence between the DSM and the International Classification of Diseases (ICD) put out by the World Health Organization (WHO).

8. Reports and letters from 1974 and 1975 can be found in the APA Archives, Arlington, VA, DSM Coll. No further identification is possible, here and elsewhere, because at the time I consulted the archives they were not catalogued.

9. See also Spitzer's letter of September 30, 1974, to John J. Schwab, Chair of the Council on Research and Development, Archives, DSM Col.

10. John J. Schwab, "Official Actions," *American Journal of Psychiatry*, Vol. 132, No. 4, April 1975, p. 480.

11. Interview with Paula Clayton, M.D., who was both a medical student and psychiatry resident at Washington University, and later a full-time faculty member.

12. E-mail from Paula Clayton, February 16, 2007. Endicott had given this information to Clayton.

13. Robert L. Spitzer, Jean Endicott, Eli Robins, Judith Kuriansky, and Barry Gurland, "Preliminary Report of the Reliability of Research Diagnostic Criteria Applied to Psychiatric Case Records," in Abraham Sudilovsky, Samuel Gershon, and Bernard Beer, eds., *Predictability in Psychopharmacology: Preclinical and Clinical Correlations*. New York: Raven Press, 1975; Robert L. Spitzer, Jean Endicott, and Eli Robins, "Clinical Criteria for Psychiatric Diagnosis and DSM-III," *American Journal of Psychiatry*, Vol. 132, No. 11, November 1975, pp. 1187–1192.

14. Grand rounds, PI, January 6, 2006.

15. Grand rounds, PI, January 6, 2006.

16. Spitzer and Wilson, "DSM-II Revisited."

17. Judith P. Kuriansky, E. W. Deming, and Barry J. Gurland, "On Trends in the Diagnosis of Schizophrenia," *American Journal of Psychiatry*, Vol. 131, 1974, pp. 402–408; R. L. Spitzer and J. L. Fleiss, "A Reanalysis of the Reliability of Psychiatric Diagnosis," *British Journal of Psychiatry*, Vol. 125, 1974, pp. 341–347.

18. Robert L. Spitzer, "On Pseudoscience in Science, Logic in Remission and Psychiatric Diagnosis: A Critique of Rosenhan's 'On Being Sane in Insane Places,'" *Journal of Abnormal Psychology*, Vol. 84, 1975, pp. 442–452; Robert L. Spitzer, "More on Pseudoscience in Science and the Case for Psychiatric Diagnosis: A Critique of D. L. Rosenhan's 'On Being Sane in Insane Places' and 'The Contextual Nature of Psychiatric Diagnosis,'" *Archives of General Psychiatry*, Vol. 33, 1976, pp. 459–470.

19. Spitzer, Endicott, et al., "Preliminary Report," p. 1.

20. Spitzer, Endicott, and Robins, "Clinical Criteria," p. 1190.

21. DSM-III had categories of "Not Elsewhere Classified" for a given diagnosis if a patient did not fit into a precise diagnosis within the larger category.

22. Spitzer, Endicott, and Robins, "Clinical Criteria," p. 1191.

23. Interview with Spitzer, June 3, 2006.

24. Spitzer, Endicott, et al., "Preliminary Report," p. 44.

25. Spitzer, Endicott, et al., "Preliminary Report," pp. 43, 46.

26. Spitzer, Endicott, et al., "Preliminary Report," pp. 8, 44.

27. Spitzer, Endicott, and Robins, "Clinical Criteria," p. 1189.

28. Spitzer, Endicott, and Robins, "Clinical Criteria," p. 1191.

29. "Introduction," DSM-III, p. 11.

30. I have taught such psychiatric residents and presented to them the course of illness of a famous psychiatric patient and asked for their reaction to her situation. Instead of comments or discussion, I have received knee-jerk responses on how to code the patient ("Axis I" or "Axis II" in current psychiatric language). However, Spitzer said he was not surprised by this outcome. (Interview June 2, 2006).

    Yet see also Nancy C. Andreasen, "DSM and the Death of Phenomenology in America: An Example of Unintended Consequences," Schizophrenia Bulletin, Vol. 33, No. 1, 2007, pp. 108–112.

31. Although if Nancy Andreasen is correct in her recollections, the possibility of DSM-III assuming the role of a textbook had crossed the minds of the Task Force.

32. Robert L. Spitzer, Jean Endicott, and Eli Robins, "Research Diagnostic Criteria: Rationale and Reliability," Archives of General Psychiatry, Vol. 35, June 1978, pp. 773–782.

33. "Validity" refers to the accuracy and usefulness of a diagnosis, or is the diagnosis a valid one?

34. Spitzer, Endicott, and Robins, "Research Diagnostic Criteria," pp. 774, 775, 779, 781. Spitzer continued to work and publish on the RDC while immersed in the development of DSM-III.

35. Jean Endicott and Robert L. Spitzer, "A Diagnostic Interview: The Schedule for Affective Disorders and Schizophrenia," Archives of General Psychiatry, Vol. 35, July 1978, p. 844.

36. Other members of the Task Force also undertook the task of educating the profession about what to expect in DSM-III. An example of the numerous papers at the time with this aim is one in which Nancy Andreasen, whose area of concentration was schizophrenia, joined Spitzer and Endicott. Their article in the specialty journal, Schizophrenia Bulletin, was meant to spread the word on what was being developed about psychotic disorders by the DSM-III Advisory Committee on Schizophrenic, Paranoid, and Affective Disorders as well as by the Task Force, which coordinated the work of all the advisory committees. See Robert L. Spitzer, Nancy C. Andreasen, and Jean Endicott, "Schizophrenia and Other Psychotic Disorders in DSM-III," Schizophrenia Bulletin, Vol. 4, No. 4, 1978, pp. 489–494.

37. Payne Whitney is the psychiatric division of the New York Hospital and is staffed by the psychiatry department of the Weill Cornell College of Medicine.

38. Letter from Roy H. Hart, M.D., to Spitzer, November 2, 1974, Archives, DSM Coll.

39. Kirk and Kutchins, p. 102. Spitzer added that "the Task Force would be glad to meet with representatives of your group to further discuss [black representation] or any other matter relevant to DSM-III."

40. Letter from Spitzer to John J. Schwab, Chair of the Council on Research and Development, January 20, 1975, Archives, DSM Coll.

41. Report to the Council on Research and Development from the Task Force on Nomenclature and Statistics, 3/18/75, Archives, DSM Coll. Whereas in March 1975 Spitzer could say that "over half" of the disorders had been described, this is a half only "in progress" because the number of disorders on the record then was nowhere near the 265 disorders that eventually appeared in DSM-III.

42. Letter of Spitzer to Lester Grinspoon, Chair of the Council on Research and Development, July 27, 1978, Archives, DSM Coll. Spitzer wrote to Grinspoon six months later requesting

$60,000 again for 1980, not for the DSM-III itself but for various projects that Spitzer considered important outgrowths of DSM-III, including starting to prepare for DSM-IV. See letter of Spitzer to Grinspoon, January 16, 1979, Archives, DSM Coll. and a formal proposed budget also in Box 100904.

43. Council on Research and Development Budgets for 1975–1978, Archives, DSM Coll.

44. Letter from Louis Jolyon West to Henry H. Work, September 15, 1975, Archives, DSM Coll.

45. Kirk and Kutchins, in *The Selling of DSM*, cite (without an adequate source) the remarks of an unknown commentator about Spitzer's handling of questions at the 1975 APA panel: "Spitzer fielded an onslaught of objections with genial flexibility. A number of times he accepted suggestions of critics on the spot, promising changes with comments such as, 'That's a good idea. We haven't thought of that.'" Then, as part of their quotation, Kirk and Kutchins include the following comment, not in quotations: *Spitzer's political style is one of accommodation. Rather than turn his dissenters into enemies he prefers to join them.* See pp. 105–106. If this material is to be trusted, I would observe that depending on the nature of the questions at the panel, this appraisal may have been accurate. Spitzer was always ready to make small adjustments and clarifications in various parts of DSM-III as long as they did not undo his basic philosophical positions. However, the provenance of the entire account by Kirk and Kutchins is cloudy.

Kirk and Kutchins also state that Janet B. W. Williams, Spitzer's text editor, published a regular column, "Questions and Answers About DSM-III," in *Hospital and Community Psychiatry*, but I have been unable to verify this assertion. See *The Selling of DSM*, p. 105.

46. Letters from John E. Fryer, M.D., to Spitzer, May 18, 1975, and August 18, 1975; Judd Marmor, M.D., June 2, 1975; Justin D. Call, M.D., August 15, 1975, Archives, DSM Coll. Spitzer attempted to "sooth [Fryer's] frayed nerves" (and failed) in a letter of July 24, 1975, Archives, DSM Coll.

47. Letter from Richard Green, M.D., to Spitzer, December 14, 1976, Archives, DSM Coll.

48. Letters from Tina Strobos, M.D., Date not legible, either June 10, 15, or 18, 1975; Adrien L. Coblentz, M.D., June 12, 1975; Herbert Dorken, Ph.D. (a psychologist), July 2, 1975, Archives, DSM Coll.

49. Letters from Ellen McDaniel, M.D., and Herbert S. Gross, M.D., June 11, 1975; George F. Schnack, M.D., August 18, 1975; John A. Talbott, M.D., October 2, 1975 (if the records are complete, Talbott seems to have been the first prominent psychiatrist to write to Spitzer); letter from Francis J. Gurgin, M.D., October 14, 1975. These letters addressed other complaints in addition to the lack of neurosis in the classification. All letters are found in Archives, DSM Coll.

50. Letter from Theodore Millon to Spitzer, September 18, 1974, Archives, DSM Coll.

51. Robert L. Spitzer and Paul T. Wilson, "Nosology and the Official Psychiatric Nomenclature," in Alfred M. Freedman, Harold I. Kaplan, and Benjamin I. Sadock (eds.), *Comprehensive Textbook of Psychiatry*, Chapter 14: Classification in Psychiatry. Baltimore: Williams and Wilkins, 1975, pp. 826–845. Paul Wilson was the same psychiatrist who had been second author with Spitzer of the 1969 article evaluating DSM-II and proposing the steps to be taken when putting together DSM-III.

52. Spitzer and Wilson, p. 841.

53. One has also to wonder if there was a failure of Spitzer's three own analyses, to deal in a satisfying way with his expectations of resolving certain problems, that affected his thinking. Spitzer was certainly disenchanted with his Reichian analyst and left his second one (Abram Kardiner) because of his prolonged analytic silences. Whatever problems Spitzer

encountered with his last analyst, Arnold Cooper, are not clear. At first, Spitzer was very taken with Cooper's theories on narcissism and masochism. Resentment against their analysts has been the case with disillusionment experienced by other analyzed psychiatrists in our story.

54. Letter from John A. Talbott to Spitzer, October 2, 1975, Archives, DSM Coll.

55. Letter from Spitzer to Talbott, October 7, 1975, Archives, DSM Coll. Eventually, DSM-III included Neurotic Disorders under Affective, Anxiety, Somatoform, Dissociative, and Psychosexual Disorders.

56. See John A. Talbott, "An In-Depth Look at DSM-III: An Interview with Robert Spitzer," *Hospital and Community Psychiatry*, Vol. 31, No. 1, Jan. 1980, p. 25.

57. Erik Essen-Möller and S. Wohlfahrt, "Suggestions for the Amendment of the Official Swedish Classification of Mental Disorders," *Acta Psychiatrica Scandinavica*, Vol. 47 Supplement, 1947, pp. 551–555. Essen-Möller followed up his 1947 paper with two further articles: "On Classification of Mental Disorders," *Acta Psychiatrica Scandinavica*, Vol. 37, No. 2, 1961, pp. 119–126, and "Suggestions for Further Improvement of the International Classification of Mental Disorders," *Psychological Medicine*, Vol. 1, 1971, pp. 308–311.

58. Criteria Committee, New York Heart Association, *Diseases of the Heart and Blood Vessels: Nomenclature and Criteria for Diagnosis* (6th ed.). Boston: Little, Brown, 1964.

59. Michael Rutter, Serge Lebovici, Leon Eisenberg, et al, "A Tri-axial Classification of Mental Disorders in Childhood: An International Study," *Journal of Child Psychology and Psychiatry*, Vol. 10, 1969, pp. 41–61. Rutter, David Shaffer, and M. Shepherd also evaluated the diagnostic system in "An Evaluation of the Proposal for a Multi-axial Classification of Child Psychiatric Disorders," *Psychological Medicine*, Vol. 3, 1973, pp. 244–250.

60. "Proposed Multiaxial System for DSM-III," Archives, DSM Coll.

61. Interview with Robert Spitzer, June 3, 2006.

62. "Proposed Multiaxial System for DSM-III," Archives, DSM Coll.

63. John S. Strauss, "A Comprehensive Approach to Psychiatric Diagnosis," *American Journal of Psychiatry*, Vol. 132, No. 11, Nov. 1975, pp. 1193–1197.

64. World Health Organization, *Reports of the Fourth and Sixth WHO Seminars on Psychiatric Diagnoses, Classification, and Statistics*. Geneva: WHO, 1968 and 1970. See also World Health Organization, *Report of the Seventh WHO Seminar on Standardization of Psychiatric Diagnosis, Classification and Statistics of Personality and Drug Dependence*, Tokyo, 1971.

65. We shall see that one of Spitzer's goals for the revised manual was that it could be used as a counter to the popularity of the social studies of science with its spawn of "cultural relativism."

66. Additional possible codes were (1) Unspecified mental disorder (nonpsychotic); (2) No diagnosis or condition on Axis I; (3) Diagnosis or condition deferred.

67. Spitzer and Wilson, "Nosology, and the Official Psychiatric Nomenclature," p. 836, and Talbott, "An In-Depth Look," 1980.

68. Robert L. Spitzer, "A Response to the Threat of a Classification Scheme for the Psychosocial Disorders: Some Specific Suggestions," *American Journal of Orthopsychiatry*, Vol. 41, 1971, pp. 838–840.

69. Spitzer and Wilson, "Nosology," p. 836.

70. Robert L. Spitzer, "A Proposal About Homosexuality and the APA Nomenclature: Homosexuality as an Irregular Form of Sexual Behavior [not a disorder] and Sexual Orientation Disturbance as a Psychiatric Disorder," *American Journal of Psychiatry*, Vol. 130, No. 11, November 1973, p. 1216. The reference to mental illness as a "myth"

is clearly in response to Thomas Szasz's assertion of the "myth" of mental illness (1961).

71. Robert L. Spitzer, Michael Sheehy, and Jean Endicott, "DSM-III: Guiding Principles," in Vivian M. Rakoff, Harvey C. Stancer, and Henry B. Kedward (eds.), *Psychiatric Diagnosis*. New York: Brunner/Mazel, 1977, p. 3.

72. Henry Pinsker, Memo to Members of the Task Force on Nomenclature & Statistics, June 4, 1975, Archives, DSM Coll.

73. Letter from Spitzer to Pinsker, February 3, 1976. Archives, DSM Coll.

74. *1975 definition*:

    1. The manifestations of the condition are primarily psychological and involve alterations in behavior. However, it includes conditions manifested by somatic changes, such as psycho-physiologic reactions, if an understanding of the cause and course of the condition is largely dependent on the use of psychological concepts, such as personality, motivation, and conflict.

    2. The condition in its full-blown state is regularly and intrinsically associated with subjective distress, generalized impairment in social effectiveness or functioning, or voluntary behavior that the subject wishes he could stop because it is regularly associated with physical disability or illness.

    3. The condition is distinct from other conditions in terms of the clinical picture and, ideally, follow-up, family studies, and response to treatment.See Spitzer and Wilson, "Nosology," 1975, p. 829.

    1977 definition:A medical disorder is a relatively distinct condition resulting from an organismic dysfunction which in its fully developed or extreme form is directly and intrinsically associated with distress, disability, or certain other types of disadvantage. The disadvantage may be of a physical, perceptual, sexual, or interpersonal nature. Implicitly there is a call for action on the part of the person who has the condition, by the medical or its allied professions, and society.

    A mental disorder is a medical disorder whose manifestations are primarily signs or symptoms of a psychological (behavioral) nature, or if physical, can be understood only when using psychological concepts.

    See Robert L. Spitzer and Jean Endicott, "Medical and Mental Disorder: Proposed Definition and Criteria," in Robert L. Spitzer and Donald Klein (eds.), *Critical Issues in Psychiatric Diagnosis*. New York: Raven Press, 1978, p. 18.

75. Spitzer and Klein, pp. 16–17.

76. The authors of DSM-5 are engaged in partly undoing the strict categorization of DSM-III and IV in favor of a spectrum (continuum) approach, as in Autism Spectrum Disorders and Personality Disorders. This is somewhat in keeping with the traditional psychoanalytic view.

77. Robert L. Spitzer Memo to the Task Force and Childhood and Adolescence Subcommittee, July 19, 1976, Archives, DSM Coll.

78. The DSM-III states: "The term Paraphilia [which had been adopted by Spitzer] is preferable because it correctly emphasizes that the deviation (para) [lies] in that to which the individual is attracted (philia)." American Psychiatric Association, *Diagnostic and Statistical Manual of Mental Disorders* (3rd ed., *DSM-III*). Washington, DC: American Psychiatric Association, 1980, pp. 266–267.In DSM-I (1952) there was a category "Sexual Deviation" listed under "Sociopathic Personality Disturbance." In DSM-II (1968) eight

subtypes of Sexual Deviations were listed under "Personality Disorders and Certain Other Non-Psychotic Mental Disorders."

The term *paraphilia* was originally coined by the Viennese psychoanalyst, Wilhelm Stekel (1868–1940), in the 1920s.

79. Letter from Leon L. North, M.D., to Spitzer, July 30, 1975, Archives, DSM Coll.

80. Letter from Spitzer to Leon L. North, August 1, 1975, Archives, DSM Coll. There is also an interesting letter from John Talbott, a prominent member of the New York County District Branch to Charles Socarides, who loudly complained about the decision to take homosexuality out of DSM-II. (Socarides (1922–2005) was a psychoanalyst and one of the most outspoken in his conviction that homosexuality was a mental disorder.) Talbott rebutted him firmly and said the issue of homosexuality as pathological had been reviewed at every level of the APA and the issue would not be reopened. Letter from John A. Talbott to Charles W. Socarides, M.D., October 2, 1975, Archives, DSM Coll.

Interestingly enough, Socarides went on to write a book, *Homosexuality: A Freedom Too Far. A Psychoanalyst Answers 1000 Questions About Causes and Cure and the Impact of the Gay Rights Movement on American Society* (Phoenix: Adam Margrave Books, 1995) about his beliefs. In it he asserted that the removal of homosexuality from DSM-II in 1974 was instrumental in bringing about the AIDS epidemic.

In an ironic twist, Socarides had a son who is openly gay, Richard Socarides (b. 1954), a lawyer and Democratic commentator who was an advisor to President Bill Clinton on gay and lesbian civil rights issues from 1993 to 1999.

81. Letter to Spitzer from Robert J. L. Waugh, M.D, July 11, 1975, Archives, DSM Coll.

82. Letter from Spitzer to Waugh, July 24, 1975, Archives, DSM Coll.

83. Letter from Charles B. Wilkinson to Spitzer, June 24, 1975, Archives, DSM Coll. Wilkinson was Executive Director of the Greater Kansas City Mental Health Foundation and a dean at the UM-KC School of Medicine.

84. Letter of Spitzer to Wilkinson, July 24, 1975, Archives, DSM Coll. Spitzer concluded that "the failure to include racism as a diagnostic category should in no way imply that psychiatrists are unaware of the harmful effects of racism on the racist and on society at large."

Later that year, Spitzer received a report from the Committee of Black Psychiatrists of the Council on National Affairs regarding the inclusion of racism as a diagnostic category in DSM-III. See Archives, DSM Coll. Spitzer's reply is not in the Archives.

85. Spitzer to Committee of Black Psychiatrists, December 29, 1975, quoted in Kirk and Kutchins, 1992, p. 102.

86. Letter from Spitzer to John A. Talbott, October 7, 1975, Archives, DSM Coll.

87. Letters to Spitzer from William E. Holt, M.D., and Charles K. Hofling, M.D., representing the St. Louis Psychoanalytic Society, December 12, 1975, and Merl M. Jackel, M.D., representing The Psychoanalytic Association of New York, January 2, 1976, Archives, DSM Coll. It should be noted that next to the two names of the analysts writing from St. Louis someone (Spitzer? A colleague to whom he had shown the letter?) had written in "well-known non-entity" (next to William E. Holt) and "amiable anacronism" (sic) (next to Charles K. Hofling). Hofling was the author of a well-known 1966 study on obedience to authority.

88. Letters from Spitzer to William E. Holt and Charles K. Hofling and to Merl M. Jackel, January 29, 1976.

89. Task Force on Nomenclature and Statistics of the American Psychiatric Association, "Progress Report on the Preparation of DSM-III," March 1976, pp. 11–12. Hereafter referred to as "Progress Report." Archives, DSM Coll.

90. Spitzer did not explicitly say so, but by "situation" he had to have meant usual hetero- or homosexual sexual activity.

91. The important "DSM-III in Midstream" Conference was about to meet in two weeks. See memo from Spitzer to Members and Consultants of the Sex Subcommittee, May 28, 1976, Archives, DSM Coll. However, the last sentence in the quotation is confusing because two months earlier the participants of the conference had already been sent the "Progress Report" which contained "this revision," i.e., renouncing the requirement for subjective distress.

92. This information comes from Summary of Conference on "Improvements in Psychiatric Classification and Terminology: A Working Conference to Critically Examine DSM-III in Midstream." Summarized and Edited by Ivan W. Sletten, M.D., Robert L. Spitzer, M.D., and James L. Hedlund, Ph.D., p. 1. Hereafter referred to as "Summary." The documents relating to the planning of, participation in, events at, and summary of the Midstream Conference were found dispersed among the Archives, DSM Coll.

93. Again, the unstated "usual activity with another person" should be inserted here.

94. Spitzer memo to the Task Force and the Childhood and Adolescence Subcommittee, July 19, 1976, pp. 7–8, Archives, DSM Coll.

95. Spitzer's memo to the Sex Subcommittee, Dr. Robert Arnstein (Childhood and Adolescent Disorders), and Drs. Howard Berk, Harvey Bluestone, and Hector Jaso (members of the APA Assembly of District Branches Liaison Committee to the DSM-III Task Force), July 30, 1976, p. 1, Archives, DSM Coll.

Chapter 8

1. Ivan W. Sletten, M.D., Robert L. Spitzer, M.D., and James L. Hedlund, Ph.D. (Summarizers and Editors), "Summary of Conference on 'Improvements in Psychiatric Classification and Terminology: A Working Conference to Critically Examine DSM-III in Midstream,'" June 10 and 11, 1976, St. Louis Hilton, St. Louis, Missouri, p. 1. (Unpublished document sent to Melvin Sabshin, M.D., Medical Director, APA, September 24, 1976, Archives, DSM Coll.) Hereafter "Summary."

2. Memo from Spitzer to Jolly West, Chair of the APA Council on Research and Development, July 23, 1975, "Minutes of Committee to Plan Conference on Psychiatric Classification, Standardization & Terminology," June 20, 1975, Archives, DSM Coll.

3. "Progress Report on the Preparation of DSM-III, by the Task Force on Nomenclature and Statistics of the American Psychiatric Association," March 1976, p. 10, Archives, DSM Coll. Hereafter "Progress Report."

4. The actual schedule of the conference, with a breakdown of times, topics, and main speakers, can be found in Archives, DSM Coll.

5. "Summary," pp. 2–3.

6. "Summary," p. 5.

7. "Summary," pp. 5–7, 9.

8. Arieti's *Handbook* was published in two editions whose volumes had various printing dates. The first edition with three volumes appeared between 1959 and 1966, and the second edition, six volumes, first appeared in 1974.

9. "Summary," pp. 7–9. As we shall see, this took many months to happen.

10. "Summary," p. 8.

11. Robert L. Spitzer and Jean Endicott, "Medical and Mental Disorder: Proposed Definition and Criteria," in Robert L. Spitzer and Donald Klein (eds.), *Critical Issues in Psychiatric Diagnosis*. New York: Raven Press, 1978, p. 36. Spitzer also reported that a former President of the American Psychological Association had said two months before the Midstream meeting that DSM-III was "turning every human problem into a disease, in anticipation of the shower of health plan gold that is over the horizon."

12. "Summary," p. 10.

13. "Summary," p. 9.

14. "Summary," p. 9.

15. "Summary," pp. 11–13.

16. See p. 9 of "The Nomenclature" of DSM-II.

17. In Chapter 6, in the context of diagnostic reliability studies at the time the Task Force began meeting, I referred to two articles by Kuriansky et al. and Strauss et al., on schizophrenia. See also the then contemporary article by Arthur Falek and Hanna M. Moser, "Classification in Schizophrenia," *Archives of General Psychiatry*, Vol. 32, Jan. 1975, pp. 59–67. Recall also the classic paper about achieving diagnostic validity for the diagnosis of schizophrenia: Eli Robins and Samuel B. Guze, "Establishment of Diagnostic Reliability in Psychiatric Illness: Its Application to Schizophrenia," *American Journal of Psychiatry*, Vol. 126, 1970, pp. 983–987.

18. "Summary," pp. 14–33. The breakdown is as follows: Schizophrenia, pp. 14–16; Personality Disorders, pp. 17–19; Childhood Disorders, pp. 20–22; Mood Disorders, pp. 23–26, Sexual Disorders, pp. 27–31; Organic Mental Disorders, pp. 32–34.

19. Yet the word *neurosis* was used well over a century before Sigmund Freud adopted it and linked it to his theory of unconscious conflict. The word is often still used throughout the world without any connection to a psychoanalytic etiology.

20. "Summary," pp. 36–40.

21. "Summary," 40–41.

22. Robert Spitzer and Michael Sheehy, "DSM-III: A Classification System in Development," *Psychiatric Annals*, Vol. 6, Sept. 1976, pp. 102–109.

23. *Psychiatric Annals*, Vol. 6, No. 9: *Classification of Psychiatric Disorders*, September 1976.

24. Memo from Spitzer's secretary, Harriet, to Spitzer, December 20, 1976. Archives, DSM Coll.

25. Spitzer and Sheehy, pp. 103–104.

26. Spitzer started out by using Mandel Cohen's term of "operational" but ultimately this was changed to "diagnostic."

27. Spitzer and Sheehy, p. 105.

28. Spitzer and Sheehy, p. 109, Table 3. Under discussion were separate systems for adults and children.

29. "Summary," pp. 59–60, Archives, DSM Coll.

30. Spitzer and Sheehy, p. 109.

31. Spitzer and Sheehy, p. 109.

32. Vivian M. Rakoff, Harvey C. Stancer, and Henry B. Kedward, *Psychiatric Diagnosis*. New York: Brunner/Mazel, 1977.

33. Robert L. Spitzer, Michael Sheehy, and Jean Endicott, "DSM-III: Guiding Principles," in Vivian M. Rakoff, Harvey C. Stancer, and Henry B. Kedward (eds.), *Psychiatric Diagnosis*. New York: Brunner/Mazel, 1977, p. 2.

34. Spitzer, Sheehy, and Endicott, "DSM-III: Guiding Principles," pp. 14–15.
35. Spitzer, Sheehy, and Endicott, "DSM-III: Guiding Principles," pp. 15, 17.

    Spitzer's decision was to have one manual for both clinicians and researchers. But in the years since DSM-III appeared, some psychiatrists have argued that this accommodation is impossible and have put forward designs for separate manuals for research and clinical practice. It has even been suggested that there be three manuals: one for researchers, one for clinicians, and a third that would contain the diagnostic and procedure codes used for collecting payments from insurance companies.

36. Spitzer, Sheehy, and Endicott, "DSM-III: Guiding Principles," pp. 3–4.
37. Spitzer, Sheehy, and Endicott, "DSM-III: Guiding Principles," pp. 12–14.
38. Spitzer, Sheehy, and Endicott, "DSM-III: Guiding Principles," pp. 16–17.
39. Rakoff et al., *Psychiatric Diagnosis*, pp. 208–210.
40. Rakoff et al., *Psychiatric Diagnosis*, p. 210.
41. Rakoff et al., *Psychiatric Diagnosis*, p. 213.
42. Rakoff et al., *Psychiatric Diagnosis*, p. 216.
43. Rakoff et al., *Psychiatric Diagnosis*, p. 215.
44. Rakoff et al., *Psychiatric Diagnosis*, pp. 207–226.
45. Rakoff et al., *Psychiatric Diagnosis*, pp. 216, 219.
46. Rakoff et al., *Psychiatric Diagnosis*, pp. 226–228.

Chapter 9

1. Letter and memo from Howard E. Berk to Spitzer, June 2, 1976, eight days before the Midstream meeting. Archives, DSM Coll. (The first two pages of the memo are missing.)
2. "Progress Report on the Preparation of DSM-III," March, 1976, Table of Contents, and pp. 2, 11, 55–56.
3. Report of the Assembly Liaison Committee to the DSM-III Task Force to the Assembly of District Branches, APA at the meeting of October 29–31, 1976, Archives, DSM Coll.
4. Interview with Roger Peele, M.D., July 31, 2010.
5. Berk's letter to Spitzer, June 29, 1976. Archives, DSM Coll. There may have been a misunderstanding. Spitzer later wrote to Berk that only invited speakers spoke at the final session, and he said Berk was not on the list of invitees. But the question remains: Why was Berk sitting on the platform if he hadn't been invited?
6. Berk was the first Chair of the Assembly Liaison Committee. Later the Liaison Committee was enlarged, and Hector Jaso became Chair.
7. Berk and Jaso backdated their protest June 11, 1976, and labeled it as if they had presented their remarks to the final plenary session of the conference. They did not actually send out the letter June 11, but much later.
8. Letter from Spitzer to participants at the Midstream meeting, July 7, 1976, Archives, DSM Coll. Interestingly, the Archives contain a polite letter from Gerald Klerman to Berk thanking him for his letter but telling Berk that he did not share his negative view of the conference and voicing his hope that the Assembly and other components of the APA would discuss the issues further. Letter from Klerman to Berk, July 6, 1976, Archives, DSM Coll.
9. Spitzer's memo to Robert Campbell, Edward J. Sachar, John A. Talbott, and Jolly West, July 7, 1976, Archives, DSM Coll.
10. Spitzer memo to DSM-III Task Force, July 19, 1976. Archives, DSM Coll.
11. Letter from Spitzer to Berk, August 3, 1976, Archives, DSM Coll.

12. Memo from Spitzer to Berk, Jaso, and Bluestone, September 14, 1976, Archives, DSM Coll.

13. Memo from Spitzer to the Task Force and to Bernard C. Glueck, Edward J. Sachar, Louis Jolyon West, and Henry H. Work, October 15, 1976, Archives, DSM Coll.

14. Letter of Berk to a "Dr. G_____," February 19, 1977, Archives, DSM Coll. This was a handwritten letter and the recipient's name is unreadable.

15. See "DSM-III Materials for Assembly of District Branches Meeting, October 29–31, 1976," Archives, DSM Coll.

16. Report of the Assembly Liaison Committee, p. 11.

17. Memo from Spitzer to the Task Force and Robert Arnstein, Everett Dulit, Bernard Glueck, Jr., Gerald L. Klerman, Eli Robins, Melvin Sabshin, Edward J. Sachar, Louis Jolyon West, and Henry H. Work, November 5, 1976, Archives, DSM Coll.

18. Letter from Spitzer to Berk, Bluestone, and Jaso, April 8, 1977, Archives, DSM Coll.

19. Assembly DSM-III Task Force Report to the Assembly, Toronto, April 1977, Archives, DSM Coll.

20. Nevertheless, there are two documents that point to the continued activity of the committee and its interaction with the Task Force and Spitzer. When the Task Force held one of its infrequent meetings, in Atlanta in May 1978, the Assembly Liaison Committee was sent a copy of the minutes of that meeting. See Memo from Janet B. W. Forman, M.S.W., to Members of the Task Force and Assembly Liaison Committee, Archives, DSM Coll. There is also a letter from Spitzer to Jaso. See letter of May 25, 1978, Archives, DSM Coll.

21. Letter from Charles A. Kiesler, Ph.D., executive officer of the American Psychological Association, to Spitzer, October 7, 1976, Archives, DSM Coll.

22. Spitzer to Charles A. Kiesler, October 22, 1976, Archives, DSM Coll.

23. Letter of Kiesler to Spitzer, February 1, 1977, Archives, DSM Coll.

24. Robert L. Spitzer and Jean Endicott, "Medical and Mental Disorder: Proposed Definition and Criteria," In Donald F. Klein and Robert L. Spitzer (eds.), *Critical Issues in Psychiatric Diagnosis*. New York: Raven Press, 1978, pp. 15–39.

25. Letter from Spitzer to Drs. Maurice Lorr, Leonard Krasner, Peter E. Nathan, and Arthur Centor, Archives, DSM Coll.

26. The APPA had an elite quality. One could not just join but had to be approved by the Council of the APPA in order to become a member.

27. "Preface," Spitzer and Klein, *Critical Issues in Psychiatric Diagnosis*, p. v.

    Spitzer and Endicott, in their paper, offered these definitions: "A medical disorder is a relatively distinct condition resulting from an organismic dysfunction which in its fully developed or extreme form is directly and intrinsically associated with distress, disability, or certain other types of disadvantage. The disadvantage may be of a physical, perceptual, sexual, or interpersonal nature. Implicitly there is a call for action on the part of the person who has the condition, the medical or its allied professions, and society."

    "A mental disorder is a medical disorder whose manifestations are primarily signs or symptoms of a psychological (behavioral) nature, or if physical, can be understood only using psychological concepts." See p. 18.

28. "Draft of a statement to be considered for inclusion in DSM-III," 5/23/77. Archives, DSM Coll. Spitzer later stated that he had had input into the drafting of this statement.

29. Letter from Theodore H. Blau to Robert Gibson, President of the APA, August 8, 1977.

    The appendage listed the following disorders as learned: Simple Phobias, Generalized Anxiety Disorder, Somatization Disorder, Conduct Disorders of Childhood and Adolescence, and eight Personality Disorders.

30. Letter from Melvin Sabshin, Medical Director of the APA, to Spitzer, October 11, 1977, Archives, DSM Coll.

31. Letter of Joan S. Zaro to Spitzer, October 21, 1977, Archives, DSM Coll.

32. Spitzer to Melvin Sabshin, October 26, 1977, Archives, DSM Coll.

33. Memo from Spitzer to the Task Force on Nomenclature and Statistics, Assembly Liaison Committee, Dr. Lester Grinspoon, Dr. Edward Sachar, November 14, 1977, Archives, DSM Coll.

34. Letter from Blau to Weinberg, December 6, 1977. Quoted in Stuart A. Kirk and Herb Kutchins, *The Selling of DSM: The Rhetoric of Science in Psychiatry*. New York: Walter de Gruyter, 1992, pp. 114–115.

35. Letter from Zaro to Spitzer, February 15, 1978. Attached to Zaro's letter was "Summary of Final Report, APA Phase I Task Force on Descriptive Behavioral Classification, January 1978." The psychologists' classification seemed to be heading in the same direction as DSM-III. "Intrapsychic processes [were to be] minimized....Level of inference is to be kept as low as possible." One of the stated goals was to promote communication among mental health professionals, lay persons, and clients. However, such a manual was never published.

36. Theodore Millon, "The DSM-III: An Insider's Perspective," *American Psychologist*, Vol. 38, 1983, p. 806.

37. The May 7, 1978 minutes state: "*Medical Model Reference*: The group agreed that no mention was better than any mention. The Psychological American [sic] Association Liaison Committee will be informed of this. The Foreword will contain a description of the distinction between conditions and disorders and will give further details about the notion of a disorder in our classification, without specific reference to a medical model." Memo from Janet B. W. Forman, M.S.W., to the Task Force and the Assembly Liaison Committee, Archives, DSM Coll.

38. Memo from Janet B. W. Forman, M.S.W., to the Task Force and the Assembly Liaison Committee, May 7, 1978, Archives, DSM Coll.

39. E-mails from Jean Endicott, May 14 and 15, 2012; Telephone interview with Theodore Millon, May 8, 2012; E-mail from Janet Williams, May 10, 2012; Telephone conversation with Robert Spitzer, May 10, 2012.

40. Memo from Spitzer to the Liaison Committee of the American Psychological Association, May 26, 1978. Archives, DSM Coll.

41. Memo from Maurice Lorr to Spitzer, July 12, 1978, Archives, DSM Coll.

42. Memo from Lorr to Spitzer, November 3, 1978.

    Perhaps the Archives of the American Psychological Association contain additional documents to shed light on Spitzer's capitulation to the demands of that organization during the months of 1978.

43. "Introduction," *Diagnostic and Statistical Manual of Mental Disorders* (3rd ed., *DSM-III*), p. 4.

44. "Introduction," DSM-III, p. 6.

45. Memo from Janet Forman to the Task Force and Assembly Liaison Members re Minutes of the May 7, 1978 meeting of the Task Force.

46. Because of the overuse of schizophrenia diagnoses in the United States, Spitzer wanted to reduce their high volume, rattling those who had their favorite subtype, that is, latent schizophrenia or simple schizophrenia. But this issue was less controversial because of recent unambiguous research showing that schizophrenia was overdiag-

nosed in the United States, while affective disorders were overdiagnosed in the United Kingdom.

47. Letter from Aaron T. Beck, M.D., to Spitzer, July 22, 1975, Archives, DSM Coll. Beck is now famous for his development of cognitive behavior therapy (CBT).

48. Letter from Donald B. Rinsley, M.D., to Spitzer, May 18, 1976, Archives, DSM Coll.

49. Adolph Stern, "Psychoanalytic Investigation of and Therapy in the Borderline Group of Neurosis," *Psychoanalytic Quarterly*, Vol. 7, 1938, pp. 467–489.

50. Robert P. Knight, "Borderline States," *Bulletin of the Menninger Clinic*, Vol. 17, 1953, pp. 1–12.

51. Letter from Spitzer to Rinsley, June 3, 1976, Archives, DSM Coll.

52. Memo From Spitzer to the Task Force and Childhood and Adolescence Subcommittee, July 19, 1976; Letter from Spitzer to Rinsley, July 19, 1976; Letter from Spitzer to John G. Gunderson, M.D., July 19, 1976. All in Archives, DSM Coll. Gunderson, still alive, is an expert on BPD.

53. Letter from Spitzer to Alex Kaplan, M.D., July 19, 1976, Archives, DSM Coll.

54. DSM-II, 1968, p. 34.

55. As Theodore Millon, who was on the Personality Disorders Advisory Committee, put it, "Borderline [means] at best, a level of severity and not a descriptive type. As [Allen] Frances [also on the Committee] has noted, unless the word is used to signify a class that borders on something, then it has no clinical or descriptive meaning at all." "Borderline Personality Disorders," 6/28/78, Archives, DSM Coll.

56. Memo from Spitzer to the Task Force on Nomenclature and Statistics and Dr. Paul Wender, December 21, 1976, Archives, DSM Coll. Wender was one of the psychiatrists doing work on borderline schizophrenia. He had been at the 1976 Toronto Symposium on psychiatric diagnosis.

57. Robert L. Spitzer, Jean Endicott, and Miriam Gibbon, "Crossing the Border into Borderline Personality and Borderline Schizophrenia: The Development of Criteria," *Archives of General Psychiatry*, Vol. 36, January 1979, pp. 17–24.

58. Memo from Michael Sheehy, M.D., to Spitzer, January 25, 1977, Archives, DSM Coll.

59. Wender made the same point about "schizoid" because it "carries the implication of long term social isolation and withdrawal." Borderlines don't have such a history, he went on. See letter from Paul H. Wender to Spitzer, January 24, 1977, Archives, DSM Coll.

60. Letter from Otto F. Kernberg, M.D., to Spitzer, January 25, 1977, Archives, DSM Coll.

61. Letter from Donald W. Goodwin, M.D., to Spitzer, January 27, 1977, Archives, DSM Coll.

62. Memo from Spitzer to Drs. Otto Kernberg, John Gunderson, Roy R. Grinker, Sr., Rachel Gittelman, William Frosch, and Advisory Committee on Personality Disorders, October 31, 1978, Archives, DSM Coll. Gittelman and Frosch (an analyst) were on the Task Force, and Grinker was a senior psychiatrist and analyst of great repute.

63. Memo from John Gunderson to Drs. Robert L. Spitzer, Otto Kernberg, Roy R. Grinker, Sr., Rachel Gittelman, William Frosch, and Advisory Committee on Personality Disorders, November 9, 1978; Memo from Dr. Donald Klein to Dr. Robert Spitzer, November 9, 1978; Memo from Michael Sheehy, M.D., to Robert L. Spitzer, M.D., November 13, 1978; Memo from Roger A. Mackinnon, M.D., to Advisory Committee on Personality Disorders, November 15, 1978; Memo from Michael Sheehy, M.D., to Robert L. Spitzer, M.D., November 16, 1978; Letter from Otto Kernberg, M.D., to Robert Spitzer, M.D., November 28, 1978; Letter from Allen Frances, M.D., to Robert L. Spitzer, M.D., November 29, 1978;

Letter from John Frosch, M.D., to Dr. Robert Spitzer, December 4, 1978. All memos and letters in Archives, DSM Coll.

64. Letter from Allen Frances to Spitzer, November 29, 1978, Archives, DSM Coll. Frances argued bluntly: "I still think that 'borderline' is a lousy, nondescriptive, misleading term, but realize that I am outvoted by the experts in the field." Later, as leader of the Task Force for DSM-IV, Frances put a great premium on the precise and clear use of language. He continues to stress this matter today, often saying there is unclear language in the drafts of DSM-5.

65. Spitzer wrote to Gunderson, and Gunderson replied, even though both men were locked into opposing views on the validity of Schizotypal PD, Spitzer's new diagnosis. Gunderson did not believe there was evidence to separate out Schizotypal and Borderline PDs. See Spitzer, Endicott, and Gibbon, "Crossing the Border into Borderline Personality and Borderline Schizophrenia," 1979, pp. 17–24; Larry J. Siever and John G. Gunderson, "Genetic Determinants of Borderline Conditions," *Schizophrenia Bulletin*, Vol. 5, No. 1, 1979, pp. 81–83; Robert L. Spitzer and Jean Endicott, "Justification for Separating Schizotypal and Borderline Personality Disorders," *Schizophrenia Bulletin*, Vol. 5, No. 1, 1979, pp. 95–104.

66. John G. Gunderson and Margaret T. Singer, "Defining Borderline Patients: An Overview," *American Journal of Psychiatry*, Vol. 132, No. 1, January 1975, pp. 1–10.

67. Letter from Spitzer to Gunderson, January 4, 1979, Archives, DSM Coll.

68. Letter from Gunderson to Spitzer, January 12, 1979, Archives, DSM Coll. Not everyone agreed with Gunderson about including brief psychotic episodes in the diagnostic criteria of BPD, just one more indication of the variety of opinions about what constituted the disorder. See Memo from Michael Sheehy, M.D. (member of the Task Force), "Schizoaffective Disorder" [sic], November 16, 1978, Archives, DSM Coll.

69. Letter from Spitzer to Gunderson, January 22, 1979, Archives, DSM Coll.

70. DSM-III, pp. 321–322.

71. Memo from Spitzer to Members of the Advisory Committee on Personality Disorders, September 20, 1977, Archives, DSM Coll.

72. Memo from Spitzer to the Personality Disorders Committee, April 24, 1978, Archives, DSM Coll.

73. "Task Force on Nomenclature and Statistics October 4 Agenda," Archives, DSM Coll.

74. Letter from Roger A. Mackinnon to Spitzer, February 6, 1979, Archives, DSM Coll.

75. Memo from Spitzer to Drs. Allen Frances and Arnold Cooper, May 3, 1979, Archives, DSM Coll. Frances recalls that Spitzer called on him to write criteria for Narcissistic Personality Disorder and to edit the criteria for other personality disorders "to make them clearer and more consistent." E-mail from Allen Frances, October 23, 2012.

It is George Vaillant's opinion that Spitzer included Narcisisstic and Borderline Personality Disorders in DSM-III in order to buy off the analysts, although, matter these two PD subtypes actually should not have been included. Telephone interview with Dr. George E. Vaillant, October 19, 2012.

Chapter 10

1. "Somatoform Disorders," DSM-III, pp. 241, 249, 251.
2. "Psychological Factors Affecting Physical Condition," DSM-III, p. 303.
3. Letter from Samuel B. Guze to Spitzer, April 19, 1977, Archives, DSM Coll.

4. Letter from Guze to Spitzer, July 27, 1977, Archives, DSM Coll.
5. Memo from Paula J. Clayton to Spitzer, July 18, 1977, Archives, DSM Coll. There is also a fragment of an earlier memo from Clayton to Spitzer, July 6, 1977, relating to one of Clayton's patients with an irrational fear of breast cancer.
6. Letter from David A. Soskis, M.D., to Spitzer, March 16, 1978, Archives, DSM Coll.
7. Memo from Spitzer to the Factitious and Somatoform Disorders Committee, plus Drs. Donald Klein, Nancy Andreasen, Bish (Z. J.) Lipowski, Jean Endicott, and Lee Robins, March 27, 1978, Archives, DSM Coll.
8. Memo from Steven E. Hyler, M.D., "Soskis' Proposed Draft of Hypochondriasis," 4/6/78, Archives, DSM Coll. We can tell from a letter Soskis wrote to Spitzer at a later date that Donald Klein had also responded to Spitzer's request for comments. However, Klein's response is not in the Archives.

   Hyler was fond of making jokes about people presenting with ostensibly unappealing characteristics. He not only served on the Factitious and Somatoform Disorders Advisory Committee but also on the Personality Disorders Committee. In this latter capacity, Hyler proposed as a joke a new personality disorder, "Chronic Complaint Disorder," clearly never intending this to be a real diagnosis at all but to bring some levity to the sometimes tense proceedings. Hyler wrote: "To be included in this category are persons who heretofore were known by the synonyms: "kvetch" [and] "noodge." ... There also appears to be an ethnic association with this disorder in that it is found predominantly in persons of Eastern-European ancestry. In these cases, the pathognomonic expression becomes, 'Oy vay, don't ask.'"

   This memo is quoted by Christopher Lane in his book *Shyness: How Normal Behavior Became a Sickness* (New Haven and London: Yale University Press, 2007). Lane's book is clearly critical of DSM-III and Spitzer, and he has allowed his dislike to color his reaction to material in the APA Archives. After quoting Hyler's memo Lane concludes, with total seriousness, that "the task force had to reject these and related proposals because it could not decide on their validity or distinct criteria" (Lane, p. 67). Patently the memo was written in jest, and should not be taken seriously.
9. Letter from Soskis to Spitzer, October 30, 1978, Archives, DSM Coll.
10. Memo from Spitzer to Members of the Task Force and Assembly Liaison Committee, May 25, 1978, Archives, DSM Coll.
11. Memo from J. Brophy, M.D., to Spitzer re "Somatoform Disorders," January 29, 1979, Archives, DSM Coll.
12. There was no such committee. Brophy was on the Psychosomatic Disorders Committee.
13. Memo from Brophy to Spitzer, April 20, 1979, Archives, DSM Coll.
14. Letter from Spitzer to Brophy, May 3, 1979, Archives, DSM Coll. "Psychological Factors Affecting Physical Condition" became a stand-alone diagnosis in DSM-III.
15. Although Spitzer rejected the use of the fundamental psychoanalytic conceptions of "unconscious conflict" and "neurosis" and stopped carrying out psychoanalytic treatment with patients, he nevertheless had been trained as an analyst and never lost some of his psychoanalytic thinking. This crops up in isolated sections of DSM-III. For example, he retained Conversion Disorder under Somatoform Disorders (pp. 244–247) and introduced Psychological Factors Affecting Physical Condition (pp. 303–304), although in the diagnostic criteria for the latter he was very careful not to imply etiology. But his general discussion of the disorder is telling.
16. Letter from Guze to Spitzer, April 16, 1979, Archives, DSM Coll. In DSM-III, thirty-seven different symptoms are listed in the criteria for Somatization Disorder, of

which women must have at least fourteen and men twelve for the diagnosis to be made. These symptoms are almost identical with the ones in the draft of April 25, 1979 in Archives, DSM Coll.

See also the letter from Lee Robins, the epidemiologist at Washington University and a member of the Substance Abuse Disorders and Personality Disorders Advisory Committees, who ran a statistical check for reliability on both the Feighner criteria and the proposed DSM-III criteria for Somatization Disorder with somewhat muddy results. Letter from Robins to Spitzer and Janet Forman (later Williams), DSM-III text editor and field trials coordinator, April 10, 1979, Archives, DSM Coll.

17. Letter from George Saslow, M.D., to Spitzer, "Criteria for Somatization Disorder," April 2, 1979, Archives, DSM Coll.

18. DSM-III, "Somatization Disorder," pp. 243–244

19. Memo from Spitzer to the Task Force and Sam Guze, Lee Robins, and John Helzer, a psychiatrist whose professional roots were strongly set in Washington University, "Criteria for Somatization Disorder," May 3, 1979, Archives, DSM Coll.

20. Memo from Pinsker to Spitzer, "Somatization disorder," Archives, DSM Coll.

21. The documentation on the controversy is unusually large, so a brief description of these sources is called for. All of it was produced in the years 1976 to 1982. There are two secondary sources: an article by Spitzer and a book by Ronald Bayer, who at the time was a researcher at the Hastings Center, a nonpartisan and nonprofit bioethics research institute. See Robert L. Spitzer, "The Diagnostic Status of Homosexuality in DSM-III: A Reformulation of the Issue," *American Journal of Psychiatry*, Vol. 138, No. 2, February 1981, pp. 210–215; Ronald Bayer, *Homosexuality and American Psychiatry*. New York: Basic Books, 1981, especially pp. 169–178. Bayer is currently a professor at the Mailman School of Public Health at Columbia University.

Then there is an edited version of the correspondence generated by the dispute that was compiled by Bayer and Spitzer jointly. See Ronald Bayer and Robert L. Spitzer, "Correspondence on the Status of Homosexuality in DSM-III," *Journal of the History of the Behavioral Sciences*, Vol. 18, 1982, pp. 32–52.

Finally, there are the original documents in the DSM-III Archives. I have collated the documents from the Archives with the Bayer–Spitzer edited correspondence to create an extended chronological bank of primary data. Bayer's book adds some useful factual information.

22. Judd Marmor (ed.), *Sexual Inversion: The Multiple Roots of Homosexuality*. New York: Basic Books, 1965; "'Normal' and 'Deviant' Sexual Behavior," *JAMA: The Journal of the American Medical Association*, Vol. 217, No. 2, July 1971, pp. 165–170.

23. Letter from Richard Green, M.D., to Spitzer, December 14, 1976, Archives, DSM Coll.

24. Letter from Spitzer to Green, December 27, 1976, Archives, DSM Coll.

25. Bayer, *Homosexuality and American Psychiatry*, pp. 171–172.

26. Judd Marmor, M.D., to Richard C. Pillard, M.D., March 15, 1977, Archives, DSM Coll.

27. N.B. The first official draft was actually dated 4/15/77, however.

28. Richard Green to Richard Pillard, May 9, 1977, Archives, DSM Coll.

29. Pillard to Spitzer, May 10, 1977, Archives, DSM Coll.

30. Letter from Judd Marmor to Spitzer, May 12, 1977, Archives, DSM Coll.

31. Letter from Green to various psychiatrists, June 27, 1977, in Bayer and Spitzer, "Correspondence on Status of Homosexuality," p. 41.

32. Spitzer to members of the Psychosexual Disorders Committee and other psychiatrists involved in Bayer and Spitzer, p. 42.

33. Many years later, Money became notorious for some of his sex-change advice.

34. John Money, Ph.D., to Spitzer, August 8, 1977, Archives, DSM Coll. Interestingly, Money's term "Gender Dysphoria" has been adopted by the makers of DSM-5 as their new diagnostic title for the former "Gender Identity Disorder." It is hoped the new term will reduce the stigma for transgendered individuals and put emphasis less on the "disorder" and more on any distress being experienced by the transgendered person.

35. Spitzer to Marmor, September 1, 1977, in Bayer and Spitzer, p. 43.

36. Marmor to Spitzer, September 9, 1977, in Bayer and Spitzer, p. 43.

37. Memo from Michael Mavroidis, M.D., to the Task Force on Nomenclature and Statistics, Advisory Committee on Psychosexual Disorders, and Assembly [Liaison to the] Task Force, October 31, 1977, Archives, DSM Coll. Mavroidis copied his memo widely to Marmor, Melvin Sabshin (Medical Director of the APA), Jack Weinberg (President of the APA), other relevant psychiatrists, and Franklin Kameny of the Mattachine Society.

   Mavroidis, as a psychiatry resident, held an APA fellowship that assigned him to the DSM-III Task Force. As a resident, he played an active role in DSM-III matters. We will see this particularly with regard to an undertaking known as "Project Flower," which Spitzer ultimately adopted.

   Mavroidis' five-page single-spaced memo makes allusion to several pieces of correspondence that appear neither in the Archives nor in Bayer and Spitzer's article.

38. Spitzer to Green, September 23, 1977, in Bayer and Spitzer, p. 44.

39. Spitzer to Robert J. Stoller, M.D., September 23, 1977, Archives, DSM Coll.

40. Stoller to Spitzer, September 30, 1977, in Bayer and Spitzer, pp. 44–45.

41. Memo from Spitzer to the Members of the Advisory Committee on Psychosexual Disorders and to Judd Marmor October 5, 1977, in Archives, DSM Coll. Another form of the memo appears in Bayer and Spitzer, p. 46.

42. Memo from Spitzer to the Task Force on Nomenclature and Statistics, October 18, 1977, in Bayer and Spitzer, pp. 46–47.

43. Memo from Donald Kline [sic] to Spitzer, November 3, 1977, in Ibid., pp. 47–49.

   Although a November 9, 1977, memo from Spitzer to Klein (Archives, DSM Coll) seems to indicate that Klein first formulated "ego-dystonic homosexuality," Spitzer assured me in a telephone interview that he was the author. In the November 9 memo, Spitzer seems to prefer Homosexual Conflict Disorder.

44. Memo from Jon K. Meyer, M.D., to Spitzer, November 7, 1977, in Bayer and Spitzer, pp. 49–50.

45. Letter from Stoller to Spitzer, November 15, 1977, Archives, DSM Coll.

46. Memo from Spitzer to Participants in Homosexual Conflict Disorder Category, November 22, 1977, Archives, DSM Coll.

47. Letter from Green to Spitzer, November 23, 1977, Archives, DSM Coll.

48. Letter from Spitzer to Green, December 8, 1977, Archives, DSM Coll.

49. Draft of 12/20/77 for 302.01 [DSM-III code] Ego-dystonic Homosexuality, in Bayer and Spitzer, pp. 50–52.

50. Bayer and Spitzer, p. 51.

   By contrast, the draft of March 25, 1977, which was released on April 15, 1977, listed under the Paraphilias (sexual deviations), 302.00 Dyshomophilia (Homosexuality):

"Predisposing Factors. Since homosexuality predisposes to Dyshomophilia, factors which predispose to Homosexuality probably also predispose to Dyshomophilia. There is some evidence that such factors include a family constellation in which the same sexed parent is distant and a poor role model, and the relation with the opposite sexed parent is disturbed in various ways. There is also some evidence that boys who label themselves as unmasculine because of an aversion to same-sexed peer-group activities, such as rough-and-tumble play, or who manifest significant degrees of feminine behavior are predisposed to the development of homosexuality as adults." See pp. L:17 and L:18 of the draft.

51. L. Psychosexual Disorders—Paraphilias," p. L:18, 4/15/77 draft of DSM-III.

52. Ballots on Ego-dystonic Homosexuality submitted by Task Force member Rachel Gittelman and Advisory Group member John Money, Archives, DSM Coll.

53. Green to Spitzer, December 27, 1977, in Bayer and Spitzer, p. 52.

54. Marmor to Spitzer, January 6, 1978, in Bayer and Spitzer, p. 52.

55. Letter from Pinsker to Spitzer, January 16, 1978, in Archives, DSM Coll.

56. DSM-III, "Psychosexual Disorders," p. 282.

57. Ronald Bayer, *Homosexuality and American Psychiatry*. New York: Basic Books, 1981, p. 177.

58. Robert L. Spitzer, "Can Some Gay Men and Lesbians Change Their Sexual Orientation? 200 Participants Reporting a Change from Homosexual to Heterosexual Orientation," *Archives of Sexual Behavior*, October 2003, pp. 403–417.

59. Benedict Carey, "Psychiatry Giant Sorry for Backing Gay 'Cure,'" *New York Times*, May 19, 2012, p. A1.

60. Wayne Besen, "Dr. Robert Spitzer Retracts 'Ex-Gay' Study and Apologizes to the LGBT Community," *Truth Wins Out*. http://www.youtube.com/watch?v=glifMxPcRnI

61. Letter to Ann Laycock Chappell, M.D., from Elaine Hilberman, May 26, 1977; Letter from Pauline B. Bart, Ph.D., to Spitzer, June 3, 1977; Letter from Carol C. Nadelson, M.D., to Chappell, June 13, 1977. All letters are in Archives, DSM Coll.

62. Letter from Nadelson to Chappell June 13, 1977, Archives, DSM Coll.

63. Letter from Nadelson to Chappell June 13, 1977, Archives, DSM Coll.

64. Letter from Spitzer to Chappell, June 21, 1977, Archives, DSM Coll.

65. Letter from Chappell to Spitzer, June 29, 1977, Archives, DSM Coll.

66. Letter from Chappell to Spitzer, July 13, 1977, Archives, DSM Coll.

67. Letter from Spitzer to Chappell, July 21, 1977, Archives, DSM Coll.

68. Letter from Spitzer to the Advisory Committee on Gender Identity, July or August, 1977, Archives, DSM Coll. The letter has no date, but Spitzer asked for the committee's comments by September 1.

69. Memo from Spitzer to Drs. Jon Meyer, Richard Green, Anke Ehrhardt, Arthur Zitrin and Ann Chappell, October 4, 1977, Archives, DSM Coll.

70. "Gender Identity Disorder of Childhood," *Diagnostic and Statistical Manual of Mental Disorders*, Third Edition, prepared by the Task Force on Nomenclature and Statistics of the American Psychiatric Association. DSM-III Draft, 1/15/78, First Printing, pp. L: 4–7. The date for this particular section is 12/1/77.

71. Letter from Elisssa P. Benedek, M.D., Chair of the APA Committee on Women, to Spitzer, March 8, 1978; Letter from Nancy Felipe Russo, Ph.D., administrative officer of Women's Programs of the American Psychological Association, to Spitzer, May 17, 1978, Archives, DSM Coll.

72. Letter from Stoller to Spitzer, August 10, 1978, Archives, DSM Coll.

73. DSM-III, "Gender Identity Disorder of Childhood," pp. 265–266.

74. However, there was some criticism after the publication of the new manual. See, for example, the *American Psychologist* issue of July 1983, which ran a forum, "The Issue of Sex Bias in DSM-III." There were four articles: "A Woman's View of DSM-III," pp. 786–792, by Marcie Kaplan; "A Critique of 'A Woman's View of DSM-III,'" pp. 793–798, by Janet B. W. Williams and Robert L. Spitzer; "An Empirical Study of the Issue of Sex Bias in the Diagnostic Criteria of DSM-III Axis II Personality Disorders," pp. 799–801, by Frederic Kass, Robert L. Spitzer, and Janet B. W. Williams; and "Comments on the Articles by Spitzer, Williams, and Kass," pp. 802–803, by Marcie Kaplan.

Chapter 11

1. There was also a liaison committee from the American Academy of Psychoanalysis, but the committee from the Psychoanalytic Association either dominated the negotiations or spoke for the Academy.

2. Memo from Spitzer's secretary, December 20, 1976, Archives, DSM Coll.

3. Memo from Spitzer to the American Psychoanalytic Association and American Academy of Psychoanalysis Liaison [sic] Committees. The only record in the Archives is a draft of the memo with no date. Archives, DSM Coll.

4. Interview of Leo Madow by Ronald Bayer, May 26, 1982. Ronald Bayer and Robert L. Spitzer, "Neurosis, Psychodynamics, and DSM-III," *Archives of General Psychiatry*, Vol. 42, Feb. 1985, p. 189.

5. Bayer and Spitzer, p. 189.

6. Ad Hoc Committee on DSM-III, American Psychoanalytic Association: Report to the Executive Council, April 28, 1977. Summarized and quoted in Bayer and Spitzer, pp. 189–190.

7. Telegram from Herbert S. Gaskill, M.D., President, and Kenneth T. Calder, President-elect of the American Psychoanalytic Association, to Louis J. West, M.D., April 29, 1977, Archives, DSM Coll. There are numerous misspellings in the telegram that I have not reproduced here.

8. Letter from Louis Jolyon West, M.D., to Herbert S. Gaskill, M.D., President, American Psychoanalytic Association, May 17, 1977, Archives, DSM Coll. West added that the analysts could also communicate directly with the President of the APA, Jack Weinberg, M.D., with copies to Melvin Sabshin, M.D., Medical Director, and to Spitzer and Grinspoon.

9. Bayer and Spitzer, "Neurosis, Psychodynamics, and DSM-III," p. 190.

10. Letter from Spitzer to Madow, Chairman, Ad Hoc Committee on DSM-III, the American Psychoanalytic Association, June 6, 1977, Archives, DSM Coll.

11. Letter from Madow to Spitzer, June 10, 1977, Archives, DSM Coll.

12. Interview with Roger Peele, M.D., July 31, 2010. Peele remains a supporter of psychodynamic treatment as one possible modality among others, to be used when appropriate.

13. Letter from Irwin H. Marill, Donald F. Bogdan, Gene Gordon, Allen E. Marans, all M.D.s, to Peele, June 6, 1977, Archives, DSM Coll. Peele had sent the draft sections to the analyst on May 20.

14. An interesting side note to the censure in this letter is that the analysts pointed out that, paradoxically, the description of Conversion Disorder in the draft acknowledged "the etiologic role of unconscious conflict." Spitzer, who probably was sent this letter by Madow,

took out the psychodynamic language. This deletion can be seen by a comparison of the 1977 draft version with the actual published version of DSM-III.

15. Letter from Spitzer to Madow, July 11, 1977, Archives, DSM Coll.

16. In just one letter to an analyst, trying to arrange for feedback, Spitzer asked for "detailed and specific critiques," "a detailed critique," "specific suggestions for change," and "specific input." See a letter from Spitzer to Thomas Lynch, M.D., President, Baltimore-District of Columbia Society for Psychoanalysis, July 8, 1977, Archives, DSM Coll.

17. The Archives contain only the first two pages of Dr. Rockland's proposals, which offer only a very limited look at his suggestions. See "DSM-III: 'Anxiety Disorders'—Suggested Modifications," L. Rockland, M.D. No date. Archives, DSM Coll.

18. Memo from Spitzer to the Task Force on Nomenclature and Statistics with copies to the Assembly [of Delegates] Liaison Committee, the Liaison Committee of the American Academy of Psychoanalysis, and the Liaison Committee of the American Psychoanalytic Association, September 20, 1977, Archives, DSM Coll. Leo Madow's accompanying letter and the suggestions from Dr. Rockland are not included in the Archives.

   Spitzer's four alternatives to the Task Force were as follows: If you believe that this kind of material should be included in DSM-III, should it only be included if it is possible to have such material for all the appropriate diagnostic categories?

   If you believe that such material should not be included, should there be an explanation of why such material is not being included?

   If you believe that such an explanation should be included, please suggest an appropriate paragraph.

   If you believe that such material should be included, but in a form other than proposed by Dr. Rockland, please indicate how.

19. Bayer and Spitzer, "Neurosis, Psychodynamics and DSM-III," p. 190.

20. Letter from Madow to Spitzer, November 2, 1977, Archives, DSM Coll.

21. Letter from Spitzer to Madow, November 7, 1977, Archives, DSM Coll.

22. Letter from Spitzer to Madow, December 8, 1977, Archives, DSM Coll.

23. Letter from Spitzer to Madow, January 30, 1978, Archives, DSM Coll.

24. Letter from Spitzer to Rockland, December 8, 1977, Archives, DSM Coll.

25. Letter from John L. Schimel, M.D., President of the American Academy of Psychoanalysis, to Spitzer, December 6, 1977, and Letter from Spitzer to Schimel, December 8, 1977, Archives, DSM Coll.

26. Letter from Spitzer to Madow, January 30, 1978, Archives, DSM Coll.

27. In the Archives there is a two-page document, undated, that appears to be either Spitzer's or the analysts' rewriting of the Anxiety Disorders category and a section of the Psychosexual Disorders category. The caption at the head of the document reads "Psychodynamic material that had been included in a draft of Anxiety Disorders and Paraphilias but will not be included in the next draft of DSM-III." Archives, DSM Coll.

28. In the Archives there is an undated, informal request from Spitzer to Donald Klein, asking his help in composing a paragraph for the Introduction of DSM-III "indicating the impossibility of including a comprehensive discussion of mechanisms involved in the mental disorders." Archives, DSM Coll.

29. Letter from Madow to Spitzer, January 4, 1978, Archives, DSM Coll.

30. Letter from Madow to Spitzer, January 4, 1978, Archives, DSM Coll.

31. Letter from Spitzer to Madow, January 30, 1978, Archives, DSM Coll.

32. Telephone interview with Dr. George E. Vaillant, October 19, 2012.

33. "Theoretical Hierarchy of Adaptive Ego Mechanisms: A 30-Year Follow-up of 30 Men Selected for Psychological Health," *Archives of General Psychiatry*, Vol. 24, 1971, pp. 107–118; "The Evolution of Adaptive and Defensive Behaviors During the Adult Life Cycle," abstracted in the *Journal of the American Psychoanalytic Association*, Vol. 19, 1971, pp. 110–115.

34. George Vaillant, "Editorial: Lifting the Field's 'Repressions' of Defenses," *American Journal of Psychiatry*, Vol. 169, No. 9, September 2012, pp. 885–887.

35. Memo from Spitzer to the Task Force, "Coping Styles and Multi-Axial Diagnosis," undated, Archives, DSM Coll.

36. Memo from David Shaffer, M.D., to Spitzer, "Coping Styles," April 5, 1978, Archives, DSM Coll. Shaffer sat on the Infancy, Childhood, and Adolescence Disorders and the Multiaxial Advisory Committees.

37. Letter from Madow to Spitzer, April 11, 1978, Archives, DSM Coll.

38. Minutes of the Task Force and Assembly Liaison Committee, May 7, 1978, Atlanta, GA, Archives, DSM Coll.

39. *Diagnostic and Statistical Manual of Mental Disorders* (3rd ed.), p. 24.

40. Memo from Spitzer to Task Force; Dr. Vaillant; Glossary Committee; Multiaxial Committee; Assembly Liaison Committee American Psychoanalytic Association; Academy of Psychoanalysis; American Psychological Association, "Axis for Etiological Formulation," March 28, 1978, Archives, DSM Coll.

41. Minutes of the "Open Meeting on DSM-III" September 8, 1978, Archives, DSM Coll.

42. Twelve ballots returned plus Madow's vote in his letter to Spitzer, April 11, 1978, Archives, DSM Coll.

43. Minutes of a meeting of the Task Force and the Assembly Liaison Committee, May 7, 1978, Atlanta, GA, Archives, DSM Coll.

44. Questionnaire from Spitzer to field trial participants, "Some Hot Issues for you to Think About," May 5, 1978, Archives, DSM Coll.

45. The March 28 memo, on the axis for etiological formulations, was one place where Spitzer's argument occurs, but it is found strewn in many of his communications.

46. Rockland wrote: "DSM-III is most strongly anti-psychoanalytic in its very attempts to be fair to all competing schools.…It is unreasonable …to treat equally the carefully reproduced work of thousands of psychoanalysts and psychodynamic clinicians, and the relatively recent learning theories, or esoteric fantasies about the etiology of psychopathology.…It is an abandonment of common sense and reasonableness to state that since there are different opinions among the various schools, therefore all should be left out." Of course, the psychoanalytic insistence that psychoanalysis is superior to all other forms of psychological explanation must have grated on the nerves of the representatives of other etiological schools. Archives, DSM Coll.

47. Letter from Paul J. Fink, M.D., to Lester Grinspoon, M.D., May 15, 1978, and letter from Madow to Grinspoon, May 18, 1978, Archives, DSM Coll. Fink became President of the APA, 1988–1989. To this day he remains angry over Spitzer's actions. Telephone interview with Fink in 2010.

48. Letter from Grinspoon to Fink, June 28, 1978, Archives, DSM Coll.

49. "Open Meeting on DSM-III Minutes" September 8, 1978, Archives, DSM Coll.

50. NIMH-sponsored Field Trial Questionnaire Number 1 with 36 questions. 271 Responses as of 9/5/78, Archives, DSM Coll.

51. See, for example, Stuart A. Kirk and Herb Kutchins, *The Selling of DSM: The Rhetoric of Science in Psychiatry.* New York: Aldine de Gruyter, 1992.

52. Interview with Theodore Shapiro, M.D., January 29, 2007.

53. Actually, in Chinese, it was a hundred flowers.

54. Melvin Sabshin, *Changing American Psychiatry: A Personal Perspective.* Arlington, VA: American Psychiatric Publishing, 2008.

55. Bayer and Spitzer, "Neurosis, Psychodynamics, and DSM-III," p. 191.

56. Minutes of the Executive Council. Washington, DC, American Psychoanalytic Association, December 1978 in Bayer and Spitzer, p. 191.

57. Letter from Robert Michels, M.D., to Peter C. Whybrow, M.D., October 16, 1978, Archives, DSM Coll.

58. Draft "Response to Michels letter," undated, Archives, DSM Coll.

59. Letter from Whybrow to Spitzer, November 2, 1978, Archives, DSM Coll.

60. Letter from Spitzer to Whybrow, November 17, 1978, Archives, DSM Coll.

61. Letter from Spitzer to Douglas L. Lenkoski, M.D., President of the American Association of Chairmen of Departments of Psychiatry, February 1979, Archives, DSM Coll.

62. Letter from Spitzer to Lenkoski, February 14, 1979, Archives, DSM Coll.

63. Of course, one cannot but think how little input and guidance Spitzer had actually allowed the Assembly's Liaison Committee to have.

64. Memo from Spitzer to the Task Force on Nomenclature and Statistics, "Appendix Designed for Psychiatrists with a Psychodynamic Orientation," November 16, 1978, Archives, DSM Coll.

65. Allen Frances and Harold Pincus. "Remembrance: Mel Sabshin Was Truly a Man for All Seasons," *Clinical Psychiatry News,* June 28, 2011. http://www.clinicalpsychiatrynews.com.

66. Letter from Spitzer to Alan A. Stone, M.D., November 16, 1978, Archives, DSM Coll.

67. Memo from Henry Pinsker to Spitzer, November 27, 1978, Archives, DSM Coll.

68. Letter from Jaso to Stone, December 1, 1978, Archives, DSM Coll.

69. Letter from Sabshin to Spitzer, February 14, 1979, Archives, DSM Coll.

70. Letter from Offenkrantz to Sabshin, February 19, 1979, Archives, DSM Coll.

71. "DSM-III & Psychodynamic Psychiatry" (contributed by the Joint DSM-III Committee of the American Psychoanalytic Association & the American Academy of Psychoanalysis; William Offenkrantz, M.D., Chair), Draft of the Appendix, Undated, in Archives, DSM Coll.

72. Letter from Spitzer to Offenkrantz, March 27, 1979, Archives, DSM Coll.

73. Letter from Michael Mavroidis, M.D., to Spitzer, June 6, 1978, Archives, DSM Coll.

74. Memo from Spitzer to the Task Force, "Project Flower," July 26, 1978, Archives, DSM Coll.

75. Letter from Mavroidis to Madow, September 19, 1978, Archives, DSM Coll.

76. Letter from Madow to Mavroidis, September 25, 1978, Archives, DSM Coll.

77. Letter from Spitzer to Alex Kaplan, M.D., Joe Yamamoto, M.D., Iver F. Small, M.D., Allen E. Kazdin, Ph.D., Murray Bowen, M.D., and Donald F. Williamson, Ph.D., October 30, 1978, Archives, DSM Coll.

78. Letter from Spitzer to Brewster Smith, Ph.D., October 30, 1978, Archives, DSM Coll.

79. Memo from Spitzer to the Task Force, "Appendix Designed for Psychiatrists with a Psychodynamic Orientation," November 16, 1978; Letter from Spitzer to Grinspoon, November 16, 1978; Letter from Spitzer to Stone, November 16, 1978. All correspondence in Archives, DSM Coll.

80. Letter from Jaso to Stone, December 1, 1978, Archives, DSM Coll.

81. Letter from Spitzer to George Tarjan, M.D., December 13, 1978, Archives, DSM Coll.

82. Letter from Spitzer to Grinspoon, December 13, 1978; Letter from Grinspoon to Spitzer, December 26, 1978. Both letters are in Archives, DSM Coll.

83. Letter from Kaplan to Spitzer, January 22, 1979, Archives, DSM Coll. The members of the psychoanalytic committee ("Sub Committee" of the American Psychoanalytic Association, as Kaplan called it) were William Offenkrantz (Chair), Sol Altschul, Arnold Cooper, Gene Gordon, Allen Frances, and Allan Rosenblatt. Robert Michels was a consultant.

84. Letter from Spitzer to Kaplan, February 5, 1979, Archives, DSM Coll.

85. Letters from Spitzer to Joan Zaro, Ph.D., February 2, 1979, and Peter E. Nathan, Ph.D., Archives, DSM Coll.

86. Letter from Spitzer to Kaplan, February 5, 1979, Archives, DSM Coll.

87. Letter from Zaro to Spitzer, February 15, 1979, Archives, DSM Coll. Spitzer also wrote to Sabshin asking for his advice in this thorny situation, noting Zaro's "poignant letter." Spitzer to Sabshin, February 27, 1979, Archives, DSM Coll.

88. Letter from Kaplan to Zaro, March 6, 1979, Archives, DSM Coll.

89. Letter from Kaplan to Spitzer, March 6, 1979, Archives, DSM Coll.

90. Letter from Spitzer to Zaro, March 22, 1979, Archives, DSM Coll.

91. Robert L. Spitzer, "Prospectus on DSM-III and Evaluation for Treatment Planning Book," Undated document but perhaps July 1979, Archives, DSM Coll.

92. Letter and Chapter Summary from William Offenkrantz, M.D., to Sabshin, February 19, 1979, Archives, DSM Coll.

93. Spitzer, "Prospectus," p. 1.

94. Letter from Spitzer to Rebecca Solomon, M.D., May 23, 1979, Archives, DSM Coll.

95. Memo From Spitzer to the Task Force, May 23, 1979, Archives, DSM Coll.

96. Memo From Spitzer to the Task Force, May 23, 1979, Archives, DSM Coll.

97. Letter from Spitzer to John M. Davis, M.D., September 21, 1979, Archives, DSM Coll.

98. Memo from Offenkrantz to DSM-III Committee, August 31, 1979, Archives, DSM Coll.

99. Memo from Donald G. Langsley, M.D., to Members of the Reference Committee, September 14, 1979, Archives, DSM Coll. See also Memo from Spitzer to John M. Davis, M.D., September 21, 1979, Archives, DSM Coll.

100. Memo from Spitzer to Keith Brodie, M.D., Lew Robbins, M.D., and John A. Talbott, M.D., December 27, 1979, Archives, DSM Coll. See also the related memo from Lew L. Robbins to Keith Brodie, January 9, 1980, Archives, DSM Coll.

101. Letter from Lawrence Hartmann, M.D., to Carolyn B. Robinowitz, M.D. January 22, 1980, Archives, DSM Coll.

102. Letter from Keith Brodie, M.D., to Alan A. Stone, M.D., February 12, 1980, Archives, DSM Coll.

103. Letter from Sanford I. Finkel, M.D., to Sabshin, May 29, 1980, Archives, DSM Coll.

104. Memo from Jeanne Robb to Dr. Sabshin, "Assembly [of Delegates] Discussion of Project Flower," October 31, 1980, Archives, DSM Coll. Accompanying this memo are three loose pages containing the discussion in the Assembly of Project Flower on October 26, 1980.

105. "Introduction," *Diagnostic and Statistical Manual of Mental Disorders* (3rd ed.), p. 11.

106. Gene Usdin and Jerry M. Lewis (eds.), *Treatment Planning in Psychiatry*. Washington, DC: American Psychiatric Association Press, 1982.

Chapter 12

1. Robert L. Spitzer, Principal Investigator, NIMH Contract #278–77–0022 (DB), "DSM-III Field Trials," $93, 286.00, September 19, 1977 to March 18, 1980.
2. "Field Trial Questionnaire Number 1," June 28, 1978, Archives, DSM Coll.
3. David J. Barry, M.D., and J. Richard Ciccone, M.D. "The Experience of Using DSM-III in a Court Clinic Setting: II Practicality and effect of DSM-III on a Court Clinic's Work with the Legal System," *Bulletin of the American Academy of Psychiatry and the Law*, Vol. 6, No. 1, 1978, pp. 26–30.
4. Stuart A. Kirk and Herb Kutchins, *The Selling of DSM: The Rhetoric of Science in Psychiatry*. New York: Aldine de Gruyter, 1992.
5. "Revised response to request for proposal for field test of DSM-III submitted to the National Institute of Mental Health by the American Psychiatric Association," July 18, 1977. NIMH DB 77–0022.
6. "Revised response," 1977.
7. A draft of a "Dear Colleague" letter Spitzer used for recruiting institutions can be found in the Archives, DSM Coll. An example of a specific letter based on this draft is that sent to Walter H. Wellborn, Jr., M.D., of the National Association of Private Psychiatric Hospitals, dated August 11, 1976, Archives, DSM Coll.
8. Letter from Spitzer to Sabshin, June 26, 1979, Archives, DSM Coll.
9. Letter and Instructions to Diagnosticians Participating in DSM-III Field Trials from Robert L. Spitzer, M.D., and Michael Sheehy, M.D. [new Task Force member], January 7, 1977; Instructions for DSM-III Field Trial Coordinators, January 7, 1977, Archives, DSM Coll.
10. There are numerous letters, memos, and instructions in the Archives, with updates. The two earliest are a memo from Spitzer to field trial coordinators, "Psychic Factors in Physical Conditions," January 14, 1977, just one week after the initial letters and instructions, and letters from Spitzer to field trial coordinators and to diagnosticians, March 10, 1977, Archives, DSM Coll.
11. Draft of a letter, probably from Spitzer and Forman, to a Mr. Miller at the NIMH, undated, but most likely in summer 1979, asking for an extension of 6 months to finish the analysis of all the results of the field trials. Archives, DSM Coll.
12. "Appendix F: DSM-III Field Trials, Project Staff and Participants in Facilities and Participants in Private Practice," in *Diagnostic and Statistical Manual of Mental Disorders* (3rd ed.), 1980, pp. 473–481.
13. "Introduction," DSM-III, p. 5.
14. NIMH-Sponsored DSM-III Field Trial Procedure Manual—Phase One, undated, but probably in the late spring or summer 1977, Archives, DSM Coll.
15. Letters from Spitzer and Forman to Field Trial Participants, March 20, 1978, and May 5, 1978, Archives, DSM Coll.
16. Barry and Ciccone, p. 27.
17. Barry and Ciccone, p. 28.
18. For the final version of this see DSM-III, pp. 331–334.
19. Barry and Ciccone, pp. 28–29.
20. Barry and Ciccone, pp. 29–30.
21. Appendix F, "DSM-III Field Trials: Interrater Reliability and List of Project Staff and Participants," pp. 465–481.

22. Letter from Boyd L. Burris, M.D., to "Dear Doctors" [presidents, affiliate societies, American Psychoanalytic Association], March 21, 1979, Archives, DSM Coll.

23. "Appendix F," DSM-III, pp. 473–481.

24. Letter from Spitzer and Steven E. Hyler [member of three Advisory Groups], August 14, 1978; survey from Spitzer and Forman, September 21, 1978; questionnaire from Spitzer and Forman, undated, but probably November or December, 1978, all from Archives, DSM Coll; "Micro-D," new draft of 1/2/79, Archives, DSM Coll.

25. "Field Trial Questionnaire Number 2 (and the last!)," March 30, 1979, Archives, DSM Coll.

26. "Introduction," DSM-III, p. 5. Of course, this statement is at odds with what he told the NIMH, that the main goal was to get the bugs out of the DSM-III drafts.

27. See, for example, the "Questionnaire #1—Supplement on Reliability Study," undated, but clearly around June 1978; or Phase 2 Questionnaire, Question #4, 3/30/79, Archives, DSM Coll.

28. Stuart A. Kirk and Herb Kutchins, "The Myth of the Reliability of DSM," http://www.academyanalyticarts.org/kirk&kutchins.htm.

29. Robert L. Spitzer, Janet B. W. Forman, and John Nee, "DSM-III Field Trials: I. Initial Interrater Diagnostic Reliability," American Journal of Psychiatry, Vol. 136, No. 6, June 1979, p. 816.

30. Spitzer et al., p. 817; Appendix F, DSM-III, p. 468; Robert L. Spitzer and Joseph L. Fleiss, "A Reanalysis of the Reliability of Psychiatric Diagnosis," British Journal of Psychiatry, Vol. 125, 1974, p. 344. This last article presents a useful comparison of kappa for several disorders in studies from 1956 to the early 1970s.

31. Kirk and Kutchins, The Selling of DSM, p. 129, and "Field Trial Questionnaire Number 1," June 28, 1978, Archives, DSM Coll.

32. Kirk and Kutchins, pp. 41–45.

33. Kirk and Kutchins, pp. 122, 128–130, 157.

34. "Use of This Manual," DSM-III, p. 23.

35. Robert L. Spitzer and Janet B. W. Forman, "DSM-III Field Trials, II: Initial Experience with the Multiaxial System," American Journal of Psychiatry, Vol. 136, No. 6, June 1979, pp. 820, 818.

36. "Use of This Manual," DSM-III, p. 26.

37. Spitzer and Forman, "Initial Experience with the Multiaxial System," p. 819.

38. Spitzer and Forman, pp. 819–820.

39. "Use of This Manual," DSM-III, p. 26.

40. The documents are under the headings "Proposed Multiaxial System for DSM-III;" "Axis V"; "Glossary of Terms"; "Multiaxial System (Adults)"; "Global Ratings," January, 1976; and "Master," March, 1976. They include both drafts and final copies. Undated documents appear to have come from late 1975 and early 1976. Archives, DSM Coll.

41. Or it could have been a meeting involving the written work of the U.K. experts recorded in the minutes along with the opinions of the committee present in the United States.

42. Memo from Spitzer to APA Task Force Members and Drs. Glueck, Sachar, West, Work, October 15, 1976, Archives, DSM Coll.

43. Letter from Spitzer to A. James Morgan, M.D., August 31, 1977, Archives, DSM Coll.

44. "Axis IV. Severity of Psychosocial Stressors," DSM-III Draft, 4/15/77, p. 2:6, 3/10/77 [the date this section was put into the draft as opposed to its public issuance].

    But of course, there could be any of a host of stressors, which he tried to spell out with many examples in the final version of DSM-III. See "Use of This Manual," p. 28.

45. "Axis IV," DSM-III Draft, 4/15/77, p. 2:5.
46. "Use of This Manual," DSM-III, p. 26.
47. "Use of This Manual," DSM-III, pp. 26–27.
48. Letter from Frederic W. Infeld Jr., M.D., to Spitzer, September 28, 1977, Archives, DSM Coll.
49. "Axis IV Types of Psychosocial Stressors," Ilfeld draft, 9–77, Archives, DSM Coll.
50. Memo from Spitzer to Ilfeld, "Distribution of Psychosocial Stressor Proposal," October 7, 1977, Archives, DSM Coll.
51. Memo from Spitzer to Members of the Advisory Committee on Multiaxial Disorders, "Dr. Ilfeld's Psychosocial Stressor Proposal," October 7, 1977, and Memo from Spitzer to Task Force Members; Members of the Advisory Committee on Childhood and Adolescence Disorders, "Psychosocial Stressor Proposal," October 7, 1977, Archives, DSM Coll.
52. Memo from Spitzer to Bruce Dohrenwend, Ph.D., "DSM-III Axis IV," October 7, 1977, Archives, DSM Coll.
53. Memo from Spitzer to Drs. Ilfeld, Juan Mezzich, David Shaffer, Rachel Gitelman, Donald Klein, Dennis Cantwell, "Newport Beach Meeting on Psychosocial Stressors and Multiaxial Diagnosis in Children," October 31, 1977, Archives, DSM Coll. The meeting was held November 13, 1977.
54. DSM-II, 1968, p. 45.
55. News article, *Psychiatric News*, June 4, 1975.
56. Letter from Adrien L. Coblentz, M.D., June 12, 1975, Archives, DSM Coll.
57. Letter from Nakhleh P. Zarzar, M.D., to Spitzer, January 6, 1976, Archives, DSM Coll.
58. See, for example, Jerome H. Jaffe, M.D., "Tobacco Use as a Mental Disorder: The Rediscovery of a Medical Problem," In *Research on Smoking Behavior*, Publication of the National Institute on Drug Abuse (NIDA), 1977, pp. 202–217.
59. M. D. Neuman, A. Bitton, S. A. Glantz, "Tobacco Industry Influence on the Definition of Tobacco Related Disorders by the American Psychiatric Association," *Tobacco Control*, Vol. 14, 2005, pp. 328–337. Accessed online December 31, 2009.
60. Memo from William L. Dunn, principal scientist at Philip Morris to various executives and other scientists at PM, October 28, 1976, quoted in Neuman et al., pp, 2–3 of the online version.
61. Memos from Horace R. Kornegay to Committee of Counsel, November 4, 1976, and November 18, 1976, quoted in Neuman et al., p. 3 of the online version.
62. Letter from Richard C. Proctor, M.D., to Spitzer, December 7, 1976, Legacy Tobacco Documents Library at the University of California at San Francisco, http://legacy.library. ucsf.edu/action/document/page?tid=zvn85d00.
63. See also Proctor's letter to Spitzer, January 4, 1977, located on http://legacy.library.ucsf. edu/action/document/page?tid=xyn85d00. DSM-5 will contain the diagnosis "Binge Eating Disorder."
   There are eating disorders in DSM-III listed under "Disorders Usually First Evident in Infancy, Childhood, or Adolescence."
64. Letter from Spitzer to Proctor, January 11, 1977, located on http://legacy.library.ucsf.edu/ action/document/page?tid=wyn85d00.
65. Proctor, "Who's Mentally Ill?," *Psychology Today*, January 1978, quoted in Neuman et al., "Tobacco industry influence," online, p. 4.
66. Neuman et al., "Tobacco industry influence," online, p. 4.
67. Letter from Leonard Cammer, M.D., to Spitzer, January 17, 1977, Legacy Tobacco Documents Library at the University of California at San Francisco, http://legacy.library. ucsf.edu/tid/xso18c00/pdf.

68. Neuman et al, "Tobacco industry influence," see especially Table 1. In one notable instance, Proctor wrote to George Tarjan, M.D., President-elect of the APA, October 22, 1980; see p. 6 of the online version.

69. DSM-5, due out in 2013, will no longer use the term *dependence*. Here is their rationale: "The Substance-Related Disorders Work Group has proposed to eliminate the current category of Substance-Related Disorders, and replace it with a new category, Substance Use and Addictive Disorders. This category will include the substance use disorders (e.g., alcohol use disorder), in place of separate designations for substance abuse and dependence. One reason for dropping the term "dependence" in this revision is that the term can be misleading and is frequently confused with the term "addiction." The tolerance and withdrawal that patients experience with dependence are normal responses to prescribed medications that affect the central nervous system and do not necessarily indicate the presence of an addiction. By revising and clarifying these criteria, the work group hopes to alleviate some of the widespread misunderstanding around these issues." Taken from "Q&A with Dr. William Narrow, Research Director for the DSM-5 Task Force," January 30, 2012. See http://www.post-gazette.com/pg/12030/1206972–114–0.stm?cmpid=news.xml.

70. J. Kasanin, "The Acute Schizoaffective Psychoses," *American Journal of Psychiatry*, Vol. 90, 1933, pp. 97–126.

71. Robert L. Spitzer, Nancy C. Andreasen, and Jean Endicott, "Schizophrenia and other Psychotic Disorders in DSM-III," *Schizophrenia Bulletin*, Vol. 4, No. 4, 1978, pp. 489–494.

72. Carpenter went on to a distinguished career in schizophrenia studies. He is currently Chair of the Psychotic Disorders Work Group developing DSM-5 and is a member of the prestigious Institute of Medicine of the National Academy of Sciences. He is also editor-in-chief of *Schizophrenia Bulletin*.

73. William T. Carpenter, Jr., "Schizophrenia and Psychoses Not Classified Elsewhere," 4/13/78, Archives, DSM Coll.

74. Memo from Spitzer to Drs. Nancy Andreasen, Jean Endicott, Donald Klein, Lyman Wynne, and Arthur Rifkin, "Schizoaffective and Affective Disorders," April 20, 1978, Archives, DSM Coll.

75. "Mood-Congruent psychotic features: Delusions or hallucinations whose content *is entirely consistent* with either a depressed or manic mood. If the mood is depressed, the content of the delusions or hallucinations *would* involve themes of either personal inadequacy, guilt, disease, death, nihilism, or deserved punishment..... Mood-Incongruent psychotic features: Delusions or hallucinations whose content *is not consistent* with either a depressed or manic mood. In the case of depression, a delusion or hallucination whose content *does not* involve themes of either personal inadequacy, guilt, disease, death, nihilism, or deserved punishment." Italics added. Appendix B, "Glossary of Technical Terms," DSM-III, p. 364.

76. Memo from Dr. Donald Klein to Dr. Robert Spitzer, April 25, 1978, Box 100904; Memo from Jean Endicott to DSM-III Schizoaffective "Conferees," Re: "RDC Criteria for Schizoaffective Disorders and other comments," and "Changes in the Criteria," no date; Memo from Paula J. Clayton, M.D., to Robert L. Spitzer, "Schizoaffective," October 5, 1978; Letter from Nancy C. Andreasen, M.D., to Robert L. Spitzer, M.D., November 2, 1978, Archives, DSM Coll.

77. Minutes of the Task Force Meeting of October 4, 1978, October 12, 1978, Archives, DSM Coll.

78. Memo from Spitzer to the Members of the APA Task Force on Nomenclature and Statistics, "Schizoaffective Disorder," November 3, 1978, Archives, DSM Coll.

79. Memo from Spitzer to the Task Force on Nomenclature and Statistics, "Further Thoughts on Schizoaffective Disorder," November 16, 1978, Archives, DSM Coll.

80. "295.70 Schizoaffective Disorder," 11/20/78, Archives, DSM Coll.

81. Letter from Spitzer to Lester Grinspoon, M.D. April 2, 1979, Archives, DSM Coll.

82. "Field Trial Questionnaire Number 2 (and the last!)" Archives, DSM Coll.

83. Memo from Spitzer to Klein, "Your April 17th Schizoaffective memo," May 7, 1979, Archives, DSM Coll. At the time he was writing to Klein, Spitzer was deeply enmeshed in trying to defend DSM-III before the APA Board of Trustees.

84. Letter from Spitzer to Roger Mesmer, M.D., June 4, 1979.

85. Letter from A. L. Halpern, M.D., to Spitzer, October 26, 1976, Archives, DSM Coll.

86. "General Comments" of the DSM-III Committee of the American Academy of Psychiatry and the Law, June 12, 1977. The Committee cited a ruling that upheld this principle, *McDonald v. United States*, 312 F. 2d 847 (D.C. Cir. 1962.)

87. "Introduction," DSM-III, p. 12.

88. "Cautionary Statement," DSM-IV, 1994, p. xxvii.

89. The conditions are found under "Disorders of Impulse Control Not Elsewhere Classified" in Section 0 in the draft of 4/15/77.

90. I own a copy of this draft, and it also can be found on Google Books.

91. DSM-I, 1952, pp. 40–42.

92. DSM-II, 1968, pp. 49–50.

93. William Frosch, one of the analysts on the Task Force, says that his suggestion that childhood disorders be placed first in the new manual was the only significant way he affected the revision. Interview with William A. Frosch, M.D., January 27, 2007.

94. Yiddish term for those possessing special knowledge or expertise.

95. Memo from Spitzer to Drs. Paul Wender, Rachel Gittelman, Dennis Cantwell, Judith Rapoport, Donald Klein, and Michael Sheehy, April 20, 1978, Archives, DSM Coll.

96. Memo from Spitzer to Drs. Paul Wender et al., April 20, 1978, Archives, DSM Coll.

97. Memo from Judith Rapoport to Drs. Bob Spitzer, Paul Wender, Donald Klein, and Rachel Gittelman, April 24, 1978, Archives, DSM Coll.

98. Perhaps this topic could be further researched—if there are those interested in this specific piece of history—by interviewing some of the Advisory Group members still living.

99. Letter most likely from Dennis P. Cantwell at the Neuropsychiatric Institute at UCLA to Spitzer, July 24, 1978, Archives, DSM Coll.

100. Before Cantwell died at age 58 he had established himself as an expert on family genetic studies of ADHD.

101. Letter from Wender to Spitzer, November 2, 1978, Archives, DSM Coll.

102. Memo from Drs. Robert L. Spitzer, Joaquim Puig-Antich, Rachel Gittelman to Attention Deficit Disorder Mavens: Drs. Cantwell, Field Marshall Wender (Wender had adopted military sobriquets in his dealings with Spitzer), [David] Shaffer, Rapoport, [Richard] Jenkins, March 2, 1979, Archives, DSM Coll.

103. Letter from Field Marshall Paul Wender to Attention Deficit Disorder Mavens: Drs. Cantwell, Commander in Chief Spitzer, Shaffer, Rapoport, Jenkins, Puig-Antich, Rachel Gittelmen, March 13, 1979, Archives, DSM Coll.
    "Hyperkinetic Reaction of Childhood (or Adolescence)" was a diagnosis in DSM-II.

104. Memo from Field Marshall Paul Wender to Commander in Chief, "Regarding your memo of March 20, 1979," March 28, 1979, Archives, DSM Coll.

105. Memo from Field Marshall Paul Wender to Commander in Chief, March 28, 1979.

106. Wender has spoken and published frequently on adult ADD. See, for example, his *ADHD: Attention-Deficit Hyperactivity Disorder in Children, Adolescents, and Adults.* New York: Oxford University Press, 2000.

107. A full account of this is contained in Wilbur J. Scott, "PTSD in DSM-III: A Case in the Politics of Diagnosis and Disease," *Social Problems*, Vol. 37, No. 3, August 1990, pp. 294–310.

108. Shatan's, Lifton's, Haley's, and Talbott's publications are listed in Scott's references. The International Society for Traumatic Stress Studies has established the Sarah Haley Award for Clinical Excellence in Haley's honor. The first award went to Shatan in 1994.

109. DSM-III, "Anxiety Disorders," p. 238.

110. John E. Helzer, Lee N. Robins, and D. H. Davis, "Antecedents of Narcotic Use and Addiction: A Study of 898 Vietnam Veterans," *Drug and Alcohol Dependence*, Vol. 1., 1976, pp. 83–90; Helzer, Robins, and Davis, "Depressive Disorders in Vietnam Returnees," *Journal of Nervous and Mental Disease*, Vol. 168, 1976, pp. 177–185.

Chapter 13

1. Letter from Boyd L. Burris to Spitzer, January 22, 1979, quoted in Ronald Bayer and Robert L. Spitzer, "Neurosis, Psychodynamics, and DSM-III," *Archives of General Psychiatry*, Vol. 42, February 1985, p. 191.

    Dr. Burris declined to be interviewed.

2. Letter from Boyd L. Burris to "Dear Doctors" (presidents of the psychoanalytic societies affiliated with the American Psychoanalytic Association), March 21, 1979, Archives, DSM Coll.

3. Letter from F. A. Silva, M.D., to Jules R. Masserman, M.D., January 30, 1979, Archives, DSM Coll. Silva based his letter on a detailed report on the DSM-III draft of 1/15/78 by a member of his Association. She had written persuasively: "Grouping conditions together simply because of shared phenomenology—because they superficially 'look alike' suggests a regressive trend away from increased understanding of a disease entity." See letter from Marilyn M. Skinner, M.D., to Millard Jensen, M.D., January 15, 1979, Archives, DSM Coll.

4. Letter from Richard P. Goldwater, M.D., to unknown addressee, February 3, 1979, Archives, DSM Coll. Indeed, now in the United States, the lion's share of psychotherapy is being done by psychologists, social workers, and counselors.

5. Letter from John Racy, M.D., to Spitzer, March 5, 1979, Archives, DSM Coll.

6. Letter from William Offenkrantz, Chair of the analysts DSM-III Subcommittee, to Lester Grinspoon, Chair of the APA Council of Research and Development, March 5, 1979, Archives, DSM Coll.

7. The full citation of the Bayer and Spitzer article is in Note 1 above.

8. Letter from Offenkrantz to Grinspoon, March 5, 1979, and attached untitled statement, Archives, DSM Coll.

9. Memo from John J. McGrath, M.D., legislative representative, Area III to Boyd L. Burris, M.D., President, Baltimore-DC Psychoanalytic Society, "DSM-III: The Omission of the Neuroses," March 13, 1979, Archives, DSM Coll.

10. Letter from Burris to "Dear Doctors," March 21, 1979.

11. Bayer and Spitzer, "Neurosis, Psychodynamics, and DSM-III," 1985, p. 192.

12. Letter from Roger Peele to Spitzer, March 12, 1979, quoted in Bayer and Spitzer, p. 192.

13. Bayer and Spitzer, p. 192.

14. Bayer and Spitzer, p. 192.
15. Memo from Spitzer to Assembly Liaison, Joint American Psychoanalytic Association and American Academy of Psychoanalysis Committees, "April 7th meeting and possible neurotic peace treaty," March 27, 1979, Archives, DSM Coll.
16. Letter from Spitzer to Offenkrantz, March 27, 1979, Archives, DSM Coll.
17. Memo from Spitzer to Assembly Liaison and Joint Association and Academy Committees, March 27, 1979.
    The Archives also contain a last minute revision of the section on neurotic disorders, 10:15 AM, April 7, 1979, Archives, DSM Coll.
18. Letter from Roger Peele, M.D. (Assembly Liaison Committee) to Spitzer, April 4, 1979, Archives, DSM Coll.
19. Donald Klein, "Memorandum to the Task Force on Nomenclature and Statistics," March 30, 1979, quoted in Bayer and Spitzer, p. 192.
20. Memorandum to the Task Force on Nomenclature and Statistics, March 30, 1979, in Bayer and Spitzer, p. 193.
21. Letter from Spitzer to Grinspoon, April 2, 1979, Archives, DSM Coll.
22. Letter from Spitzer to Sabshin, April 6, 1979, Archives, DSM Coll.
    One additional point to note is that at the meeting with Sabshin, Spitzer broached the still problematic subject of including in DSM-III a discussion of the concept of mental disorder, and Sabshin supported this idea. A definition of a mental disorder appeared in the Introduction on page 6.
23. Informal letter from Peele to Spitzer, April 4, 1979, Archives, DSM Coll.
24. Letter from Burris to Masserman, April 18, 1979, Archives, DSM Coll.
25. Letter from Burris to Hector C. Jaso, Chairman Task Force on DSM-III of the Assembly of District Branches, April 9, 1979, Archives, DSM Coll.
26. Jaso wrote up the minutes and in the 1980s probably possessed a copy that Spitzer had access to.
27. Telephone interview with Roger Peele, September 9, 2011. Peele has been a valuable source of information about the last few months before the Assembly's vote as well as about other psychiatric matters relevant to DSM-III.
28. Bayer and Spitzer, p. 193.
29. Telephone interview with Peele.
30. Letter from Burris to Jaso, April 9, 1979.
31. Letter from Kurt Nussbaum. M.D., chief consultant in Psychiatry and Neurology, Social Security Administration, to Lee. C. Park, M.D., President, Maryland Psychiatric Society, April 4, 1979, Archives, DSM Coll.
32. Letter from William Offenkrantz to Dear Dr. (Trustees of APA), with the attached two page statement sent to Spitzer February 28, April 9, 1979, Archives, DSM Coll.
33. Board of Trustees Agenda Item 13-B, April 21–22, 1979, "Diagnostic & Statistical Manual—III," Archives, DSM Coll.
34. Letter from Spitzer to Jaso, April 18, 1979, and letter from Spitzer to Grinspoon, April 18, 1979, Archives, DSM Coll.
35. Letters of Masserman to Keith Brodie, M.D., chair of an ad hoc committee that the Board of Trustees had created to prepare a report on DSM-III because of a number of stated dissatisfactions with it, April 24, 1979, and April 26, 1979, Archives, DSM Coll.
36. American Psychiatric Association, American Society for Group Therapy, American Association for Social Psychiatry, American Society for Biological Psychiatry, and

American Academy of Psychoanalysis. In 1980, *Current Biography* referred to him as "a unifying force in a field fraught with divergent schools and tendencies." See *New York Times* obituary, November 15, 1994, http://www.nytimes.com/1994/11/15/obituaries/ju les-masserman-89-leader-of-psychiatric-group-is-dead.html.

37. Burris puts one in mind of Sir Edward Grey, the British Foreign Secretary on the eve of World War I, with his prognostication that "the lamps are going out all over Europe. We shall not see them again lit in our time."

38. Letter from Burris to Masserman, April 18, 1979, Archives, DSM Coll.

39. Trustees Agenda Item 13-B, "Diagnostic & Statistical Manual—III," April 21–22, 1979.

40. Memo from Spitzer to Task Force Members, "Our travails never seem to end," April 25, 1979, Archives, DSM Coll.

41. Memo from Spitzer to Task Force Members, April 25, 1979.

42. The ad hoc committee's report to the full Board was soon moved up to occur before, rather than after, the Assembly's vote.

Spitzer was later able to see the official minutes of the Board of Trustees' meeting. In his 1985 article with Ronald Bayer, he thus explained the decision to form an ad hoc committee: the Board was sympathetic to Offenkrantz's complaint—"some members out of theoretical sympathy, some out of weariness with [all] the controversies [and] some out of a desire to end the divisive threats to the APA. When the depths of dissatisfaction became clear, the board realized it was confronted with a serious crisis, at once political, institutional, and theoretical." See Bayer and Spitzer, 1985, p. 194.

43. The committee members were Robert Campbell, M.D., Lewis Robbins, M.D., and John Talbott, M.D.

44. Letter from Masserman to Brodie, April 24, 1979, Archives, DSM Coll.

45. Memo from Masserman to Ad Hoc Committee on DSM-III, April 25, 1979, Archives, DSM Coll. The attachment in the Archives is only in reference to the version that was being considered by the ad hoc committee: Masserman's "A Critique of the Current Version of DSM-III."

46. This was a reference to the infamous fifteenth century treatise on witches that had eventually given support to the sixteenth and seventeenth centuries witch trials and killings.

47. Bayer and Spitzer (1985) identify the other letters from Board members, M. A. Bartusis, A. Hostetter, and C. B. Wilkinson. See p. 196, Notes 61 and 62. Their letters are not in the DSM-III Archives.

48. Letter from Judd Marmor to Brodie, April 26, 1979, Archives, DSM Coll.

49. Memo from Keith H. Brodie, M.D., to Drs. Jules Masserman, Robert Campbell, Lewis Robbins, John Talbott, "Meeting of the Ad Hoc Committee of the Board of Trustees Charged to Review DSM-III," April 26, 1979, Archives, DSM Coll.

The Archives contain the statement of opinion of only one Board member, Peter A. Martin, M.D., who voted for the approval of DSM-III with some slight caveats. Letter from Peter A. Martin, M.D., to Keith H. Brodie, M.D., secretary [of the Board], April 28, 1979, Archives, DSM Coll.

50. Memo from Spitzer to the Ad Hoc Committee of the Board of Trustees to Review DSM-III, "Additional materials for your review," April 27, 1979, Archives, DSM Coll.

51. Letter from Roger Peele, M.D., to Dear Colleague, April 25, 1979, Archives, DSM Coll. Letters went to all Area Representatives, Area Deputies, District Branch Representatives, and District Deputies.

52. It may be remembered that the sociologist Ervin Goffman spent a year in 1954 at St. Elizabeth's observing the workings of the institution and based his book *Asylum* on his observations. The book played an important part in the antipsychiatry movement of the 1960s.

53. E-mail from Peele, September 14, 2011.

54. Personal interview with Roger Peele, July 31, 2010.

55. E-mail from Peele, September 14, 2011.

56. E-mail from Peele, September 14, 2011.

57. The diagnoses Reactive depression or Depressive reaction were also to be included under "Depressive neurosis." Involutional Melancholia and Manic-Depressive Illness were to be distinguished from Depressive neurosis.

58. Peele has commented that in the years since DSM-III came into being, psychiatrists rarely use the terms *mild* or *moderate* to describe a disorder, with an eye that such a word might deny insurance coverage. Telephone interview with Peele, September 9, 2011.

59. Letter from Spitzer to "Dear Colleague," April 30, 1979, Archives, DSM Coll.

60. Ultimately, this was "(Depressive neurosis)" in DSM-III.

61. Telephone interview with Peele, September 9, 2011.

62. It is not clear on exactly which days the ad hoc committee met, May 7–8 or May 8–9.

63. Letter from Brodie to Spitzer, May 9, 1979, Archives, DSM Coll.

64. Letter from Brodie to Spitzer, May 9, 1979, Archives, DSM Coll.

65. Talbott went on to become President of the APA five years later, in 1984.

66. Bayer and Spitzer, 1985, p. 194.

67. Spitzer wrote letters to the following, all on May 9, 1979: Henry B. Bracklin, Jr., M.D.; Peter A. Martin, M.D.; Jules H. Masserman, M.D.; Nancy Roeske, M.D.; William B. Spriegel, M.D.; David Starrett, M.D.; and Alan A. Stone, M.D. All letters are in the Archives, DSM Coll.

68. A mailgram was a new variety of a Western Union telegram that was sent electronically from the sender to a post office and then printed and delivered to the recipient by the postal service. It was a speedy means of communication, lower in cost than a conventional telegram, and could be sent to multiple recipients.

69. Letter from Burris to Brodie, May 10, 1979, Archives, DSM Coll.

70. "Talbott Plan (as of May 9, 1979)," Archives, DSM Coll.

71. Minutes of the Meeting of the Assembly DSM-III Task Force, Thursday and Friday, May 10 and 11, 1979, Chicago, Illinois, Archives, DSM Coll.

72. It is relevant to note that the DSM-III Liaison Committee of the American Academy of Psychiatry and the Law, in its response to the April 15, 1977 draft of DSM-III, had recommended that "in deference to the very large number of psychiatrists who could not possibly live comfortably with a diagnostic classification which excludes 'neurosis,' it would seem desirable to put in parentheses following 'Anxiety Disorders,' 'Somatoform Disorders,' 'Dissociative Disorders,' the words 'Neurotic Disorders,' thus indicating that 'Neurotic Disorders' is specified in ICD-9." "General Comments," June 12, 1977, submitted to Spitzer by the Chair of the Liaison Committee, A. L. Halpern, M.D. At this point, two years away from the APA approval of DSM-III, Spitzer ignored these comments.

73. This "alternative" (Figure 13.7) had to have made it more palatable for many psychodynamically oriented psychiatrists to accept the unfamiliar terminology in the classification.

However, Peele's memory may not be accurate as to just *when* Spitzer agreed to this sentence since it does not appear in the May 11 minutes of the Assembly Liaison Committee.

74. Bayer and Spitzer, 1985, p. 194.
75. Bayer and Spitzer, 1985, p. 194.
76. Agenda, "Assembly, May 11–13, 1979, New Material—Packet # 3 – May 12, 1979 – Third Plenary Session, Item 5.G – Assembly Liaison DSM-III Committee Proposal (Modified Talbott Plan)," Archives, DSM Coll.
77. Personal interview with Peele, July 31, 2010.
78. Personal interview with Peele, July 31, 2010.
79. For this detailed setting of the scene and the events at the meeting of the Assembly, I am indebted to Dr. Peele, with whom I not only spoke on the phone but who, on September 12, 2011, wrote out a detailed recollection including a diagram of the room and its occupants. Afterwards I asked for clarification of some information in an e-mail, and Peele answered me in an e-mail of September 14, 2011.
80. Peele's e-mail of September 14, 2011.
81. Peele's e-mail of September 14, 2011.
82. Bayer and Spitzer, 1985, p. 194.
83. Telephone interview with Peele, September 9, 2011.
84. Telephone interview with Peele, September 9, 2011.
85. Letter from Peele of September 12, 2011.
86. Personal and telephone interviews with Peele. At the first interview in 2010, Peele said Spitzer was "appalled" when he received the news.

Conclusion

1. Thomas Kuhn, *The Structure of Scientific Revolutions*. 1962. (First published as a monograph in the *International Encyclopedia of United Science*.) See Thomas Kuhn, *The Structure of Scientific Revolutions*. Chicago: University of Chicago Press, 1970.
2. Robert K. Merton, *On the Shoulders of Giants: A Shandean Postscript*. New York: Free Press, 1965. A famous expositor of this idea was Isaac Newton (1643–1727). He said in a letter at age 33, by which time he had formulated his theories of calculus, optics, and gravitation: "If I have seen a little further it is by standing on the shoulders of Giants."
3. See, for example, the assertion of a Harvard psychologist in 1935: "The course for psychology is clear. We must examine and sift the meanings of its concepts in accordance with operational procedures....We must define the criteria by which we determine the applicability of a term in a given instance." S.S. Stevens, "The Operational Basis of Psychology," *American Journal of Psychology*, Vol. 47, No. 2, 1935, p. 330.
4. Mandel Cohen and Paul Dudley White, "Life Situations, Emotions and Neurocirculatory Asthenia (Anxiety Neurosis, Neurasthenia, Effort Syndrome)," Proceedings, Association for Research in Nervous and Mental Diseases, In *Life Stress and Bodily Disease*, Vol. 29. Baltimore: Williams and Wilkens, 1950, p. 832; E. O. Wheeler, P. D. White, E. W. Reed, and M. E. Cohen, "Neurocirculatory Asthenia (Anxiety Neurosis, Effort Syndrome, Neurasthenia): 20-year Follow-up Study of 173 Patients," *JAMA*, Vol. 142, 1950, pp. 876–889.
5. Spitzer repeatedly argued the former in various formats, and Nancy Andreasen stressed the latter. See Nancy C. Andreasen, "DSM and the Death of Phenomenology in America:

An Example of Unintended Consequences," *Schizophrenia Bulletin*, Vol. 33, No. 1, 2007, p. 110. The analysts answered that they did pay attention to signs and symptoms since symptoms were a consequence of the patient's underlying neurotic anxiety.

6. John S. Strauss, "Comments" on the article by Roger K. Blashfield, "Feighner et al., Invisible Colleges, and the Matthew Effect," *Schizophrenia Bulletin*, Vol. 8, No. 1, 1982, p. 8. See also R. E. Kendell, "Comments" in *Schizophrenia Bulletin*, Vol. 8, No. 1, 1982, p. 11.

7. For his views at the time DSM-III was being developed see Melvin Sabshin, M.D., "Editorial: On Remedicalization and Holism in Psychiatry," *Psychosomatics*, October 1977, pp. 7–8. For fuller views see Melvin Sabshin, "Turning Points in Twentieth-Century American Psychiatry," *American Journal of Psychiatry*, Vol. 147, No. 10, 1990, pp. 1267– 1274, and Melvin Sabshin, M.D., *Changing American Psychiatry: A Personal Perspective*. Arlington, VA: American Psychiatric Publishing, 2008.

8. Washington University School of Medicine, Oral History Project, "Transcript: Samuel B. Guze, 1994," Interview 3. http://beckerexhibits.wustl.edu/oral/transcripts/guze1994. html.

9. Memo from Edward Shorter to Spitzer, March 3, 2004. Personal copy.

10. Significantly, Roger Peele, knowing Spitzer over the years and certainly at odds with him at times, reached the conclusion that he was flexible, saying that many people did not recognize this aspect of Spitzer's thinking. Peele points specifically to the time in 2003 when he spoke against continuing the multiaxial system, and Spitzer said to him: "Roger, you've done a lot of bad things, but this is the worst." Then, quite publicly at the 2004 APA annual meeting, Spitzer told an audience: "Roger is right, it is time for the Multiaxial system to go." Letter from Peele, September 12, 2011.

11. I am willing to consider the possibility that the Task Force did not play such a prominent role, since the Archives do not record the numerous phone calls and personal conversations that took place. But based on the archival documents, my conclusion about their major role is correct. This deduction is supported by Spitzer's own report in the 1985 article he wrote with Ronald Bayer, "Neurosis, Psychodynamics, and DSM-III."

12. Personal interview with Peele, July 31, 2010.

13. And even with this, David Riesman in *Faces in the Crowd* assessed Henry Friend's personality and prospects quite favorably.

14. Eli Robins and Samuel B. Guze, "Establishment of Diagnostic Validity in Psychiatric Illness: Its Application to Schizophrenia," *American Journal of Psychiatry*, Vol. 126, no. 7, January 1970, pp. 983–987. This was the paper that proclaimed, "In medicine, and hence in psychiatry, classification is diagnosis." Robins and Guze slammed current "diagnostic schemes …based upon a priori principles [read psychoanalysis] rather than upon systematic studies" (p. 983). The five steps they believed necessary to establish a valid diagnosis were clinical description, laboratory studies, delimitation from other disorders, follow-up studies, and family study. DSM-III in many respects came to value reliability more than validity, Spitzer departing from the Wash. U. thinking.

15. Published interview with Spitzer, "Psychological Warfare: The DSM-5 Debate." http:// www.hcplive.com/publications/mdng-Neurology/2011/february_2011/dsm_5.

16. "Introduction," DSM-III, pp. 9–10.

17. Letter from Spitzer to Madow, June 6, 1977, Archives, DSM Coll.

18. Letter from Madow to Spitzer, June 10, 1977, Archives, DSM Coll. Madow did add that they had rethought the issue and decided that there was "value in our input." But he did

not mean for his committee at that time. Instead he reported that he has "encouraged Dr. Kenneth Calder, our President, to look into this in order to participate as helpfully as possible in this work that you are undertaking." Either Calder got back to Madow or Madow's committee eventually reconsidered their options three months later. See following text.

19. Letter from Spitzer to Lawrence Rockland, M.D., December 8, 1977, Archives, DSM Coll.

20. Letter from Spitzer to Madow, December 8, 1977, Archives, DSM Coll.

21. Letter from Michael L. Mavroidis, M.D., APA Falk Fellow, to Madow, September 19, 1978, Archives, DSM Coll.

22. Letter from Madow to Mavroidis, September 25, 1978, Archives, DSM Coll.

23. See Jerry M. Lewis and Gene Usdin (eds.), *Treatment Planning in Psychiatry*. Washington, DC: American Psychiatric Association, 1982. The two editors presumably were selected because they had just published a large volume on *Psychiatry in General Medical Practice* (1979.)

24. To the extent that DSM-5 provides clear measurements of severity, this problem may be minimized.

25. When etiologies are known, there will be less comorbidity and more accurate single diagnoses.

26. There is the option of using ICD codes, although that alternative is usually not the choice of psychiatrists and other mental health professionals.

27. "Use of This Manual," DSM-III, p. 23.

28. See R. E. Kendell, J. E. Cooper, A. J. Gourlay, J. R. Copeland, and B. Gurland, "Diagnostic Criteria of American and British Psychiatrists," *Archives of General Psychiatry*, Vol. 25, 1971, pp. 123–130; R. E. Kendell, "Psychiatric Diagnosis in Britain and the United States," *British Journal of Psychiatry*, Vol. 9, 1975, pp. 453–461.

29. M. D. Neuman, A. Bitton, S. A. Glantz, "Tobacco Industry Influence on the Definition of Tobacco Related Disorders by the American Psychiatric Association," *Tobacco Control*, Vol. 14, pp. 328–337.

30. The exact phrase was coined by the psychoanalyst Frieda Fromm-Reichmann (1889–1957) in 1948, but the idea goes back earlier. However, the phrase and the notion became especially popular for two or three decades after.

31. In 1979, a physician, Raphael Osheroff, who had been hospitalized for insomnia and suicidal depression at well-known and analytically oriented Chestnut Lodge in Rockville, MD, sued the institution for lack of effective treatment. Osheroff had been treated only with intensive psychotherapy for seven months, while his depression worsened. Ultimately he was treated elsewhere with antidepressants, to which he responded well in a few weeks; he then resumed his medical practice. Chestnut Lodge eventually settled Osheroff's suit out of court. The case shook up the analytic world, and afterwards an analyst could only disregard illness that required a biological treatment at his or her peril.

32. David J. Kupfer and Darrel A. Regier, "Neuroscience, Clinical Evidence, and the Future of Psychiatric Classification in DSM-5," *American Journal of Psychiatry*, Vol. 168, July 1, 2011, pp. 672–674.

33. Steven Hyman, "The Diagnosis of Mental Disorders: The Problems of Reification," *Annual Review of Clinical Psychology*, Vol. 6, April 2010, pp. 155–179.

34. Nancy C. Andreasen, Editorial: "Diversity in Psychiatry: Or, Why Did We Become Psychiatrists?" *American Journal of Psychiatry*, Vol. 158, May 2001, p. 674.

Andreasen's words were recently echoed by two eminent psychiatrists, Paul R. McHugh and Phillip Slavney. See "Mental Illness—Comprehensive Evaluation or Checklist?," *New England Journal of Medicine*, Vol. 366, 2012, pp. 1853–1855. http://www.nejm.org/doi/full/10.1056/NEJMp1202555.

35. Allen Frances. "Epidemiology Mis-Counts: Systematic Bias Leads to Misleading Rates," *Psychology Today*, September 15, 2011. http://www.psychologytoday.com/blog/dsm5-in-distress/201109/epidemiology-mis-counts.

36. Recent research has shown that the psychoanalytic roots of CBT, developed by Aaron T. Beck (b. 1921), who was trained as an analyst, are stronger than was realized. See Rachel I. Rosner, "Aaron T. Beck's Drawings and the Psychoanalytic Origin Story of Cognitive Therapy," *History of Psychology*, Vol. 15, No. 1, February 2012, pp. 1–18. This article stems from Rosner's unpublished doctoral dissertation, "Between Science and Psychoanalysis: Aaron T. Beck and the Emergence of Cognitive Therapy" (1999).

37. Christopher Lane, *Shyness: How Normal Behavior Became a Sickness*. New Haven: Yale University Press, 2007; Allan V. Horwitz and Jerome C. Wakefield, *The Loss of Sadness: How Psychiatry Transformed Normal Sorrow into Depressive Disorder*. New York: Oxford University Press, 2007.

38. Frances' expression of these ideas was frequent and can easily be found online. Many of his articles and blogs appeared in *Psychiatric Times*, *Psychology Today*, and the *Huffington Post*. Frances' new book, *Saving Normal* (HarperCollins, 2013), recounts his time as Head of the DSM-IV Task Force and develops his critique of the DSM-5 process and decisions. Christopher Lane again voiced his concerns about the proposed diagnosis of Social Anxiety Disorder in DSM-5. An excellent summary of Frances' arguments and counterarguments by David Kupfer, Chair of the DSM-5 Task Force, appeared online in a "Medscape Special Report," June 5, 2012. http:/www.medscape_10-ctg0ieb6saamcliqkaj7sbh446o2abjq@mp.medscape.com.

39. See comments from the *British Medical Journal*, the *British Journal of Psychiatry*, and an Open Letter from Psychologists (belonging to sections within the American Psychological Association.)

40. Kupfer and Regier, "Neuroscience, Clinical Evidence, and the Future of Psychiatric Classification in DSM-5," 2011.
    See also "Medscape Special Report," June 5, 2012, in Note 38.

41. Jeffrey Lieberman, "Counter-argument: Changes to DSM-V Bring Needed Improvements," http://www.foxnews.com/health/2012/05/22/counter-argument-changes-to-dsm-v-bring-needed-improvements/#ixzz1vuUS2Ufh.

42. See, for example, James H. Scully, Medical Director of the APA, "DSM-5 Inaccuracies: Setting the Record Straight," *Huffington Post*, May 31, 2012, http://www.huffingtonpost.com/james-h-scully-jr-md/dsm-5_b_1560280.html.

43. American Psychiatric Association (1994). *Diagnostic and Statistical Manual of Mental Disorders* (4th ed., *DSM-IV*). Washington, DC: American Psychiatric Publishing, p. 538. (Gender Identity Disorder is found on pp. 532–538).

44. But for an additional view, see Ronald Bayer, *Homosexuality and American Psychiatry: The Politics of Diagnosis*. Princeton, NJ: Princeton University Press, 1981, pp. 168–178. I am indebted to Jack Drescher, M.D., for calling my attention to this.

INTERVIEWS

PERSONAL INTERVIEWS

Paula J. Clayton, M.D., January 29, 2007

Jean Endicott, Ph.D., January 26, 2007

William A. Frosch, M.D., January 27, 2007

Robert M.A. Hirschfeld, M.D., March 2008

Donald F. Klein, M.D., January 26, 2007

Robert Michels, M.D., January 30, 2007

Roger Peele, M.D., July 31, 2010

Theodore Shapiro, M.D., January 29, 2007

Robert L. Spitzer, M.D., June 2 and 3, 2006

Janet B. W. Williams, Ph.D., June 3, 2006

TELEPHONE INTERVIEWS

Louise Albert, July 7, 2009

Nancy C. Andreasen, M.D., February 17, 2012

Paula F. Clayton, M.D., October 5, 2009

Anne Hamlen Cohen, M.D., March 11, 2012

Paul J. Fink, M.D., 2010

Allen J. Frances, M.D., June 28, 2010 and October 26, 2012

Theodore Millon, Ph.D., May 8, 2012

William Offenkrantz, M.D., March 19, 2012

Roger Peele, M.D., September 9, 2011

Henry Pinsker, M.D., August 1, 2009

Robert L. Spitzer, M.D., June 11, 2009

George E. Vaillant, M.D., October 19, 2012

N.B.   With several of the individuals in both lists I have also had an ongoing, fruitful
e-mail correspondence.

BIBLIOGRAPHY

Ackerknecht EH (1968) [1959]. *A Short History of Psychiatry*. Trans. S. Wolff. New York & London: Hafner.

American Heritage Medical Dictionary (2007). New York: Houghton Mifflin.

American Journal of Psychiatry, (1969). Supplement. Cross-National Study of the Mental Disorders, *125*(10): 1–46.

American Psychiatric Association (1964). *Training the Psychiatrist to Meet Changing Needs* (Report of the Conference on Graduate Psychiatric Education, held in December 1962). Washington, DC: American Psychiatric Association.

American Psychiatric Association (1968). *Diagnostic and Statistical Manual of Mental Disorders*, Second Edition (DSM-II). Washington, DC: American Psychiatric Association.

American Psychiatric Association (1973). Summary Report of the Special Policy Meeting of the Board of Trustees, Atlanta, Ga., February 1–3, 1973. *American Journal of Psychiatry*, *130*(6): 732–738.

American Psychiatric Association (1980). *Diagnostic and Statistical Manual of Mental Disorders*, Third Edition (DSM-III). Washington, DC: American Psychiatric Publishing.

American Psychiatric Association (1994). *Diagnostic and Statistical Manual of Mental Disorders*, Fourth Edition (DSM-IV). Washington, DC: American Psychiatric Publishing.

Andreasen, Nancy Coover, National Medal of Science. *Wikipedia*, http//en.wikipedia.org/wiki/Nancy_Coover_Andreasen..

Andreasen NC (1984). *The Broken Brain: The Biological Revolution in Psychiatry*. New York: Harper & Row.

Andreasen NC (2001). Editorial: Diversity in Psychiatry: Or, Why Did We Become Psychiatrists? *American Journal of Psychiatry*, *158* (May): 673–675.

Andreasen NC (2001). *The Brave New Brain: Conquering Mental Illness in the Era of the Genome*. New York: Oxford University Press.

Andreasen NC (2005). *The Brave New Brain: Conquering Mental Illness in the Era of the Genome*. New York: Dana Press.

Andreasen NC (2007). DSM and the Death of Phenomenology in America: An Example of Unintended Consequences. *Schizophrenia Bulletin 33*(1): 108–112.

Arana G (2012). My So-Called Ex-Gay Life. *The American Prospect*. April 11. http://prospect.org/article/my-so-called-ex-gay-life

Arieti S, ed. (1974). *American Handbook of Psychiatry*, 2nd Edition. New York: Basic Books.

Arkonac O & Guze SB (1963). A Family Study of Hysteria. *New England Journal of Medicine*, *268*: 239–242.

Ash P (1949). The Reliability of Psychiatric Diagnosis. *Journal of Abnormal and Social Psychology*, *44*: 272–276.

Atkinson R (Dec. 2003). Interview with George Saslow, M.D. *Oregon Health Sciences University History Program, Oral History Project*. Transcript on deposit in OHSU library under call number W19 038 no. 90 2003.

Bailey P (1956). The Great Psychiatric Revolution. *American Journal of Psychiatry*, *113*(5): 387–406.

Barry DJ & Ciccone JR (1978). The Experience of Using DSM-III in a Court Clinic Setting: II. Practicality and Effect of DSM-III on a Court Clinic's Work with the Legal System, *Bulletin of the American Academy of Psychiatry and the Law*. *6*(1): 26–30.

Bayer R (1981). *Homosexuality and American Psychiatry: The Politics of Diagnosis*. New York: Basic Books.

Bayer R & Spitzer RL (1982). Correspondence on the Status of Homosexuality in DSM-III. *Journal of the History of the Behavioral Sciences*, *18*: 32–52.

Bayer R & Spitzer RL (1985). Neurosis, Psychodynamics, and DSM-III, *Archives of General Psychiatry*, *42*(February): 187–195.

Beck AT (1962). Reliability of Psychiatric Diagnoses: 1. A Critique of Systematic Studies. *American Journal of Psychiatry*, *119*: 210–216.

Beck AT, Ward CH, Mendelson M, Mock J, & Erbaugh J (1961). An Inventory For Measuring Depression. *Archives of General Psychiatry*, *4*(June): 561–571.

Beck AT, Ward CH, Mendelson M, Mock JE, & Erbaugh JK (1962). Reliability of Psychiatric Diagnoses: 2. A Study of Consistency of Clinical Judgments and Ratings, *American Journal of Psychiatry*. *119*: 351–357.

Becker HS (1963). *Outsider: Studies in the Sociology of Deviance*. New York: Free Press.

Bergler E (1949). *The Basic Neurosis: Oral Regression and Psychic Masochism*. New York: Grune and Stratton.

Berlim MT, Fleck MPA, & Shorter E (2003). Notes on Antipsychiatry, *European Archives of Psychiatry and Clinical Neuroscience*, *25*: 61–67.

Bernfeld S (1944). Freud's Earliest Theories and the School of Helmholtz, *Psychoanalytic Quarterly*, *13*: 341–362.

Berrios GE & Porter R, eds, (1995). *A History of Clinical Psychiatry: The Origin and History of Psychiatric Disorders*. London and New Brunswick: Athalone Press.

Besen W (2012). Truth Wins Out http://www.youtube.com/watch?v=gIifMxPcRnI [Re: Spitzer Apology].

Bettelheim B (1943) Individual and Mass Behavior in Extreme Situations, *Journal of Abnormal and Social Psychology*, *38*: 417–452.

Bindra D (1959). Experimental Psychology and the Problem of Behavior Disorders, *Canadian Journal of Psychology*, *13*: 135–150.

Blashfield RK (1982). Feighner et al., Invisible Colleges, and the Matthew Effect, *Schizophrenia Bulletin*, *8* (1): 1–6. Comments on the article by John S. Strauss, 8–9 and R.E. Kendell, 11–12.

Bleuler E (1950). *Dementia Praecox or the Group of Schizophrenias*. Transl. Joseph Zankin. Foreword Nolan D.C. Lewis. New York: International Universities Press.

Breuer J & Freud S (1955) [1895]. Studies on Hysteria, *The Standard Edition of the Complete Psychological Works of Sigmund Freud*. Vol. II. Ed. & Transl. James Strachey, Anna Freud, Alix Strachey, and Anna Tyson. London: Hogarth Press.

Bridgman, PW (1932). *The Logic of Modern Physics*. New York: The Macmillan Company.

Brodie HKH & Sabshin M (1973). An Overview of Trends in Psychiatric Research: 1963–1972, *American Journal of Psychiatry*, *130* (12): 1309–1318.

Burch C, Van Atta W, & Blain D, eds., (1968*). National Commission on Mental Health Manpower Careers in Psychiatry*. New York: Macmillan.

Cadoret R, Winokur G, Dorzab J, & Baker M (1972). Depressive Disease: Life Events and Onset of Illness, *Archives of General Psychiatry*, *26*: 133–136.

Carey B (2012). Psychiatry Giant Sorry for Backing Gay "Cure," *The New York Times*, May 18.

Cassidy WL, Flanagan NB, Spellman M, & Cohen ME (1957). Clinical Observations in Manic-Depressive Disease: Quantitative Study of One Hundred Manic-Depressive Patients and Fifty Medically Sick Controls, *J.A.M.A.*, *164*: 1535–1546.

Clayton PJ (1998). George Winokur: a personal memoir, *Journal of Affective Disorders, 50* (2): 77–78.

Clayton PJ (2006). Training at the Washington University School of Medicine in Psychiatry in the late 1950's, from the perspective of an affective disorder researcher, *Journal of Affective Disorders, 92*: 13–17.

Cloninger CR, ed. (2001). In Memoriam—Samuel Barry Guze (October 18, 1923-July 19, 2000), *Annals of Clinical Psychiatry, 13* (1): 1–10.

Cohen AH, ed. (2003). In Memoriam—Mandel E. Cohen, *Annals of Clinical Psychiatry, 15* (3/4): 149–159.

Cohen ME (1995). In Memoriam and Memorial Service, Eli Robins, *Annals of Clinical Psychiatry, 7* (1): 3.

Cohen ME & and White PD, (1950). Life Situations, Emotions and Neurocirculatory Asthenia (Anxiety Neurosis, Neurasthenia, Effort Syndrome), Proceedings, Association for Research in Nervous and Mental Diseases, In *Life Stress and Bodily Disease* Vol. 29. Baltimore: Williams &Wilkins.

Colby KM (1960). *An Introduction to Psychoanalytic Research*. New York: Basic Books, Inc.

Compton WM & Guze, SB (1995). The neo-Kraepelinian Revolution in Psychiatric Diagnosis, *European Archives of Psychiatry and Clinical Neuroscience*, *245*(4–5): 196–201.

Cooper JE, Kendell RE, Gurland BJ, Sharpe L, Copeland JRM, & Simon R (1972). *Psychiatric Diagnosis in New York and London*. Maudsley Monograph Series, No. 20. London: Oxford University Press, Inc.

Cranefield PF (1966). Freud and the School of Helmholtz, *Gesnerus, 23*: 35–39.

Crossley N (1998). R.D. Laing, and the British Anti-Psychiatry Movement: A Socio-Historical Analysis, *Social Science and Medicine, 47* (7): 877–889.

Decker HS (1977). *Freud in Germany: Revolution and Reaction in Science, 1893–1907*. New York: International Universities Press.

Decker HS (2007). How Kraepelinian was Kraepelin? How Kraepelinian are the neo-Kraepelinians? – from Emil Kraepelin to DSM-III, *History of Psychiatry, 18* (3): 337–360.

Decker HS (2004). The Psychiatric Works of Emil Kraepelin: A Many-Faceted Story of Modern Medicine, *Journal of the History of the Neurosciences, 13* (3): 248–276.

Decker HS, Operational Criteria. Unpublished paper.

Deutsch A (1948). *The Shame of the States*. New York: Harcourt, Brace and Company.

Doering CR & Raymond AF (1934). Reliability of Observation in Psychiatric and Related Characteristics, *American Journal of Orthopsychiatry, 4*: 249–257.

Doidge N (2007). *The Brain that Changes Itself: Stories of Personal Triumph from the Frontiers of Brain Science*. New York: Viking Penguin.

Dorland's Medical Dictionary for Health Consumers (2007). Philadelphia: Saunders.

Drescher J (2003). An Interview with Robert L. Spitzer, *Journal of Gay and Lesbian Psychotherapy, 7* (3): 97–111.

Ellenberg JH (1997). A Conversation with Morton Kramer, *Statistical Science, 12* (2): 103–107.

Endicott J & Spitzer RL (1978). A Diagnostic Interview: The Schedule for Affective Disorders and Schizophrenia, *Archives of General Psychiatry, 35* (7): 837–844.

Endicott J, Spitzer RL, Fleiss JL, & Cohen J (1976). The Global Assessment Scale: A Procedure for Measuring Overall Severity of Psychiatric Disturbance, *Archives of General Psychiatry, 33*: 766–771.

Engstrom EJ (1995). Kraepelin, Social Section, In Berrios, GE & Porter, R (Eds.), *A History of Clinical Psychiatry: The Origin and History of Psychiatric Disorders*. London and New Brunswick, NJ: Athlone Press, 292–301.

Engstrom EJ (2003). *Clinical Psychiatry in Imperial Germany: A History of Psychiatric Practice*. Ithaca: Cornell University Press.

Engstrom EJ, Burgmair W, & Weber MM (2002). Emil Kraepelin's Self Assessment. Clinical Autobiography in Historical Context (Classic Text No. 49). *History of Psychiatry, 13*: 89–118.

Engstrom EJ & Weber MM (2005). The Directions of Psychiatric Research: Introduction, *History of Psychiatry, 16*: 345–364.

Ennis BJ (1972). *Prisoners of Psychiatry: Mental Patients, Psychiatrists and the Law*. New York: Harcourt Brace Jovanovich.

Essen-Möller E (1961). On Classification of Mental Disorders, *Acta Psychiatrica Scandinavica, 37* (2): 119–126.

Essen-Möller E (1971). Suggestions for Further Improvement of the International Classification of Mental Disorders, *Psychological Medicine, 1*: 308–311.

Essen-Möller E & Wohlfahrt S (1947). Suggestions for the Amendment of the Official Swedish Classification of Mental Disorders, *Acta Psychiatrica Scandinavica, 47* (Supplement): 551–555.

Falek A & Moser HM (1975). Classification in Schizophrenia, *Archives of General Psychiatry, 32* (Jan.): 59–67.

Feighner JP (1989). The Advent of the Feighner Criteria. This Week's Citation Classic, *Current Contents, 43* (October 23): 14.

Feighner JP, Robins E, Guze SB, Woodruff Jr. RA, Winokur G, & Munoz R (1972). Diagnostic Criteria for Use in Psychiatric Research, *Archives of General Psychiatry, 26* (January): 57–63.

Fine GA & Martin DD (1990). A Partisan View: Sarcasm, Satire, and Irony as Voices in Goffman's Asylums, *Journal of Contemporary Ethnography, 19*: 89–115.

First MB, Spitzer RL, Gibbon M, & Williams JBW (1995). The Structured Clinical Interview for DSM-III-R Personality Disorders (SCID II), Part I: Description, *Journal of Personality Disorders, 9* (2): 83–91.

First MB, Spitzer RL, Gibbon M, Williams JBW, Davies M, Borus J, Howes MJ, Kane J, Pope HG, & Rounsaville B (1995). The Structured Clinical Interview for DSM-III-R Personality Disorders (SCID II): Part II. Multi-site Test-retest Reliability Study, *Journal of Personality Disorders, 9* (2): 92–104.

Foulds GA (1956). The Reliability of Psychiatric, and the Validity of Psychological, Diagnosis, *Journal of Mental Science. 7* (Sept.): 1305–1312.

Frances A (2011). Epidemiology Mis-Counts: Systematic Bias Leads to Misleading Rates, *Psychology Today*, September: 15. http://www.psychologytoday.com/blog/dsm5-in-distress/201109/epidemiology-mis-counts

Frances A & Kupfer DJ (2012). Medscape Special Report, June 5. <medscape_10-ctg0ieb6saa mcliqkaj7sbh446o2abjq@mp.medscape.com> (Accessed June 6, 2012).

Frances A & Pincus H (2011). Remembrance: Mel Sabshin Was Truly a Man for All Seasons, *Clinical Psychiatry News*, June 28, 2011. http://www.clinicalpsychiatrynews.com.

Freud S (1960). The Psychopathology of Everyday Life in *The Standard Edition of the Complete Psychological Works*, Vol. 6, London: The Hogarth Press.

Garfield E (1989). A Tribute to Eli and Lee Robins—Citation Superstars. A Citationist Perspective on Biological Psychiatry, *Current Comments, 46* (November 13): 321–329.

Garrison FH (1929). *An Introduction to the History of Medicine*, 4th edition. Philadelphia & London: Saunders.

Gatfield PD & Guze SB (1963). The Prognosis and Differential Diagnosis of Conversion Reactions: A Follow-up Study, *Diseases of the Nervous System*, *23*: 623–631.

Goffman E (1961). *Asylums: Essays on the Social Situation of Mental Patients and Other Inmates.* Chicago: Aldine Publishing Co.

Goleman D (1978). Who's Mentally Ill? *Psychology Today*, *11* (8): 34–41.

Goleman D (1985). Social Workers Vault Into a Leading Role in Psychotherapy, *The New York Times*, Science Section: April 30.

Goodwin DW, Guze SB, & Robins E (1969). Follow-Up Studies in Obsessional Neurosis, *Archives of General Psychiatry*, *20* (February): 182–187.

Griesinger W (1965). [1845] *Mental Pathology and Therapeutics. A Facsimilie of the English Edition of 1867.* Introduction E.H. Ackerknecht. New York: Hafner.

Grinker RR, Sr. (1965). The Sciences of Psychiatry: Fields, Fences and Riders, *The American Journal of Psychiatry*. *122* (4): 367–376.

Grob G (1991). Origins of DSM-I: A Study in Appearance and Reality, *American Journal of Psychiatry*, *148* (4): 421–431.

Grob GN (1987). The Forging of Mental Health Policy in America: World War II to the New Frontier, *Journal of the History of Medicine and Allied Sciences*, *42*, (4): 410–446.

Grob GN (2011). The Attack of Psychiatric Legitimacy in the 1960s: Rhetoric and Reality, *Journal of the History of the Behavioral Sciences*, *47* (4): 398–416.

Grob GN & Goldman HH (2006). *The Dilemma of Federal Mental Health Policy: Radical Reform or Incremental Change?* Rutgers, NJ: Rutgers University Press.

Grossman JB (2001). Images in Psychiatry: Dennis Patrick. Campbell, M.D., 1939–1997, *American Journal of Psychiatry*, *158* (4): 546. (Accessed online, January 27, 2012.)

Group for the Advancement of Psychiatry (1948). *Medical Education*, Report 3. New York.

Group for the Advancement of Psychiatry (1950). *The Social Responsibility of Psychiatry: A Statement of Orientation*, Report 13. New York.

Group for the Advancement of Psychiatry (1955). *Trends and Issues in Psychiatric Residency Programs*, Report 31. New York.

Gunderson JG & Singer MT (1975). Defining Borderline Patients: An Overview, *American Journal of Psychiatry*, *132* (1): 1–10.

Guze SB (1967). The Diagnosis of Hysteria: What Are We Trying to Do? *American Journal of Psychiatry*, *124*: 491–498.

Guze SB (1970). The Need for Toughmindedness in Psychiatric Thinking, *Southern Medical Journal*, *63*, (June): 662–671.

Guze SB (1970). The Role of Follow-up Studies: Their Contribution to Diagnostic Classification as Applied to Hysteria, *Seminars in Psychiatry*, *2* (4): 392–402.

Guze SB (1978). Validating Criteria for Psychiatric Diagnosis: The Washington University Approach. In Akiskal, HS, & Webb, WL, eds. (1978). *Psychiatric Diagnosis: Exploration of Biological Predictors.* New York: Spectrum Publications., 47–59.

Guze SB (1992). *Why Psychiatry is a Part of Medicine.* New York: Oxford University Press.

Guze SB (1994). Oral History Project of the Washington University School of Medicine, Interview 4. http://beckerexhibits.wustl.edu/oral/transcripts/guze1994.html

Guze SB (1995). In Memoriam and Memorial Service Eli Robins February 22, 1921-December 21, 1994, *Annals of Clinical Psychiatry*, *7* (1): 7.

Guze SB (1997). Obituary for George Winokur, MD, 1925–1996, *Archives of General Psychiatry*, *54* (6): 574–575.

Guze SB & Murphy GE (1963). An Empirical Approach to Psychotherapy: The Agnostic Position, *American Journal of Psychiatry*, *120*: 53–57.

Guze SB & Perley MJ (1963). Observations on the Natural History of Hysteria, *American Journal of Psychiatry*, *119*: 960–965.

Harris P (2001). Obituary: Dr. Samuel B. Guze, *Psychiatric Bulletin*, *25*, 77–78.

Healy D (1996). *The Psychopharmacologists: Interviews*, Vol. I. London: Chapman & Hall.

Healy D (1998). *The Psychopharmacologists, II: Interviews*. London: Chapman & Hall.

Healy D (2000). *The Psychopharmacologists, III: Interviews*. London: Arnold; New York: Oxford University Press.

Healy D (2007). Mandel Cohen and the Origins of the Diagnostic and Statistical Manual of Mental Disorders, Third Edition: DSM-III, *History of Psychiatry*, *13*: 209–230.

Helzer JE, Robins LN, & Davis DH (1976). Antecedents of Narcotic Use and Addiction: A Study of 898 Vietnam Veterans, *Drug and Alcohol Dependence*, *1*: 83–90.

Helzer JE, Robins LN, & Davis DH (1976). Depressive Disorders in Vietnam Returnees, *Journal of Nervous and Mental Disease*, *168*: 177–185.

Hoff P (1998). Emil Kraepelin and Forensic Psychiatry, *International Journal of Law and Psychiatry*, *21*: 343–353.

Horwitz AV (2002). *Creating Mental Illness*. Chicago and London: The University of Chicago Press

Horwitz AV & Wakefield JC (2007). *The Loss of Sadness: How Psychiatry Transformed Normal Sorrow into Depressive Disorder*. New York: Oxford University Press.

Hudgens RW (1993). The Turning of American Psychiatry, *Missouri Medicine*, *90* (6): 283–291.

Hudgens RW (2001). In C. Robert Cloninger (ed.) In Memoriam—Samuel Barry Guze (October 18, 1923-July 19, 2000), *Annals of Clinical Psychiatry*, *13* (1): 4.

Hunt WA, Wittson CL, & Hunt EB (1953). A Theoretical and Practical Analysis of the Diagnostic Process, In P. Hoch and J. Zubin, (eds.), *Current Problems in Psychiatric Diagnosis*. New York: Grune & Stratton, Inc.

Hyman S (2010). The Diagnosis of Mental Disorders: The Problems of Reification, *Annual Review of Clinical Psychology*, *6*: 155–179.

It's Different in Men [In reference to Purtell, Robins, & Cohen, 1951] (1952). *TIME*, (Monday, June 9).

Jaffe JH (1977). Tobacco Use as a Mental Disorder: The Rediscovery of a Medical Problem, In *Research on Smoking Behavior*, Publication of the National Institute on Drug Abuse (NIDA): 202–217.

Jenkins RL (1953). Symptomatology and dynamics in diagnosis: A medical perspective, *Journal of Clinical Psychology*, *9*: 149–150.

Jones E (1953). *The Life and Work of Sigmund Freud*, 1. New York: Basic Books.

Kannel WB, Dawber TR, & Cohen ME (1959). The electrocardiogram in neurocirculatory asthenia (anxiety neurosis or neurasthenia): A Study of 203 Neurocirculatory Asthenia Patients and 757 Healthy Controls in the Framingham Study, *Annals of Internal Medicine*, *49*: 1351–1360.

Kaplan M (1983). A Woman's View of DSM-III, *American Psychologist*, July: 786–792.

Kaplan M (1983). Comments on the Articles by Spitzer, Williams, and Kass, *American Psychologist*, July: 802–803.

Kasanin J (1933). The Acute Schizoaffective Psychoses, *American Journal of Psychiatry*, *9*: 97–126.

Kass F, Spitzer RL, & Williams JBW (1983). An Empirical Study of the Issue of Sex Bias in the Diagnostic Criteria of DSM-III Axis II Personality Disorders, *American Psychologist*, July: 799–801.

Katz MM, Cole JO, & Barton WE, eds. (1967). *The Role and Methodology of Classification in Psychiatry and Psychopathology*. Proceedings of a Conference held in Washington, DC, November 1965 under the Auspices of The American Psychiatric Association and the Psychopharmacology Research Branch of the National Institute of Mental Health. Public Health Service Publication No. 1584. Washington, DC: U.S. Government Printing Office.

Katz MM & Klerman GL [Co-chairs of the NIMH-Clinical Research Branch Collaborative Program on the Psychobiology of Depression], (1979). Introduction: Overview of the Clinical Studies Program, *American Journal of Psychiatry*, *136* (1): 49–51.

Kendell RE (1975). Psychiatric Diagnosis in Britain and the United States, *British Journal of Psychiatry*, *9*: 453–461.

Kendell RE, Cooper JE, Gourlay AJ, Copeland JR & Gurland B (1971). Diagnostic criteria of American and British psychiatrists, *Archives of General Psychiatry*, *25*: 123–130.

Kendler KS, Munoz RA, & Murphy G (2010). The Development of the Feighner Criteria: A Historical Perspective, *American Journal of Psychiatry*, *167* (2): 134–142.

Kety SS (1961). The Academic Lecture: The Heuristic Aspects of Psychiatry, *American Journal of Psychiatry*, *118*: 385–397.

Kirk SA & Kutchins H (1992). *The Selling of DSM: The Rhetoric of Science in Psychiatry*. New York: Aldine De Gruyter.

Kirk SA & Kutchins H. (1994). The Myth of the Reliability of DSM, *Journal of Mind and Behavior*, *15* (1&2): 71–86. http://www.academyanalyticarts.org/kirk&kutchins.htm

Klein DF (1978). A Proposed Definition of Mental Illness, in Robert L. Spitzer and Donald Klein (eds.), *Critical Issues in Psychiatric Diagnosis*. New York: Raven Press, 41–71.

Klerman GL (1972). Psychotropic Hedonism vs. Pharmacological Calvinism, *Hastings Center Report*, *2* (4): 1–3.

Klerman GL (1978). The Evolution of a Scientific Nosology, in John C. Shershow (ed.) *Schizophrenia: Science and Practice*. Cambridge: Harvard University Press.

Klerman GL (1986). Historical Perspectives on Contemporary Schools of Psychopathology, In Theodore Millon and Gerald L. Klerman (eds.), *Contemporary Directions in Psychopathology: Toward the DSM-IV*. New York and London: Guilford Press.

Klerman GL, Weissman MM, Rounsaville BJ, & Chevron ES (1984). *Interpersonal Psychotherapy of Depression*. New York: Basic Books.

Knight RP (1953). Borderline States, *Bulletin of the Menninger Clinic*, *17*: 1–12.

Kraepelin E (1907) [1904]. *Clinical Psychiatry*. Abstracted and Adapted from the 7th edition of *Psychiatrie* by A.R. Diefendorf. New York and London: Macmillan; Reprinted Bristol, England: Thoemmes Press, 2002.

Kraepelin E (1913). *Lectures on Clinical Psychiatry*. Authorized Translation from the Second German Edition. Revised and Edited by Thomas Johnstone, Third English Edition. New York: William Wood & Company.

Kraepelin E (1919) [1913]. *Dementia Praecox and Paraphrenia*. Transl. R Mary Barclay. Edinburgh: E. & S. Livingstone; Reprinted Bristol, England: Thoemmes Press, 2002.

Kraepelin E (1921). *Manic-Depressive Insanity and Paranoia*. Transl. R. Mary Barclay (from the 8th German edition of the *Text-Book of Psychiatry*.) Ed. George M. Robertson. Edinburgh: E. & S. Livingstone; Reprinted Bristol, England: Thoemmes Press, 2002.

Kraepelin E (1962) [1917]. *One Hundred Years of Psychiatry*. Transl. W. Baskin. New York: Citadel Press.

Kraepelin E (1974) [1920]. Patterns of Mental Disorder, Transl. H. Marshall. In S.R. Hirsch and M. Shepherd (eds.), *Themes and Variations in European Psychiatry*. Bristol: John Wright & Sons, 7–30.

Kraepelin E (1987). *Memoirs*, Ed. H. Hippius, G. Peters, and D. Ploog. Transl. C. Wooding-Deane. Berlin: Springer Verlag.

Kraepelin E (1992) [1920]. The Manifestations of Insanity, Transl. D. Beer, (Classic text No. 12), *History of Psychiatry*, 3: 509–529.

Kramer M (1952). Statistical Reporting, Section IV: 52–72 and Statistical Classifications of Mental Disorder, Section V: 73–86. In American Psychiatric Association, *Diagnostic and Statistical Manual of Mental Disorders, DSM-I*, Washington, DC.

Kramer M (1961). Some Problems for International Research suggested by Observations of Differences in First Admission Rates to Mental Hospitals of England and Wales and the United States, *Geriatrics*, 16: 151–160.

Kramer M (1968). Introduction: The Historical Background of ICD-8; Statistical Tabulations, Section 4: 53–63; and Comparative Listing of Titles and Codes, Section 5: 64–82. In American Psychiatric Association, *Diagnostic and Statistical Manual of Mental Disorders, DSM-II*. Washington, DC.

Kramer M (1969). Cross-National Study of Diagnosis of Mental Disorders: Origin of the Problem, *American Journal of Psychiatry*, 25 (Supplement): 1–11.

Kramer Y, Rabkin R, & Spitzer RL (1958). Whirling as a Clinical Test in Childhood Schizophrenia, *Journal of Pediatrics*, 52: 295–303.

Kuhn TS (1962). The Structure of Scientific Revolutions. *International Encyclopedia of Unified Science*; 2nd edition (1970) University of Chicago Press.

Kupfer DJ & Regier DA (2011). Neuroscience, Clinical Evidence, and the Future of Psychiatric Classification in DSM-5, *American Journal of Psychiatry*, 168 (July 1): 672–674.

Kuriansky JB, Deming WE, & Gurland BJ (1974). On Trends in the Diagnosis of Schizophrenia, *American Journal of Psychiatry*, 131 (4): 402–408.

Laing RD (1960). *The Divided Self: A Study in Sanity and Madness*. Chicago: Quadrangle Books.

Laing RD (1967). *The Politics of Experience*. New York: Pantheon Books.

Laing RD & Esterson A (1970 [1964]). *Sanity, Madness, and the Family: Families of Schizophrenics*. Penguin Books: Harmondsworth, England; Baltimore, Maryland; Victoria, Australia.

Lane C (2007). *Shyness: How Normal Behavior Became a Sickness*. New Haven and London: Yale University Press.

Langfeldt G (1960). Diagnosis and Prognosis of Schizophrenia, *Proceedings of the Royal Society of Medicine*, 53 (Section of Psychiatry. June 14): 1047–1052.

Lewis JM & Usdin GL eds. (1982). *Treatment Planning in Psychiatry*. Washington, DC: American Psychiatric Association Press.

Lieberman J (2012). Counter-argument: Changes to DSM-V Bring Needed Improvements, http://www.foxnews.com/health/2012/05/22/counter-argument-changes-to-dsm-v-bring -needed-improvements/#ixzz1vuUS2Ufh, May 22.

Lorr M (1961). Classification of the Behavior Disorders, *Annual Review of Psychology*, 12: 195–216.

Luft EVD (2001). Thomas Szasz, MD: Philosopher, Psychiatrist, Libertarian, *Upstate Medical University Alumni Journal*, Summer. This also can be found at http://www.szasz.com/ alumnijournal.html.

Luhrmann TM (2000). *Of Two Minds: The Growing Disorder in American Psychiatry*. New York: Alfred A. Knopf.

Maisel AQ (1946). Bedlam, *Life, 20*: 102–118.

Marmor J, ed. (1965). *Sexual Inversion: The Multiple Roots of Homosexuality*. New York: Basic Books.

Marmor J (1971). "Normal" and "Deviant" Sexual Behavior, *JAMA: The Journal of the American Medical Association, 217* (2): 165–170.

Marmor J (1975). *Psychiatrists and Their Patients: A National Study of Private Office Practice*. Washington, DC: Joint Information Service of the APA and the NIMH.

Masserman JH & Carmichael HT (1938). Diagnosis and Prognosis in Psychiatry: With a Follow-Up Study of the Results of Short-Term General Hospital Therapy of Psychiatric Cases, *The Journal of Mental Science, 84* (333, Nov.): 893–946.

Mayer-Gross W, Slater E, & Roth M (1954). *Clinical Psychiatry*. London: Cassell and Company, 1954.

McCracken J (n.d.) In Memoriam, Dennis P. Cantwell, Neuropsychiatric Institute UCLA, http://www.universityofcalifornia.edu/senate/inmemoriam/DennisP.Cantwell.htm (Accessed online, January 27, 2012.)

McHugh PR & Slavney P (2012). Mental Illness—Comprehensive Evaluation or Checklist? *New England Journal of Medicine, 366*: 1853–1855. Accessed online May 17, 2012. http://www.nejm.org/doi/full/10.1056/NEJMp1202555

McNally K (2009). Eugen Bleuler's Four As, *History of Psychology, 12* (2): 43–59.

Meehl P (1959). Some Ruminations on the Validation of Clinical Procedures, *Canadian Journal of Psychology, 13*: 102–128.

Mehlman B (1952). Reliability of Psychiatric Diagnosis, *Journal of Abnormal and Social Psychology, 47*: 577–578.

Menninger K, Mayman M, & Pruyser P (1964). *The Vital Balance: The Life Process in Mental Health and Illness*. New York: The Viking Press.

Merton RK (1965). *On the Shoulders of Giants: A Shandean Postscript*. New York: Free Press.

Meyer A. (1896) Review of Kraepelin E. *Psychiatrie: Ein Lehrbuch für Studierende und Aertze*, Fünfte Auflage. *American Journal of Insanity, 53*, 298–302.

Meyer A (1927). In Memorium: Emil Kraepelin. *American Journal of Psychiatry, 151* (6 Suppl.): 140–143.

Millon T (1981). *Disorders of Personality, DSM-III: Axis II*. New York: John Wiley & Sons.

Millon T (1983). The DSM-III: An Insider's Perspective, *American Psychologist, 38* (7): 804–814.

Millon T (1986). On the Past and Future of DSM-III: Personal Recollections and Projections, In Theodore Millon and Gerald L. Klerman (eds.) *Contemporary Directions in Psychopathology: Toward the DSM-IV*. New York and London: The Guilford Press, 29–70.

Millon T (1990). *Toward a New Personology: An Evolutionary Model*. New York: Wiley-Interscience.

Millon T (2002). A Blessed and Charmed Personal Odyssey, *Journal of Personality Assessment, 79* (2): 171–194.

Millon T, Biography http://www.millon.net/content/tm_bio.htm

Millon T. Personalized Assessment: Clinical Personality Instruments, http://www.millon.net/content/instrumentation.htm

Millon T & Davis RO (1996). *Disorders of Personality: DSM-IV and Beyond* (2nd ed.). Oxford: John Wiley & Sons.

Millon T & Klerman GL, eds. (1986). *Contemporary Directions in Psychopathology: Toward the DSM-IV*. New York: Guilford Press.

Mora G (1965). The Historiography of Psychiatry and Its Development: A Re-evaluation, *Journal of the History of the Behavioral Sciences*, *1*: 43–52.

Morel BA (1857). *Traité des Dégénérescences Physiques, Intellectuelles et Morales de l'Espèce Humaine*. Paris: J.B. Baillière.

Mulligan K (2003). Carter Commission Legacy Still Reaping Benefit, *Psychiatric News*, *38* (5): 14.

Murray RM (1979). A Reappraisal of American Psychiatry, *The Lancet*, February 3.

Narrow W (2012). Q&A with Dr. William Narrow, Research Director for the DSM-5 Task Force, January 30. See http://www.post-gazette.com/pg/12030/1206972–114–0.stm?cmpid=news. xml Accessed Feb. 1, 2012.

Neuman MD, Bitton A, & Glantz SA (2005). Tobacco industry influence on the definition of tobacco related disorders by the American Psychiatric Association, *Tobacco Control*, *14*: 328–337. Accessed online 12/31/2009.

New York Heart Association, Criteria Committee (1964). *Diseases of the Heart and Blood Vessels: Nomenclature and Criteria for Diagnosis*, 6th edition. Boston: Little, Brown and Co.

Noll R (2011). *American Madness: The Rise and Fall of Dementia Praecox*. Cambridge, MA: Harvard University Press.

Norris V (1959). *Mental Illness in London*, Maudsley Monographs, (6). London: Chapman and Hall, Ltd.

Oregon Health and Science University (2004). George Saslow, Ph.D., M.D., Academic Contributions. http://www.ohsu.edu/psychiatry/faculty/saslow.htm.

Pace E (1994). Obituary: Jules Masserman, 89, Leader of Psychiatric Group is Dead, *The New York Times*, November 15. http://www.nytimes.com/1994/11/15/obituaries/jules-masserm an-89-leader-of-psychiatric-group-is-dead.html

Paris J (2005). *The Fall of an Icon: Psychoanalysis and Academic Psychiatry*. Toronto: University of Toronto Press.

Pasamanick B, Dinitz S & Lefton M (1959). Psychiatric Orientation and its Relation to Diagnosis and Treatment in a Mental Hospital, *American Journal of Psychiatry*, *116*: 127–132.

Pasamanick B, Scarpitti FR, & Dinitz S. (1967). *Schizophrenics in the Community: An Experimental Study in the Prevention of Hospitalization*. New York: Appleton-Century-Crofts.

Perley MJ & Guze SB (1962). Hysteria—The Stability and Usefulness of Clinical Criteria: A Quantitative Study Based on a Follow-up Period of Six to Eight Years in 39 Patients, *The New England Journal of Medicine*, *266* (9): 421–426.

Pines M (1983). The Foundations' Fund for Research in Psychiatry and the growth of research in psychiatry, *The American Journal of Psychiatry*, *140*, 1–10.

Pinsker H (1997). *A Primer of Supportive Psychotherapy*. Hillsdale, NJ: The Analytic Press.

Pinsker H & Spitzer RL (1977). Classification of Mental Disorders: DSM-III, in B. Wolman (ed.), *International Encyclopedia of Neurology, Psychiatry, Psychoanalysis, and Psychology*. New York: Van Nostrand, Reinhold.

President's Commission on Mental Health, *Report to the President* (1978). Vol. 1: Number 040–000–00390–8. Washington, D.C.: U.S. Government Printing Office.

Psychiatry in American Life: The Freudian Revolution (1961*). The Atlantic Monthly, A Magazine of Literature, Science, Art and Politics*. Boston: The Atlantic Monthly Company, Vol. CCVIII, July—September.

Purtell JJ, Robins E, & Cohen ME (1951). Observations on Clinical Aspects of Hysteria: A Quantitative Study of 50 Hysteria Patients and 156 Control Subjects, *J.A.M.A.* (*Journal of the American Medical Association*), *146* (July 7): 902–909.

Puschmann T (1966) [1889]. *A History of Medical Education from the Most Remote to the Most Recent Times*. Trans. & ed. E.H. Hare. London: Lewis, 1891; New York: Hafner.

Rakoff VM, Stancer HC, & Kedward HB (1977). *Psychiatric Diagnosis*. New York: Brunner/Mazel.

Rattigan D (2012). Spitzer: "I Owe the Gay Community an Apology," Ex-Gay Watch, April 26. http://www.exgaywatch.com/wp/2012/04/spitzer-i-owe-the-gay-community-an-apology/

Reich W (1948). *The Discovery of the Orgone. II: The Cancer Biopathy*. New York: Orgone Institute Press.

Reich W (1951) [1945]. *The Sexual Revolution*. 4th English Edition. Transl from the German by Theodore P. Wolfe. London: Peter Nevill, Vision Press.

Reich W (1973) [1940]. *The Function of the Orgasm*. New York: Farrar Straus & Giroux.

Rich CL (2003). Editorial: Swan Song, *Annals of Clinical Psychiatry*, *15* (3/4): 143–144.

Riesman D (1950). *The Lonely Crowd: A Study of the Changing American Character*. New Haven: Yale University Press, 1950.

Riesman D (1965). *Faces in the Crowd: Individual Studies in Character and Politics* in collaboration with Nathan Glazer. Abridged Edition. New Haven and London: Yale University Press.

Rissmiller DJ & Rissmiller JH (2006). Evolution of the Anti-Psychiatry Movement into Mental Health Consumerism, *Psychiatric Services*, *57* (6): 863–866.

Robins E (1967). Antisocial and Dyssocial Personality Disorders, in Alfred M. Freedman and Harold I.Kaplan (eds.) *Comprehensive Textbook of Psychiatry*. Baltimore: Williams & Wilkins, 951–958.

Robins E (1977). New Concepts in the Diagnosis of Psychiatric Disorders, *Annual Review of Medicine*, *28*: 67–73.

Robins E (1981). *The Final Months: A Study of the Lives of 134 Persons Who Committed Suicide*. New York, Oxford: Oxford University Press.

Robins E & Guze SB (1970). Establishment of Diagnostic Validity in Psychiatric Illness: Its Application to Schizophrenia, *American Journal of Psychiatry*, *126* (7): 983–987.

Robins E & Guze SB (1972). Classification of Affective Disorders: The Primary-Secondary, the Endogenous-Reactive, and the Neurotic-Psychotic Concepts, *Recent Advances in the Psychobiology of the Depressive Illnesses: Proceedings of a Workshop*, 283–293.

Robins LN (1966). *Deviant Children Grown Up: A Sociological and Psychiatric Study of Sociopathic Personality*. Baltimore: Williams & Wilkins.

Rogow A (1990). *The Psychiatrists*. New York: Putnam.

Rosenhan DL (1973). On Being Sane in Insane Places, *Science*, *179* (January 19): 250–258.

Rosner RI (2012). Aaron T. Beck's Drawings and the Psychoanalytic Origin Story of Cognitive Therapy, *History of Psychology*, *15* (1): 1–18.

Rubin EH, Zorumski EF, & Guze SB (1986). Somatoform Disorders, in Theodore Millon and Gerald L. Klerman (eds.), *Contemporary Directions in Psychopathology: Toward the DSM-IV*. New York and London: Guilford Press.

Rutter M, Lebovici S, Eisenberg L, Sneznevskij AV, Sadoun R, Brooke E, & Lin T-Y (1969). A Tri-axial Classification of Mental Disorders in Childhood: An International Study, *Journal of Child Psychology and Psychiatry*, *10*: 41–61.

Rutter M, Shaffer D, & Shepherd M (1973). An Evaluation of the Proposal for a Multi-axial Classification of Child Psychiatric Disorders, *Psychological Medicine*, *3*: 244–250.

Sabshin M (1977). Editorial: On remedicalization and holism in psychiatry, *Psychosomatics*, October: 7–8.

Sabshin M (1990). Turning Points in Twentieth-Century American Psychiatry, *American Journal of Psychiatry*, *147* (10): 1267–1274.

Sabshin M (2008). *Changing American Psychiatry: A Personal Perspective*. Arlington, VA: American Psychiatric Publishing, Inc.

Saghir MT & Robins E (1969). Homosexuality: I. Sexual Behavior of the Female Homosexual, *Archives of General Psychiatry*, *20* (February): 192–201.

Saghir MT & Robins E (1969). Homosexuality: II. Sexual Behavior of the Male Homosexual, *Archives of General Psychiatry*, *21* (August): 219–229.

Scheff TJ (1964). Social Conditions for Rationality: How Urban and Rural Courts Deal with the Mentally Ill, *American Behavioral Scientist*, March: 21–24.

Scheff TJ (1964). The Societal Reaction to Deviants: Ascriptive Elements in the Psychiatric Screening of Mental Patients in a Midwestern State, *Social Problems*, No. 4, Spring.

Scheff TJ (1966). *Being Mentally Ill: A Sociological Theory*. Chicago: Aldine Publishing: 401–413.

Schilpp PA ed., (1957). *The Philosophy of Karl Jaspers*. New York: Tudor.

Schmidt HO & Fonda CP (1956). The Reliability of Psychiatric Prognosis, *Journal of Abnormal and Social Psychology*, *52*: 262–267.

Schwab JJ (1975). Official Actions, *American Journal of Psychiatry*, *132* (4): 480.

Scott WJ (1990). PTSD in DSM-III: A Case in the Politics of Diagnosis and Disease, *Social Problems*, *37* (3): 294–310.

Scully JH (2012). DSM-5 Inaccuracies: Setting the Record Straight, *Huffington Post*, May 31. http://www.huffingtonpost.com/james-h-scully-jr-md/dsm-5_b_1560280.html

Siever LJ & Gunderson JG (1979). Genetic Determinants of Borderline Conditions, *Schizophrenia Bulletin*, *5* (1): 81–83.

Slater E (1936). The Inheritance of Manic-Depressive Insanity, *Proceedings of the Royal Society of Medicine*, *29*, (Section of Psychiatry, February 11): 981–990.

Slater ETO (1961). Obituary: W. Mayer-Gross, M.D., F.R.C.P., *British Medical Journal*, *1*: February 25: 5225.

Socarides C (1995). *Homosexuality: A Freedom Too Far. A Psychoanalyst Answers 1000 Questions About Causes and Cure and the Impact of the Gay Rights Movement on American Society*. Phoenix: Adam Margrave Books.

Spiegel A (2002). This American Life, Chicago Public Radio Jan. 18, online at http://www.this americanlife.org/Radio_Episode.aspx?episode

Spiegel A (2003). NPR News, "All Things Considered," Profile: Effort by Robert Spitzer in 1974 to revise and update the Diagnostic and Statistical Manual for the American Psychiatric Association, and its impact on the understanding of human emotions. (August 18).

Spiegel A (2005). Annals of Medicine. The Dictionary of Disorder: How One Man Revolutionized Psychiatry. *The New Yorker* (January 3.)

Spitzer RL (1959). A Clinical Trial of Monosodium Glutamate (L-Glutavite) on Hospitalized Elderly Male Psychotic Patients, *American Journal of Psychiatry*, *115*: (April): 936–938.

Spitzer RL (1966). Mental Status Schedule: Potential Use as a Criterion Measure of Change in Psychotherapy Research, *American Journal of Psychotherapy*, *20*:156–167.

Spitzer RL (1973). A Proposal About Homosexuality and the APA Nomenclature: Homosexuality as an Irregular Form of Sexual Behavior [not a disorder] and Sexual Orientation Disturbance as a Psychiatric Disorder, *American Journal of Psychiatry, 130* (11): 1214–1216.

Spitzer RL (1975). On Pseudoscience in Science, Logic in Remission and Psychiatric Diagnosis: A Critique of Rosenhan's "On Being Sane In Insane Places," *Journal of Abnormal Psychology, 84*: 442–452.

Spitzer RL (1976). More on Pseudoscience in Science and the Case for Psychiatric Diagnosis: A Critique of D.L. Rosenhan's "On Being Sane in Insane Places," *Archives of General Psychiatry, 33* (April): 459–470.

Spitzer RL (1981). The Diagnostic Status of Homosexuality in DSM-III: A Reformulation of the Issue, *American Journal of Psychiatry, 138* (2): 210–215.

Spitzer RL (1982). Letters to the Editor, *Schizophrenia Bulletin, 8* (4): 592.

Spitzer RL (2001). Images in Psychiatry, *American Journal of Psychiatry, 158* (July): 1019.

Spitzer RL (2003). Can Some Gay Men and Lesbians Change Their Sexual Orientation? 200 Participants Reporting a Change from Homosexual to Heterosexual Orientation, *Archives of Sexual Behavior, 32* (5): 403–417.

Spitzer RL (2005). Wilhelm Reich and Orgone Therapy: The Story of Robert L. Spitzer's Paper, "An Examination of Wilhelm Reich's Demonstrations of Orgone Energy," *The Scientific Review of Mental Health Practice, 4* (1). http://www.srmhp.org/0401/spitzer. html.

Spitzer RL (2006). DSM and Psychiatric Institute: A (Very) Personal History. Department of Psychiatry Grand Rounds, New York State Psychiatric Institute (January 6).

Spitzer RL (2011) Psychological Warfare: The DSM-5 Debate, http://www.hcplive.com/ publications/mdng-Neurology/2011/february_2011/dsm_5.

Spitzer RL (2012). Dr. Robert Spitzer Retracts "Ex-Gay" Study and Apologizes to the LGBT Community.

Spitzer RL, Andreasen NC, & Endicott J (1978). Schizophrenia and Other Psychotic Disorders in DSM-III, *Schizophrenia Bulletin, 4* (4): 489–494.

Spitzer RL & Cohen J (1968). Common Errors in Quantitative Psychiatric Research, *International Journal of Psychiatry, 6*: 109–118.

Spitzer RL, Cohen J, Fleiss JL, & Endicott J (1967). Quantification of Agreement in Psychiatric Diagnosis: A New Approach, *Archives of General Psychiatry, 17* (July): 83–87.

Spitzer RL & Endicott J (1968). DIAGNO, a Computer Program for Psychiatric Diagnosis Utilizing the Differential Diagnostic Procedure, *Archives of General Psychiatry, 18*: 746–756.

Spitzer, RL & Endicott, J (1969). DIAGNO II: Further Developments in a Computer Program for Psychiatric Diagnosis, *American Journal of Psychiatry, 125*: (January Supplement): 12–21.

Spitzer RL & Endicott J (1970). Automation of Psychiatric Case Records: Boon or Bane? *International Journal of Psychiatry, 9*: 604–621.

Spitzer RL & Endicott J (1970). Automation of Psychiatric Case Records: Will It Help the Clinician? *Diseases of the Nervous System,* GWAN Supplement, *31*: 45–46.

Spitzer RL & Endicott J (1971). An Integrated Group of Forms for Automated Psychiatric Case Records, *Archives of General Psychiatry, 24*: 540–547.

Spitzer RL & Endicott J (1974). Can the Computer Assist Clinicians in Psychiatric Diagnosis? *American Journal of Psychiatry, 131*: 523–530.

Spitzer RL & Endicott J (1974). Computer Diagnosis in Automated Record-Keeping Systems: A Study of Clinical Acceptability. In J. Crawford, D. Morgan, and D. Gianturco (eds.) *Progress in Mental Health Information Systems: Computer Applications*. Cambridge: Ballinger Publishing Company, 73–105.

Spitzer RL & Endicott J (1975). Assessment of Outcome by Independent Clinical Evaluators. In I.E. Waskow and M.B. Parloff (eds.) *Psychotherapy Change Measures: Report of the Clinical Research Branch Outcome Measures Project*. Rockville, MD: National Institute of Mental Health, 222–232.

Spitzer RL & Endicott J (1975). Computer Applications in Psychiatry, In Silvano Arieti, (ed.), *American Handbook of Psychiatry*, Vol. VI, Second Edition. New York: Basic Books, 811–839.

Spitzer RL & Endicott J (1975). Psychiatric Rating Scales, in A. Freedman, H. Kaplan, and B. Sadock (eds.), *Comprehensive Textbook of Psychiatry*, Vol. II, Second Edition. Baltimore: Williams & Wilkins, 2015–2031.

Spitzer RL & Endicott J (1978). Medical and Mental Disorder: Proposed Definition and Criteria, in Robert L. Spitzer and Donald Klein (eds.) *Critical Issues in Psychiatric Diagnosis*. New York: Raven Press.

Spitzer RL & Endicott J (1979). Justification for Separating Schizotypal and Borderline Personality Disorders, *Schizophrenia Bulletin*, 5 (1): 95–104.

Spitzer RL, Endicott J, Cohen J, & Fleiss JL (1974). Constraints on the Validity of Computer Diagnosis, *Archives of General Psychiatry*, 31 (August): 197–203.

Spitzer RL, Endicott J, & Gibbon M (1979). Crossing the Border into Borderline Personality and Borderline Schizophrenia: The Development of Criteria, *Archives of General Psychiatry*, 36 (January): 17–24.

Spitzer RL, Endicott J, & Robins E (1975). Clinical Criteria for Psychiatric Diagnosis and DSM-III, *American Journal of Psychiatry*, 132: 1187–1192.

Spitzer RL, Endicott J, & Robins E (1975). Research Diagnostic Criteria, *Psychopharmacology Bulletin*, 11: 22–25.

Spitzer RL, Endicott J, & Robins E (1978). Research Diagnostic Criteria: Rationale and Reliability, *Archives of General Psychiatry*, 35 (June): 773–782.

Spitzer RL, Endicott J, Robins E, Kuriansky J, & Gurland B (1975). Preliminary Report of the Reliability of Research Diagnostic Criteria Applied to Psychiatric Case Records, In Abraham Sudilovsky, Samuel Gershon, and Bernard Beer, eds., *Predictability in Psychopharmacology: Preclinical and Clinical Correlations*. New York: Raven Press.

Spitzer RL & Fleiss JL (1974). A Reanalysis of the Reliability of Psychiatric Diagnosis, *British Journal of Psychiatry*, 125: 341–347.

Spitzer RL, Fleiss JL, Burdock EL, & Hardesty AS (1964). The Mental Status Schedule: Rationale, Reliability and Validity, *Comprehensive Psychiatry*, 5: 384–395.

Spitzer RL & Forman JBW (1979). DSM-III Field Trials, II: Initial Experience with the Multiaxial System, *American Journal of Psychiatry*, 136 (6): 818–820.

Spitzer RL, Forman JBW, & Nee J (1979). DSM-III Field Trials: I. Initial Interrater Diagnostic Reliability, *American Journal of Psychiatry*, 136 (6): 815–817.

Spitzer RL, Gibbon M, Williams JBW, & Endicott J (1996). The Global Assessment of Functioning (GAF) Scale, In L.I. Sederer and B. Dickey, *Outcomes Assessment in Clinical Practice*. Baltimore: William & Wilkins.

Spitzer RL & Gilford LM (1968): UPDATE: A Computer Program for Converting Diagnoses to the New Nomenclature of the American Psychiatric Association, *American Journal of Psychiatry*, 125: 395–396.

Spitzer RL & Klein DF, eds. (1976). *Evaluation of Psychological Therapies: Psychotherapies, Behavior Therapies, Drug Therapies, and Their Interactions.* Baltimore: Johns Hopkins University Press.

Spitzer RL & Klein DF, eds. (1978). *Critical Issues in Psychiatric Diagnosis.* New York: Raven Press.

Spitzer RL, Kramer Y, & Rabkin R (1958). The Neck Righting Reflex in Children, *Journal of Pediatrics, 52*: 149–151.

Spitzer RL, Kroenke K, Linzer M, Hahn SR, Williams JBW, deGruy FV, Brody D, & Davies M (1995). Health Related Quality of Life in Primary Care Patients with Mental Disorders: Results of the PRIME-MD 1000 Study, *JAMA, 274*: 1511–1517.

Spitzer RL, Rabkin R, & Kramer Y (1959). The Relationship Between "Mixed Dominance" and Reading Disabilities, *Journal of Pediatrics, 54*: 76–80.

Spitzer RL & Sheehy M (1976). DSM-III: A Classification System in Development, *Psychiatric Annals, 6* (9): 102–109.

Spitzer RL, Sheehy M, & Endicott J (1977). DSM-III: Guiding Principles, in Vivian M. Rakoff, Harvey C. Stancer, and Henry B. Kedward (eds.), *Psychiatric Diagnosis.* New York: Brunner/ Mazel.

Spitzer RL, Williams JBW, Gibbon M, First MB (1992). The Structured Clinical Interview for DSM-III-R (SCID) I: History, Rationale, and Description, *Archives of General Psychiatry, 49*: 624–629.

Spitzer RL, Williams JBW, Kroenke K, Linzer M, de Gruy III, FV, Hahn SR, & Brody D (1994). Utility of a New Procedure for Diagnosing Mental Disorders in Primary Care: The PRIME-MD 1000 Study, *JAMA, 272* (22): 1749–1756.

Spitzer RL & Wilson PT (1968). A Guide to the New Nomenclature, *American Journal of Psychiatry, 124* (12): 1619–1629.

Spitzer RL & Wilson PT (1969). DSM-II Revisited: A Reply, *International Journal of Psychiatry, 7*: 421–426.

Spitzer RL & Wilson PT (1975). Nosology and the Official Psychiatric Nomenclature, In A. Freedman, H. Kaplan, and B. Sadock (eds.), *Comprehensive Textbook of Psychiatry*, Vol. I, Second Edition. Baltimore: Williams and Wilkins, 826–845.

Staub ME (2011). *Madness is Civilization: When the Diagnosis Was Social, 1948–1980.* Chicago: University of Chicago Press.

Stephens JH, Astrup C, & Mangrum JC (1966). Prognostic Factors in Recovered and Deteriorated Schizophrenics, *American Journal of Psychiatry, 122* (April): 1116–1120.

Stern A (1938). Psychoanalytic Investigation of and Therapy in the Borderline Group of Neurosis, *Psychoanalytic Quarterly, 7*: 467–489.

Stevens SS (1935). The Operational Basis of Psychology, *American Journal of Psychology, 47* (2): 323–330.

Stewart MA, Drake F, & Winokur G (1965). Depression Among Medically Ill Patients, *Diseases of the Nervous System, 26*: 479–484.

Stone AA (1976). Psychiatry: Dead or Alive? *Harvard Magazine*, Dec.: 17–23.

Stone L (1954). The Widening Scope of Indications for Psychoanalysis, *Journal of the American Psychoanalytic Association, 2*: 567–594.

Stone L (1961). *The Psychoanalytic Situation: An Examination of Its Development and Essential Nature.* New York: International Universities Press.

Strack S & Kinder W, eds. (2006). *Pioneers of Personality Science.* New York: Springer.

Strauss JS (1975). A Comprehensive Approach to Psychiatric Diagnosis, *American Journal of Psychiatry, 132* (11): 1193–1197.

Strauss SS, Carpenter Jr., WT, & Bartko JJ (1974). The Diagnosis and Understanding of Schizophrenia, Part III, *Schizophrenia Bulletin*, No. 11 (Winter): 61–80.

Szasz TS (1961). *The Myth of Mental Illness: Foundations of a Theory of Personal Conduct.* Boston: Harper & Row.

Szasz TS (1973). *The Second Sin.* New York: Doubleday.

Szasz TS, Knoff WF, & Hollender MH (1958). The Doctor-Patient Relationship and Its Historical Context, *American Journal of Psychiatry*, 115: 522–528.

Talbott JA (1974). Radical Psychiatry: An Examination of the Issues, *American Journal of Psychiatry*, 131 (2): 121–128.

Talbott JA (1980). An In-Depth Look at DSM-III: An Interview with Robert Spitzer, *Hospital and Community Psychiatry*, 31 (1): 25–32.

Tanguay PE (1997). Dennis P. Cantwell, M.D. (1939–1997), Obituary, *Journal of the American Academy of Child and Adolescent Psychiatry*, 36, October 1.

Tanna V, Winokur G, Elston R, Go RC (1976). "A Linkage Study of Depression Spectrum Disease: The Use of the Sib-Pair Method," *Neuropsychobiology*, 2: 52–62.

Thompson GN (1954). The Society for Biological Psychiatry, *American Journal of Psychiatry*, 111 (5): 389–391.

Torrey EF (1974). *The Death of Psychiatry.* Radnor, PA: Chilton.

Tsuang MT (1999). Images in psychiatry, George Winokur, M.D. 1925–1996, *American Journal of Psychiatry*, 156 (3): 465–466.

Vaillant GE (1962). The Prediction of Recovery in Schizophrenia, *Journal of Nervous and Mental Disease*, 135 (1): 617–627.

Vaillant GE (1964). Prospective Prediction of Recovery in Schizophrenia, *Archives of General Psychiatry*, 11 (November): 509–518.

Vaillant GE (1971). Theoretical Hierarchy of Adaptive Ego Mechanisms: A 30-Year Follow-up of 30 Men Selected for Psychological Health, *Archives of General Psychiatry*, 24: 107–118.

Vaillant GE (1971). The Evolution of Adaptive and Defensive Behaviors During the Adult Life Cycle, *Journal of the American Psychoanalytic Association*, 19: 110–115.

Vaillant GE (1977). *Adaptation to Life.* Boston: Little, Brown.

Vaillant GE (2012). Editorial: Lifting the Field's 'Repressions' of Defenses, *American Journal of Psychiatry*, 169: 885–887.

Veith I (1965). *Hysteria: The History of a Disease.* Chicago & London: University of Chicago Press.

Von Feuchtersleben E (1847) [1845]. *The Principles of Medical Psychology: Being the Outlines of a Course of Lectures.* Trans. H.E. Lloyd. Rev. & ed. B.G. Babington. London: Sydenham Society.

Ward MJ (1946). *The Snake Pit.* New York: Random House.

Weber MM & Engstrom EJ (1997), Kraepelin's Diagnostic Cards: The Confluence of Empirical Research and Preconceived Categories, *History of Psychiatry*, 8: 375–385.

Weissman MM (2006). *A Brief History of Interpersonal Psychotherapy*, 36 (8): 553–557.

Wender P (2000). *ADHD: Attention-Deficit Hyperactivity Disorder in Children, Adolescents, and Adults.* New York: Oxford University Press.

Wheeler EO, White PD, Reed EW & Cohen ME (1950). Neurocirculatory asthenia (anxiety neurosis, effort syndrome, neurasthenia): 20 year follow-up study of 173 patients, *JAMA*, 142: 876–889.

Williams JBW, Gibbon M, First MB, Davies M, Borus J, Howes MJ, Kane J, Pope HG, Rounsaville B, & Wittchen H (1992). The Structured Clinical Interview for DSM-III-R (SCID) II: Multi-site Test-retest Reliability, *Archives of General Psychiatry*, 49: 630–636.

Williams JBW & Spitzer RL (1983). A Critique of "A Woman's View of DSM-III," *American Psychologist*, July: 793–798.

Wilson M (1993). DSM-III and The Transformation of American Psychiatry: A History, *American Journal of Psychiatry*, 150 (3): 399–410.

Wing JK (1970). A Standard Form of Psychiatric Present State Examinations (PSE) and a Method of Standardizing the Classification of Symptoms, In E.H. Hare and J.K. Wing (eds.), *Psychiatric Epidemiology*. London: Oxford University Press.

Wing JK ed. (1976). Classification of Psychiatric Disorders, *Psychiatric Annals*, 6 (9).

Winokur G (1970). Genetic Findings and Methodological Considerations in Manic Depressive Disease, *British Journal of Psychiatry*, 117: 267–274.

Winokur G (1973). The Types of Affective Disorders, *Journal of Nervous and Mental Disease*, 156: 83–96.

Winokur G (1974). Division of Depressive Illness into Depressive Spectrum Disease and Pure Depressive Disease, *International Pharmakopsychiatrie*, 9: 5–13.

Winokur G (1974). Genetic and Clinical Factors Associated with Course in Depression, *Pharmakopsychiatrie Neuro-Psychpharmak*, 7: 122–126.

Winokur G (1979). Unipolar Depression: Is It Divisible Into Autonomous Subtypes? *Archives of General Psychiatry*, 36 (1): 47–52.

Winokur G, Cadoret R, Baker M, & Dorzab J (1975). Depressive Spectrum Disease vs Pure Depressive Disease: Some Further Data, *British Journal of Psychiatry*, 127: 75–77.

Winokur G, Cadoret R, Dorzab J, & Baker M (1971). Depressive Disease, a Genetic Study, *Archives of General Psychiatry*, 24: 135–144.

Winokur G & Clayton PJ (1967). Family History Studies I: Two Types of Affective Disorders Separated According to Genetic and Clinical Factors," in J. Wortis (ed.), *Recent Advances in Biological Psychiatry*. New York: Plenum Press.

Winokur G & Clayton PJ, (1967). Family History Studies: II. Sex Differences in Primary Affective Illness, *British Journal of Psychiatry*, 113: 973–979.

Winokur G, Clayton PJ, & Reich T (1969). *Manic Depressive Illness*. Saint Louis: The C.V. Mosby Company.

Winokur G & Morrison J (1973). The Iowa 500: Followup of 225 Depressives, *British Journal of Psychiatry*, 123: 543–548.

Winokur G & Pitts Jr., FN (1964). Affective Disorder: I. Is reactive depression an entity? *Journal of Nervous and Mental Disease*, 138: 541–547.

Winokur G & Pitts Jr., FN (1965). Affective Disorder: VI. A Family History Study of Prevalence, Sex Differences, and Possible Genetic Factors, *Journal of Psychiatric Research*, 3: 113–123.

Winokur G & Pitts Jr., FN (1965). Affective Disorder: V. The Diagnostic Validity of Depressive Reactions, *Psychiatric Quarterly*, 39: 727–728.

Winokur G & Reich T (1970). Two Genetic Factors in Manic Depressive Disease, *Comprehensive Psychiatry*, 11: 93–99.

Winokur G & Tsuang MT (1996). *The Natural History of Mania, Depression, and Schizophrenia*. Washington DC: American Psychiatric Press.

Winokur G, Zimmerman M, & Cadoret R (1988). "Cause the Bible Tells Me So," *Archives of General Psychiatry*, 45 (July): 683–684.

Winston, A, Rosenthal, RN, & Pinsker, H (2004*). Introduction to Supportive Psychotherapy*. Washington, DC: American Psychiatric Publishing, Inc, 2004.

Woodruff, Jr. RA, Goodwin DW, &. Guze, SB (1974). *Psychiatric Diagnosis*. New York: Oxford University Press.

Woodruff Jr., RA, Pitts Jr., FN, & Winokur G (1964). Affective Disorder: II. A Comparison of Patients with Endogenous Depressions with and without Family History of Affective Disorder, *Journal of Nervous and Mental Disease, 139*: 49–52.

World Health Organization, *Report of the Fourth WHO Seminar on Psychiatric Diagnoses, Classification, and Statistics.* Geneva: WHO, 1968.

World Health Organization, *Report of the Seventh WHO Seminar on Standardization of Psychiatric Diagnosis, Classification and Statistics of Personality.* Geneva: WHO, 1971.

World Health Organization, *Report of the Sixth WHO Seminar on Psychiatric Diagnoses, Classification, and Statistics.* Geneva: WHO, 1970.

Zilboorg G (1941). *A History of Medical Psychology.* New York, W.W. Norton.

ABOUT THE AUTHOR

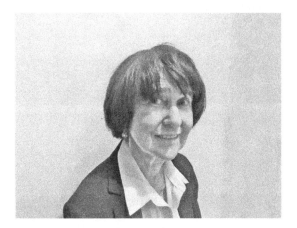

Hannah S. Decker is a cultural historian of psychiatry and professor of history at the University of Houston. She is also adjunct professor in medical history in the Menninger Department of Psychiatry at the Baylor College of Medicine and an adjunct faculty member at the Center for Psychoanalytic Studies (Houston). Her publications include *Freud in Germany: Revolution and Reaction in Science, 1893–1907* and *Freud, Dora, and Vienna 1900.* In 2007 she received the Carlson Award from the Cornell University Medical College for "extraordinary contributions to the history of psychiatry and psychoanalysis." She is married and has two grown children.

INDEX

Page numbers followed by *t* or *f* indicate a table or figure/photo respectively.

CPSIA information can be obtained
at www.ICGtesting.com
Printed in the USA
LVHW051953180722
723790LV00006B/348